MEDICAL TRANSCRIPTION

Techniques and Procedures

SEVENTH EDITION

MARCY O. DIEHL
BVE, CMA-A, CMT, AHDI-F

Professor Emeritus
Medical Transcriptionist Specialist Curriculum
Grossmont Community College
El Cajon, California

ELSEVIER
SAUNDERS

3251 Riverport Lane
St. Louis, Missouri 63043

MEDICAL TRANSCRIPTION TECHNIQUES AND PROCEDURES   ISBN: 978-1-4377-0439-6
Copyright © 2012, 2007, 2002, 1997, 1991, 1984, 1979 by Saunders, an imprint of Elsevier Inc.

Notices

Knowledge and best practice in this field are constantly changing. As new research and experience broaden our understanding, changes in research methods, professional practices, or medical treatment may become necessary.

Practitioners and researchers must always rely on their own experience and knowledge in evaluating and using any information, methods, compounds, or experiments described herein. In using such information or methods they should be mindful of their own safety and the safety of others, including parties for whom they have a professional responsibility.

With respect to any drug or pharmaceutical products identified, readers are advised to check the most current information provided (i) on procedures featured or (ii) by the manufacturer of each product to be administered, to verify the recommended dose or formula, the method and duration of administration, and contraindications. It is the responsibility of practitioners, relying on their own experience and knowledge of their patients, to make diagnoses, to determine dosages and the best treatment for each individual patient, and to take all appropriate safety precautions.

To the fullest extent of the law, neither the Publisher nor the authors, contributors, or editors, assume any liability for any injury and/or damage to persons or property as a matter of products liability, negligence or otherwise, or from any use or operation of any methods, products, instructions, or ideas contained in the material herein.

ISBN: 978-1-4377-0439-6

Publishing Director: Andrew Allen
Senior Acquisitions Editor: Jennifer Janson
Developmental Editor: Kelly Brinkman
Publishing Services Manager: Julie Eddy
Senior Project Manager: Laura Loveall
Designer: Jessica Williams

Printed in the United States

Last digit is the print number: 9 8 7 6 5 4 3 2

This edition of this textbook is dedicated to
all those patient, kind, forgiving, instructive women and men
who have guided me or befriended me and with whom
I have worked with, worked for, or taught during my
professional career in medical transcription that I began in 1966.

Preface

This is the seventh edition of a book that has had an exciting transformation each time it has been updated—and, of course, I believe that this time it is particularly enhanced and special. It is my hope that, if you are picking up this text for the first time as a student or an instructor, you will be as pleased with it as I am. If you have used previous editions of the book, I hope you will find this edition more interesting and even easier to work with.

The textbook is designed for the student who plans to major in medical transcription and seek eventual employment in a medical transcription service, private physician's office, clinic, or hospital, or be self-employed and freelance. There continues to be a serious shortage of well-trained medical transcriptionists, resulting from the problems of training, the increase in the quantity of dictation because of longer reports and a larger number of diagnostic studies, the fact that documentation must show medical necessity and correspond to reimbursement, and the demand by hospitals for quality reports. The advent of the electronic medical record and the enhanced capabilities of speech recognition technology have further required formal instruction and guidelines for the beginner. The textbook is appropriate for a first-semester medical transcription class after completion of a medical terminology course. Legal-secretary and court-reporting students will also find the book a useful introduction to medical terms and practices.

The book is designed to be used in the community college or vocational-technical institute, for in-service training in the hospital or private medical office, or in extension programs. It is a very useful core text for a one- or two-semester online course and may also be used for independent home study if no formal classes are available in the community. The textbook may also be used by practicing medical or legal assistants who want to upgrade their skills but unable to attend class. Finally, the book serves as a reference for the working medical or legal transcriptionist.

The general format of the book is the same as in previous editions so that both students and instructors

can use it in ways that are most convenient to them. Each chapter begins with a list of objectives to let students and instructors know exactly what will be taught. Instructors may test with the objectives in mind to see how well the objectives have been met.

Because medical transcriptionists work in a variety of settings, I have tried to address the responsibilities of the private office-based transcriptionist, the home-based entrepreneur, the hospital professional, and those employed by transcription services.

A reference section, Appendix B, consists of tear sheets (perforated pages) that may be used in each student's personal transcriptionist's notebook. The section consists of additional data, some tables that appear within chapters, and popular reference information found in several appendices in past editions. Having all of this information in one location makes it possible to access reference data easily and quickly. This enhancement gives students a good start for their collections and encourages use of reference materials.

Appendix C on Evolve is a collection of actual transcripts from a variety of medical specialties and facilities that show the wide variation of styles used. Students will enjoy seeing genuine documents and can even search for errors that have inadvertently occurred during transcription.

All the material included in the exercises and Appendix C is authentic medical dictation or writing. The facts in the examples have been altered only to the extent necessary to prevent identification of the cases or parties involved. No evaluation of medical practice, no medical advice, and no recommendations for treatment are to be inferred from the selections. Actual medical documents illustrating format and content are used liberally throughout the major chapters.

Basic English rule books and style manuals form the backbone of the rules and guidelines, with my own experience, that of reviewers and colleagues, and field research determining which methods are most frequently and consistently used when there is a variety of choices. Changes in the way professionals do things are reflected in modification in rules and format.

Major changes with this edition include:

- ▶ Additional practice exercises
- ▶ An updated chapter on technology with emphasis on speech recognition technology and the electronic medical record
- ▶ A new chapter concerning the transition to speech recognition editor with actual speech recognition dictation drafts for practice
- ▶ An enhanced section in Chapter 16 on working from home
- ▶ The legal ramifications and responsibilities of working with medical documents
- ▶ A complete rule synopsis at the end of Chapters 3, 4, and 5, as well as new information to enhance the understanding of concepts involved as they apply to the style of current medical transcription
- ▶ The addition of 100 new actual physician-dictated medical documents

EVOLVE COMPANION WEBSITE

A variety of supplemental materials are available to the student and the instructor.

For the Student

The Evolve companion website offers a resource that allows students to harness the power of the Internet. Dictation practice, chapter quizzes, chapter-specific web links, and certification examination preparation materials are available. Instructors can download supplemental teaching materials.

This edition includes over 10 hours of authentic medical dictation to provide application to the skills taught in the text. Speech recognition dictated reports allow students to edit files developed using the software and assume the role of a medical editor.

A PIN code is required to access the Evolve website. A sticker with this PIN code may be found on the inside front cover of this book.

For the Instructor

- ▶ Instructor's Resource Manual (ISBN: 978-1-4377-2683-1): An Instructor's Resource Manual, available for use with this text, assists in the establishment of a transcription course and gives the teacher some ideas about how to use the text as an adjunct to an online class or regular classroom setting. The manual provides a complete syllabus, features answers to each chapter's review exercises and answer keys to the audio/student dictations, and gives additional exercises for which answers are not provided in the text. There are many examples of critical thinking problems for classroom or Internet discussion. Performance evaluation sheets for review tests are included for those who wish to use them.
- ▶ Evolve Companion Website: The Evolve companion website offers an electronic version of the Instructor's Resource Manual, as well as access to Evolve content for students. The TEACH Lesson Plan Manual is also available to instructors on the Evolve website (http://evolve.elsevier.com/Diehl/transcription/).
- ▶ TEACH Online: TEACH is a complete curriculum solution package that provides the instructor with a customizable series of lesson plans, curriculum guides, and instructor development resources. TEACH enhances existing text ancillaries such as test banks, instructor resource manuals, and image collections. TEACH offers straightforward lesson plans that save valuable time and help fully engage students in classroom discussions. TEACH is accessible to instructors online through the Evolve companion website.

Drake and Drake's *Pharmaceutical Word Book,* Drake's *Sloane's Medical Word Book, Dorland's Illustrated Medical Dictionary,* and a variety of word books are publications that may be obtained from Elsevier.

Acknowledgments

A debt of appreciation is owed to many individuals for their participation in making this new edition special. Sharon B. Allred, CMT, AHDI-F, VP of Operations Opti-Script, Inc., instructor, and quality assurance expert, made sure that proper medical transcription format and style were followed as she reviewed each textbook and IRM chapter. Her helpful suggestions and sample documents enhanced each chapter. With her meticulous attention to detail and her talent for consistency, Dr. Barbara L. Halliburton, copy editor, gave the text the polish and professional editing that it deserves. I owe my artist friend, Gail Niebrugge, my heartfelt thanks for bringing "Joy" to our chapter opening pages.

Thanks go to the staff at Elsevier. Jennifer Janson, Senior Acquisitions Editor, deserves the credit for steering this edition to final production. Thanks also go to Kelly Brinkman, Developmental Editor; Laura Loveall, Senior Project Manager; and Jessica Williams, who designed the book.

In addition, the following professionals submitted many valuable suggestions, provided details on equipment and format, or reviewed materials: Paul-Kip Otis-Diehl; Marlene M. DeMers, clinical laboratory scientist and medical technologist, Biology Department, San Diego State University, Georgia Green, CMT, AHDI-F, Transcription Supervisor, Grays Harbor Community Hospital, and Peg Nelson, CMT-R, past corporate director of quality control.

I also acknowledge the professionals who provided valuable input to this revision during the pre-revision review process.

Marcy O. Diehl, BVE, CMA-A, CMT, AHDI-F
Professor Emeritus, Grossmont College
El Cajon, California

Contents

CHAPTER 1

The Medical Transcriptionist's Career, Including Ethical and Legal Responsibilities

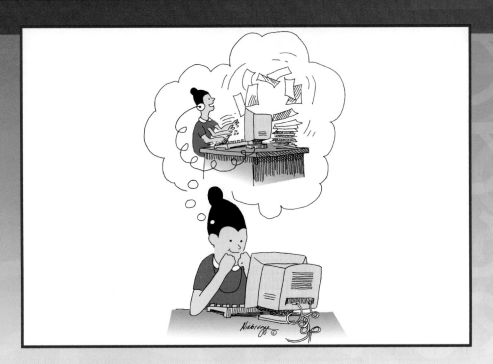

OBJECTIVES

After reading this chapter and working the exercises, you should be able to

1. Specify the background and importance of medical records.
2. Explain the variety of skills that a medical transcriptionist (MT) must have.
3. Identify opportunities for physically challenged transcriptionists.
4. List the certification levels a MT may obtain in this career.
5. Define and explain the purpose of a medical report or record.
6. Describe the importance of the emerging use of electronic health records (EHRs).
7. Identify specific Health Insurance Portability and Accountability Act of 1996 (HIPAA) regulations that affect MTs.
8. Explain the importance of HIPAA regulations for patients.
9. Define risk management.
10. Recognize time limits imposed on document insertion into a medical record: the turnaround time (TAT).
11. Define privileged and nonprivileged information.
12. Enumerate the guidelines for release of patient information.
13. Explain the importance of subpoenas for patient records.
14. Discuss professional issues.

15. Explain the many ways the Internet may affect a MT's job performance.
16. Describe some of the responsibilities of other healthcare workers that may affect the duties and responsibilities of a MT.
17. Assemble a reference notebook.
18. Recognize the importance of continuing education.

Note from the Author

Welcome to your new career! Even though I first began transcribing medical documents nearly 46 years ago, I have not lost my interest in or enthusiasm for this exciting endeavor. To be able to participate in patient care in this manner has continued to be exciting and challenging. To be sure, many things have changed since I began, and things will continue to change—every day. But that is something that has never had a negative impact on the work of medical transcriptionists (MTs); it has been, instead, one more facet that generates a lively interest in whatever will help us do our work well and communicate what the clinician wants to preserve in a permanent record.

One of the many things you will learn in this chapter concerns the orders from the court for medical records. The first time I had a subpoena served at the site where I worked, I had to take the records to court, appear before the judge, and swear that the record was complete. (This event was not nearly as exciting as I thought it would be. All I could think of was the time wasted and all the catching up I would have to do when I returned to work.) It was not long before I was allowed to copy the records, simply sign a statement for the court, and mail them to the attorney. Next, someone directed by the attorney's office would come in and either photocopy or microfilm the records. My role was reduced to standing there to make sure that the entire record was copied. The records I am speaking about in my career all had to do with patients who had either work injuries or accidents. Today, very few MTs have to provide records for the court, but they do have to know that every document they transcribe is a legal record and could be part of a court record at some time. This fact is of vital importance, just as you are a vital component in record preparation.

INTRODUCTION

Welcome to an exciting and vitally important career field. I hope that this text will assist you in maintaining an eager interest and excitement about the course of study you are undertaking, as well as provide you with a strong foundation as a MT to be self-employed or employed by a transcription service, a private physician's office, a hospital, or a clinic. This text has been designed to speed the beginner transcriptionists (who already know how to use a word processing program and a computer) on their way to proficiency. The more skills you bring with you, the faster you will progress. I hope that, at the same time, you will begin to experience the fascination and appreciation for medicine that MTs have come to enjoy.

With your formal education, you begin to build the structure of your career by obtaining the core knowledge to be successful. However, continuing education is your bridge to the future. Take every opportunity you can now to learn all you can outside of your formal training. Continue along these paths to broaden your knowledge base through networks of other students and professionals. You should understand right now that you must make a career-long commitment to continuing education.

Now, let's meet your textbook.

Think of your textbook as a large toolbox full of brand-new tools being presented to you to learn to use. You probably also have some perfectly good old tools (your computer, Internet research skills) that you can polish up, fit in, and add to your collection, so please look for your old tools as we examine your new tools.

Of course you know that many workers have all sorts of tools: some worn on big leather belts, some carried in tiny cloth kits, some trotted to the job in steel boxes. You can see tool sets in the hands of many different workers: a manicurist, hair stylist, watchmaker, plumber, writer, chef, chemist, computer repair worker, physician, and so on. There really is no end to the list of workers with tools, wonderful and specialized tools! Will you have tools like the ones they care for and use? Yes. Your tools will look a bit different, but they will have the same function: to enable you to carry out the many intricate and broad functions of your job in the best and most comfortable way, resulting in a finished product of which you can be proud.

As you read, I will introduce you to these tools and explain each of them to you so that you can add them to your toolbox. This might be a bit intimidating at first, but you will look at one tool at a time—as one does in any tool-based profession. At the same time, I will remind you to polish up the tools you already own and use, so that all of them, smoothly working together, not only enable but also enhance your career.

BASIC SKILLS AND INTERESTS

Before you begin this program, it is important to see what skills you already have, which are the tools you already own and are skilled at using that will help you become successful with not only your school work but also with the profession itself. Some of these skills will become enhanced as you proceed. When you read the job descriptions in the pages that follow, you will see how the following basic skills and interests fit into the competencies that will be required of you:

▶ English: spelling, grammar, and usage (high school graduate equivalency)
▶ Keyboard: speed of at least 45 words per minute after correction
▶ Computer and Word Processing: the ability to create, save, format, copy and paste documents and to install software and manage files
▶ Internet: ability to send and receive emails with attachments and to use the Internet for research purposes
▶ Attention to Details: ability to focus and problem solve, and ability to listen carefully and read carefully to spot errors and inconsistencies
▶ Interest in Medicine: the lure of the association with medicine in a "nonphysical" sense

MEDICAL COMMUNICATION

The recording of diseases and injuries goes back many centuries. This medical communication has helped bridge the gap between ancient and modern civilizations. Part of the joy of being a MT is in knowing that you are the modern communicator in the medical field. Imagine your role in today's worldwide and nearly instantaneous capability of sharing medical documentation.

JOB OPPORTUNITIES

Healthcare reform across the United States and the development of a variety of managed care systems have had a significant impact on documentation in inpatient and outpatient settings, necessitating increasingly detailed documentation to back up what is billed. Many MTs are unaware of their importance in the reimbursement chain and of how vital the documents they produce are to the correct and timely billing for services performed. Advances in computer and

telecommunications technology have caused changes in how documents are transmitted, increasing the cost of generating reports. To remain cost-efficient, smaller facilities are merging with larger ones to remain a part of the medical industry. Many more professionals in all fields, including MTs, are establishing home-based businesses that involve using a computer. Medical transcription, also known as medical dictation editing, is an excellent profession in which to successfully work independently. It is important to take all this information into account when thinking about job opportunities in the region in which you want to work. (Chapter 16 presents some of the important details to consider when you are a home-based MT.)

When you have finished your course of study and completed many hours of practice, you will be prepared to seek employment in a variety of medical settings or to become a self-employed transcriptionist (independent contractor) or telecommuter. The private physician's office, the hospital, and transcription services are exciting and interesting work environments, and the duties and responsibilities of an employee in these settings offer real challenges for the modern MT. Although transcribing correspondence, reports, and other medical documents will be your prime responsibility, you may find that you have other interesting business duties.

As more tasks are affected by computerization, career specialists have predicted that workers will become multiskilled. With a broad background in terminology and the Internet, MTs can enhance their knowledge and skills by enrolling in classes on how to edit medical documents, complete insurance claims, or become proficient in procedural and diagnostic coding (the attachment of a numeric code to services and procedures performed by caregivers). In some settings, you may be responsible as a full-time transcriptionist or as a part-time transcriptionist with records management or editing duties. Some hospital departments, such as radiology, cardiology, physical therapy, rehabilitation therapy, pathology, outpatient surgery, and emergency services, require the skills of MTs. Other possibilities include ambulatory surgery centers, imaging centers, acute care centers, and walk-in clinics.

Public health clinics, school health facilities, private insurance agencies, specialized computer and transcription agencies, large legal firms, military medical departments, and governmental agencies also offer challenging opportunities for professional transcriptionists. Medical research is conducted in many settings, and as a MT, you may have the opportunity to participate in this forum. You might decide to work for a private transcription service. In this setting, you could be working on several accounts, and each account might have different criteria.

JOB DESCRIPTIONS

You will always be working with others who have chosen the field of medicine in some similar way, and you will find that you are a vital part of the team wherever you are employed. Therefore, it is important that you also learn to respect and appreciate the duties of the other personnel with whom you work. To avoid confusion, note the differences in the duties of some of the other professionals with whom you may work:

1. A *medical administrative assistant* is a professional who
   ▸ Sets up medical records and accounting forms
   ▸ Prepares letters from drafts by using proper mechanics
   ▸ Does "light" transcribing of letters and chart notes
   ▸ Completes workers' compensation and state disability forms
   ▸ Writes letters to follow up insurance claims, orders supplies, collects monies, and so on
   ▸ Responds to requests for data from life insurance companies.

2. A *medical office administrator* is a professional who
   ▸ Has mastery of all medical business office skills (such as appointment making, telephone procedures, accounting, completion of insurance claims, collection of accounts, banking, payroll, mail processing, filing, maintenance of patient records, and office maintenance)
   ▸ Has knowledge of medical terminology, as well as excellent grammar skills
   ▸ Demonstrates ability to assume responsibility without direct supervision
   ▸ Exercises initiative and judgment
   ▸ Makes decisions within the scope of assigned authority
   ▸ Writes letters over his or her signature or that of his or her employers
   ▸ Abstracts medical records and reports
   ▸ Edits and revises documents for employers.

3. A *medical scribe* (also known as a *health information assistant*) is a professional who
   ▸ Has excellent word processing skills
   ▸ Is highly knowledgeable about human anatomy, physiology, medications, laboratory values, and pathophysiology
   ▸ Has knowledge of medical transcription guidelines and practices
   ▸ Has excellent spelling, editing, and proofreading skills
   ▸ Has a good command of English grammar, structure, and style
   ▸ Has a thorough knowledge of medical terminology as it relates to medical and surgical procedures, drugs, instruments, and laboratory tests
   ▸ Is able to work independently
   ▸ Has excellent listening skills
   ▸ Has a thorough understanding of the electronic health record (EHR) platform and the requirements for data input
   ▸ Is able to directly assist in patient care by documenting the patient's medical story during the patient's visit, thus reducing physician time per patient. (The clinician examines, diagnoses, and treats the patient while the scribe enters information into an EHR.)
   ▸ Reviews medication lists with the patient when necessary
   ▸ Reviews and reinforces instructions from the physician with the patient
   ▸ Is able to transcribe any dictated material from the physician

4. A *medical transcriptionist* or *medical dictation editor* is a professional who
   ▸ Has excellent word processing skills
   ▸ Is highly knowledgeable about human anatomy, physiology, medications, laboratory values, and pathophysiology
   ▸ Has knowledge of medical transcription guidelines and practices
   ▸ Has excellent spelling, editing, and proofreading skills
   ▸ Has a good command of English grammar, structure, and style
   ▸ Has a thorough knowledge of medical terminology as it relates to medical and surgical procedures, drugs, instruments, and laboratory tests
   ▸ Is able to use the Internet for reference, along with traditional reference materials
   ▸ Is able to work independently
   ▸ Has excellent listening skills
   ▸ Is able to recognize legal and ethical requirements pertaining to medical documents
   ▸ Is an indispensable assistant to physicians, surgeons, dentists, and other medical professionals in producing medical reports, which become permanent records of medical, scientific, and legal value

Other allied personnel you may work with include a registered health information administrator (or RHIA, a professional with a 4-year degree who oversees healthcare documentation in a hospital or clinic) and a registered health information technician (or RHIT, a professional with a 2-year degree who works in health information management in a hospital or clinic).

The Association for Healthcare Documentation Integrity (AHDI) guidelines describes a MT as one who interprets dictation by physicians and other healthcare professionals and records the content in either print or electronic form while editing simultaneously to produce

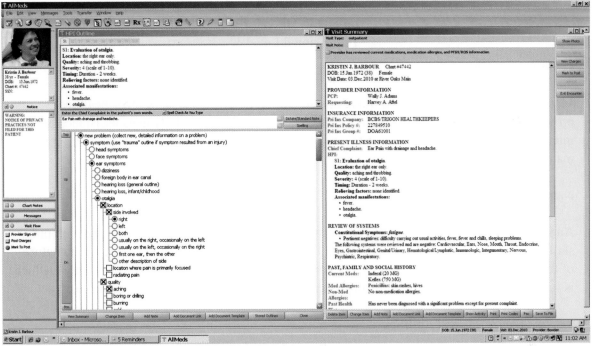

A screen shot of the exam screen, which allows documentation of all body systems. Documents, drawings, or notes can be added to augment the information. This platform is used by the health information assistant/medical scribe accessing the EHR. (Used with permission; courtesy of AllMeds, Inc., Oak Ridge, Tenn.)

a grammatically correct document. The dictation is commonly related to patient assessment, workup, diagnostic and therapeutic procedures, treatment and clinical course, prognosis, and patient instructions. The resulting documentation is the record of patient care that is necessary to facilitate delivery of healthcare services.

Because the role of a MT requires knowledge, skills, and performance standards, the AHDI developed a model job description. The complete description of all levels is in Chapter 15. See Figure 1-1, which is a list of just the Professional Level 1 responsibilities. This list of duties and responsibilities is not complete, but it may be useful as a guideline in the development of a job description by an employer.

Betty Honkonen, CMT, AHDI-F, former president of AHDI, describes the skills of this career thus:

"knowledge workers behind the keyboard who ensure an accurate, concise, and billable legal document that meets the integrity standard."

The subsequent chapters in this book will help you develop the skills outlined in the job description. Because medicine is always changing, and because people and their problems are interesting, I can assure you that you will never get bored. In fact, the demand for medical business personnel is increasing. There is no age limit, provided that you work proficiently and maintain an acceptable standard of performance. The earning potential for high-quality professionals is excellent, depending on experience and locality, of course.

As you embark on this profession, you may be interested in where this career may lead. You can further your education and obtain a liberal arts degree or enroll in courses, such as English, communications, journalism, professional writing, editing, or education. With experience and background, a MT can find work as a medical quality assurance manager, writer, editor, or publications coordinator. Literally hundreds of professional training courses are available on the Internet for continuing education in the field of medical transcription and related fields.

TRANSCRIPTION SKILLS

As you begin this book, think about when you finish it at Chapter 16. What skills do you think you will need in the workplace, and what do you plan to do to get them? Reading this book will help you obtain the tools you need so you can discover the facts you need to be successful in the workplace. As you continue to study, you might even change your ideas about your ultimate goal and be eager to learn all the possibilities available to you.

Model Job Description
Professional Level 1

Position Summary

Medical language specialist who transcribes dictation by physicians and other healthcare providers in order to document patient care. The incumbent will likely need assistance to interpret dictation that is unclear or inconsistent or need to make use of professional reference materials.

Nature of Work

An incumbent in this position is given assignments that are matched to his or her developing skill level, with the intention of increasing the depth and/or breadth of exposure or the nature of the work performed (type of report or correspondence, medical specialty, originator), which is repetitive or patterned, not requiring extensive depth and/or breadth of experience.

Knowledge, Skills, and Abilities

- Basic knowledge of medical terminology, anatomy and physiology, disease processes, signs and symptoms, medications, and laboratory values. Knowledge of speciality (or specialities) as appropriate.
- Knowledge of medical transcription guidelines and practices.
- Proven skills in English usage, grammar, punctuation, style, and editing.
- Ability to use designated professional reference materials.
- Ability to operate word processing equipment, dictation and transcription equipment, and other equipment as specified.
- Ability to work under pressure with time constraints.
- Ability to concentrate.
- Excellent listening skills.
- Excellent eye, hand, and auditory coordination.
- Ability to understand and apply relevant legal concepts (e.g., confidentiality).

FIGURE 1-1 The *AHDI Model Job Description: Professional Level 1.* This document is a practical, useful compilation of the basic job responsibilities of a MT. It is designed to assist human resource managers, department managers, supervisors, and others in recruiting, supervising, and evaluating persons in medical transcription positions.

Medical transcription is both an exacting science and an artistic accomplishment. MTs are not "typists." Rather MTs are amazingly skilled technicians and medical language specialists who transform a voice file into a complete document. The payment cycle or revenue cycle is initiated with this transcribed document. In simple terms, doctors alone do not generate revenue. Documents generate revenue, and when payments for services occur, the payments are based on these documents. Quality records play the key part in this process. After the dictator signs off the completed document, coding experts go through it and assign billing and diagnostic codes to it. Then the document proceeds to the billing department.

MTs require a combination of skills, including a knowledge of correct document and letter formats; an understanding of medical content, drugs, and disease processes; competence in spelling and in English grammar, structure, and style; proficiency in medical terminology; competence in keyboarding and computer programs; and the ability to proofread both on-screen documents and printed copy. The successful MT has accuracy and speed; a broad knowledge of anatomy; and a thorough knowledge of medical, surgical, drug, and laboratory terms. The MT also knows how to use all the standard reference materials, medical dictionaries, wordbooks, abbreviation reference books, specialty reference books, standard English dictionaries, and drug reference books. MTs must be Internet experts, able to recognize and use accurate and valid websites and to use search engines online. MTs must learn to coordinate their hearing (listening closely) with the keyboards under their fingers and the pedals under their feet. Additionally, they must train their eyes to read the transcribed content to verify accuracy. They must be critical thinkers and problem solvers.

As you proceed through the exercises in this text, you will become more aware of terms that may sound alike but are spelled differently because they specify areas located in different parts of the body. MTs need to pay close attention to the context of a medical report to select the proper word with the meaning intended by the dictator. Greek terms are sometimes more difficult to spell than Latin terms. You will learn how to pluralize Greek and Latin words. In Chapter 8, you will find exercises that will help you use a medical dictionary and other reference materials effectively. Other practice sets will develop your skills in punctuating and capitalizing, in using abbreviations, and in typing symbols.

In Chapter 2, you will be introduced to the equipment used by the transcriptionist, such as computers, transcribing equipment, speech recognition systems, modems, facsimile equipment, photocopiers, and scanners.

It is vital for medical professionals to understand the ethical and legal implications of handling medical records. Confidentiality issues and the individual needs of clients must be considered at all times. Experience in medical transcription brings with it the ability to interpret, translate, and edit medical dictation for content and clarity, as well as the ability to use deductive reasoning and detect medical inconsistencies in dictation. Critical thinking skills are vital to this task.

TRANSCRIPTION SPEED

Unless copy is perfect, speed is worthless. You should always strive for accuracy. At the same time, earnings are often based on the number of pages, characters, or lines that are typed or edited, and so speed also becomes a skill to achieve. However, some employers pay by the hour or provide a monthly salary. Opinions vary in regard to how many lines per hour an experienced professional should transcribe. One suggested goal is 130 lines per hour, with a 6-inch line as the average. Depending on the speed of the person giving dictation, a 15-minute dictation has an average of approximately 150 lines, and a 30-minute dictation has an average of 300 to 400 lines. However, a production goal in one

situation cannot be applied to another because of a wide range of variables, such as type of hospital (local community, large metropolitan, Veterans Affairs, university teaching medical center); person giving dictation (medical students, residents, persons whose native language is not English, persons with regional accents); type of equipment (computer-linked equipment, off-site printing); use of speech recognition technology, macros, templates, and word expanders; additional duties besides transcription; resource materials available; definition of a "line" or other measure of production (words, keystrokes by page, minutes of dictation, characters typed per day; and whether blank lines, half lines, spaces, and punctuation are included); and standards of quality.

One method of determining a production goal is using the 65-character line that includes all letters, numbers, symbols, and formatting codes used to maintain and reproduce a document, including the space bar, shift key, and use of boldface. A contrasting recommendation is the visual-black-character (VBC) method. This character can be seen with the naked eye. With this counting scheme, spaces and hidden formatting instructions (such as returns and the use of boldface or underline) are not counted. This can be counted on a very basic character-counting application to bill for medical reports.

Another variable that affects line count is the familiarity of the dictation. An established MT will be able to produce more lines for an account than would a new person transcribing. As all experienced MTs know, speed and accuracy occur together only with constant practice.

If you do not know your keyboarding speed at the beginning of the course and want to take a timed test, ask the instructor for assistance. Your instructor might want to time you with familiar and unfamiliar work.

PHYSICALLY CHALLENGED TRANSCRIPTIONISTS

Persons who have impaired vision or who must use a wheelchair have done office work since the invention of the typewriter. When transcribing equipment came into use, many new career paths developed for persons who are blind or vision impaired, making it possible for them to be in positions in management. Persons with limited dexterity use special equipment; for example, a stenotype machine interfaced with a word processor or computer with voice technology or enlarged print. A person with one hand can be as productive as a person with both hands. Speech recognition has provided many possibilities for workers with limited keyboard abilities. With the need for professional MTs and the shortage that is always apparent in most communities, training of persons who are physically challenged has been started in private and community colleges across the United States. Many medical terminology textbooks have been printed in Braille and recorded on cassettes or compact disks to make learning easier and faster.

If a person who has a physical impairment needs training or assistive devices, he or she should contact the appropriate state department of vocational rehabilitation. In addition to the Braille Institute, many other sources of help are available, such as the AHDI, the American Heart Association, the United Way, and the Easter Seals program. See Chapter 2 for materials and equipment developed specifically for persons who are physically challenged.

Because listening and keyboarding are the two most important skills in medical transcription, this field usually is not suitable for a person who has a significant hearing impairment.

ASSOCIATION FOR HEALTHCARE DOCUMENTATION INTEGRITY

The AHDI (formerly the American Association for Medical Transcription [AAMT]), founded in 1978, is the largest association for MTs in the world. The overall mission of the AHDI is to promote the integrity of healthcare documentation through development of an educated, prepared workforce in clinical documentation; to lead and direct the evolution of medical transcription; to represent and advance the profession and its practitioners; and to protect patients through documentation by setting standards of education and practice in the field of medical transcription. The purpose of the AHDI is to set and uphold standards for education and practice in the field of clinical documentation to ensure the highest level of accuracy, privacy, and security of healthcare documentation for the U.S. healthcare system and to protect public health, increase patient safety, and improve quality of care for healthcare consumers. See Figure 1-2, which lists the Bill of Rights for a MT.

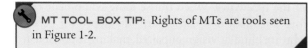

MT TOOL BOX TIP: Rights of MTs are tools seen in Figure 1-2.

The AHDI Code of Ethics for Medical Transcriptionists

The AHDI code of ethics sets forth standards of conduct and ethical principles for MTs that all members of the AHDI and individuals holding the designation of registered medical transcriptionist (RMT) and certified medical transcriptionist (CMT) are expected to follow. MTs are vigilant advocates for quality patient documentation and adhere to the highest privacy and security provision. They uphold the moral and legal rights of patients, safeguard patients' privacy, and collaborate with care providers to ensure patient safety, public health, and quality of care to the fullest extent possible, through the practice of medical transcription.

Members understand that membership and/or certification may be revoked by the AHDI for failure to act in accordance with the provisions of the AHDI Code of Ethics.

Medical transcription professionals

▶ Maintain confidentiality of all patient information
▶ Implement and maintain standards of professional transcription practice
▶ Respect the rights and dignity of all individuals
▶ Continue professional growth-enhancing knowledge and skills
▶ Strive to provide accurate and timely information
▶ Exercise integrity in professional practices, including work or professional experience, credentials, affiliations, productivity reporting, billing charges, and payment practices
▶ Comply with all laws, regulations, and standards governing the practice of patient documentation
▶ Strive to advance the goals and purposes of the AHDI and work for the advancement and good of the profession

Membership

The AHDI has many membership categories, including student and postgraduate. To qualify for student membership, a person must be enrolled in a medical transcription program. A student can be a member for up to 2 years. In addition to the national organization, many large communities have local chapters, as do many states. An online chapter exists that a person can join in addition to belonging to the national organization or local chapter. Membership in the AHDI includes a subscription to both of the organization's professional journals: *Plexus* and *Health Data Matrix*, published bimonthly. The website www.ahdionline.org contains information on joining the AHDI. Two more journals for the health information profession are *For The Record* (biweekly, subscriptions@gvpub.com) and the free online journal *ADVANCE for Health Information Professionals* (1-800-355-5627, or http://health-information.advanceweb.com). Also free is the online newsletter: www.ahdisa.org.

Certification for Medical Transcriptionists

At some time in your career, you may decide to prove to yourself that you truly have mastered the essentials of medical transcription and you want to be recognized

A Medical Transcriptionist's Bill of Rights

Whereas, the medical transcriptionist contributes significantly to the delivery and quality of patient care, while also helping to assure appropriate reimbursement, promote research integrity, and fulfil provider's legal obligations through documentation of health services.

Be it therefore declared that each medical transcriptionist has the following rights:

- The right to full disclosure of the basis on which pay is determined.
- The right to fair pay, including overtime pay, and to benefits, including sick pay, holiday pay, vacation pay, and health insurance.
- The right to non-discrimination on any basis, including gender, age, disability, race, religion, sexual orientation, and ethnicity.
- The right to a safe work environment that promotes prevention, identification, and treatment of work-related injuries and disabilities.
- The right to communicate with others in order to assist or be assisted, including feedback on performance and inquiries made regarding dictation or transcription.
- The right to edit dictation as necessary and appropriate to produce a clear, concise, and accurate document, correcting grammar, punctuation, and spelling, drawing attention to inaccuracies, inconsistencies, incomprehensible dictation, and potential risk-management concerns.
- The right to professional resources (print, video, audio, electronic) that facilitate the preparation of accurate and complete documents.
- The right to environmental resources (space, equipment, furniture, lighting, and supplies) that promote the efficient and effective accomplishment of responsibilities.
- The right to professional development and continuing education opportunities.
- The right to professional association membership and participation.
- The right to participate in the development of, to be informed of, and to adopt professional guidelines and standards for medical transcription.
- The right to respect and recognition as a professional, as a medical language specialist, and, for those who have earned the designation, as a certified medical transcriptionist (CMT).
- The right to participate fully as a healthcare professional in the preparation of patient care documentation in order to enhance the quality of that documentation and thereby the quality of patient care.

FIGURE 1-2 A Medical Transcriptionist's Bill of Rights. (Modified from the Association for Healthcare Documentation Integrity MT Bill of Rights.)

as a professional. The RMT and CMT are the professional designations awarded to individuals who have met certification requirements as specified by the AHDI. The AHDI mastery-level CMT examination has been established to recognize individuals with specialized advanced transcription competencies. The AHDI has published both an RMT and a CMT review guide to help prepare candidates for the examinations. Two years of practical experience are required before the CMT examination can be taken. (However, it is a good idea to start preparing immediately to take the examination, working to acquire the skills you need to pass.)

The AHDI has also established an entry-level examination to encourage recent graduates of MT programs to measure their competencies as well. A study guide to help you prepare for the examination is available from the AHDI. The new Level 1 examination (for RMTs) is set up in two parts: In the written part of the multiple-choice, timed examination, approximately 40% concerns terminology; 20% anatomy/physiology;

5% disease processes; and 12% grammar. The remainder of the test covers medical records, medicolegal aspects of risk management, and professional concerns. In part II of the examination, audio technology is used for a dictation/transcription examination; about 55% involves transcribing brief bits of medical reports; 30% involves proofreading; and 15% editing. Testing includes units of measure, medical symbols, typos, spelling, abbreviations, English words, difficult grammar, and punctuation. Neither spellcheckers nor references are available during testing. Testing is done at centers all over the country run by Thomson Prometric. The company has more than 400 test centers in the United States and Canada (www.prometric.com). Candidates are informed of pass-fail status immediately upon completion of the test.

An overview of the certification process and self-assessment tools is available at the AHDI website. Candidates who pass both parts of the examination (written and practical) become RMTs or CMTs. A CMT is recognized as a professional MT who participates in an ongoing program of continuing medical education to increase his or her knowledge of medicine and improve skills in medical transcription. CMTs are required to accrue 30 continuing education credits in each 3-year period after certification. The certification of Fellow of AHDI is awarded to CMT certificate holders who are involved in civic, association, and community activities. In the 5 years preceding an application for the fellow designation, the MT must obtain a CMT, be a member of AHDI, write articles for professional journals, serve on AHDI committees, attend professional meetings, make industry-specific presentations, and assume mentor and leadership roles.

Belonging to a professional association has other benefits besides certification. As a student member, you will get to meet others in the field and learn how they cope with certain on-the-job problems. When attending local or online meetings, you receive further education from guest speakers on pertinent topics of current interest. From the professional publications you receive, you will learn what is current in the field. Sometimes part-time or full-time job opportunities are mentioned in the publications, and this information can lead to employment. Local chapter meetings are often a resource for job openings. Most important, you will become acquainted with those in your chosen profession and will feel more professional by belonging to a group.

For more information regarding membership, certification, recertification, and self-assessment products, contact:

> Association for Healthcare Documentation Integrity
> 4230 Kiernan Avenue, Suite 130
> Modesto, CA 95356
> Telephone: 800-982-2182 and 209-527-9620
> Fax: 209-527-9633
> Email: AHDI@AHDI.org
> Website: www.ahdionline.org

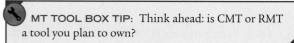

MT TOOL BOX TIP: Think ahead: is CMT or RMT a tool you plan to own?

Health Professions Institute

Health Professions Institute is a private publishing company that has provided services to the MT industry since 1965. In addition to publishing the SUM Medical Transcription program and transcription modules, they provide a free online medical transcription student network and a free online journal, *e-Perspectives on the Medical Transcription Profession*. This journal features professional articles by experts in the medical transcription field. One of the special features is a list of the newest medical terms, "Update: What's New in Medicine." It is a good idea to download these terms and add them to your notebook. See Figure 1-3 for a sample look at the Update. Other offerings include an online newsletter, practice work sheets, and online seminars. Further information is available at the Health Professions Institute website, www.hpisum.com.

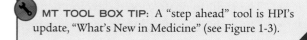

MT TOOL BOX TIP: A "step ahead" tool is HPI's update, "What's New in Medicine" (see Figure 1-3).

ETHICAL AND LEGAL RESPONSIBILITIES

Before you begin work as a MT, it is wise to have some basic knowledge of ethical and legal responsibilities as they pertain to the medical profession and to MTs. Ethics are not laws but are standards of conduct. The AHDI adopted a code of ethics on July 10, 1995. Current copies of the code are available from the AHDI (see preceding contact information). If you become employed by a transcription service, you also should adhere to the code of ethics and standards developed by the Medical Transcription Industry Alliance (MTIA) (Figure 1-4).

Confidentiality

Preserving the confidentiality of information, protecting the integrity of the information, and ensuring the availability of the information are moral and legal obligations for the transcriptionist. The MT must prevent unauthorized disclosure of confidential information.

Update

What's New in Medicine

APPEAR technique – an anterior perineal plane for ultra-low anterior resection of the rectum, a technique to effect an ultra-low sphincter-saving anastomosis, when this is not possible by conventional surgery.

CG Future ring and band system – a trigone-to-trigone semirigid anuloplasty band for mitral valve repair. CG stands for Colvin-Galloway, the designers of the band.

CIAP (continuous monitoring of intra-abdominal pressure) – a simple means of measuring intra-abdominal pressure using a standard 3-way bladder catheter.

COBAS TaqMan HBV test – a laboratory test kit that measures the amount of hepatitis B viral DNA in the blood of an individual infected by the hepatitis B virus.

Crowded right atrium – a form of vascular congestion.

DSAEK (descemet-stripping automated endothelial keratoplasty) – procedure used to correct severe bullous keratopathy.

DT-MRI (diffusion tensor magnetic resonance imaging) **tractography** – an imaging technique designed to construct global connectivity of white matter tracts in the brain.

Ductal lavage – a diagnostic procedure to detect breast cancer. It involves collecting cell samples from the lining of milk ducts in a minimally invasive outpatient procedure. Laboratory tests then can determine if the cells are normal, irregular or malignant. The procedure also allows physicians to 'bookmark' suspicious milk ducts and retest those sites at a later date.

ESD (endoscopic submucosal dissection) – a technique that uses specially developed endoscopic knives for en bloc resection of esophageal squamous-cell carcinoma that measures 20 mm or more in diameter.

Interosseous suture endobutton – a minimally invasive technique that eliminates the need for implant removal, as opposed to traditional interfragmental screw fixation, used to stabilize Lisfranc fracture dislocations.

Intrapleural perfusion

hyperthermo-chemotherapy – a method of inducing apoptosis of tumor cells in patients with malignant pleural mesothelioma.

NOTES (natural orifice transluminal endoscopic surgery) – a procedure by which an endoscope is inserted through a natural body opening, rather than through an internal incision in the stomach, vagina, bladder or colon. This avoids any external incisions or scars. (Example: An appendix removed through the mouth.)

Pedicled tensor fascia lata flap – an alternative option for the stable repair of pelvic floor defects to prevent radiation injury.

P-Mate disposable urine director – a device that allows women to urinate standing up.

Reading man procedure – a technique for repair of resultant defects after surgical removal of circular skin lesions. The technique uses the extra skin relaxation gained with an unequal Z-plasty maneuver in favor of the defect closure. It is called 'the reading man' procedure

FIGURE 1-3 Sample from Update, published in e-Perspectives. (Courtesy Health Professions Institute, available at www.hpisum.com, accessed February 5, 2010). *Continued*

because its surgical design resembles the silhouette of a man who is reading a book held in his hand.

ROLL (radio-guided occult lesion localization) – for nonpalpable breast carcinomas.

SAVI applicator – a single-entry, multi-catheter breast cancer radiation treatment device that allows customization of the radiation dose depending on the patient's anatomy and precise configuration of the surgical site. It is said to have minimal side effects for women who do not qualify for breast conservation therapy using a previously available balloon device.

SVR (surgical ventricular restoration) – a procedure combined with coronary atery bypass grafting (CABG) in patients with advanced heart failure to

remold the heart to a near-normal size, by cutting and suturing together stretched muscle and scar tissue resulting from the initial attack.

TBA (transluminal balloon accessotome) – a device used for transmural drainage of pancreatic pseudocysts. The TBA device is inserted through a therapeutic duodenscope and the pseudocyst punctured at the point of maximal bulge. The needle-knife and handle of the TBA are withdrawn after the cyst cavity is entered and a guidewire inserted. The TBA balloon is inflated to dilate the tract, and a pigtail catheter inserted for drainage.

Time-SLIP (time spatial labelling inversion pulse) – a technique used in noncontrast magnetic resonance angiography to

better illustrate the lower extremity vessels where blood flows more slowly.

Uresta pessary – the first pessary made available over the counter to women. The Uresta pessary is shaped like a bell and works much like a tampon. It comes in three sizes. Once inserted, it sits under the urethra and provides mechanical support.

FIGURE 1-3, cont'd.

> **MT TOOL BOX TIP:** Safeguard tools should always be in place to ensure data is not compromised.

Transcription services must have written policies and formal employee awareness training on an ongoing basis. Computer service technicians should have a signed security and confidentiality agreement in place, and the agreement should be reviewed any time a hard drive recorded with stored medical documents leaves the service center.

Most employers require MTs to sign a confidentiality agreement (Figure 1-5). A comprehensive monograph addressing confidentiality, privacy, and security of patient care documentation through the process of medical dictation and transcription can be obtained from AHDI.

Health Insurance Portability and Accountability Act of 1996

The federally mandated Health Insurance Portability and Accountability Act of 1996 (HIPAA) requires healthcare providers to safeguard an individual's

protected health information (PHI). PHI refers to any part of an individual's identifiable health information that is collected by the healthcare provider and is maintained or transmitted by electronic media. This material includes (but is not limited to) print and electronic patient records, daily schedules, surgery lists, patient sign-in sheets, computer files of any type (document, database, or voice), external removable drives, analog audiotapes, and digital voice files. PHI is defined as follows: the patient's name, family names, birthday, age, address, telephone numbers, fax numbers, email addresses, Social Security number, occupation, diagnosis, results of physical examination, treatment plans, admission date, discharge date, date of death, medical records number, health plan number, account number, certificate number, license number, vehicle identifiers (serial number and license plate), Internet addresses, device identifiers, fingerprints, voiceprints, full-face photographs, and any data that can reasonably be used to identify the patient.

To *de-identify* health information when it is no longer protected, all PHI must be removed or *scrubbed* from the document.

Code of Ethics

The goal of the Medical Transcription Industry Association (MTIA) is to promote superior performance standards for medical transcription service companies, and to provide a forum for industry representatives to exchange information.

Members of MTIA subscribe to the Code of Ethics and Standards adopted by the organization in Chicago on May 2, 1992:

We pledge to provide medical transcription service of the highest professional standards to our clients in order to contribute to the quality and efficiency of the healthcare industry.

We pledge to conduct ourselves and our businesses in a dignified, honorable manner that benefits the medical transcription profession and industry.

We pledge to deal with our clients with the highest standards for integrity and honesty, and to communicate clearly our standards for:

- Protection of confidentiality
- Quality of transcription
- Turnaround time
- Billing practices that include definable, verifiable units of measurement.

We pledge to protect and promote the dignity of our employees:

- To respect them as individuals.
- To honor their right to privacy.
- To encourage and reward continuing education.
- To uphold the highest professional standards for confidentiality and quality work.
- To respect employee rights as reflected in federal, state, and local laws.

We pledge to follow the highest ethical principles and procedures in relationships with colleagues in the medical transcription industry.

We pledge to achieve and maintain the highest attainable levels of professional competence in medical transcription businesses.

© 1999-2010 MTIA, 4230 Kiernan Ave, Ste 130, Modesto, CA 95356 1-800-543-MTIA

FIGURE 1-4 Clinical Documentation Integrity Association (CDIA) formerly known as Medical Transcription Industry Association (MTIA) Code of Ethics and Standards. (© 1999-2010 MTIA, 4230 Kiernan Ave, Ste 130, Modesto, CA 95356 1-800-543-MTIA, available at www.mtia.com/CodeOfEthics.cfm, accessed February 5, 2010.)

Care providers must address both privacy and security issues in maintaining and transmitting patient information. You probably became aware of HIPAA as it pertains to the confidentiality of your own medical records when you made a visit to your own private physician's office, emergency department, or other medical facility.

Because many MTs are independent contractors or business owners, they are acting on behalf of a healthcare provider and must implement clear policies and

Medical Record Confidentiality Agreement

As a condition of my employment with _____

I agree to the following provisions:
- All information received that relates to patients of this facility will be considered private, confidential, and privileged.
- Patient information will not be accessed unless needed in order to perform my job.
- No patient information will be removed from the premises in any form without permission.
- E-mail and fax transmission of patient data will be restricted to that permitted by the facility.
- Computer passwords will be safeguarded and not posted in any public place or where they could be misplaced.
- Computer passwords will not be shared with any other employee for any reason.
- Computer passwords of other employees will not be used to log on for any reason.
- Patient information obtained while an employee of this facility will continue to remain private, privileged, and confidential even upon cessation of employment with the facility.
- HIPAA policies and regulations will be complied with at all times.

I understand that violation of any part of this agreement could result in termination of employment.

Signed _____ Date _____
Printed name _____ Witness _____

FIGURE 1-5 Example of a confidentiality agreement that should be used by a facility when a new employee is hired. *HIPAA,* Health Insurance Portability and Accountability Act of 1996.

procedures that ensure appropriate safeguards are in place to protect PHI. MTs are affected by HIPAA regulations, regardless of whether the MTs are employees or independent contractors. All business associates are directly subject to HIPAA regulations. (The employment terms *employee, statutory employee,* and *independent contractor* are discussed in Chapter 16.)

You must adhere to the federal HIPAA regulations that affect your responsibility for patient confidentiality, and you must understand that disclosure of PHI is prohibited except as required to fulfill your contractual obligations. You must abide by individual state laws that may further provide legal protection of medical documents. Some state laws take precedence over HIPAA regulations if the state laws are more stringent than the privacy rules. Everyone must comply with security standards and procedures so that patient data is protected. Written policies and

procedures must be in place with security awareness and training.

Here are some important guidelines for all professionals who have access to PHI:
- Know that you may disclose PHI only if you have the patient's written consent to do so.
- Observe confidentiality issues with regard to sending and receiving email messages; use password protection, encryption, and authentication in transmission of patients' records. Data security must be ensured. Do not send protected documents by email without written permission to do so from the provider. (Patients must acknowledge that they understand the risks of sending information by email.)
- Save and log all fax transmissions and receipt confirmations.
- Fax only to machines located in a secure area of a business or office that is inaccessible to any individual

not bound to a HIPAA compliance contract. The area should be locked when the fax machine is unattended. Do not fax to machines in mail rooms, office lobbies, or other open areas unless the machines are secured with passwords. Use a transmittal sheet with each fax transmission that includes a statement about the receiving of confidential information and that includes language clearly outlining the confidential nature of the data being transmitted. Do not use patient identifiers in the subject field.

▶ Have the patient sign a properly completed authorization form for release of confidential medical information if such data must be faxed. Do not fax protected documents without written permission to do so by the provider. Anytime a hardcopy document is faxed, all attempts should be made using a fax machine with industry standard secure fax capabilities. In general, when sending a secure fax, a password (usually a four digit number) is generated at the sending machine by the user. This password must then be separately transmitted, e.g., by phone or secure email, to the recipient. Upon receipt, the user enters the password to retrieve the fax from the local machine. This also adds a layer of protection in case the fax was accidentally sent to the wrong number, as without the password, the unintended recipient would be unable to retrieve the misdirected fax. In some fax machines, the password also serves as an encryption key that provides limited protection from unintended disclosure during fax transmission and while on the fax machine's hard drive. Every office should have written policies and procedures, or standard operating procedures, regarding secure fax transmission and receipt.

▶ Verify the telephone number and make arrangements with the recipient for a scheduled time of transmission or send the fax to a coded mailbox to maintain confidentiality, and notify the authorized recipient immediately upon receipt of a fax record. Do not leave messages containing PHI on answering machines or voice mail.

▶ Be aware that all paper records and media records must be stored, transmitted, secured, and labeled according to HIPAA regulations at all times. Retain health information only as long as it is necessary for verification, distribution, and billing purposes. (The healthcare provider is the appropriate caretaker of patient files.) Make sure computer hard drives are completely purged of PHI.

▶ Make sure that an obvious measure, such as shredding PHI when the information is no longer needed, is documented as policy.

▶ Be aware that it is inappropriate to include one patient's name in another patient's document.

▶ Know that it is permitted to disclose protected information for treatment, payment, or healthcare operations.

▶ Know that you may provide access to those who perform quality assurance or record review of your medical transcripts as long as a contract is in place with the reviewer of the records that outlines permission to access.

▶ Seek out training on updates on policies and procedures by attending lectures and seminars on HIPAA.

▶ Make yourself knowledgeable about HIPAA issues so you can make appropriate modifications to your business.

▶ Keep all papers, tapes, disks, and removable drives in a locked fireproof container or file cabinet. Do not leave any patient document unattended on a desk or work space. Cover such documents when an unauthorized person enters the work area.

▶ Use a bonded courier for transporting medical records. The records should be sent in a sealed and tamper-proof container with no patient data information visible to the courier or any other third party.

▶ Make sure the computer you use for work is not accessible to unauthorized individuals and make sure your computer screen is protected from unauthorized viewing by persons passing your work station; use firewall protection software on your computer when working from home. Use software that makes the computer's IP address "invisible" to anyone who might try to access it through an uninterrupted Internet connection. Utilize encryption software and password protection when transferring files via direct connection to another computer.

▶ Remember that being compliant with HIPAA regulations is an ongoing process. Utilize password management, keep workstations secure, keep transmissions secure, have unique user identification for all files, monitor all log-in to records, keep things private that should remain private. See Figure 1-5 for a sample confidentiality agreement you could use to protect your business.

 MT TOOL BOX TIP: HIPAA Rules: tools for everyone.

NOTE: For further information, order "HIPAA for MTs: Considerations for the Medical Transcriptionist as Business Associate (with Sample HIPAA Business Associate Agreement)" from the AHDI (800-982-2182), or research online at www.hipaa.org.

Risk Management

A risk management department is established to prevent situations that can lead to liability. An organization must do as much as possible to identify and prevent potential risks to patients, visitors, and personnel. Organizations must develop policies and procedures to ensure patient safety, first and foremost. Risk managers identify potential problems, forestall incidents, and are charged with making sure that healthcare documents are complete and accurate. The managers coordinate and manage claims and settlements in conjunction with administrative and hospital legal personnel, receive legal documents related to hospital liability, act as liaisons to hospital and medical staff for hospital policy and for state and federal legislative requirements, review managed care contracts, and assess losses in hospital activities and future ventures.

MTs must be aware of their role in risk management by being compliant with all industry standards for privacy and security. Some hospital regulations should be carried over into clinics and private practice facilities (e.g., see Chapter 5, section on abbreviations). MTs are a vital link in patient safety and must understand and clearly and accurately transcribe what is dictated to them. One must be alert to dictated material that may be incorrect or inaccurate and be responsible for reporting this situation to the supervisor. (Specific scenarios will be addressed in later chapters when you work directly with "patient" records.) MTs must pay attention to the administrative policies and procedures of the organization for which they work. Because the medical document is the foundation of the revenue cycle and also serves as the first line of defense for risk management, patient safety, and continuity of care, MTs must learn to abide by all patient safety regulations even when not required by law to do so. It is important to participate in quality control activities and maintain the highest possible standards. The top two national patient safety goals are to improve the accuracy of patient identification and to improve the effectiveness of communications among caregivers.

If you are employed by a health facility that has a policy manual or office procedure manual, familiarize yourself with its rules for the release of information. However, in a situation for which you do not have the answer, consult your supervisor or risk management department regarding hospital regulations. If you are working in a private medical office or as an independent transcriptionist, consult the local medical society or your employer's attorney if an unusual problem arises. You are under the jurisdiction of *respondeat superior* ("let the master answer"), which means that the physician/dictation provider is liable in certain cases for the wrongful acts of assistants or employees.

Laws governing the medical profession are constantly changing as advances in medical care occur; therefore, it is essential for you to stay current in this area. Medical records are a tremendous source for research, and to protect patients' privacy, some authorities have suggested that a patient's name be used only once: at the introduction of the record, where it can be located easily and removed when the document is used for research. It is the responsibility of the person dictating, of course, to make this decision about where to place a patient's name. Be aware of this issue and keep in mind the seriousness of patient confidentiality.

As I further discuss the ethical and legal implications in regard to medical records, refer to the following vocabulary list to assist you in better understanding some of the difficult legal terms.

Vocabulary

Advanced directive: A power of attorney that permits someone to make decisions for a patient who is incompetent to do so. Also called *advance directive*.

Americans with Disabilities Act: Title I of the Americans with Disabilities Act of 1990 that prohibits private employers, state and local governments, employment agencies, and labor unions from discriminating against qualified individuals with disabilities in job application procedures, hiring, firing, advancement, compensation, job training, and other terms, conditions, and privileges of employment.

Breach of confidential communication: In a medical setting, the unauthorized release of information about a patient.

Confidentiality: Treatment of a patient's medical information as private and not for publication.

Custodian of records: A person put in charge of medical records.

Damages: Compensation to those who have been injured as a result of another's negligence or incompetence.

Defamation: A common tort; injury to reputation—that is, slander or libel.

Documentation: The supplying of written or printed official information that can be used for evidence.

Do-not-resuscitate order (DNR): Specifics concerning what should and should not be done to revive (and continue care for) a patient who has experienced cardiac or pulmonary arrest.

Electronic signature: A process whereby a document is legally signed by computer directive.

Ethics: Moral principles and standards in the ideal relationships between physicians and patients or other physicians.

Etiquette: Customs, rules of conduct, courtesy, and manners of the medical profession.

Fraud: A criminal misrepresentation by an individual for benefit to himself or herself or to another.

Gross negligence: Extreme departure from standard of care.

Healthcare directive: A statement made by a competent individual outlining preferences for medical treatment in the event that he or she is unable to make decisions at the time care is needed. *See also* Advanced directive.

Independent contractor: A person who is not an employee but is hired to perform a specific job for the employer and is free to perform the work the contractor chooses. (See Chapter 16 for a comprehensive description of an independent contractor.)

Informed consent: An agreement to permit something to happen after the patient is informed of the risks involved and advised of alternatives for care. (Obtaining informed consent before an operative procedure and some diagnostic procedures is standard practice.)

Invasion of right to privacy: Unwarranted exploitation of another's personality or personal affairs with which one has no legitimate concern in such a way as to cause mental anguish or humiliation.

Libel: A false written or graphic statement to a third person that damages the reputation of a patient or subjects a patient to ridicule.

Life-sustaining procedure: A medical procedure in which artificial means are used to sustain life and postpone death.

Malpractice: Negligence or incompetence in the performance of duties to a client that results in injury or death.

Medical record: Written or computer-stored information (medical reports), tissue samples, log books, or x-ray films. (See "Medical Reports and Records" following this vocabulary list.)

Medical report: Written or computer-stored information about a patient's medical history. The report is part of the medical record.

Negligence: Injury or death due to failure to exercise reasonable care or the care required by the circumstance; failure to do something to prevent death or injury.

Protected health information (PHI): Any part of an individual's identifiable health information that is collected by the healthcare provider and is maintained or transmitted by electronic media, including (but not limited to) print and electronic patient records, daily schedules, surgery lists, patient sign-in sheets, computer files of any type (document, database, or voice), external removable drives, analog audiotapes, and digital voice files.

Release of information: Medical information given out to a third party with the written authorization of the patient.

Respondeat superior: "Let the master answer." A physician is liable in certain cases for the wrongful acts of his or her assistants or employees.

Risk management: A department to prevent situations that can lead to liability. (An organization must do as much as possible to identify and prevent potential risks to patients, visitors, and personnel. Organizations must develop policies and procedures to ensure patient safety, first and foremost. Risk managers identify potential problems, forestall incidents, and are charged with making sure that healthcare documents are complete and accurate.)

Slander: A false spoken statement made in the presence of others that damages a person's reputation or subjects a person to ridicule.

Statutory employee: Basically an independent contractor who is treated as an employee. (See Chapter 16 for a discussion of statutory employee, employee, and independent contractor.)

Subpoena duces tecum: A subpoena that requires the appearance of a witness with his or her records at a deposition, trial, or other legal proceeding. Usually the court permits these records to be professionally copied and verified so that someone other than the physician or medical record custodian presents them to the court.

Verbatim: Word for word.

MEDICAL REPORTS AND RECORDS

Records must be maintained in a manner that follows all applicable regulations, including accreditation, professional practice, and legal standards. The Joint Commission (JC; formerly the Joint Commission on Accreditation of Healthcare Organizations) is an independent not-for-profit organization that accredits and certifies more than 15,000 healthcare organizations. The commission was formed to improve the quality of care and services provided in organized healthcare settings through a voluntary accreditation process. Accreditation standards are continually updated and published in the *Comprehensive Accreditation Manual for Hospitals (CAMH): The Official Handbook.* The JC conducts surveys of hospitals to measure and encourage compliance with the standards. When these standards are met, the commission awards accreditation to the healthcare facility. The chapter on medical record services in the handbook describes standards that require certain entries, information, and signatures to be entered into the medical record as determined by a prescribed format.

A *medical record* is information to authenticate evidence of facts and events, and it is a legal document in all cases of litigation. The MT is responsible only for the accuracy of the transcribed medical report and for ensuring that the report remains confidential. A *medical report* is a permanent legal document that formally states the results of an investigation.

Three main purposes of medical records are to

1. Assist in the diagnosis and treatment of a patient by communicating with the attending physician and other medical personnel working with the patient
2. Aid and advance the science of medicine
3. Comply with laws and serve in support of a claim

The accreditation manual states requirements for medical report completeness, signatures, abbreviations, deadlines, and dates of documents. Details of this information are mentioned in the following sections.

Authentication of Documents

MANUAL SIGNATURES

All medical reports dictated by a physician must be signed by the physician responsible for the dictated material. In an instance in which an intern, a nurse practitioner, or a physician's assistant performs the physical examination of the patient and the attending physician dictates the history and physical examination, the attending physician may be the person who signs the report. For use of rubber signature stamps on medical reports, state regulations and statutes, system security, and system reliability must be considered carefully before such use is adopted. The individual whose signature the stamp represents (a signed statement must be placed in the hospital administration office attesting that only the physician responsible for the dictated material will use the stamp), may use rubber signature stamps. For pathology and laboratory reports, a laboratory technician must sign, initial, or stamp the reports that he or she completes. A pathologist's signature is required only on work the pathologist performs or provides, such as tissue, cytology, autopsy, and consultation reports. For radiology reports, the radiologist must authenticate the examinations he or she interprets in transcribed reports.

ELECTRONIC SIGNATURES

Many facilities have reports generated via computer, and an electronic signature is possible. An electronic signature on a document has the same legal bearing as a handwritten signature. The person dictating uses an identification system, such as a series of letters or numbers (alphanumeric computer key entries), electronic writing, voice, or fingerprint transmissions (biometric system) to authenticate parts of the medical record. The author of the document signs off the dictation by entering a unique code and the "signature" appears on the document. For transcribed medical reports, the JC and Medicare guidelines require that signatures, electronic or other, be written or entered by the physician and not be delegated. The legal requirements for electronic signatures can be found in federal law, state law, and the accreditation standards of the JC.

MEDICARE SIGNATURE REQUIREMENTS

Federal law requires physician signatures in a medical record for hospital compliance with Medicare Conditions of Participation and to qualify for reimbursement under the Prospective Payment System. A handwritten signature, initials, or computer entry is allowed. For Medicare reimbursement, an electronic signature is permitted when the physician attests to the patient's diagnosis only if the fiscal intermediary (entity responsible for reimbursement) has approved the system. If the attestation is transmitted by fax, the physician must keep in the files the hard copy of the original signature.

State laws vary; therefore, it is important for you to know the legal requirements in your state so that you can comply with those laws.

JOINT COMMISSION SIGNATURE REQUIREMENTS

The JC accreditation standards for hospitals require that all entries into a medical record be authenticated and dated. A method must be established to identify the authors of entries in the medical record. This identification may be a written signature, initials, or a computer key. A rubber stamp is allowed if the physician has executed a statement of exclusive possession and use of the stamp. Always consult with the JC before implementing any other electronic signature systems.

ABBREVIATIONS, ACRONYMS, AND SLANG

The JC requires that the medical staff of each hospital approve abbreviations and symbols that may be used in the hospital's medical records. Each abbreviation must have a definition. In the diagnosis section of a report, "Diagnoses and procedures are written in full, without the use of symbols or abbreviations." The list of abbreviations and symbols varies between healthcare facilities, and it is important for the MT to review the appropriate list before beginning work. Because physicians tend to dictate their own preferred abbreviations, it is the MT's responsibility to use only the abbreviations approved by the medical institution whenever possible.

Abbreviations dictated by the physician and approved by the medical facility may be transcribed as abbreviations or transcribed in full, depending on the physician's preference, the medical facility's policies, or the transcriptionist's style. Abbreviations dictated by the physician but not approved by the institution must be spelled out. Each healthcare facility updates the approved abbreviation and symbol list from time to time, so it is important to make sure you have the current list for reference. See Chapter 5 for a list of abbreviations and symbols that have been banned by the JC for use in medical records.

Deadlines and Turnaround Time for Medical Reports

The turnaround time (TAT) is the elapsed time between the completion of dictation and the return of the transcribed report for authentication.

 MT TOOL BOX TIP: Turnaround Time—VIP tool for document completion.

The JC states the following in regard to deadlines for medical reports:

Physical Examination "The physical assessment shall be completed within the first 24 hours of admission to inpatient services." This document has priority when several items are pending.

Discharge Summaries "The records of discharged patients shall be completed within a period of time that will in no event exceed 30 days following discharge; the period of time shall be specified in the medical staff rules and regulations."

Operative Reports "Operative reports should be dictated or written in the medical record immediately after surgery."

Diagnostic or Therapeutic Procedures "Reports of pathology and clinical laboratory examinations, radiology and nuclear medicine examinations or treatment, anesthesia records, and any other diagnostic or therapeutic procedures should be completed promptly and filed in the record, within 24 hours of completion if possible."

Consultation Reports and Progress Reports These reports could be urgent, but they have no JC-referenced deadline. They could be the key communication between providers involving changes in condition as well as plans for a new or modified course of treatment. Be aware of the timeliness of these reports when you transcribe them.

Autopsy Reports "When a necropsy is performed, provisional anatomic diagnoses should be recorded in the medical record within three days, and the complete protocol should be made part of the record within 60 days."

TURNAROUND TIME EXPECTATIONS

TAT expectations on all documents not subject to deadlines vary not only by work type but also by method of creation or transmission of the report and by the type of authentication used. Dictated reports spend more time in a queue waiting to be delivered to the MT than in any other process. Wait time constitutes the bulk of document TAT. Certainly, timely TAT enhances patient care and empowers clinical decision making. It is paramount to complete all work as

if there were a mandated deadline. Finally, the quality of the document must always be considered and cannot be ignored. For example, do you complete a quality document only to have it available after it is needed for patient care or a document delivered on time with blanks and errors that could result in compromised patient care? Therefore, both quality and appropriate TAT are needed for patient safety. What really matters is whether a quality report was where it was supposed to be when it was needed.

 MT TOOL BOX TIP: Complete, accurate, and timely documentation—a tool to own.

DATES OF DOCUMENTS

Reports should include three dates: the date when care was provided, the date when the document was dictated, and the date when the document was transcribed. When the date is given for a letter or medical report, the date used is the day the material was dictated, *not* the day it was transcribed. A person dictating might ask to have the date on a report other than the actual date of care or dictation, to make it appear that the report was completed in a timely manner. The date *should not* be changed. This insistence on the correct date is very important for several reasons. Comments made in the document could reflect on the date when the care was provided. If the document should be entered as evidence in a court proceeding, it might be discovered that the date was changed, the physician's credibility might be questioned, and accusations of concealment, tampering, fabricating, and so forth could be made.

Completeness of Medical Reports

It cannot be overemphasized that if medical records are completed promptly after the physician sees the patient, there is less chance of an omission. In a physician's office, it is the office assistant's job to ensure that an entry is made in a patient's chart each time the patient is seen and that all procedures are documented according to the reimbursement codes used for that service. In a hospital setting, it is the medical records personnel who alert the physician to complete a medical record.

A medical record is complete "when the required contents are assembled and authenticated, including any required clinical resume or final progress note; and when all final diagnoses and any complications are recorded, without use of symbols or abbreviations. Completeness implies the transcription of any dictated record content and its insertion into the medical record." For the record to be considered complete, all medical information must be entered into the record and all signatures entered within 30 days after the patient's discharge. Experts base their opinions on the substance of the record. The following is an important adage to remember: If you didn't document it, it didn't happen. Again, the signature authenticates the record, so the record must be signed.

OWNERSHIP

Medical records are the property of the physician, corporation, or institution that provided care, and the owner is legally and ethically obligated to protect them. The Code of Hospital Ethics adopted by the American Hospital Association and the American College of Surgeons states, "It is the responsibility of the hospital and its personnel to safeguard the clinical records of the patients and to see that such records are available only to properly authorized individuals or bodies." This statement also applies to physicians and other healthcare providers. Normal property rights do not apply to patients' medical records because providers of care have a right to the information. Patients do have privacy rights to protect and control access to their records.

Information received from other hospitals and physicians about a patient's history or treatment is for informational use and is not considered the property of the hospital that receives it. Correspondence or social service information, which also may be filed in the hospital medical record, is not considered part of the medical record. When a patient is referred to a radiologist for x-ray films, the films belong to the radiologist and not to the referring physician.

CORRECTIONS

Medicolegal problems sometimes occur, so it is important to know how to correct medical reports. If a patient's medical record is presented in court as evidence in a professional liability case and the records have been sloppily corrected, a prosecuting attorney might win a case if it is proved that the records have been intentionally altered. Correcting errors on an electronically signed report requires an addendum explaining the change needed from the previous report. The new report is then signed within the electronic medical file.

See Chapter 11 for detailed information on how to make corrections on transcribed, signed paper documents.

Medical Records

Today, medical records are a vital key in patient care, medical research, and reimbursement compensation to the provider of care. If the records are kept neat, thorough, and accurate, and if the data are recorded promptly, the records help the physician in the treatment of the patient and aid in future research on diseases and their management. As you have learned

earlier in this chapter, properly kept and transcribed records can help eliminate medicolegal problems. On occasion, attorneys, employers, other physicians, insurance companies, and courts see records, and so the importance of keeping records correctly cannot be overemphasized. The professional transcriptionist types material that makes sense to him or her or asks for assistance to clean up inconsistencies by flagging the appropriate section for clarification. Therefore, it is important for you to understand medical terminology, disease processes, and laboratory terminology and to recognize accurate (or inaccurate) medical content. Material or information that is unclear, incomplete, or questionable is never transcribed until the data have been thoroughly confirmed. Discrimination skills are vital here.

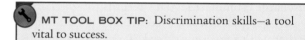

MT TOOL BOX TIP: Discrimination skills—a tool vital to success.

ELECTRONIC HEALTH RECORD

With EHRs, the medical record becomes part of a huge, shared database repository that the care provider (doctor, nurse, social service worker, and so on) is able to access to document findings, make reports, and leave orders in real time at the point of care. A patient's electronic record is composed of all clinical information: the patient's entire medical history (past and present) and all treatment received from every provider of care, including all medications and procedures. When the patient is seen in the emergency department, is admitted to the hospital, visits a consultant, or sees a new physician, all these data are available to the provider of care through the EHR database.

An EHR allows complete interaction among providers and instant retrieval of information from any source (e.g., pathology department, pharmacy, oncology department, or laboratory). This shared information helps providers improve quality of care by providing a means to track disease prevalence, learn of successful methods for care, obtain clinical decision support, exchange electronic health information and integrate such information from other sources, and so on. Security and patient privacy are maintained and protected by using technical coding tools to limit access to the records. The complete record is available 24 hours a day, a practice that eliminates delays in retrieval because the record is not stored on any single computer. The provider has access through his or her computer only as long as needed, that is, until the user logs off. The goal of using EHRs is to move away from paper records, and hospitals that have changed to EHRs will, over time, scan their paper records into the system. Having so-called backup paper records would defeat the purpose of the EHR, because this practice could allow an opportunity for errors to occur. The goal of the American Recovery and Reinvestment Act of 2009 is that each person in the United States will have an electronic medical record by 2014. Massive amounts of medical information will exist in a new form. Transition from paper to EHRs is central to health care reform. You will continue to hear more and more about this and how you will fit in to the picture of implementing and contributing to the change. New technology increases our value to the continuum of care.

ELECTRONIC MEDICAL RECORD

An electronic medical record is a software database in which caregivers use a series of drop-down menus to select entries such as patient complaints, procedures, allergies, medications, drug interactions, diagnoses, plans for care, laboratory procedures, and so on. The provider of care can use handheld equipment, such as a Palm device. This versatility gives caregivers the ability to prepare documents no matter where caregivers are.

The system is commonly used as a paperless chart. Fully functional electronic medical records add electronic ordering and full history and exam notes. The technology is a good idea, but most physicians do not want to do direct data entry—it takes too much time and they are not fast, resulting in a decrease in the number of patients they can see in a period of time, so a decrease in productivity occurs. Some transcription providers can assist a medical practice with document management as part of the transcription service. Often the physician just wants a paperless chart and the capability to get clinical notes online and to search for a patient online. Or the physician wants to support better billing and coding, so the MT will need to integrate the transcription system with billing functions. The features of the plan can be a business opportunity for the MT because the EMR does not save the physician time; it could, in fact, be a time waster with a decrease in productivity. The transcribed narrative is the vital information that forms the basis for reimbursement, proves that care was carried out, and provides the foundation for the initiation of orders. Transcribed documents can be imported directly into the EMR. (See Medical Scribe, page 4.)

RIGHT TO PRIVACY

The invasion of the right to privacy is the "unwarranted exploitation of another's personality or personal affairs with which one has no legitimate concern—particularly, intrusions into another's affairs in such a way as to cause mental anguish or humiliation." An example is publishing a patient's photograph (from which the patient could be easily identified) without the consent of the patient.

PRIVILEGED COMMUNICATION

Privileged communication is a confidential communication that may be disclosed only with the patient's permission. The right to the protection of the confidentiality of information in medical records belongs to the patient, not the physician. The MT should never mention the name of a patient or discuss a patient's condition within hearing distance of others. Everything a MT sees, hears, or reads about patients should remain confidential and should not leave the place of employment *under any circumstances*. Records, appointment books, charts, and ledgers should not be left where unauthorized people can see them. According to the "need to know" rule, you should not be accessing any medical document for any information unless you need to know the information to complete your own work product.

There are a few exceptions to the right to privacy and privileged communication. These include the records of physicians employed by insurance companies (especially for industrial cases); reports of communicable diseases, child abuse, gunshot wounds, and stabbings resulting from criminal actions; and records of diseases and ailments of newborns and infants.

In some instances, particularly sensitive information has been granted specific legislative protection by federal and state laws. Examples include information related to infection with human immunodeficiency virus (HIV), mental health treatment, drug and alcohol treatment, and reporting of child and domestic abuse. A patient's healthcare record *must* be vigilantly guarded.

RELEASE OF MEDICAL RECORDS

Information in medical records falls into two classifications: nonprivileged (not confidential) and privileged (confidential). The two can be defined as follows:

1. *Nonprivileged (or nonconfidential) information* is unrelated to the treatment of the patient. The patient's authorization is not needed to disclose these facts to anyone unless the record is in a specialty hospital or in a special service of a general hospital, such as the psychiatric unit. Even so, discretion must be used at all times, and care must be taken to make certain that the inquiry is a proper one that protects the best interests of the patient. Nonconfidential or nonprivileged information includes the following:
   ▶ Dates of treatment
   ▶ Dates of admission and discharge
   ▶ Number of times and dates when the physician attended the patient

- Fact that the patient was ill or underwent surgery
- Complete name of the patient
- Patient's address at the time the physician saw the patient or at the time the patient was admitted to the hospital
- Name of relative or friend given at the time the patient was first seen in the physician's office or at the time of admission to the hospital

2. *Privileged (confidential) information* is related to the treatment and progress of the patient and can be given out only on the written authorization of the patient or guardian (Figure 1-6). A patient can also sign an authorization to "release" only selected facts and not the entire record.

GUIDELINES FOR RELEASE OF INFORMATION

The following are guidelines for the release of information.

- The MT should become thoroughly familiar with state laws and HIPAA regulations concerning release of medical information.
- Whenever a patient fails to keep an appointment or does not follow the physician's advice, a letter should be sent to the patient, because documentation is necessary in the medical record.
- Requests from physicians concerned with patient care are honored with the written consent of the patient.

AUTHORIZATION FOR DISCLOSURE OF CONFIDENTIAL INFORMATION

I hereby authorize and request Dr. _____ to furnish

information or copy of my medical records to:

_____
_____
_____

about medical findings and treatment about my illness and/or treatment

during the period from _____to_____

I understand that this is a required consent and I must voluntarily and knowingly sign this authorization before any records may be released, and that I may refuse to sign, but in that event the records will not be released.

I further release my physician from any liability arising from the release of information to the individual(s)/agency designated herein.

Signed_____   Witness_____

Address_____   Date_____

_____

Optional statements may include:
I agree that a photocopy of this form may be used in lieu of the original.

This authorization will automatically expire one year from the date signed or is effective until_____.

FIGURE 1-6 Example of authorization for disclosure of confidential information.

▶ Requests from insurance companies, attorneys, and others concerned from a financial point of view are honored *only* with the written consent of the patient. (If the attorney cannot read the physician's handwriting, an appointment is made with the physician. The attorney should pay for the office call.) The MT should not attempt to interpret a medical record.

▶ When litigation is involved, information should *not* be released in the absence of a subpoena unless the patient has authorized the release. Never accept a subpoena or give records to anyone without the physician's prior authorization. In the instance of a subpoena or interrogatories (questions directed to a physician who is being sued), records should not be released until you have verified the records with the physician and had him or her correct any inaccuracies. Usually there is time to review such records, and any problems should be referred to the physician's lawyer before the records are released.

▶ Government and state agencies may have access to records pertaining to federal government sponsored and state-sponsored programs, but these records should not be released without explicit consent of the patient.

▶ Information of a psychiatric nature may present special or delicate problems. In general, the psychiatrist or another attending physician concerned with the case should be consulted before any data are released. Usually the computer system gives limited electronic access to these records so that no one will be able to view the records without permission to do so.

▶ Special care should be exercised in the release of any information to an employer, even with the consent of the patient.

▶ Exercise care in permitting laypersons to examine records. In this way, misunderstandings of technical terms are avoided. However, according to the Privacy Act of 1974, certain patients, such as those receiving Medicare and Civilian Health and Medical Program of the Uniformed Services (CHAMPUS/TriCare) benefits, have a right to their records, because the provisions of the act bind federal agencies. If the physician determines that the release may not be in the patient's best interests, most states allow release to a representative of the patient. The only way a physician can prevent patients from gaining access to privileged information in their own medical records is by noting that he or she believes knowledge of the contents would be detrimental to the patients' best interests. This entry, however, must be made before the patient makes his or her request. The courts usually uphold a physician's judgment under these circumstances. It is also a good idea to have the patient sign a receipt for any x-ray films.

Only the paper that the records are typed on is the physician's.

▶ Care must be exercised in the release of any information for publication, because such release also constitutes an invasion of the patient's right to privacy and can result in legal action against the physician or health facility that releases the information.

▶ Always obtain the patient's authorization in writing specifying exactly information may be released. (See Figure 1-7.)

▶ If the signed authorization form is a photocopy, it is necessary to state that the patient approves the photocopy, or to write to the patient and obtain an original signed document.

▶ Any transfer of records from hospital to hospital, physician to physician, or hospital to nursing home should be authorized in writing by the patient. If the patient is physically or mentally incapacitated, the next of kin or legal guardian may approve the transfer.

▶ You cannot justifiably refuse to provide information to another physician just because a patient has a large outstanding bill with your facility.

▶ Oral requests are handled by asking the caller to put the request in writing and to include the patient's signature for release of information.

▶ In an industrial injury (workers' compensation) case, the contract exists between the physician and the insurance carrier. When an insurance adjuster requests information by telephone, verify to whom you are speaking before giving out medical information. Such cases do not require a patient to have a signed release-of-information form on file.

If you are working in a physician's office, seek legal counsel if a patient who has a positive HIV test result or acquired immunodeficiency syndrome (AIDS) applies for life or health insurance and requests that the physician or hospital send medical records to the insurance company. Some state laws allow AIDS information to be given only to the patient's spouse. In a hospital setting, patients infected with HIV must sign an informed written consent before any medical information is released. The release of information from records of patients who have HIV infection or those tested for HIV must be handled very carefully, especially in states with restricted access to health records, because information about test results may appear in many sections of the health record. If state law says test results may be placed separate from the patient's medical record, a file for cases (e.g., HIV infection or alcohol or substance abuse) that require special release of information forms may be established. The *International Classification of Disease, 9th Revision, Clinical Modification* (ICD-9-CM) code 795.71 reflects a positive HIV test result, and so this information must be considered confidential.

CHAPTER
1

NAME OF FACILITY
Consent for Release of Information

DATE_____

1.   I hereby authorize_____to release the
         Name of Institution
         following information from the health record(s) of
         _____
         Patient Name
         _____
         Address
         covering the period(s) of hospitalization from:
         Date of Admission_____
         Date of Discharge_____
         Hospital #_____Birthdate_____

2.   Information to be released:
         [ ] Copy of (complete) health record(s)   [ ] Discharge Summary
         [ ] History and Physical   [ ] Operative Report
         [ ] Other_____

3.   Information is to be released to_____
         _____

4.   Purpose of disclosure_____
         _____

5.   I understand this consent can be revoked at any time except to the
         extent that disclosure made in good faith has already occurred in
         reliance on this consent.

6.   Specification of the date, event, or condition upon which this consent
         expires.
         _____

7.   The facility, its employees and officers and attending physician are
         released from legal responsibility or liability for the release of the
         above information to the extent indicated and authorized herein.
         Signed_____
                         (Patient or Representative)
         _____
                         (Relationship to Patient)
         _____
                         (Date of Signature)

FIGURE 1-7 Consent for release of information form. (Reprinted with permission from the American Health Informa-tion Management Association, Chicago, Ill.)

The American Health Information Management Association has suggested the use of a form for granting consent for release of information (Figure 1-7). Besides filling in the blanks, it is important to list the extent or nature of the information to be released (e.g., HIV test results, diagnosis, and treatment with inclusive dates of treatment). After authorized release of patient infor-mation, the signed authorization should be retained in the health record with notation of the specific informa-tion released, the date of release, and the signature of the person who released the information. All informa-tion released at the request of a patient with a diagnosis of HIV infection should be clearly stamped with a state-ment prohibiting redisclosure of the information to another party without the prior consent of the patient. The party receiving the information should also be requested to destroy the information after the stated need is fulfilled.

SPECIAL GUIDELINES FOR RELEASE OF HOSPITAL INFORMATION

In general, certain information is not available from the medical record for release to third parties. This infor-mation includes details of psychiatric examinations, personal history of the patient or the patient's family, and information controlled by state law. If a question occurs about the content of the medical information to be released, the attending physician should be consulted about the accuracy or interpretation of the information. Hospitals prefer to release information by the use of summaries or abstracts or on standard forms recommended by the American Hospital Association or local hospital groups. Duplicating an entire record is expensive; furthermore, control of the record by the hospital would be lost, and the copy might be misused. If the attending physician wishes information from the hospital record, an abstract or a copy can be given without the patient's written permission, as long as the information is for the physician's own use.

RETENTION OF RECORDS

The length of time medical records must be kept by an organization is determined on the basis of law or regulation and of the use of the records for patient care, treatment and services, legal, research, and operational purposes, and educational purposes. Each organization's policies as well as state and federal law or regulation would determine record retention. Many states set a minimum of 7 to 10 years for keeping records. In general, most physicians retain medical records of their patients for an indefinite period for research or for historical significance. In the case of minors, records should be retained 3 to 4 years beyond the age of majority.

SUBPOENA DUCES TECUM

Subpoena duces tecum ("Under penalty you shall bring with you") requires a witness to appear and to bring certain records to a deposition, trial, or other legal proceeding. Usually, the records are sent by certified mail, and the physician or custodian of the records is not required to appear in court. A subpoena is a legal document signed by the clerk of the court (Figure 1-8). In cases in which a "pretrial of evidence" or deposition is set up, the subpoena may be issued by a notary public, in which event it is called a *notary subpoena*. If an attorney signs a notary subpoena, he or she must validate it in the name of a judge, the court clerk, or another proper officer.

A subpoena duces tecum must be served to the prospective witness in person. If the subpoena is accepted by someone authorized to receive it, the acceptance is the equivalent to personal service. A subpoena cannot be left on a desk; it must be served.

Here are some points to remember if a subpoena is served and you are given permission to receive it.

▶ Determine which physician the subpoena is addressed to. Get the name of the custodian of records for that particular physician if you are not the custodian. Ask to see the subpoena so that you know what action to take.

▶ After receiving a subpoena for a trial, verify with the court that the case is on the calendar. If the subpoena is for a deposition, verify the date and place to appear with the attorney.

▶ You will have a prescribed time in which to produce the records. It is not necessary to show them at the time of service of the subpoena unless the court's order so states. In general, a professional copy service appears to copy the record and verify that it is complete. Otherwise, telephone the attorney who ordered the subpoena and request permission to mail a copy of the record. If the attorney agrees, send the copy by certified mail with return receipt requested. If you do not comply with a subpoena, you may be in contempt of court and subject to fine or imprisonment.

▶ Never give records to anyone or permit the records to be copied without prior permission. When a subpoena is served, an authorization form for release of records signed by the patient is not required. Read the record to see that it is complete and that signatures and initials are identifiable.

▶ Remove the records to a safe place so that they cannot be stolen or tampered with before the legal proceeding. Make copies of the records if you are in doubt about their safety. Copying may be expensive, but it can prevent total loss of the records and facilitate discovery of any altering of them while they are outside your custody. It also provides you with the record in case the patient is treated before the original is returned.

▶ If you must appear in court with records, comply with all instructions given by the court. Do *not* give up possession of records unless instructed to do so by the judge. Do *not* permit examination of the records by anyone who has not been identified in court. When you leave the records in the court in the possession of the judge or jury, obtain a receipt for them.

▶ If you have additional questions, call the patient's attorney or the physician's attorney.

PROFESSIONALISM

> 🔧 **MT TOOL BOX TIP:** Professionalism—knowing what it means is a helpful tool towards success.

Some ethical issues and professional behavioral issues are not covered by legal statutes. However, these issues are important. To be regarded as a professional, you

Name, Address and Telephone No. of Attorney(s)

Space Below for Use of Court Clerk Only

Mitchell & Green
210 W. "A" Street
Los Angeles, California 90014
(213) 232-7461

Attorney(s) for **Defendants**

SUPERIOR COURT OF CALIFORNIA, COUNTY OF LOS ANGELES

ALBERT   OTTO

Plaintiff(s) vs.

ROY M. LEDFORD, RALPH
WALLACE, et al.,

Defendant(s)

(Abbreviated Title)

CASE NUMBER

353 957

SUBPENA DUCES TECUM
(Civil)

THE PEOPLE OF THE STATE OF CALIFORNIA, to ___Dr. J. Brown___ ,

You are ordered to appear in this court, located at ___111 No. Hill Street, Los Angeles, Ca.___ ,
(Street Address of Court and City)

on ___Feb. 8, 20XX___ at ___9___ a.m., ___Department 1___ , to testify as a witness in this action,
(Date) (Time) (Department, Division or Room No., if any)

You must appear at that time unless you make a special agreement to appear another time, etc., with:

___R. Mitchell, Esq.___ at ___232-7461___
(Name of Attorney or Party Requesting This Subpena Duces Tecum) (Telephone Number)

You are also ordered to bring with you the books, papers and documents or other things in your possession or under your control, described in the attached declaration or affidavit, which is incorporated herein by reference.

Disobedience of this subpena may be punished as contempt by this court. You will also be liable for the sum of one hundred dollars and all damages to such party resulting from your failure to attend or bring the books, etc., described above.

Dated ___Jan. 31, 20XX___

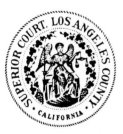

Clarence E. Cabell

CLARENCE E. CABELL, County Clerk and Clerk
of the Superior Court of California, County of Los
Angeles.

(To be completed when the subpena is directed to a California highway patrolman, sheriff, marshal or policeman, etc.)

This subpena is directed to a member of _____
(Name of Employing Agency)

I certify that the fees required by law are deposited with this court.

Receipt No._____   Amount Deposited $_____

CLARENCE E. CABELL, County Clerk   By _____ , Deputy

NOTE: The original declaration or affidavit must be filed with the court clerk and a copy served with this subpena duces tecum.

(See reverse side for Proof of Service)

SUBPENA DUCES TECUM (Civil)

C.C.P. §§1985-1997; Evid. C. §§1560-1566;
Gov. C. §§68097.1–68097.4; 35c.

FIGURE 1-8 Example of a subpoena duces tecum (civil).

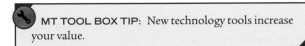

should have a desire and determination to do the following:

▶ Stay on the cutting edge. Learn not just the practice of transcription itself but also the newest technology.

> **MT TOOL BOX TIP:** New technology tools increase your value.

▶ Read the professional journals produced for this field.
▶ Accept fair or even unfair criticism with equanimity, and criticize others with fairness and gentleness.
▶ Seek continuing education. Use the Internet to learn the names of new drugs, words, procedures, and instruments. Learn more than you need to know to do your job professionally.
▶ Forsake company politics and care genuinely for those with whom you work and for whom you serve.
▶ Be self-confident, and have respect for yourself.
▶ Remember in dealing with people that you should try to understand rather than try to be understood.
▶ Mentor incoming members of the profession when you are established.
▶ Have the ability to adapt to change.
▶ Network with other professionals.
▶ Dress professionally whenever you represent your career in public.
▶ Be considerate and do not sort through dictation and reject jobs that you know are difficult and try to pick out the quick and easy material, leaving the more difficult items for others. (This practice is called "cherry picking"; it causes a lot of ill will and is counterproductive.)
▶ Be dependable and responsible in terms of completing work and completing it quickly and accurately. Be flexible to accommodate shift changes.
▶ Belong to and participate in your professional organization. Study to become an RMT or CMT.
▶ Respect fellow transcriptionists' accounts.
▶ Have an absolute unwillingness to take part in office gossip.
▶ Be flexible and teachable and keep a questioning mind. Adapt to new situations.
▶ Be able to say easily and without embarrassment, "I don't know."
▶ Work very hard to make others look good. Then your initials at the bottom of any document will say, "This is my work, and I am proud of it."

> **MT TOOL BOX TIP:** Good tools set you apart from the competition.

In the world of work, there are two classifications of work: *jobs* and *careers*.

Jobs are work-for-cash arrangements that people make to earn money, pay bills, and buy food—to get by. Jobs seldom provide opportunity for great personal growth or major advancement. Wages tend to range from low to moderate, and job workers are rarely allowed to experiment with many of their own ideas.

Careers are the employment of one's specialized knowledge and skills to meet the specialized needs of the community or industry. Broad employment opportunities exist in the industries of vocational trades, technology, and service. Management seeks meaningful input from skilled employees and provides them with growth and advancement opportunities. A lifetime of career-directed employment is a rewarding experience.

TRANSCRIPTIONIST'S NOTEBOOK OR FILE

As you prepare for your future career as a MT, you should organize two notebooks. One should be an alphabetically tabbed, pocket-sized notebook and the other a standard-size, three-ring binder, with or without index tabs. These notebooks can become valuable tools. The alphabetically tabbed notebook is for writing down any new or unfamiliar words or phrases heard while you listen to dictation (Figure 1-9). You might want to make a special page listing Internet search engines that provide the quickest and best solutions. Try *not* to make keeping your notebooks a chore, or you will not be consistent.

> **MT TOOL BOX TIP:** Your personal notebook is one of your most valuable reference tools.

Make it a rule to add any word that you had to research because of spelling, capitalization, or usage. In this way, when you hear the word again, you will be able to find it with ease. It is always easier to locate a word in your own guide, even when you know the word can be found elsewhere. Write in the word with no definitions; just include a few hints from time to time, such as the following:

▶ An (a) or (n) after an adjective or a noun term

EXAMPLE
mucous (a) mucus (n)

▶ An (s) or a (p) after a singular or plural word

EXAMPLE
bronchus (s) bronchi (p)

```
            M

m-AMSA


Manschot (implant)

Mantoux

maxilla (s)
maxillae (p)


medication-resistant

M-End Max

milieu (mee-Loo)

mill-house murmur



mucous (a)
mucus (n)
```

FIGURE 1-9 Page M from an alphabetically tabbed, pocket-sized transcriptionist's notebook, showing the following entries: unusual abbreviation for a drug name, eponym for a medical device, eponym for a test, singular-plural guide with a word pair, compound, brand name drug, French term with pronouncing help, unusual term, and adjective-noun guide with word pair. Capital letters are underlined to remind the MT that the letter is a capital letter.

▸ An extra word to complete a complicated pair

EXAMPLE

pleural poudrage or poudrage, pleural

▸ A line under a capital letter so that you will not wonder later whether it is correct

EXAMPLE

pH

▸ A source clue that could help you to determine later that you have the correct word

EXAMPLE

CABG (cardio) "cabbage"

▸ The phonetic spelling of a word with a reference to the correct spelling

EXAMPLE

▸ "sinkable": see syncopal

EXAMPLE

"sinkable episode": see syncopal episode (fainting)

Some transcriptionists prefer to indicate which physician dictated the word or term by placing the physician's initials after the word. Any other hints you can think of to help you may certainly be incorporated, because this is your reference book. As your material accumulates, be sure you carefully recopy it in strict alphabetical sequence. You can use a scanner, which provides you with a copy that you can easily sort alphabetically. You can print the sorted copy out on sticky-backed paper and overlay the copy on the original. An alternative reference method is to prepare an index file of 3 × 5 inch cards with alphabetical dividers and to use the cards in the way mentioned previously. A standard-sized binder can be used to store commonly needed information for quick reference, such as lists of new words in a particular specialty, drugs frequently prescribed, particular preferences of the institution you work for, such as restrictions of the use of certain symbols such as "°", superscript, subscript, the use of bold, abbreviations permitted, and so forth.

Throughout this text/workbook, notations appear that give you instructions to insert special data sheets into your standard notebook. Your instructors may provide additional lists and data sheets as you progress. When you are employed, you will often come across articles or lists in journals or other publications that serve as excellent reference guides. The lists of new words found in *e-Perspectives on the Medical Transcription Profession*, published by HPI, as mentioned previously, are very valuable. Handouts and printouts from speakers at professional meetings can be excellent reference materials along with the names of reliable websites you have discovered or been given. Students often collect unusual reference materials at work-study sites and from mentors. A well-filled binder is an excellent tool for you to take to a job interview.

Now you are ready to begin Self-Study 1-1, on your way to becoming a MT.

1-1 SELF-STUDY

DIRECTIONS: Let's add a terrific tool to your collection by beginning your own reference notebook. Obtain an easy-to-handle, 1/2-inch thick, three-holed ring binder about 4 x 7 inches with 25 sheets of lined paper and A-Z index guides. If it is difficult to locate a set of 26 alphabetical index tabs, obtain the two-letter combined alphabetical index tabs. As you come to words in the text that you have difficulty spelling or that you want to be able to refer to quickly, place them under the correct alphabet letter for easy reference. Write in any unusual words or abbreviations that appear in your examples or exercises.

Here is a start.

Start with your first entry under "W." Record websites that are authentic and trustworthy. (Remember to add to the list.)

▶ http://www.adhionline.org (AHDI, the medical transcription professional organization)
▶ http://www.hpisum.com (Health Professions Institute) Recall that this is the site mentioned earlier that publishes e-Perspectives, which includes the helpful list as shown in Figure 1-3.
▶ http://mtia.com (Medical Transcription Industry Association)
▶ www.tlbb.com (The Little Blue Book, which lists names and addresses of physicians and hospitals) If you can obtain a print copy for your area, please add it to your book collection.
▶ http://www.rxlist.com/interact.htm (drug list and abbreviations used with drugs)
▶ http://www.doctordirectory.com (for doctor's names and addresses)
▶ http://www.healthgrades.com (for doctor's names and addresses)
▶ http://mtdesk.com (a reference and style guide for medical transcriptionists)
▶ http://www.mtchat.com/ubbthreads/ubbthreads.php (Medical transcription forum)
▶ http://google.com (yes, this seems to work for almost anything!)
▶ http://medlineplus.gov (a store of health information)

Beginning with Chapter 3, look for some words to place in your notebook.

NOTE: If you would like to make an electronic version of the reference notebook using Excel, your instructor has some hints in the Instructors Reference Manual to help you get started with it.

1-2 REVIEW TEST

DIRECTIONS: Complete the following statements by filling in the blanks or selecting the correct answer.

1. According to the standards of the Joint Commission, what is the deadline for completion of a physical examination report on an inpatient?

   _____

2. State at least four skills that a successful transcriptionist should have.

   a. _____   b. _____

   c. _____   d. _____

3. In transcribing, what is even more important than speed? _____

4. Written or typed information set down for the purpose of preserving memory that authenticates evidence of

   facts and events is a/an _____

5. Briefly list three main purposes of medical records.

a. _____

b. _____

c. _____

6. Who owns the patient's medical records? _____

7. Name two classifications of information contained in medical records.

a. _____

b. _____

8. Name the federal entity that provides specific guidelines for patient privacy.

_____

9. How would you alert the document author if you found a critical error or discrepancy in a dictation?

_____

10. If your state has laws protecting patient confidentiality that are stricter than the federal guidelines, to which do you conform?

_____

11. Is the risk manager responsible for patients, visitors, or employees of a facility?

_____

12. What is the main hazard in using the Internet for research?

_____

13. What, if any, is the value of becoming a CMT or RMT?

_____

14. When may you disclose protected health information? _____

15. What is an advanced directive? _____

16. The transcriptionist recognized the name of a patient as that of the son of a friend of hers. The report indicated a good prognosis for the child. Because the mother had been depressed and uneasy for her child, the transcriptionist felt it was all right to telephone her and reassure her.

Was this action correct? _____

Why? _____

17. Name one main difference between a job and a career. _____

18. At this point, which area of medical transcription appears the most interesting to you?

_____

19. If a surgeon dictates the operative report before the time of surgery, it is
a. None of the transcriptionist's business
b. A matter for utilization review
c. Discussed with risk management
d. Pointed out to the surgeon

20. In which of the following instances can the medical records of a patient be released to a third party without the patient's written permission?
    a. Under no circumstances
    b. With a subpoena duces tecum
    c. Upon request of the police or prison officials
    d. On the hospital administrator's authority only

21. Your aunt is visiting and complains to you that she cannot get her physician to return her phone calls and she desperately wants to know if her recent biopsy finding is positive or negative. What would you do?

    _____

22. Your hospital administrator was just admitted to an inpatient facility in a nearby community. He has not been at work for more than two weeks and no one knows where he is or what is wrong with him. You know because you have a part-time job transcribing for this remote site. What would you do?

    _____

23. If you work as an "independent" contractor doing medical transcription, you become exempt from the HIPAA privacy restrictions. T___F___

    Comment on the question_____

24. One would not consider it a breach of HIPAA if you completed your medical transcription from your home. T___F___

    Comment on the question_____

25. Where are electronic medical records stored?
    a. In the transcriptionist's computer
    b. In the dictator's computer
    c. On the Internet
    d. In the computer where they were downloaded
    e. None of the above

26. When you have successfully delivered your transcript, your downloaded files and paper files should be
    a. Kept indefinitely
    b. Shredded or purged from your equipment
    c. Converted into an electronic file
    d. Mailed to a secure repository

27. There is an "unwritten rule" in medicine that if you did not document it, _____

28. A signed confidentiality statement should be
    a. Attached to every patient's records
    b. Attached to every employee's personnel records
    c. Displayed in the office of each care provider
    d. Included as part of every contract for services

29. Turn-around-time (TAT) concerns
    a. Your billing for the transcript
    b. Security of the medical record
    c. Conforming to HIPAA regulations.
    d. Joint Commission regulations

30. What does the reimbursement chain refer to?
    a. The fact that documents you transcribe generate revenue.
    b. Your payment for transcription based on lines transcribed or the visible black character (VBC).
    c. The encryption of the medical record for billing.
    d. A report being returned for authentication.

HIPAA REVIEW TEST

DIRECTIONS: Circle the letter identifying the answer that you think is correct.

NAME: _____   SCORE:_____

1. What does PHI stand for?
   a. Private Health Information
   b. Personal Health Information
   c. Protected Health Information
   d. Protected Hospital Information.

2. If you stumble upon a breach of PHI, whom should you notify regarding the breach?
   a. Your company's compliance officer
   b. Your unit manager
   c. The IT Department
   d. Both a and b

3. When asking your family member for help in understanding a difficult dictation, the recording should not be played over the speakers. Why not?
   a. Speakers muffle the sound quality.
   b. No family member should have access to any voice or text file, or PHI.
   c. Your family member may know the patient.
   d. Using speakers distracts others in the home.

4. You would like to maintain a file of sample reports for reference, you should:
   a. Remove all PHI and print the report for your use.
   b. Print the reports and store them in a safe place in your home.
   c. Copy the reports as a document file on your personal computer.
   d. None of the above.

5. You just transcribed a report on one of your neighbors who is in the hospital. You should:
   a. Call and tell your neighbor what his/her doctor dictated in the report.
   b. Call your friends and let them know what is going on with your neighbor.
   c. Refuse to transcribe the report; ask your supervisor to assign it to someone else.
   d. Go visit your neighbor and give him/her medical advice.

6. You decide it's time to take your 30-minute lunch break. You should:
   a. Ensure your password-protected screen saver is active.
   b. Exit all open programs.
   c. Leave all programs up and running.
   d. a and b only.

7. When disposing of specimen cups or IV bags that include patient names, a hospital should:
   a. Use a permanent marker to mark out any PHI before throwing in the trash.
   b. Remove the labels and place them in confidential trash to be shredded.
   c. Place the items in biohazard trash.
   d. Any of the above.

8. Which of the items listed below is *not* considered PHI?
   a. Date of birth
   b. Patient's name
   c. State where patient resides
   d. Social Security number

9. You are a MT or a QA editor and you keep a manual log of each report that you have worked on for the day in order to verify line counting. You should:
   a. Shred or burn the log when you are finished with it.
   b. Store the log in a filing cabinet indefinitely.
   c. Keep it out on your desk so you can add to it easily.
   d. Email a copy of it to your unit manager.

10. When you are in the waiting room of a doctor's office and the nurse says your name aloud to call you into the doctor's office for your appointment, is this a violation of the Privacy Rule? Yes or No

11. When asking a question about a report via instant messaging, it is permissible to include PHI in the message. True or False

12. According to the HIPAA Privacy Rule, there is no requirement that patients sign an authorization to obtain copies of their own records. True or False

13. Can patients be given a copy of their records on CD instead of in paper format? Yes or No

14. Are medical facilities required by the HIPAA Privacy Rule to notify patients of accidental disclosures of PHI? Yes or No

15. You had an appointment with your family physician. This physician just happens to dictate reports to the medical transcription company that you work for, and you are one of the MTs who work on that site. You go into the system at work and open up the report to see who transcribed your report and to read the report. Is this in violation of HIPAA? Yes or No

16. You just transcribed a progress note on someone who is in your prayer group at church and the situation is gravely serious. You can:
   a. Give the patient a call and tell her you're praying for her.
   b. Go visit her and show your concern.
   c. Call your pastor to let him know.
   d. None of the above.

17. You would like to maintain a file of sample reports from various doctors on your account. You can legally:
   a. Remove all PHI and print the report for your use.
   b. Print the reports and store them in a safe place in your home.
   c. Copy the reports as a document file on your personal computer.
   d. None of the above.

18. You have requested email feedback from your QA editor regarding some of the more challenging dictators on your account. This is appropriate if your QA editor:
   a. Removes all PHI from the report before sending.
   b. Sends the report using encryption software.
   c. Only emails the sentence with the blank.
   d. All of the above.

19. You are a MT working for a medical transcription company. You come across a breach of PHI and should report it immediately to:
   a. Human Resources
   b. Your company's compliance officer
   c. Your unit manager
   d. The IT department

20. When the privacy officer has been notified of a privacy breach, he/she must:
   a. Investigate the situation and find out exactly what transpired.
   b. Notify the appropriate unit manager, the site, and all other appropriate individuals involved in the investigation.
   c. Write up a HIPAA disclosure documenting what transpired, who was involved, what impact it had, and corrective measures taken to prevent it from happening again.
   d. All of the above.

21. You receive copies of patient schedules from your employer in order to verify correct spellings of patient names, etc. These copies should be handled in what manner:

a. They should be saved for 60 days as a reference to be used to verify patient names in the future.

b. They should be kept in a locked drawer when not in use and shredded or burned when you are done with dictation from that day's visits.

c. They may be kept indefinitely as long as they are electronic and the computer is secure from access by others.

d. They may be kept on your desk in the file folder for that date in order for you to have easy access.

CHAPTER 2

Equipment and Technology

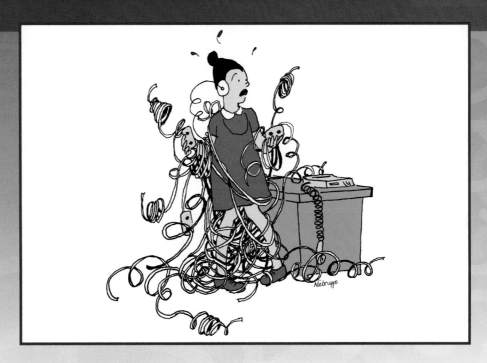

OBJECTIVES

After reading this chapter and completing the exercises, you should be able to

1. Describe the different types of dictation and transcription equipment.
2. Describe abbreviation expansion programs.
3. Explain various methods to manage and store computer data.
4. Identify types and features of printers.
5. State the purpose of a modem.
6. Apply correct ergonomic habits in your work environment.
7. Name two categories of speech-recognition systems.
8. Demonstrate proper equipment maintenance.
9. Perform the steps of transcription preparation.
10. Identify equipment for physically challenged persons.
11. Explain how fax machines can be used in the transcription process.
12. Explain why and how to dispose of electronic media.

Note from the Author

Chapter 2 is a fantastic chapter! You will learn about some of the latest technology available for medical transcriptionists (MTs) and medical editors (MEs). Of course, by the time this book is in your hands, there will be even more new and wonderful items to explore, but you have to start somewhere. You must learn as much as possible about today's technology to be prepared to follow industry trends and to market your skills in the future. Do not for a moment forget that you are the brain behind the equipment and that your role in producing the document is crucial. You are not simply getting words on paper—you are also making a personal contribution to patient care. Keep in mind this little quote from Abraham Lincoln, "I know of nothing so pleasant to the mind, as the discovery of anything which is at once *new* and *valuable*."

2

CHAPTER

MT TOOL BOX TIP: New technology tools increase your value.

HISTORY

Before beginning, please refer to the vocabulary list on page 56 if you encounter a new technical term.

MT TOOL BOX TIP: Organize your workstation (a collection of tools) before you start to transcribe.

Dictation

Initially, physicians made handwritten chart entries or dictated chart notes and medical reports in person to secretaries, who wrote in shorthand. This method required two people to be simultaneously engaged, a condition that was often difficult in a busy environment. The notes had to be converted quickly because a certain amount of human memory was involved. It was nearly impossible for someone other than the person who took the notes to transcribe them.

Then dictation machines, which have been traced back to Thomas Edison, became available. The physician dictated reports directly and at any time, making it possible for others with skills to transcribe the reports. These machines had cylinders made of material that would easily chip, crack, or break into pieces if dropped. Sound was of poor quality. By the 1960s, Mylar tape was used, which substantially improved the sound quality of standard cassettes. Eventually, microcassettes were introduced. The most common units available include the following:

▶ *Dictation unit,* for dictation only
▶ *Transcription unit,* designed for the transcriptionist who will transcribe the dictation (Figure 2-1)

Some transcriptionists use a *cassette-changer central recorder.* This device holds 15 to 25 cassettes that can be programmed to change automatically, either according

to the number of dictators who have access to the recorders or according to the percentage of tape used. The machine can be set up so that each person who dictates is recorded on a separate cassette. People who dictate can access the equipment from any telephone, at work or at home. These machines, although still in use in physicians' private offices, are fast giving way to digital dictation equipment. See Figure 2-2, which is a *direct-wired* or *telephone-connected transcribing unit.* See Figure 2-3, which is the Dictaphone C-Phone. It can be direct-wired or telephone-connected.

Digital dictation is a very popular dictation method that involves the computer, Windows platforms, information-processing programs, and the Internet. Physicians carry *portable dictating machines* to conventions, meetings, hospital rooms, and home (Figure 2-4). These are sometimes called *walk-a-bouts* or *handhelds.*

Digital Dictation

Digital dictation is used in many offices, clinics, and hospitals. It has eliminated the use of Mylar tapes, making voice recording much more portable and making the Internet the new carrier medium. The dictated voice is digitized and stored as data on a computer disk with identifying information (patient, dictator identification, and work type). Data are instantly and selectively accessible before, during, and after transcription. With the help of the Internet, these data can be accessed from remote sites anywhere in the world. When accessed (from a dictation/transcription station or connections telephone), the digitized voice files are converted back to analog waveform to sound the same as the original dictation (Figure 2-5). With the addition of a properly configured personal computer (PC) connected to a *local-area network* (LAN) or the Internet (a *wide-area network* [WAN]), these digital voice files can be played back directly from the computer. This method provides 100% digital sound, eliminating crosstalk and line interference. The dictator uses a handheld recorder or call-in system. The MT accesses the digital voice file via the computer. Control of voice flow is through a foot pedal attached to the computer. The dictator can insert or delete material for error-free dictation. The connections

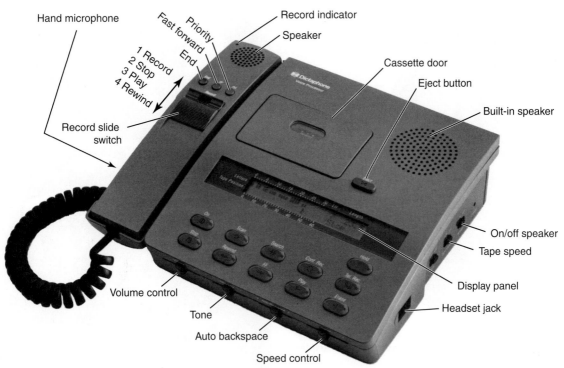

FIGURE 2-1 Dictaphone's Express Writer Plus voice processing system, a fully programmable compact desktop system. (Courtesy of Nuance, Burlington, Mass. (formerly Dictaphone Corporation). Available online at: www.nuance.com.)

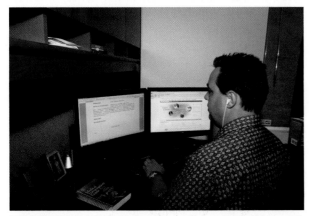

FIGURE 2-2 Medical dictation editor transcribing with companion computer providing instant Internet access.

telephone has buttons to increase or decrease the dictation speed, to increase or decrease the volume, and to adjust the bass or the treble tones. The backup feature of the foot control makes it easy to relisten to a short or a long group of words, or the MT can play back a selection and bookmark it for later reference.

Digital dictation does the following:
▸ Eliminates the need for tape
▸ Eliminates the problem of getting the dictation/transcription from place to place (e.g., from dictator to MT and then MT back to dictator)
▸ Reduces opportunity for data to be lost or damaged when moved from one place to another

▸ Saves time because the dictation arrives nearly instantaneously at its destination so the MT can begin to work with it immediately
▸ Restricts access by using encryption
▸ Provides software programs that allow the MT to manage, prioritize, and sort jobs

Considerations and problems are not eliminated. Although digital dictation sounds simple, these systems are, in fact, complex. You need to be aware of some of the potential problems, some which the MT has no control over. The dictator could forget to dock the handheld device, or the software could be inadvertently interrupted so the dictation is not sent. Devices can be dropped and damaged, lose battery power, or be stolen. The dictator may inadvertently rewind or dictate over material, and another dictator may pick up the device so work is tagged to that dictator instead of the one to whom the device is dedicated. With call-in dictation, fewer things can go wrong. The dictation is time-stamped, a job number is given to the dictation so that it can be tracked, and work types and patient identifiers are inserted.

COMPUTER SYSTEMS

Hardware

The physical components of a computer system (electronic, magnetic, and mechanical devices) are known as the *hardware*. Minimum hardware requirements are typically defined by individual software manufacturers.

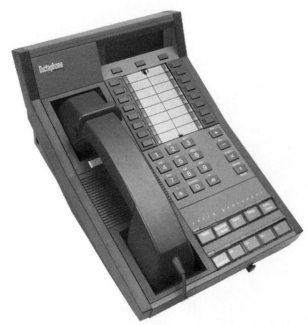

FIGURE 2-3 Dictaphone C-Phone. It can be direct-wired or telephone-connected. A lighted liquid crystal display presents demographic information.

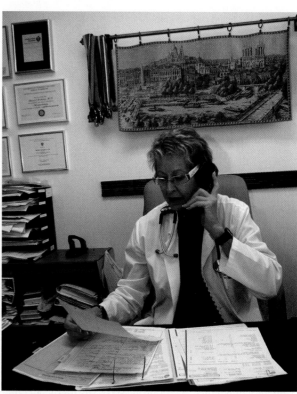

FIGURE 2-5 This physician's voice is digitized when she uses a dictation station (telephone-like device) to dictate medical reports from the hospital, emergency room, clinic, or office to the receiving device.

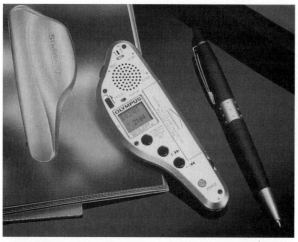

FIGURE 2-4 The Olympus V90 Digital Voice recorder is ergonomically designed to fit snugly inside the palm of the hand. It is capable of up to 90 minutes of recording time. (Courtesy of Olympus America Inc., Melville, N.Y.)

A PC should have a *mouse,* a *keyboard,* a *sound card,* a network connection (*modem, Ethernet,* or *WiFi*), and a *monitor.* Some transcriptionists use two computers, with the companion computer available for Internet research and email (see Figure 2-2).

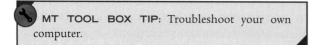

MT TOOL BOX TIP: Troubleshoot your own computer.

DATA COMMUNICATIONS AND MODEMS

The word *modem* is an acronym for *mo*dulator-*dem*odulator unit. Modems are used to communicate from one computer to another within a facility, to transmit data to another computer in a remote area, or to send data to the Internet over standard telephone lines. In today's world of high-speed Internet access, it is important to use an equally high-speed modem, such as integrated services digital network (ISDN), digital subscriber line (DSL), or cable modem. Regardless of which data communications medium you use, however, data security is vital. When transmitted over any communication medium, data are susceptible to *hacking* by someone other than the sending or receiving party.

The key to data security is to make it as difficult as possible for the hacker or eavesdropper to do anything with the data once he or she obtains the file. Therefore, a cryptosystem must be part of your Internet transfer of documents. The basic idea behind data encryption is for the sender to encrypt the data files by using a key, which is typically made up of a string of data bits (1s and 0s). The key at the receiving end is some value that allows the message to be decrypted and read. Note that the lengths of keys are described in terms of *bits* in cryptosystems. The longer the key, the more difficult it is to break an encrypted message. Secure encrypted connections are created between locations, bypassing the open networks on the Internet. Encryption can also control access at a single location to prevent unauthorized access. Many good cryptosystems are available for document protection.

Some transcription services offer telecommunication via modem. Then they can transmit correspondence or reports to an office, a clinic, or a hospital facility many miles away. Documents transmitted in this way can be revised and edited at the receiving office before they are printed out as hard copy or imported into an electronic medical record repository.

COMPUTER MAINTENANCE

Because reports and letters should be professional looking, it is essential that your equipment be maintained in good working condition. Establish a maintenance plan and delete temporary files and backups. Clean the keyboard and the central processing unit periodically with a vacuum and a slightly dampened cloth. From time to time, the computer unit should be opened and cleared of dust particles by using a series of short blasts from special pressurized cans (e.g., Dust-Off). Avoid using abrasive cleaners on any parts of your equipment.

Another important part of the file maintenance is to keep a smoothly running operating system. Over time, the hard drive can develop logical and physical errors. A utility such as ScanDisk in Microsoft Windows operating systems should be used to detect and fix any problems before they become serious. You can also use Disk Defragmenter to rearrange files and unused space on your hard disk. Defragmenting helps programs run faster. These utilities should be run at least once a month after backing up the data.

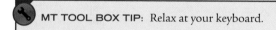

MT TOOL BOX TIP: Relax at your keyboard.

After the warranty time has expired, an annual service contract for your computer and printer is essential. Know whom to call to make repairs. If the computer is signalling that an error has occurred or performs erratically, note the error and what you were doing at the time of the error. Look in the troubleshooting section in the user manual for the computer or software causing your problem. Save any printed material that demonstrates the problem. The printout assists the service person in determining the cause of the problem. If you shut down improperly or if your computer "crashes," it may run in safe mode and will not save or print. Shut the computer down properly and restart it.

Before making a service repair call
- ▶ Check to see that all computer cables are properly connected.
- ▶ Turn the computer or printer off and then on again (to see whether the problem will clear itself).
- ▶ Check to see whether the equipment is plugged in.
- ▶ Make sure the outlet is in working order by plugging another piece of equipment in and turning that piece of equipment on and off.
- ▶ Determine whether the equipment has been turned on.
- ▶ Make sure the screen brightness has not been turned down.
- ▶ Check to make sure that another electronic device is not interfering with the computer.
- ▶ Check the equipment manual and locate the section on troubleshooting information.
- ▶ Check to see whether technical assistance is available over the telephone before calling a technician to the equipment location.

Many companies have their own help desk for resolving and tracking computer and/or software problems. Locate the machine's serial number, model, purchase date, warranty information, operating system, version of software in use, and so forth before telephoning for assistance. Keep a log of the service calls, noting the technician's name, time of call, time of arrival of technician, and resolution of the problem.

Software

All computers require an operating system that assists in managing the different hardware devices in the computer. The system manages keyboard and mouse input, video and sound output, and data storage devices such as the *hard drive*. The various compact disk (CD) drives are also managed by the operating system. The majority of computers today use a Microsoft operating system (e.g., Windows XP, Vista, Windows 7, and Windows NT). Other operating systems available are Macintosh OS (Apple Computer Operating Systems) and various versions of Linux. Today, most operating systems are capable of multitasking, meaning multiple programs can run simultaneously.

In addition, a computer typically utilizes some kind of *word processing software* to enable the transcriptionist to key, format, and edit dictation. Most computer word processors have features that make repetitive tasks easier and quicker. Some features include automatic text insertion and formatting, document templates or boilerplating, macro creation, spellchecking, word and line counting, and thesaurus research. Many more add-on software packages are available and can enhance functionality. The most common ones targeted for the medical industry are *text expanders,* which allow the MT to create text that expands into words of any length, as well as complete sentences or paragraphs (see Macros, Appendix C on Evolve). Also available are medical and pharmaceutical dictionaries and spell-checkers with tens of thousands of medical words that can be added to the standard word processor's dictionary or accessed in the spellchecking function. Be sure the software programs installed on your computer conform to copyright laws.

Speed Typing Systems

TEXT EXPANSION

The most popular method of quickly inputting data into a document is to use a text expansion application. These programs run in the "background" of a word processing program and "watch" for certain predefined abbreviations, sometimes called *short forms,* from the keyboard. Whenever the short forms are typed, the program automatically expands the characters or numbers into a predefined word, phrase, complete sentence, entire paragraph, or entire report. This feature is helpful when very long words or frequently used phrases are keyed, a common requirement in medical transcription. These programs are designed to increase production while reducing the number of keystrokes entered. Use of a program such as this may reduce the number of keystrokes 60% or more, and there is no limit to the number of entries recorded. Some programs have a built-in collection displayed in a window or "prompts" that appear when you type in a word that is available for expansion. For instance, if you type the word *history* you might see *history* and *hx* in a prompt box. Over time, you remember to use *hx* to expand to history. Imagine this situation occurring dozens of times in a paragraph, or even a sentence. You, of course, can customize the program by adding your own unique short forms and expansions. An example of what you may eventually be typing in a program could be the following:

EXAMPLE

You type: t pt is a 25 yo wd wn wm sn in t ed fng...

The text on your screen converts to: The patient is a 25-year-old well-developed, well-nourished white male seen in the emergency department following...

Figure 2-6 is a screen shot of a professional text-expansion program. Notice paragraph 3, which shows how the program assists you in cuing in a text expansion as soon as the two letters *pc* were typed.

Several software companies market text expansion products, such as InstantText, SmartType, and Speed-Type. Ask MTs who use a program to recommend one before you purchase, or ask for a 30-day demo copy before you purchase.

MT TOOL BOX TIP: Read your text expanders—a tool that keeps you from looking foolish

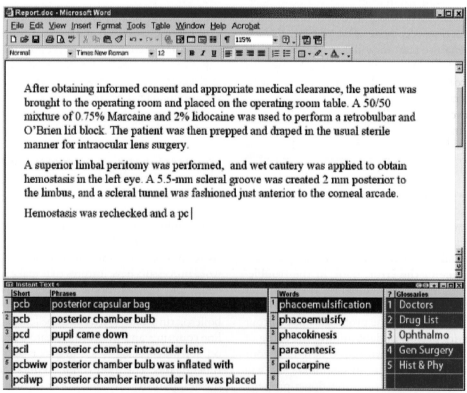

FIGURE 2-6 Sample screen showing text expansion program. (Courtesy of Instant Text by Textware Solutions.)

AUTOCORRECT

To give you an idea about how abbreviation expansion programs might work for you, try the following steps with AutoCorrect in Microsoft Word. If you are using another word processing program, you probably have a similar feature, but this example is for Microsoft Word. You will be using the AutoCorrect feature under the Tools menu. AutoCorrect is a feature of Microsoft Word that automatically corrects many commonly misspelled words as you type the words. The option is also available to automatically capitalize the next word after you type a period and capitalize the names of the days of the week.

1. Open a new document on the screen.
2. Type in a word or phrase.
3. Highlight this word or phrase.
4. From the Tools menu, select AutoCorrect. When AutoCorrect dialog box opens, the Replace With box is automatically populated with your selection and you then fill in the short form you want to use.
5. Give your word or phrase an abbreviation and add a character (code) such as an *x*. (An *x*, which is seldom used, will keep acronyms and real abbreviations from expanding).
6. Select Add and OK.
7. Return to your document and type in your new short form to see if it expands correctly. If you want a space to appear after your word, be sure to code that in as well. The *x* is convenient because you do not normally use that with abbreviations, and it is easy to remember. You might practice with a few more phrases you frequently use to get the idea. Following is a group you can practice with, or you can make up your own. You can use this AutoCorrect feature in Microsoft Word, of course, but a real abbreviation expansion program is more efficient, helps you create shortcuts, and improves your accuracy. Text expanders run at the same time as the word processing software and are simple to use and offer more flexibility.

The following are simply suggested abbreviations (feel free to make up your own, of course, and keep a list of them to refer to in the beginning).

acci	accident
accis	accidents
bec	because
becf	because of
hov	however
labo	laboratory
min	minimal
miny	minimally
neg	negative
ofi	office
ofis	offices
ofil	official
ofill	officially

Notice how important it would be to place a character code after *mini*. Otherwise you would get *minimally* when you just wanted to use the word *mini*. You could also use simply *lab* plus *x* for *laboratory* instead of *labo*. Finally, notice how the four similar *office* words are handled.

You can use AutoCorrect for symbols as well. Notice that when you place a degree symbol, for example (select this from your Symbols menu), that the symbols chart shows you the AutoCorrect menu automatically, and so all you have to insert is your code word. When you actually begin your practice transcription, start looking for words to add to your AutoCorrect utility and eventually your professional expansion program. Be careful of your spelling, and if you make a mistake, simply return to AutoCorrect and correct it. These programs also help improve accuracy by enabling the MT to create distinct abbreviations for words that frequently present spelling or fingering problems. For example, if you often type "yu" for "you," you simply teach your computer to turn "yu" into "you."

MACROS

A *macro* is typically a small program or set of instructions that the word processor uses to complete repetitive tasks. A popular task that macros are typically used for is to take an existing paragraph or a complete document and perform a "find and replace" function to insert text at a certain location in a document. Macros can be set up to be accessed by a key sequence or a mouse click. In general, a key-sequence macro is called a "keyboard macro," because the macro is activated by pressing a certain set of keys on the keyboard. You can make a macro to generate formats that have the same structure every time they are created. After you have set up a macro correctly, it can be set with a "read-only" attribute so that it cannot be changed. With this feature, new documents can be generated from it without modifying the original one accidentally. Remember that every keystroke you program into a macro or AutoCorrect is one less keystroke you have to make over and over again.

Online Information Processing Systems

In medium-sized and large companies, many users may require access to shared information on large information networks (Figure 2-7). The development of LANs, WANs, and the Internet has enabled users to share information, peripherals, email, optical character readers, and data storage devices. A network typically contains one or more large, more powerful computers called *servers* connected to several smaller computers called *workstations*. Online information processing systems take advantage of this network

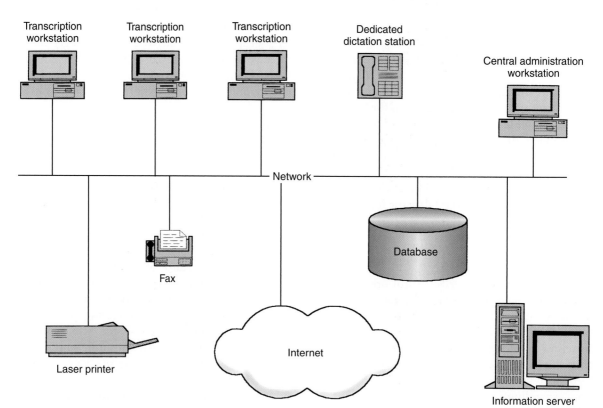

FIGURE 2-7 Online information processing system: information server, database storage, connection to the Internet, online fax system, shared printers, several transcription workstations, dedicated dictation station, and a central administration workstation.

technology by using the servers to store large amounts of information in databases that are then accessed by the users on the workstations. The information can be quite extensive, such as large databases containing electronic patient records, drug indexes, insurance information, typed and scanned documents, and digital voice files. Because all the data can be stored on the server, managing the information from one central location is much easier. The central administrator can distribute the work and produce reports, as well as archive and back up data. When dictation is recorded into the system, the dictated material can be associated with a patient record, type of dictation, and the author's name; the dictation is subsequently assigned to a transcriptionist. At the click of a mouse, the transcriptionist can access the digital voice file from the system, and all of the important information about the patient and the dictator is instantly available with the dictation. The dictated voice files can be flagged for immediacy so that the transcriptionist can prioritize the work efficiently. Once the voice file is transcribed, it can be sent to a printer or filed for later retrieval. Three popular online information processing systems in the medical industry are Dictaphone's Enterprise Express Voice System, 3M ChartScript, and Dolbey Fusion.

Data Storage

HARD DRIVE

The *hard drive,* usually located inside the computer case (internal), is the component that stores large amounts of data for quick retrieval. The hard drive gets its name from the physical characteristics of the disk inside the drive unit. These disks, or "platters," are very rigid and can withstand extremely high spin rates. Because the disk spins so fast, in order to avoid disk crashes, it is important to keep the disk very stable while it is turned on. An internal hard drive is generally not portable from one computer to another, and so the computer must be part of a network for multiple computers to be able to access the data on the hard drive.

COMPACT DISKS

A CD is much more portable than a hard drive, but CDs cannot hold as much data. CDs are used for distributing software, because after a CD is "written to," it normally cannot be changed. A CD is also more durable than a hard drive, because the CD is not a magnetic medium like the hard drive. A CD is made of a metallic sheet sandwiched by two pieces of plastic. The data are stored on the metallic sheet in the form of very small pits that are "read" by a laser. Some variations of the CD exist, such as the *compact disk–rewriteable* (CD-RW), which can be changed after it has been written to, but these disks require a special drive unit.

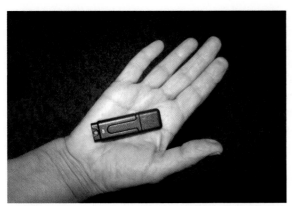

FIGURE 2-8 Flash drive/thumb drive storage device.

ZIP DRIVES, FLASH MEDIA, AND OTHER REMOVABLE DRIVES

Universal serial bus (USB) flash drives are portable storage devices that plug into a computer's USB port. These smaller drives (sometimes called *thumb* or *jump drives*) currently have a maximum storage capacity of about 64 GB (Figure 2-8).

These very convenient storage units are small (thus the "thumb drive" nickname) and lightweight; do not require an outside power source; are easy to store; and, because they are manufactured in a variety of colors, can be color coded. They are often at the end of a key chain or lanyard for ease of portability. They have no moving parts (solid-state circuitry is used) so they can be electronically erased and reprogrammed. They have a fast transfer rate, and files can be immediately copied. Data can be edited as often as necessary. When you have completed a transfer, you simply unplug the unit from the USB port on your computer (Figure 2-9).

Large USB drives (also known as *pocket hard drives*) can store up to 240 GB of data. In general, USB drives can take a little more abuse than various other types of removable drives and media.

To protect PHI and other confidential business information stored in your flash drive, remember these steps:

▶ Remove the drive from the USB port when you leave your computer.
▶ Back up the information stored in your device.
▶ Protect access with a password.
▶ Label the drive with contact information in case you misplace the drive.
▶ Secure (locked drawer, briefcase) the drive when it is not in use.

DATA BACKUP

Hard drives can crash (stop working) and CDs can be easily damaged, so making backups of your data files is very important. There are several ways to make a backup file. If you are backing up disks, make copies of

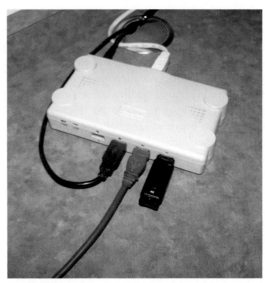

FIGURE 2-9 USB port with easy access to thumb drive and foot pedal hookup.

the disks and store the copies in an off-site location. If you are backing up your hard disk, use a tape backup or a CD to back up the data. Test your backup at least once a month to make sure the data can still be read from the media. It is most frustrating if you need to restore data from a backup and find the backup unreadable. If the system does not automatically back up the data, then you should perform manual incremental and full backups on a regular (daily, monthly) basis.

Because you will have important information stored on computer disks, it is vital to take care of them. The information is magnetically recorded; therefore, any magnetic or electromagnetic field can scramble or destroy data recorded onto a disk. Your telephone, monitor, printer, video terminal—even your electric pencil sharpener—contain magnetic fields; therefore, do not place a disk on or near this equipment. Disks should be properly stored in containers designed for electronic media. The container should be kept away from extreme heat (100° F or above) and out of direct sunlight, because the information could be destroyed or the disk could melt. Never attach rubber bands or paper clips to disks, because these could bend or damage the disks. Always label each disk before filing it in the storage box. Do not stack labels on a disk. Too many labels could cause an imbalance in the weight of the surface of the disk and may make it difficult for the computer head to read the data. Keep disks clean and out of the way of possible spills or stains. Never drink, eat, or smoke around the computer area. If a disk case must be cleaned, use a damp cloth to wipe it off.

PRINTER

The two most popular printer types are inkjet and laser. Inkjet printers shoot a very fine stream of ink at the paper. The ink is water-soluble, and therefore inkjet printers are not as desirable as laser printers. Laser printers are faster and produce much higher print quality, but they are also a bit more expensive than ink-jet printers both to operate and to purchase. Paper output from a printer is called *hard copy* and can vary greatly in quality. Paper quality is measured in weight. Heavier weight paper tends to be thicker and more expensive than lower weight paper. Laser printers are fitted with toner cartridges. Some companies sell recycled, refilled cartridges, which are less expensive than new cartridges. However, check for high-quality refill toner, and ask whether the company replaces the drum in each cartridge before the cartridge is refilled. This practice guarantees crisp, clean printouts.

In many transcription departments, printing may be done off-site. It is common for documents to be printed in another room in the building or across town or transmitted via the network to a hospital floor for accessibility. Therefore, you must read data on the screen while transcribing, because you may not get another opportunity. Some documents may never be printed and exist as electronic files. It is important for you to learn to treat your output as ready for use in any medium.

> **MT TOOL BOX TIP:** Prepare your output to be ready for use in any form.

ERGONOMICS

Ergonomics is the relationship between people and their work environments. Ergonomic problems may exist for MTs because they work in one position hour after hour and perform repetitive movements. These problems are known as *cumulative trauma disorders* or *repetitive stress injuries.* Other factors that can contribute to on-the-job injuries are indoor air pollution, electromagnetic radiation, and stress. Therefore, steps must be taken to avoid these disorders or injuries. The workstation must be in a secure and quiet environment, be free from non–work-related activities, and have adequate space for equipment and materials so that work areas remain uncluttered. Your work space must be set up for you and adjusted to meet your needs.

> **MT TOOL BOX TIP:** Provide a secure and quiet environment in which to work for a tool to success.

The height of the surface on which the computer sits is very important (Figure 2-10). Improper height can cause early fatigue and reduces productivity. You need to maintain good posture using a first-rate keyboard in front of a correctly positioned monitor. A high-quality chair is equally important and should be adjusted to the individual's height and build. A well-adjusted and properly designed chair can reduce fatigue and tension. The chair should permit you to distribute your weight evenly and allow you mobility when stretching for references, for instance. The seat should be adjustable and your knees should not brush the chair's seat. Features to look for are foldaway arms, contoured seat pads, capability for making vertical adjustments, and built-in supports. Lumbar support is very important; a rolled-up towel (see Figure 2-10) is only makeshift. Invest in a quality chair providing overall good support. Do not sit on keys, billfolds, or note pads, because these may block circulation. Sometimes a small footstool can help a short typist avoid back problems.

> **MT TOOL BOX TIP:** A good chair is a tool that can help reduce fatigue and increase productivity.

When retyping or doing copy work and to prevent fatigue, neck aches, backaches, eyestrain, or duplicating or leaving out a sentence, use an electronic copy-holder with a foot pedal control and magnifying cursor so that proper posture can be maintained and material can be easily read. To prevent frozen shoulders and carpal tunnel syndrome, use a split keyboard (one for each hand), a keyboard on the arm of a chair, or a keyboard that adjusts for your comfort. The keyboard should be placed sufficiently low so that the arms are relaxing comfortably in a neutral or downward position on the keys. Your elbows should be at a 90- to 110-degree angle and your face should be tilted down slightly 16 to 25 inches from the monitor. The monitor should be free of distractive notes and messages. Select a comfortable headset that will help absorb background noises and enhance the sound of the dictation.

> **MT TOOL BOX TIP:** Relax at your keyboard.

Match the overall brightness of your computer screen to its surroundings to protect your eyes from too much transient adaptation. Another concern is the rate of flicker on the screen, which may be diminished if the screen background is dark. If you have a white background, lower the brightness to make the flicker less noticeable. Take frequent breaks, and periodically do body and wrist stretches and focus the eyes on distant objects to eliminate eyestrain, blurred vision, headaches, dry eyes, and lowered productivity. Set a time to schedule breaks every 60-90 minutes and do

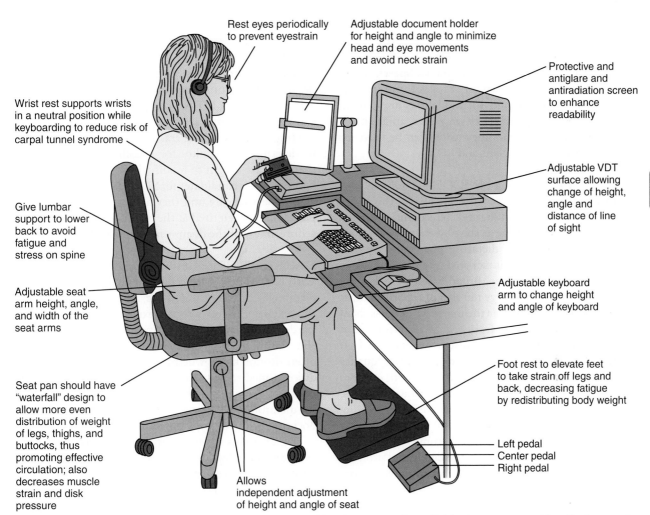

FIGURE 2-10 Ergonomic workstation, illustrating possible adjustments for individual users. *VDT*, Video display terminal. (Modified from Sloane SB, Fordney MT: *Saunders Manual of Medical Transcription*, Philadelphia, Saunders, 1994.)

some simple stretching exercises. Just resting your arms in your lap or at your sides along with shaking out your hands, clenching your fists, or extending your fingers is helpful in preventing repetitive stress injuries. Reduce exposure to low-frequency radiation and prevent glare and light reflection by installing a Polaroid-type anti-reflection screen or radiation-blocking filter over the monitor screen. A seal of acceptance by the American Optometric Association means that the filter has met its high standards. Some filters also act as a privacy protection so that people viewing a screen from either side see nothing but a blank screen but the operator seated in front of the computer terminal has a completely unobstructed view. Some software programs are designed to signal the user to stop and exercise at preferred intervals and may even give exercise hints such as suggestions to stop work and perform some hand and wrist exercises; stand up and stretch and bend your legs. If you begin to feel joint pain, apply ice to the area after work and during breaks to prevent inflammation.

An ergonomically correct workstation improves and increases productivity, minimizes illness and injury, and ensures compliance with federal privacy and security regulations.

> **MT TOOL BOX TIP:** Taking frequent breaks when you are studying and working is a tool for health.

> **MT TOOL BOX TIP:** Work safely—the first tool out of the box.

DICTATION EQUIPMENT

Speech Recognition Technology

There are two basic categories of computerized speech and voice recognition products: navigation and dictation. *Navigation* (or command control) software allows you to launch and operate software applications with spoken directions. *Dictation* software makes it possible for a computer system to recognize spoken words and to automatically convert them into text. Speech recognition (SR) is set up in two very separate and distinct modalities. These methods or modalities are defined as *front-end* and *back-end speech recognition.* In addition, speech recognition technology (SRT) can be used for dictation by both physicians and MTs.

FRONT-END SPEECH RECOGNITION

With front-end speech recognition (FESR), the physician dictates to a PC, and the speech recognition engine produces text in real time as the physician speaks. Recognizing the speech of dictating physicians is enormously challenging; it is surprising that technology can do as well as it does. Broad-based models have been developed from a large number of reports in most major specialties and cover the major work types in all settings. (Most successful front-end SR is performed in the radiology department because it's easier to design software for highly repetitive fields.) However, quality documentation begins with quality dictation. Authors must have good dictating habits. Dictating errors, improper grammar, incomplete and disorganized dictation, and excessive background noise compete with the dictator to produce a usable document. The dictator is able to edit the results immediately and produce a final document if he or she desires to do so. Errors need to be recognized and corrected immediately. Medical records are far too important to go out unedited or with undetected errors. However, not all physicians are suitable candidates for this method. (Actually some

hospitals require the radiologists to self-edit with no MEs involved. Others allow the radiologist to choose and about 70% self-edit typically). Some who find PC-based dictation feasible do not choose to self-edit because it is too time consuming, so dictation ends up being sent to the MT for completion. Initially, physicians go through a screening process whereby their existing dictations and transcribed reports are used to determine suitability for speech recognition, and then they are taught to modify their dictation styles to become better candidates for SR. Because their primary goal is patient care and they are bound to misspeak, particularly when tired at the end of a workday or procedure, many of the documents need further editing.

BACK-END SPEECH RECOGNITION

With back-end speech recognition (BESR), physicians dictate just as they always have, and a draft version of the text appears on screen. Text is automatically forwarded to the MT for correcting and final formatting, eliminating the need to type "from scratch." Dictators often do not know whether they are involved in traditional medical transcription or BESR. This method does not require any direct keyboard involvement of the dictator. See Figure 2-11 for a screen shot of a BESR document courtesy of M*Modal.

Some systems promise that dictation can be captured by traditional telephone, personal digital recorder, computer, or voice-over Internet protocol. SR takes place after the dictation is complete. As the medical dictation editor listens to the dictated audio, the matching text is displayed on screen. The editor must be a slow and deliberate listener. The speech engine can try to pick

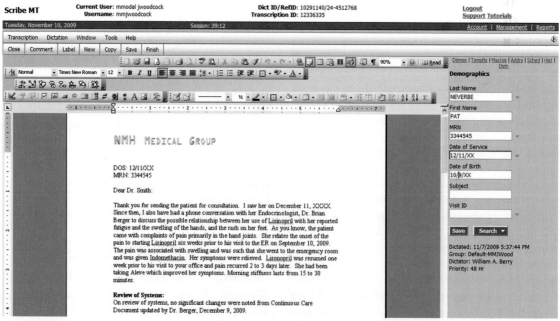

FIGURE 2-11 Sample screen of a speech recognition document. (Courtesy of M*Modal, Pittsburgh, Pa.)

up the context for a word but cannot always produce the proper word. The editor verifies and understands not only what is said but what is meant. Healthcare documentation is too complex to ever fully integrate in any system and completely eliminate the need for the final overlook of a human brain. The editor positions the cursor any place in the document, and the audio plays from that point. With a headset, the editor listens to the dictation as he or she visually reviews the written text for accuracy. A well-trained eye is vital here to catch errors, such as homonyms, missing small words, words that make no sense in the context of the document, and so on. Keystrokes are used to interrupt the voice file and to edit the text. Many SR software programs inject cues and symbols into the text to alert the editor that a

segment of the text is simply noise, an uncertainty, or a pause. The cues or symbols look like musical notes, tiny gears, squares, or other nonkeyboard symbols so that they are not confused with the actual document (Figure 2-12). A single keystroke sequence plays back the sound to any phrase or word as many times as necessary. Medical dictation editors edit the digitized text for medical accuracy as well as for grammar and punctuation. The bottom part of Figure 2-13 is the edited version of the SR document shown in the top part of the figure.

BESR is not a substitute for medical terminology and English grammar applications and cannot provide knowledge where there is none. But it is an efficiency boon to the well-trained MT. Not all physicians are suitable dictators for BESR, and not all MTs become more productive as editors. Some dictators' documents will always need to be transcribed. BESR can offer dramatic contributions to timely reports, but there must be a trained editor at the back end of the report to ensure accuracy. MTs can now act as medical language specialists and invest their time editing for accuracy and completeness rather than typing from scratch. It is not necessary for every MT to become an editor. (See the "Transitioning from MT to Speech Recognition Editor" section in Chapter 15.)

Finally, there is the opportunity for the MT to use SR at the front end. The MT listens to regular dictation and repeats it into his or her system, where it is edited and formatted properly as it is spoken by the MT.

Symbol	Description
■	Suppressed silence in dictation
♪	Filled pause in dictation (e.g., "um," "ah")
☼	Suppressed spoken punctuation in dictation (e.g., "period," "new paragraph")

FIGURE 2-12 Voice recognition technology nonkeyboard symbols, with their descriptions. These are interspersed in the document to guide the transcriptionist.

♪First of she was ready to be well be consistent causing some adverse side effects ■and ♪see ■about ■2 weeks ago had increased to the ♪b.l.d. dosing ■and ♪had been doing fine until this past week when she started to feel nauseated and ■in the ■lightheaded when she got up to quickly ■or after 2 rounds ■of she states ■that ♪he felt better his lungs he had seen in her ■belly ■and see decreased initially ■to the ■q. day dosing ♪and still continue to have symptoms ♪this past ■Saturday ■he stopped the Wellbutrin altogether ■and has now had ♪4 days ■without will be seen in continue to have ♪symptoms of nausea and lightheadedness. ♪

First off, she was worried that the Wellbutrin had been causing some adverse side effects. About 2 weeks ago, she had increased to the b.i.d. dosing and had been doing fine until this past week, when she started to feel nauseated and light-headed when she got up too quickly or after she would run. She states that she felt better as long as she had food in her belly. She decreased, initially, to the once-a-day dosing and still continued to have symptoms. This past Saturday, she stopped her Wellbutrin altogether and now has had 4 days without Wellbutrin. She continues to have symptoms of nausea and light-headiness.

FIGURE 2-13 *Top,* Sample voice recognition technology (VRT) document as it plays into the computer, showing the symbols in place for a rough draft. *Bottom,* The edited version of the paragraph. Proper lab values critical to document.

Ideally, a person dictates naturally into the computer at up to 160 words per minute. MTs who have repetitive stress injuries or congenital deformities or who lack full hand function have found SR systems to be of great help.

The advance in SR has opened the door for many MTs who may have total lack of or limited amount of keyboard ability. SR also offers a way to change the method of transcription from total keyboarding and add variety to a task. MTs who use speech recognition, however, generally try to edit as they go along, just as they do with manual transcription. They have found that their program also performs better when it is "taught" the correct way to function as documents are produced. Some SR systems are already programmed in a variety of medical specialties, a characteristic that saves time in installing a special vocabulary in your system. As a system "learns" more words, it continues to update the user file. Currently, drawbacks for SR systems are the time that the dictator must take in the beginning to properly "train" the system to recognize his or her speech and all of its nuances, the need for a quiet and controlled environment to obtain clean output, and the need for an unhurried manner and clear diction when speaking. The speech engine compares the voice and completed transcribed documents and builds vocabulary with ongoing "rewrite" to improve the vocabulary it understands. Because SR is not yet able to produce 100% reliable text, the ME must proofread and edit the documents. The output is seldom misspelled, and "sound-alike" words and true homonyms are often substituted, and words or phrases are omitted or inserted that were not dictated. In the future, when sophisticated grammar checking is part of the system, many of these problems may be overcome.

SR dictation systems suitable for the dictating physician and for the MT include the following:

Dragon
  www.dragontalk.com/NATURAL.htm
InfraWare
  www.infraware.com
Nuance Speech eScription
  www.nuance.com
M*Modal Speech Recognition
  www.scribe.com

Dictation Media

Several types of media are used in dictating machines. Media may be in the form of magnetic tapes, such as microcassettes or standard cassettes. Some machines have an adapter so that both standard and smaller sized tapes can be used. Handheld digital dictation units typically use a Flash memory card. A 2-MB Flash memory card or similar internal memory can store up to 26 minutes of digital voice files. (Much larger sized Flash memory cards are also available.) These units allow the physician to dictate from anywhere and then upload the digital voice files to the system via the Internet or any stationary dictation station. Some systems are capable of enhancing the speaker's voice, and some types of digital dictation equipment do not require any media at all.

The personal digital assistant (PDA) is a handheld mobile device that can save physicians time and provides better access to clinical information at the point of care. The physician can also record dictation in real time over a secure and wireless network. Using a PDA makes mobile point of care available, and the sooner a physician dictates, the more accurate the account of the procedure will be. Having the PDA integrated into the hospital information systems allows seamless transition of the voice file to other departments, including transcription. Voice files do not take up space on a PDA because the files are stored on a remote and secure server and not on the PDA. With PDAs connected to the hospital's network, a patient's medical record code can be attached directly to the dictation file, and the patient's demographics are accessible as well (Figure 2-14). Transcribing a voice file from a PDA in the hospital network is no different than transcribing voice files from a telephone or dictation station.

Dictation can be recorded directly into a dedicated dictation station or called into the system from any telephone in the world. Voice files are stored on a hard drive in the online information processing system.

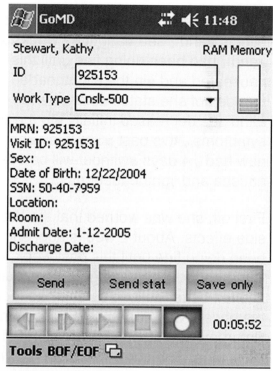

FIGURE 2-14 Sample screen on personal digital assistant (PDA).

Although magnetic tapes are still used in some small offices and clinics, digital dictation is becoming very popular in clinics and small physician practices. The high sound quality, flexibility, and portability of digital dictation systems have made digital dictation the standard in hospitals and large healthcare systems. The communications audio Waveform audio format (WAV) facilitates using your own PC as a transcription station with foot pedal, headset, and Windows interface. No specialized hardware is needed. It is easy to install the software, connect the foot pedal, and plug in the headset. You type into your word processor while listening to the voice from your PC (Figure 2-15).

Regardless of which equipment you choose, be sure to check carefully for good voice quality. Magnetic tapes, disks, cassettes, and digital recorders all allow dictators to correct their own errors so that the MT does not have to listen ahead for corrections. Most machines emit a warning tone when the end of the recording medium is approached.

HAND/FOOT CONTROL

Transcription machines have a foot pedal that starts the equipment. Pressure on the pedal causes the equipment to play; as soon as the pedal is released, the equipment stops (Figure 2-16). The pedal plugs directly into your USB port. You have complete control over how much of the dictation you hear. The control is so sensitive that you can stop and restart in the middle of a word. The pedal also has a backup feature that permits you to relisten to a few words or as much as you need to hear again before you transcribe. Some machines can be adjusted to replay a phrase or a word automatically every time you restart. This feature is called *auto rewind*. In addition, the control may have a *fast forward* feature.

Initially, you will listen to as much of a sentence as you can retain by memory, and you will type that part before listening to the next phrase. Eventually, you will learn to type as you listen, ceasing to listen only long enough to catch up to the dictation; then, just before you type the last of what you heard, start to listen again so that there is as little time as possible during which you are not typing at all.

Some dictation equipment has a speed control that should be adjusted to a natural voice sound, neither too fast nor too slow. The voice should not sound distorted. If the medical dictation editor has difficulty understanding a word or phrase, the speed control can be adjusted to slow down the voice to determine whether this change makes the voice audible or clear. However, the speed control should not be left in the slow mode; it should always be adjusted to a natural-sounding voice quality. In digital voice dictation, no sound distortion occurs when the speed of the voice is changed.

Some manufacturers make a hand control available to physically challenged MTs as an alternative accessory. The operation of the control plays a vital role in developing the essential skill of keying steadily and quickly.

DICTATION

Dictating is a communications skill, and there are good and poor dictators. Transcribing is definitely improved by good dictation. Sometimes transcriptionists can

FIGURE 2-15 GearPlayer, a personal computer–based transcriber that will play nearly all types of digital file formats. A total of 24 customizable keyboard shortcuts allow quick and easy control of the audio file from the keyboard. **A,** The GearPlayer Full Console mode display indicates the file name, file size, play progress, and time in job. A simple mouse click or keyboard shortcut allows volume, tone, and speed control change. **B,** The Slim Console mode can be easily situated in a visible place in your word processor menu while still providing a convenient view of the smaller display and control buttons.

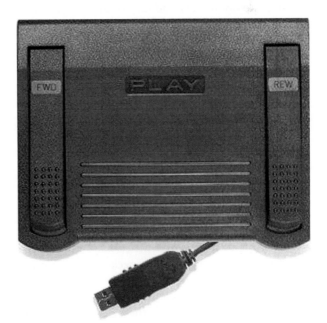

FIGURE 2-16 Typical foot pedal with plug access to USB port.

aid the authors of documents by talking about the problems encountered to determine whether there is some solution. If that approach does not work, try watching the dictator dictate. You might find the following problem-causing behaviors: eating while dictating, speaking directly into the mic and not across the mic as the dictator should, having an "intimate conversation" with the mic (resulting in a low-pitched, quiet, sultry, and inaudible voice), stretching the arms out with the microphone in one of them (resulting in fade-in and fade-out). Many dictators have no idea that they are poor dictators because no one has pointed this problem out to them. They often are also unaware of the consequences of their poor dictation habits. In addition, physicians often choose challenging environments to carry out their recording. Their "sound studio" may be the automobile (with background traffic noise), the family room (with background children's voices or TV noise), the nurse's station (with background conversation and equipment noise), and even their own office (with an open door permitting the recording of conversations, ringing telephone, children crying, and so on). A brief lecture from the salesperson who gave the original presentation on the equipment is often helpful. The equipment might have some features that the dictator has forgotten existed, has never used, or perhaps did not know about in the first place.

Many dictators neglect to use cuing, the built-in system to cue changes in the dictation; special notations to the editor; specific directions about the dictation; and so on. The medical dictation editor should explain how important these aids are and why. Some dictators do not understand how to dictate and think they have to keep up with the machine or leave it on while thinking of what to say. This practice results in poor copy. Some dictators mislead the transcriptionist by dropping their voices as if they were finished and then going on with an "and" or a "but." You may help the dictator by tactfully letting him or her know about such problems. In many settings in which there is no opportunity to interact with the dictator, the supervisor and the editor or MT might prepare a check sheet for the dictator or an orientation packet for the new dictator, giving hints, suggestions, policies, procedures, and so forth.

To make dictating easier, the transcriptionist can design a flow sheet (listing items to be covered or reminders for the order in which dictation should be given) for the physician's specialty. After seeing a patient, the physician removes the sheet from the patient's chart and places it inside a plastic sleeve. The flow sheet is combined with the dictation device so the physician can dictate at the hospital, at home, or wherever he or she may be and will not have to remove the patient's chart from the office. Dictating items out of order results in time consuming reformatting. Sometimes duplicate information is dictated under more than one heading when items are not dictated in order.

Another problem is the confusion of dictated tapes with transcribed tapes, which often results in tapes being transcribed again. With digital dictation, this problem does not occur, because the digital voice file is electronically coded for the person doing the dictation. The coding can contain information about the voice file, such as the dictator's name, patient's name, priority, and transcription status. The voice file can be prioritized in accordance with what type of dictation it contains. If a quick turnaround is required (STAT dictation), the status can be set to cue the file for immediate transcription. If the file is not transcribed within a certain time limit, it is flagged, and the department director is notified. When the transcription is started, the file status is marked "in process." Upon completion, it is marked "ready" so it can be printed and the dictator notified that it is available.

Dictators who are trained for speech recognition may or may not be better at dictating than those without such training, but they must be made aware of poor dictation habits as well. Box 2-1 provides some hints to aid the person dictating.

Table 2-1 presents information that will assist the transcriptionist in solving problem dictation.

MAINTENANCE

File Maintenance

For your word processing system to be as useful as possible, the information you record needs to be well organized. Just as you use file folders and filing cabinets to sort and store paper files, you must create a similar system to store your computer documents. There is no limit to the number of folders you can create. Create as many folders as you would like, and place subfolders within folders. You can organize your subfolders by date or category.

> 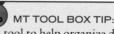 **MT TOOL BOX TIP:** Design and follow a flow chart tool to help organize dictation.

File maintenance is also important in optimal computer operation. Keeping organized and finding files easily are two reasons to perform file maintenance. If you save all your files in a single directory, you will eventually have hundreds of files to search through. You not only waste time searching for the correct file, but you also cause problems in the operating system. Plan to

BOX 2-1 Dictation Hints

- Prioritize and organize material.
- Dictate in a private and quiet environment.
- Speak clearly, slowly, and loudly. (Speaking too rapidly is perhaps at the top of the list of most MT complaints.)
- Identify yourself.
- Indicate the work type (e.g., letter, memo, report, rough draft, operative note, or medicolegal document).
- Indicate the number of copies needed, enclosures, and special paper or letterhead if required.
- Give the names of the patient and the person for whom the item is intended, and spell out the names if they are difficult to ascertain.
- Dictate the street address, city, state, and ZIP code to which the correspondence is being sent when this information is not readily available to the transcriptionist or dictation editor.
- Separate the ideas into paragraphs. Spell out any words that might be difficult to understand.
- Indicate when a word is a plural or needs quotes, parentheses ("paren open" and "paren close"), indentations, columns, and subparagraphs. However, do not dictate punctuation. It becomes tedious to hear the word "period" over and over, and often the punctuation is not correct. The MT is the punctuation specialist.
- Avoid using abbreviations unless they have been approved by the facility in which you are working. Do not abbreviate medications.
- Say the names of medications clearly and distinctly with dosage instructions.
- State lab values slowly and clearly so that it is obvious where one value stops and another begins.
- Keep a blank copy of any forms in front of you while dictating information that is to be matched to a form.
- Indicate the number of a macro or boilerplate paragraph with special care.
- Specify exactly what data the MT needs to add to your dictation before closing it off. Do not imagine that the MT knows "I always say this so it should have been included." Place instructions that expand or limit your dictation *in writing* for your protection and the protection of the MT. This step is especially important if the MT is not able to keep the voice files for backup verification.
- Eliminate extraneous sounds such as "ugh," "um," and "eh." Remember to speak slowly and clearly. Do not slur word endings.
- Avoid coughing, sneezing, yawning, clearing your throat, or blowing your nose while your microphone is open. (One can only imagine some of these noises enhanced through an earpiece.)
- Do not eat, drink, chew gum, or suck on lozenges while dictating. These items engage the tongue and distort pronunciation.
- Advise the MT when you are finished dictating that there is nothing further on the medium.
- Add a personal touch to the end of the tape by saying "thank you" to the MT. This closing will certainly make the MT feel like a valuable part of the team. Treat the MT like a professional and with respect.
- Use the pause button or key when it is necessary to stop and think.
- **Remember: Less time spent transcribing and editing equals money saved by the dictator.**

NOTE: When a MT friend reviewed this chapter, she wondered how the MT would ever get such a list to a problematic, or even any, dictator. Copy it and give it to the dictator any time there is any error caused by any of these problems. When new staff members, new residents, or new attending physicians arrive, this can be part of their orientation packet. When you take on a new client, the list can be part of your contract.

TABLE 2-1 Dictation Problem Solving

PROBLEM	SOLUTION
Fast dictation	Decrease the speed of the dictation if words and phrases are running together.
	Write out slurred phrases phonetically, and separate the syllables to try to form words.
Foreign accent	Get a copy of a report by the same physician dictated and transcribed previously, and compare words and phrases.
	Distinguish the accent, and substitute the correct sound to identify the word.
Garbled word	Increase or decrease dictation speed, and relisten.
	Relisten on audio speaker.
	Ask someone else to listen.
	Leave a blank, continue transcribing, and listen for the word to be dictated again within the transcription.
Mumbled dictation	Increase the tone control.
Dictation obscured by static	Decrease the tone control.
Unfamiliar word	Look up the word in your reference books.
	Use the Sound and Word Finder Table in Appendix B.

use several directories and subdirectories to organize your files. Using the dictator's name for a main directory and the type of document (reports, drafts, letters) or patients' names for the subdirectories is a good start. You may already have experience in naming your individual files. You may also want to code the document itself with your unique file name. This way transcribed documents can be retrieved easily and quickly when needed. You may be able to use your own file name; however, the dictator or organization may prefer that you use their unique codes. If you are able to use your own codes, here are some hints to make it simple:

- Always name the new document as soon as you create it; then save it. When you select Save as from the File menu, you not only name the document you have just begun, you also select where you will store it—that is, the name of the file folder where you want it to stay. A list of available folders is displayed as well. It is a good idea to set margins, indents, tabs, fonts, and other format elements before you save.
  1. Select format.
  2. Name and save.

- Use minimum data: identification number for the dictator, the patient's last name, date. Using too much data is confusing.
- Use letters and numbers: for dates, use just the last digit of the year and then 1 to 9 for the first nine months and *o, n, d* for the last three months. I call this system *D.P.D.,* for "dictator.patient.date."
- Use a period for a separation mark. Do not use a backward slash (\), an asterisk (*), a colon (:), a question mark (?), a forward slash (/), or greater or less than signs (<, >) as separation marks.
- Place the code as the last entry on the document.
- Use the identical code as your "save name."
- If you make changes to your document after you have saved it, be sure to change the date on your file name.

EXAMPLE: *D.P.D.*

The dictator's name is Betten. If you have two dictators whose names begin with *B,* you can give Betten code B2. He dictated a letter about a patient named Court on February 7, 20XX. Your code would be B2.Court.27X. The 2 is for February, the 7 for the day in February, the X for the year.

There are many ways to organize your files, so stick to one that makes sense to you. This practice also makes it easier and faster to back up your files.

> **MT TOOL BOX TIP:** Practice good file maintenance from the beginning (i.e., the first document you save).

Cassette Tape Transcriber

Consult the following checklist when your transcriber is not working properly:
- Is the equipment plugged in?
- Is the outlet in working order?
- Is the equipment turned on?
- Is the play button pushed down, preventing you from hearing through the headset?
- Is the foot pedal attached to the machine?
- Is the pause button pushed down?
- Is the tape inserted correctly and fully engaged?

If you have decided that your equipment needs repairs, make a note explaining the problems your machine is exhibiting, and then tape the note to the side of your machine. This way, the repair person will know what to look for even if you are not present. In a classroom, the instructor or laboratory assistant would appreciate a note to assist in ordering repairs or replacements.

TRANSCRIPTION PREPARATION

Here are some suggestions to help you organize and plan your work before you begin to transcribe and to increase your efficiency and production:

1. Gather all necessary information and materials at your desk
2. Make sure the headset, earphones, and foot control are attached to the unit and positioned comfortably for you.
3. Verify that the unit is operating properly, plugged in, and turned on.
4. Insert the medium. Priority (STAT) reports are transcribed immediately. Be aware of the TAT of the dictation in the queue. Some documents have a shorter TAT than others.
5. Listen to the instructions or cue in to see whether there are corrections by scanning the medium.
6. Adjust the volume, tone, and speed controls to your taste. Remember that too slow a speed will only distort the sound.
7. Make sure the format for margins and tabulation stops is proper before you begin to transcribe a document.
8. Mark any problems with editing codes so that the dictated report can be scanned and necessary corrections can be made.
9. Punctuate as you go.
10. Leave a blank space for words that you do not understand. A blank consists of 10 keystrokes of underlining. Make a note of where you have had to leave a blank space. Attach notes to your transcript for any unclear phrases or sentences. See Chapter 7 for help in flagging unfamiliar copy.

The more transcribing you do, the more information you will retain in memory when coordinating listening and typing.

EQUIPMENT FOR THE PHYSICALLY CHALLENGED TRANSCRIPTIONIST

Several methods have been developed to make it easier for transcriptionists who are blind or have impaired vision or who have little or no hand or arm movement to type and transcribe. A visually impaired person who wishes to take notes can use a Braille note taker. The notes can be output in electronic text, print, Braille, or synthesized speech. The MT can write and edit text, take notes privately, prepare reports, and keep track of daily schedules with Braille n Speak 2000 from Blazie Engineering, Inc. (www.blazie.co.uk) or NanoPac. The BrailleNote from HumanWare is another note taker and personal organizer that also functions as a word processor, spell-checker, calculator, and program for exploring the Internet and sending and receiving email (800-722-3393; www.humanware.com).

A variety of screen reading and speech recognition systems, screen magnifiers, Braille printers, and book scanners are available today. Freedom Scientific offers JAWS for Windows, a screen reader that uses the numeric keypad for its basic functions. Online help for JAWS is quite extensive (800-444-4443; www.freedomscientific.com).

A *screen reader* converts all text on the screen to spoken characters or words. A blind terminal user can hear the information that is displayed on the screen and can learn how to operate the machine by listening to cassette-recorded instructions or by using Braille writing. Usually, the audio output formats available on such systems include the following:

▸ *Pronounce* format. Screen contents are read in the same way as you would read a book, with each word pronounced separately but without incorporating punctuation.

▸ *Punctuate* format. Format is similar to the pronounce format. In addition, single or double spaces are identified by a sound (the number of spaces are given if more than two), and punctuation marks are also announced.

▸ *Spell* format. All words are spelled out, spaces and capital letters are identified, the number of spaces or repeated characters is given, and punctuation marks are announced.

Some machines use a keypad to control audio output. When the operator's hands are busy, an external foot switch may be used. The cursor is positioned on the screen, and then the machine reads out the row and column numbers. It reads the word at, before, or after the cursor; it may read the entire row on which the cursor is located, the row before it, or the row after it; or the complete screen may be read out. It is easy to go back and verify something not understood by backspacing and then changing the output format from pronounce to punctuate or to spell.

A low-vision MT can produce perfect letters and reports by using a *screen magnifier,* such as Zoom-Text, a product of Ai Squared (800-859-0270; www.aisquared.com), which consists of software or hardware that enlarges the characters on a computer screen and with a ZoomText USB flash drive that users can carry with them and use any time. Clearview is another popular product, available from Optelec (800-826-4200; www.optelec.com). The ClearNote Portable is a lightweight, powerful laptop magnification solution. ZeroButton converts and displays text in the user's preferred preset magnification and contrast. Optelec ClearView system magnifies images while maintaining perfect focus.

In fact, screen magnifiers and screen-reading equipment for persons who are blind, have low vision, or are reading disabled are manufactured by several companies. Some equipment uses regular Microsoft and other word processing systems and performs in much the same way but is capable of reading text from books, zooming font sizes, and providing auditory feedback from a scanned document or from the screen. Freedom Scientific produces OpenBook 7.0 (800-444-4443; www.freedomscientific.com), which features low vision products, blindness products, learning-system products, and Bluetooth Braille.

A *book scanner* easily scans books or other bound materials (e.g., magazines, photocopies, documents with multiple columns). It recognizes text, converts the text into synthesized speech, and then reads the materials aloud.

Special equipment has also been developed to produce raised-copy images, such as raised-relief maps, raised drawings, and Braille writing. Illustrations enhance the learning process, and such equipment decreases the cost and time involved in producing documents for persons who are vision impaired. Quantum Technology in Australia provides this technology with PIAF (pictures in a flash; email: quant@quantech.com.au; www.quantumtechnology.com.au).

For persons with limited hand or arm movement or only slight head movement, a Magic Wand Keyboard is available. To begin work, the user simply unplugs the existing computer keyboard, plugs in the Magic Wand Keyboard, and uses a hand or a mouthstick to touch the keys. No strength or dexterity is required. This device is manufactured by In Touch Systems, 11 Westview Road, Spring Valley, New York 10977, 800-332-6244, email: Esc@magicwandkeyboard.com (www.magicwandkeyboard.com).

Disabled MTs are not only employable but frequently are sought after. These individuals have often had to overcome many obstacles and have learned to adjust to their unique environments. They have had to overcome discrimination despite the Americans with Disabilities Act, and this experience makes them an asset and deserving of an opportunity to the extent of their capabilities.

FAX MACHINES

Fax machines are used to send and/or obtain charts, electrocardiographic (ECG) tracings, laboratory reports, referral authorizations, letters, medical reports, and insurance claims; to order supplies; and to accomplish tasks for which forms and printouts from other sources are needed. Hospitals use fax machines to transmit material within the facility, such as medical records, laboratory and pathology reports, prescriptions to the hospital pharmacy, surgical scheduling, patient admissions, patient room scheduling, ECG tracings, face sheets, medical staff committee meetings, and so forth. Pharmacies send physicians' requests and confirm orders, and physicians send prescription orders. Information can also be sent and received from medical libraries, attorneys, accountants, financial advisers, and vendors of medical and office supplies. Whenever possible, it is a good practice to abstract and fax only necessary and pertinent information, rather than entire documents. Transcription services offer faxing as a benefit for fast turnaround of medical reports. Documents can be faxed from the service to different floors within a hospital facility, from a physician's office to the hospital across town, or around the world within a few minutes. Fax capabilities can be built into your computer for ease of sending documents.

Standalone fax machines should be located in a secure or restricted area. (See the "Health Insurance Portability and Accountability Act of 1996" section in Chapter 1.) Frequently called numbers can be preprogrammed into the machine, which helps to avoid entering wrong numbers. A digital display is helpful so that the number being dialed is on view. Many fax machines generate open-document communications; therefore, someone must be assigned to secure incoming documents to provide confidentiality. Some PC-based fax boards solve the security problem for sending and receiving documents because these boards give PCs the ability to function like standalone fax machines. Thus, the documents are printed on quality bond paper and have good image quality. Although image quality is better when a document is received directly through the computer's fax board, it is still not letter quality. Therefore, it may be necessary to send the document through a courier service instead of via fax.

Many features are available for fax machines. The most useful are user and receiver confidentiality, automatic dialer, automatic document cutter, document feeder, autodialers, and delayed broadcasting for sending documents when telephone tolls are low.

Any time a hardcopy document is faxed, all attempts should be made with a fax machine with industry standard secure fax capabilities. In general, when a secure fax is sent, a password (usually a four digit number) is generated at the sending machine by the user. This password must then be separately transmitted (e.g., by phone or secure email) to the recipient. Upon receipt, the recipient enters the password to retrieve the fax from the local machine. This feature also adds a layer of protection in case the fax was accidently sent to the wrong number, because without the password, the unintended recipient would be unable to retrieve the misdirected fax. In some fax machines, the password

also serves as an encryption key to provide limited protection from unintended disclosure during fax transmission and while the document is on the fax machine's hard drive. Every office should have written policies and procedures, or standard operating procedures, regarding secure fax transmission and receipt.

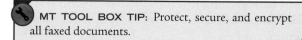

MT TOOL BOX TIP: Protect, secure, and encrypt all faxed documents.

Many medical facilities also have *scanning* capability whereby a hardcopy document is digitally scanned or reproduced and then transmitted via email or stored on a shared computer for later retrieval. The same type of protection must be afforded documents transmitted in this fashion.

When sending confidential material such as medical or legal records, telephone the recipient before faxing the information so that someone authorized to view the documents is standing by. The receiver should check back with the sender to verify receipt of the material. Incoming documents may be available for inspection by anyone at the receiving end, and the fax machine may be unstaffed. Begin every transmission with a cover sheet detailing the sender (name, telephone number, and fax number), the number of pages being sent, who is to receive the transmission (name and address), and any other information that will help get the fax to the proper person (Figure 2-17). Include a telephone number to call in case a problem occurs with the transmission, such as a lost page, dropped line, or missing text.

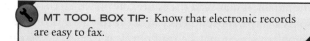

MT TOOL BOX TIP: Know that electronic records are easy to fax.

A handy hint is to make up a standard cover sheet letter on the employer's stationery and enclose it in a clear plastic sleeve (one that will allow you to fax a cover sheet within it). Fill in the information on the plastic sleeve with a dry erasable marker, using the cover sheet inside as your guide. After completing it, check to make sure the markings are dry, then fax. When the fax is complete, erase the cover information from the plastic sleeve with a blackboard eraser and put the sleeve aside for the next fax transmission.

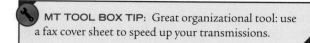

MT TOOL BOX TIP: Great organizational tool: use a fax cover sheet to speed up your transmissions.

KARL ROBRECHT, MD
Internal Medicine

ADRIANNA SACHS, MD
Cardiology

Gulf Medical Group, Inc.

800 Gulf Shore Drive
Naples, FL 33940

Telephone 813 649-1111

FAX 813 987-5121

FAX COMMUNICATION TRANSMITTAL COVER SHEET

To:_____Date:_____

Fax #_____Time:_____

Telephone #_____

Number of pages (including this one):_____

From: **Gulf Medical Group, Inc.; Karl Robrecht, MD; Adrianna Sachs, MD**

If you cannot read this fax or if pages are missing, please contact Gulf Medical Group at 813-649-1111.

Remarks:_____

_____

Note: This transmittal is intended only for the use of the individual or entity to which it is addressed and may contain information that is privileged, confidential, and exempt from disclosure under applicable law. If you are not the intended recipient, any dissemination, distribution, or photocopy of this communication is strictly prohibited. If you have received this communication in error, please notify this office immediately by telephone and mail the original fax to us at the address above. Thank you.

Instructions to the authorized receiver
Please complete this statement of receipt and return to sender via this fax number: 813-987-5121

I, _____, verify that I have received_____
        (name)   (no. of pages including cover sheet)
from **Gulf Medical Group, Inc.**

FIGURE 2-17 Example of a fax cover sheet for medical document transmission illustrating a confidentiality statement with appropriate wording. (From Diehl MO: *Medical Transcription Guide: Do's and Don'ts,* ed 3, St Louis, 2004, Saunders.)

If you are concerned about clarity, test your material by making a copy on your fax machine before you send the document. You may wish to make a photocopy of the document or enlarge the document on your copy machine and transmit the copied page. Do not use correction tape or fluid on documents to be faxed. Always remove paper clips and staples, to prevent damage to the fax machine. If the original document has copy near the left or right edge of the page, position the paper in such a way that the entire image can be reproduced. Learn your fax's error messages and how to correct the problems that caused the errors. Noise or interference from telephone lines can garble your message, requiring you to resend or to slow down the transmission rate. Be sure the transmission has been completed before you leave the fax machine.

DIGITAL SCANNERS

Digital scanners (also called *digital senders*) are replacing many fax machines because of ease of use and the widespread use of email. Scanned documents are securely transmitted to one or more email addresses, usually in the page description format. There are no long-distance charges, and the documents are less prone to unintentional disclosure (e.g., sitting in the fax machine for all to see). In combination with public key interface technology, page description format-type files may also be digitally signed, and in some jurisdictions, this signature is considered as valid as a written signature. Also with public key interface, the transmission can be encrypted to ensure that only someone with the proper password can view the document.

ELECTRONIC SIGNATURES

The *e-signature,* your name typed at the end of your email, is considered an electronic signature as is a signature that is scanned into an image and embedded in an electronic document. Such a signature is regarded as the equivalent of a handwritten signature. Verification of the signature can be made by using a unique assigned code.

The digital signature is technology known as public key infrastructure (PKI), which guarantees the signer's identity with the identification embedded in the signed document. The signer is issued a private key to sign a document, which is unique to that signature. A public key can be used to verify the signer's identity and prove data integrity. Pathology slides, radiological images, test results, and all written documents can be signed and their integrity ensured by using PKI. A patient checking in at a physician's office, with a witnessing employee present, can use an e-pad to record a one-time graphical signature. Paperwork such as routinely signing insurance claim forms, HIPAA forms, release forms, and so on can be transformed into a digital process.

DISPOSAL OF ELECTRONIC MEDIA

HIPAA security rules require the removal of PHI stored on computers and other electronic media before the media is reused or disposed of. The information can be removed by overwriting media with nonsensitive data or purging with a strong magnetic field, which disrupts the recorded magnetic information. Media may be shredded, and paper records may be shredded, burned, or pulverized. Media and computers may be destroyed by pulverizing or incinerating so that data cannot be reconstructed.

Vocabulary

Backup: A copy of a file that is kept in case the original file is destroyed.

Cassette: A magnetic tape wound on two reels encased in a plastic or metal container that can be mounted on or inserted in a tape recording or playback device. Cassettes are standard or microsized.

CD-ROM: Compact disk read-only memory: A disk on which the data is read at high speed but cannot be changed by program instructions.

Central processing unit (CPU): The part of the computer in which operations are controlled and executed.

Command key: A key that enters a particular command into a word processing system. Also called *control* or *function key*.

Compact disk (CD): A small plastic disk on which digital information is stored and from which the information can be read by using reflected laser light. *See also* CD-ROM.

C-Phone: Manufactured by Dictaphone, a direct-wired or telephone-connected transcribing unit (see Figure 2-3).

Crash: Sudden and complete failure of all or a substantial part of a system. *See also* Hard drive/head crash.

Cut and paste: Moving a piece of your copy to another place in your document or to another document.

Data: Information that can be processed or produced by a computer.

Default: A standard setting, preset for convenience, that can be changed when necessary. In word processing software, defaults define margins, tabs, page length, spacing, and other format elements.

Delete: A command in word processing that removes a specific section of text from the recording medium.

Digital dictation: The process whereby dictated voice is digitized (converted to a string of 0s and 1s, representing the audio waveform) and stored as data on a computer disk. When instantly and selectively assessed from a dictation/transcription station or telephone, the binary digits are converted back to analog waveform sound.

Digital player: Storage media for input from mobile digital dictation devices (Figure 2-18).

Digital signature: An electronic guarantee of the signer's identity.

Disk: A magnetic storage device made of rigid material (hard disk) or flexible plastic (floppy disk).

Disk drive: A device that holds a disk and retrieves and saves information on it.

Dot matrix printer: An impact printer that prints characters composed of many dots.

Earphone: An electrical device worn on the ear (or in the ear) to receive communications or listen to recordings. Also called *headset*.

Editing: Revision and correction of text (read back, scan, delete, insert, reformat) before final document printout.

Electronic signature (e-signature): Signature scanned into an image or your email signature.

Encryption: Conversion of data with a cipher or code to prevent unauthorized access.

Equipment service contract: Routine maintenance and emergency repair services provided for a set fee per year.

Ergonomics: The science of adapting working environment, conditions, and equipment to suit workers (see Figure 2-10).

Error-free: A characteristic of recording on magnetic media that allows correction of errors by recording over unwanted material; in word processing, a term used when a document with no mistakes is printed.

Fax machine: A machine connected to a telephone line and electric wall outlet that scans a document's image, transmits and/or receives the image, and prints an exact facsimile. Also called *fax*.

Fidelity: The degree of accuracy with which sound is reproduced.

File: A single stored unit of information that is given a file name so that it can be accessed.

File server: A device that controls access to separately stored files as part of a multiuser system.

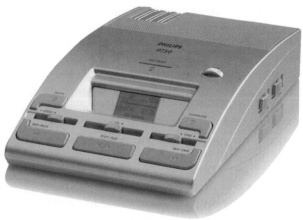

FIGURE 2-18 Philips Digital Transcription unit with visual workflow display, showing the number of files, priorities, and special instructions. It allows you to transfer dictation directly to your personal computer.

File transfer protocol (FTP): A standard for the exchange of program and data files across a network.

Flash drive: A portable storage device that plugs into a computer's USB port. Also called *jump drive or thumb drive*.

Font: The size and style of type.

Global search and replace: The ability of a word processing system to change, with one instruction, a word or other text element everywhere the word or element appears in a document. Also called *global change*.

Hard copy: Written or printed document.

Hard drive/head crash: Severe damage caused when the read-write head of a disk drive flies above the disk and strikes the surface. *See also* Crash.

Hardware: The physical components (electric, electronic, magnetic, and mechanical devices) of a computer system that, combined with software (e.g., programs, instruction), create a system.

Headset: *See* Earphone.

Information technology (IT): The use of computers and telecommunications for storing, retrieving, and sending information.

Insert: A word processing function that allows introduction of new material within previously recorded text.

Jump drive: *See* Flash drive.

Justification: Alignment of text between fixed right and left margins by the addition of spacing between the words in a line of text; alignment of text margins on both right and left sides (i.e., flush left and flush right).

Local area network (LAN): A computer network that links devices within a building or group of adjacent buildings.

Macro: A small program or set of instructions that the word processor uses to complete repetitive tasks.

Medium (plural, media): Material on which information can be recorded.

Memory: The section of the computer where instructions, data, and information are stored. Also called *storage* and *internal* or *main memory*.

Menu: Series of program options or commands displayed in a list on the computer screen that act as aids in using the word processing software. A menu may be referred to as main, mini, pull-down, or pop-up.

Merge: Document assembly, such as combining prerecorded text with keyboarded text, combining selections from prerecorded text to form a new document, and inserting names and addresses to create a number of nearly identical documents.

Modem: Acronym for modulator-demodulator unit. A modem is a device that converts data into signals for telephone transmission and then (at the receiving end) back again into data.

Navigation keys: Keyboard keys used to reposition the cursor.

Operating system: The software that supports a computer's basic functions, such as scheduling tasks, executing applications, and controlling peripherals.

Output: The final results after recorded information is processed, revised, and printed out.

Peripheral: Any input, output, or storage device (hardware) connected to the computer, such as hard disks, modems, and printers.

Playback: Listening to recorded dictation.

Ports: A socket in a computer or network into which a device can be plugged. *See* Flash drive.

Program: *See* Software.

Response time: The time a computer takes to react to given input.

Retrieve: Finding stored information in the archive.

Scanner: A machine or handheld device that converts text or a printed image into a format readable by the computer and printer. Also known as *optical character recognition (OCR)*.

Server architecture: A system to provide remote files to a client's local computer.

Software: Programs or instructions used to support a piece of equipment, as opposed to the equipment itself (hardware).

Speech recognition: The capability of a computer system (equipped with sound sensors) to translate the tones of the human voice into computer commands.

Telecommunications: Transmission of information between widely separated locations by means of electric or electromagnetic systems, such as telephone or telegraph.

Template: A preset format for a document or file so that the format does not have to be recreated each time it is used.

Thumb drive: *See* Flash drive.

Universal serial bus (USB): A connection for attaching peripheral devices to a computer providing fast data exchange. *See also* Flash Drive.

Utility program: A general-purpose software program that performs activities (e.g., initializing a disk) that are not specific to an application.

Voice activation: The capability of a machine to recognize and respond to spoken words.

Voice files: Voice transferred via the Internet. A dictator calls a service, follows prompts, and then dictates. The computer notifies the MT by email or some other method, and the MT downloads the file.

Voice synthesizer: A device that allows the computer to output artificial speech. It is used by visually impaired MTs. Also called *speech synthesizer.*

WAV system: A system that facilitates using your own computer as a transcription station with foot pedal, headset, and Windows interface.

Word wrap: A feature in which a word that has more characters than will fit at the end of a line is moved to the beginning of the next line.

2-1 REVIEW TEST

DIRECTIONS: Select some AutoCorrect shortcuts that you would like to try with your word processing system.

▶ Look at the following document and see whether there are any words or phrases that would be helpful to expand from an abbreviated form.
▶ Start out by using a highlighter to identify them and mark them.
▶ Write in the word and abbreviation expansion you might select for that word.
▶ Try it out. (Remember to type the word or phrase; highlight it; and then select Tools, AutoCorrect, and type in your abbreviation.)

November 9, 20XX

Department of Rehabilitation
1350 Frost Street, Room 4053
GrandView, XX 00010

Gentlemen:

RE: Deanna Jude

The above-named individual, a 22-year-old single, unemployed female, has been seen in these offices on several occasions beginning December 1, 200X, and ending October 30, 200X. The patient has been seen infrequently because she has been incarcerated for drug-abuse problems.

At the present time, the patient is interested in pursuing opportunities at Vocational Rehabilitation. She last used heroin one year ago. After having given up heroin, the patient has demonstrated manifest symptoms of depressive neurosis with trouble sleeping, depression, crying spells, and moodiness. She has received previous psychiatric treatment from Dr. Michael Reilly and Dr. Leonard Moon. The past medical history is otherwise normal.

The patient denies current alcohol or substance abuse. She complains of continued anxiety and depression. She was once hospitalized for a short period of time at Mesa Vista.

On mental status examination, the patient professes strong motivation to regain her self-respect and her social and occupational adjustment. She views Vocational Rehabilitation as offering an opportunity in this regard. Her mood and affect are intermittently depressed but seemingly are responding well to Triavil 2-25 t.i.d. She recognizes the need for continued psychotherapy. Insight into the fact that she is ill is present. Remote and recent memory are intact. Judgment is intermittently under the influence of her pathological emotional immaturity.

At the present time, the patient suffers from depressive neurosis. She has the capacity to return to heroin based upon psychological dependence but most likely would not return to heroin based on physical depen dence alone in view of the long gap between her last injection and the present time. It is believed that she ¯ can work with a counselor.

If I can be of further assistance, please let me know.

Sincerely yours,

William A . Berry, MD

Try this example to get started. Select the physician's name: William A. Berry, MD. Type it exactly as written. Your expansion code is pretty easy: a simple *wabx* will suffice. Notice that you do not capitalize the code abbreviation.

Word for expansion

William A. Berry, MD_____

_____

_____

_____

_____

_____

_____

_____

Code abbreviation

wabx____

_____

_____

_____

_____

_____

_____

_____

2-2 REVIEW TEST: PRACTICE FILE MANAGEMENT

There is no best way to do this, and you may have already established a method of your own. Try the system described in this chapter, p. 52. Remember the hint: D.P.D. If Dr. Berry has been given the code B1, how would you identify this document in your file management system?

CHAPTER 3

Punctuation

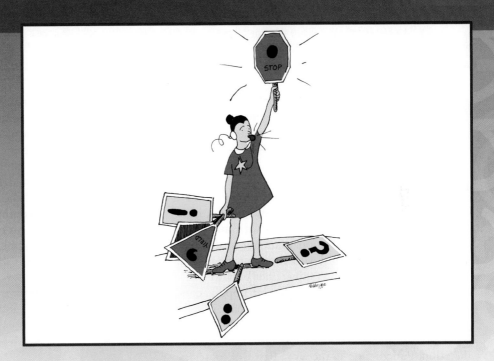

OBJECTIVES

After reading this chapter and completing the exercises, you should be able to

1. Demonstrate the ability to use reference materials to select the proper punctuation needed in new material.

2. List in your own words reasons for the accurate use of punctuation marks.

3. State grammatical terms for different parts of speech and for various parts of a sentence and match these terms with a written example.

4. Use the vocabulary of punctuation by writing the rule, using your own words and the proper terms, while working with an illustration of the rule in use.

5. Demonstrate the ability to use punctuation marks accurately by inserting punctuation into unpunctuated copy.

Note from the Author

Chapter 3 is the first of three vital chapters in your study. You may become discouraged with yourself and upset with me as you work through this chapter. But you have to trust me, and your instructor working closely with you, that progress in this chapter is critical for your success. Please learn the special vocabulary words and terms used in the rules. These are peculiar neither to "medical punctuation" nor to this text. These terms are used in any reference you consult to help you with punctuation. There *is* no such thing as medical punctuation. Students often think more commas, more apostrophes, and certainly more colons were invented for medical documents. Sorry. Not so. These rules are the very same ones used in all English language writing. Some authorities disagree on some of the "optional" rules and never exercise the option of leaving them out or putting them in. That is fine; do not worry about it; that is why they are called *optional*. Relax, take it easy, and do not rush through these lessons; stop and go back when you do not understand something. Remember that your instructor and I really do care about your success!

 MT TOOL BOX TIP: Nonmedical writing uses the same rules—same tools.

INTRODUCTION

Transcriptionists, like many other professionals, have more trouble with punctuation than with any other aspect of document preparation. Many authorities disagree with one another and with common usage. The following rules and exercises adhere not only to traditional guidelines but also to those used in popular contemporary lay magazines and medical journals; in style guides for medical writers, editors, and transcriptionists; and in the material preferred by authors of medical dictation. Punctuation is therefore based on observations of actual practice and is consistent with the style recommended by other authorities, because the use of punctuation should be guided by well-established, accepted conventions of style. However, sometimes "well-established" uses change, sometimes dramatically. In this chapter, I attempt to show you variations in practices and to alert you to possible future style changes. Often, this chapter shows current methods, but information is given on an earlier style that might be preferred in your work environment. You need to learn to follow the basic principles and *be consistent.*

 MT TOOL BOX TIP: This chapter is always going to be your best punctuation guide.

Because proper punctuation is vital in business writing and document preparation, this chapter will help you acquire good punctuation habits. Proper punctuation helps the reader understand which items belong together, when to pause, which material must be set apart, and what is being emphasized. Some of us never learned to punctuate correctly, and many keyboard operators simply add a comma when it seems time for the reader to take a breath!

Without proper punctuation, communication breaks down, meaning can be lost or distorted, or the flow of ideas is interrupted. For example, the comma is used to clarify or signal the writer's exact meaning for the reader; therefore, comma misuse may either mislead the reader or delay his or her comprehension. You have undoubtedly seen sentences in which the meaning changes when a comma is added or deleted.

 MT TOOL BOX TIP: Rules of the "road" tools are punctuation marks.

In review, remember that punctuation is often simple, but also keep in mind that it is not always subject to precise and unchanging rules. Certain punctuation marks are simply common practice, so if you rely on *common sense,* you might not always be right.

Finally, because this chapter is not, and cannot be, a guide to proper punctuation under all circumstances, a professional writer should have a comprehensive guide book in his or her desk library.

This chapter is not easy. Some of the words described in the vocabulary might not have received your attention since grade school. Please take time to review any areas that present problems before continuing. Remember that the material here will not disappear, and you might want to refer to it at some time.

Typeset marks and symbols often appear different from those made with the computer. Follow the basic rules for size and placement of symbols and characters as given.

 MT TOOL BOX TIP: Accept that policies, rules, and procedures keep your tools in perfect working order.

VOCABULARY

The following terms are used freely and without further definition in the rules that follow, so you should become quite comfortable with them. Before you begin to punctuate a sentence, review some of the vocabulary pertaining to sentence formation. You need to develop knowledge of the parts of speech and how these parts are strung together to form simple, compound, or complex sentences.

Sentence: A group of words containing a subject and a verb that forms a complete statement that is able to stand alone. The subject need not always be expressed; it may be understood.

EXAMPLES

She did not report her problem to her primary care physician.

Get this to the lab STAT. *(The subject* you *is understood.)*

The first step in acquiring sentence sense is learning to recognize verbs.

Verb: A word (or a group of words) that expresses action or otherwise helps to make a statement. It may be one word or several words that are written together or separated by other words.

Notice the verbs written in italics in the following sentences:

EXAMPLES

The patient *needs* a complete blood count.

The patient *is scheduled* for a complete blood count.

The patient *had* a complete blood count.

Send the patient to the lab for a complete blood count and *ask* him to return.

Will you *advise* the patient to have a complete blood count?

Pick out the verb in this sentence:

Instructors may be critical of students' work.

If you selected *may be,* you are correct. It expresses action. This part of the sentence is called the *predicate.*

The second step in acquiring sentence sense is learning to recognize the subjects of verbs.

Subject: The subject is the part of a sentence about which something is being said. This part is properly called the *complete subject,* but within the complete subject there is always a word or group of words that is the principal word within the complete subject and is called the *simple subject.* The subject is usually a noun or pronoun.

Noun/pronoun: The noun is the name of a person, place, or thing.

Notice the subject written in italics in the following sentences.

EXAMPLES

The *patient* needs a complete blood count.

The *patient* is scheduled for a complete blood count.

The *patient* had a complete blood count.

He had a complete blood count.

The first three examples are nouns, and the fourth example is a pronoun.

A word used in place of a noun is called a *pronoun.* Pick out the noun subject of the following sentence:

My goal is to become a certified MT.

If you picked the noun *goal,* you are correct.

Now look at this sentence, and identify the subject and then the verb.

Exactly one year ago, Janet was promoted.

If you selected *Janet* as the subject and *was promoted* as the verb, you are correct. Because the subject may appear at almost any point in a sentence, it is usually easier to identify the verb first.

We can also express a sentence as follows:

Exactly one year ago, *she* was promoted.

In this case, the pronoun *she* is used in place of the noun.

Select the subject of the following sentence:

Down the elevator on a broken wheelchair struggled my patient.

Good for you if you selected *patient* from this convoluted grouping! Did you remember to find the verb first and then ask yourself "who struggled"?

Here are some additional parts of speech that go along with nouns, pronouns, and verbs.

Adjective: A descriptive word that modifies a noun or pronoun, telling how many, what kind, and so on.

EXAMPLES

complete blood count

painful bleeding ulcer

Adverb: A word that qualifies, intensifies, or modifies a verb, an adjective, or another adverb, explaining when, where, or how and often ending in "-ly."

EXAMPLES

She breathes *slowly. (Modifies verb)*

She breathes *too* slowly. *(Modifies adverb)*

She experiences *very* shallow breaths. (Modifies adjective)

Step three in acquiring sentence sense is recognizing the independent clause or main clause in a sentence and the dependent clause when there is one.

Clause: Any group of words containing a subject and a verb.

EXAMPLE

Everyone *who is learning to transcribe* should study punctuation.

Notice that in this sentence, there are two sets of clauses. The one in italics is dependent. It contains a subject and a verb, like the remainder of the sentence, but it *depends* on the balance of the sentence to make sense.

Pick out the subject and the verb in the following sentence:

Routine laboratory studies that we carried out on admission disclosed a white count of 19,200.

If you selected *studies* (or the complete subject, *routine laboratory studies*) as the subject, you are correct. The verb is *disclosed.* What about the clause *that we carried out on admission?* That is called a *dependent clause.* Continue with your vocabulary.

Independent Clause: A group of words that contains a subject and a verb, makes a complete statement, and is able to stand alone as a complete sentence.

EXAMPLE

We found a small area of fibrotic scarring involving the right uterosacral ligament.

NOTE: In this example, *we* is the subject and *found* is the verb.

Compound Sentence: A sentence consisting of two or more independent clauses.

EXAMPLES

I understand that you will complete the history and physical for the admission, **and** *I will order the preoperative evaluation.*

Good English skills are essential to our profession, **and** *we will study hard to ensure success.*

Pick out the two independent clauses from this unpunctuated compound sentence:

The patient had a complete blood count and we agreed to mail him a copy of the results.

HINT: Remember to look for the verb first (*had* in the first clause and *agreed* in the second).

The patient had a complete blood count is the first independent clause, and *we agreed to mail him a copy of the results* is the second. Notice that each of these clauses can stand alone and that neither depends on the other to express a complete thought.

 MT TOOL BOX TIP: Good English language skills are vital to good transcripts.

Dependent Clause (This is also called a *subordinate clause*): A group of words that contains a subject and a verb and that depends on some other word or words in the sentence for completeness of meaning.

EXAMPLES

He is a patient *who must have general anesthesia because he does not respond normally to routine dental care.*

Many students find transcribing easy *because they have prepared themselves well for it.*

NOTE: *In the first example,* he is a patient *is the independent clause and* who must have general anesthesia *is the first dependent or subordinate clause. This dependent clause modifies* patient. *The group of words* because he does not respond normally to routine dental care *is the second dependent clause in the sentence; it modifies the verb* must have *in the first dependent clause.*

In the second example, *Many students find transcribing easy* is the independent clause, and *because they have prepared themselves well for it* is the dependent or subordinate clause. This is a common way sentences are formed. Notice how the dependent clause *depends* on other words for completeness of meaning.

Select the dependent clause in the following sentence:

She had a complete blood count because she was scheduled for surgery tomorrow.

The clause *because she was scheduled for surgery tomorrow* is the dependent or subordinate clause because it depends on the first part of the sentence to complete the sentence. It cannot stand alone as the first part of the sentence (an independent clause) does.

Take a close look at the following sentence. Does it contain a dependent clause?

The patient had a complete blood count and was asked to wait for the results.

No. The phrase *was asked to wait for the results* does not contain a subject. This example illustrates a *compound predicate,* or two sets of verbs after the single subject. In other words, the words in the second half of the sentence *imply* the subject. For instance it seems to read, "The patient was asked to wait for results" following "The patient had a complete blood count." See how it works and how you can recognize a compound predicate. Because this structure is very common, you need to be able to tell the differences between an independent clause, a dependent clause, and a compound predicate.

To do so, select the verb first and then find the noun that is the subject of the sentence; finally, decide whether the subject-verb combination can stand alone (independent clause) or whether it depends on the independent clause to be complete (dependent clause). If there is no subject-verb combination, then you may have the third illustrated combination: a compound predicate, which is two or more verbs with one subject. There are additional pieces of these sentences to explore.

Select the compound predicates in the following sentences. Then locate the subject that refers to both of them.

> The patient is a painter and has worked there for many years.

First predicate: *is*
Second predicate: *has worked*
Subject: *patient*

> On April 17, 20XX, he underwent an incisional biopsy and received his first course of chemotherapy shortly thereafter.

First predicate: *underwent*
Second predicate: *received*
Subject: *he*

> The patient will return in one week and was encouraged to come in for a flu shot next month.

First predicate: *will return*
Second predicate: *was encouraged*
Subject: *patient*

Introductory Phrase: A group of words that occurs at the beginning of a sentence. This phrase can be thought of as being out of order or transposed in the sentence.

EXAMPLE

By now, you should have decided what courses you will need for graduation.

NOTE: The simple order of the sentence would be *You should have decided what courses you will need for graduation by now.*

EXAMPLE

In view of the continuing excessive tone in the plantar flexor muscles, it will be necessary to continue with orthotic control.

Please select the introductory phrase from the following sentence:

> One day after beginning treatment, the patient's sense of well-being markedly improved.

There are several clues here: First, the introductory phrase appears at the beginning of the sentence;

second, the sentence is correctly punctuated with a comma after the phrase (more about this later).

At this point, do not worry too much about the words *phrase* and *clause* themselves. (Clauses have a subject and a verb; phrases do not.) The important point is to notice the action and position of these groups of words in the sentence and the impact that they have on the dynamics of the sentence itself.

Essential: A word, phrase, or clause that is vital to the meaning of the sentence. Sometimes these are called *restrictive.*

EXAMPLES

Everyone *employed in the medical records department* received a commendation from the administrator.

The patient *who was born with a meningomyelocele* underwent closure of his spinal dysraphia in the newborn period.

Nonessential: A word, phrase, or clause that is not vital to the meaning of the sentence and simply provides explanatory material. Sometimes these are called **nonrestrictive.**

EXAMPLE

Marlene Bruno, *who took medical terminology with me last semester,* is on the Dean's List.

NOTE: It is interesting that Marlene Bruno took *medical terminology* with the writer, but it is not essential or vital to the meaning of the sentence.

EXAMPLE

The patient's weight was 83.5 kg, *up presumably as a result of inactivity,* and his height was 166 cm.

Determine in the following sentences whether the words in italics are essential or nonessential (restrictive or nonrestrictive):

> Students *who wish to enroll in medical keyboarding* must be typing 45 words per minute.
> Any health plan *in which there is a broad selection of hospitals, clinics, and caregivers* stands a good chance for success.
> Our health plan, *with a broad selection of hospitals, clinics, and caregivers,* is very successful in the community.

In the first two sentences, the italics illustrate essential elements. You must know *which* students and *what* kind of plan will be successful. In the third sentence, you are told that the plan is successful, and *additional* information is provided with the words in italics.

Parenthetical Expression: An interrupting group of words that does not change or contribute to the meaning of a sentence. The words may appear at the beginning, middle, or end of the sentence and are usually nonessential.

EXAMPLES

It is important, *as you know*, for medical records to be typed accurately.

I do not question the diagnosis; *however*, the result of his urinalysis and culture is negative.

NOTE: Some very common words or groups of words used as parenthetical expressions are *therefore, however, furthermore, in my opinion, strictly speaking, for example, in the first place, on the other hand, indeed, I suppose, of course, after all, by the way, it seems,* and *to be sure*.

Select the parenthetical expression in the following sentences:

The patient will be seen, I suppose, as soon as the triage is complete.

The patient, I suppose, will be seen as soon as the triage is complete.

The patient will be seen as soon as the triage is complete, I suppose.

I suppose is the correct selection.

The expression, as you no doubt noticed, completes its purpose in a variety of places in the sentence.

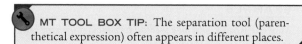 **MT TOOL BOX TIP:** The separation tool (parenthetical expression) often appears in different places.

Appositive: A noun or pronoun that closely follows another noun or pronoun to restate, rename, explain, or clarify it. It may be essential or nonessential. An appositive must always consist of a word or words that can be directly substituted for the noun or pronoun they follow. This term is unusual, but please try to remember it and its use in the sentence.

EXAMPLES

Dr Pappin, *my employer*, prefers to dictate all chart notes.

This 2-month-old male child, *a Hmong Laotian*, was admitted via the emergency room with a cough, fever, and congestion.

Please select the appositive in the following sentence:

The syringe was disposed of properly in the sharps container, the box for hazardous materials.

Your selection of *the box for hazardous materials* is correct.

 MT TOOL BOX TIP: Understand the language used by the writers of the rules—concentrate on unusual terms used in the rule itself.

Conjunction: A word used to join other words, phrases, clauses, and independent clauses.

EXAMPLES

and, or, nor, so, but, yet

▶ Joining other words: The records librarian **and** the medical transcriptionist…

▶ Joining phrases: The records librarian and the medical transcriptionist *attended the lecture* **and** *participated in the discussion*.

▶ Joining independent clauses: The records librarian and the medical transcriptionist attended the lecture, **and** they planned to participate in the discussion that followed.

Sometimes parenthetical expressions are used as conjunctions or as transitional words linking two independent clauses or sentences.

EXAMPLES

however, furthermore, therefore

The records librarian and the medical transcriptionist attended the lecture; *therefore*, they planned to participate in the discussion that followed.

Select the conjunctions in the following sentence, and decide the nature of the word or words that they are joining.

I enjoyed Chapter 1 and Chapter 2 of my textbook, but it appears that Chapter 3 may be a bit more difficult.

You are correct if you selected *but*, which joins **two independent clauses**, and *and*, which joins **two sets of words**.

3-1 SELF-STUDY

DIRECTIONS: Examine the sentences or parts of sentences that follow and write the part of the sentence or phrase that is requested on the line provided. The first exercise is completed for you. If the question does not apply to the sentence, write "none" on the blank line.

1. Furthermore, I feel that a well-trained medical transcriptionist should be very well paid.

   Subject of the sentence <u>I</u> _____

   Parenthetical expression <u>furthermore</u> _____

Independent clause <u>I feel that a well-trained medical transcriptionist should be very well paid.</u>

Appositive <u>none</u> _____

2. I appreciate my understanding of medical terminology.

   Subject of the sentence _____

   Independent clause _____

3. Please return this to Medical Records as soon as possible.

   Subject of the sentence _____

   Independent clause _____

4. After spending five hours in the operating room, the patient was sent to the recovery room.

   Introductory phrase _____

   Subject of the sentence _____

   Independent clause _____

5. The patient is a well-developed, well-nourished black female and reported that she has been well until this time.

   Subject of the sentence _____

   Independent clause _____

   Second verb clause _____

   Appositive _____

   Conjunction _____

6. Joan, the emergency department technician, and Beth, the admitting clerk, are taking an evening college course in medical ethics.

   Subject _____

   Independent clause _____

   Appositive 1 _____

   Appositive 2 _____

   Parenthetical expression _____

7. The reception room is well lighted and stocked with current literature, so the patients do not mind their wait to see Dr Jordan, who never seems to arrive on time.

   First subject _____

   Independent clause _____

   Second subject _____

   Independent clause _____

   Conjunction joining independent clauses _____

   Appositive _____

   Nonessential clause _____

8. There is overwhelming evidence, however, to prove that the ability to spell is vital to success in this field.

Independent clause _____

Parenthetical expression _____

Appositive _____

9. The Association for Healthcare Documentation Integrity, the national organization for medical transcriptionists, has a business and educational meeting every month.

Subject _____

Independent clause _____

Appositive _____

Parenthetical expression _____

Conjunction joining two independent clauses _____

10. Perfection, not speed, is the key goal in medical transcription skills.

Subject _____

Verb _____

Independent clause _____

Appositive _____

Parenthetical expression _____

Nonessential phrase _____

11. Hospital transcriptionists often need to.

Subject _____

Independent clause _____

12. When you telephone the hospital, please have the patient's complete name, address, and telephone number and the admitting diagnosis.

Subject _____

Verb _____

Independent clause _____

Nonessential phrase _____

Introductory clause _____

Conjunction joining words in a series _____

13. Appointment scheduling, contrary to what you might think, requires skill; it should be, and can be, a real art.

First independent clause _____

Second independent clause _____

Nonessential clause or phrase _____

Parenthetical expression _____

14. A perfectly typed resume, well-planned and prepared, should accompany your letter of application.

Independent clause _____

Introductory phrase _____

Nonessential phrase _____

15. He walks with his heel down with a varus tendency in the ankle but with no severe problem.

Independent clause _____

First dependent group of words _____

Second dependent group of words _____

Conjunction joining two independent clauses _____

16. In order to minimize the chance of overlooking a recurrence of the infection, a CBC and sed rate were carried out today.

Subject _____

Independent clause _____

Introductory phrase _____

Nonessential phrase _____

After you have completed the exercise, turn to p. 429 in Appendix A and check your answers. If you were unable to make a correct selection, please review the vocabulary before continuing.

THE COMMA

The comma is the most commonly used mark of punctuation and often causes the most problems for writers. At the same time, it is a very important aid in clarifying meaning for the reader. Commas should be used *appropriately* and *sparingly* when breaks are needed to avoid misinterpretation and to ease the reading of a sentence. Therefore, it is important to learn the rules for proper placement. When you have learned the basic rules, the remainder of the punctuation marks should cause little problem.

RULE 3.1a Use a comma, or a pair of commas, to set off nonessential words, phrases, or clauses from the remainder of the sentence

These nonessential words, phrases, or clauses are also called *parenthetical expressions* or *nonrestrictive phrases*. We need to examine them carefully. They interrupt the flow of thought in the sentence.

EXAMPLE: *Nonessential clause*

Paul Otis, *who had a coronary last year,* came in for an examination today.

You may test yourself to be sure this is nonessential by asking the question "Do I need to know which Paul Otis?" Unless you have several or even two patients with this name, you can say that the clause is nonessential to the meaning of the sentence. When you are in doubt, ask yourself if you need to know *which one*.

EXAMPLE: *Nonessential phrase*

Please notice, *if you will,* the depth of the incision.

EXAMPLES: *Nonessential word or words*

Yes, please type this before you leave this afternoon.

There is, *no doubt,* a reason for the failure of the electrical system.

EXAMPLE: *Parenthetical expression*

She should have, *in my opinion,* immediate surgery.

NOTE: Nonessential or nonrestrictive descriptive phrases or clauses add information that is *not* essential to the meaning of the sentence. However, do not enclose *essential* material within commas. Essential material indicates the manner, condition or who, what, why, when, or where.

EXAMPLES

I want to examine all of the children, *when they have been prepared. (Incorrect, because we need to know when)*

I want to examine all of the children when they have been prepared. *(Correct)*

Medical staff members, *who fail to attend the meeting,* will lose their consulting privileges. *(Incorrect, because we need to know which staff members)*

Medical staff members who fail to attend the meeting will lose their consulting privileges. *(Correct)*

There is no doubt that she transcribed that report. *(In this case the expression* no doubt *is essential because it adds emphasis to the statement. Commas would be incorrect.)*

Do not create a comma fault by leaving out one of the commas when a pair is required.

Her temperature, *which has been high* fell suddenly. *(Incorrect)*

Her temperature, *which has been high,* fell suddenly. *(Correct)*

NOTE: Many people often have difficulty with correct usage of *who/whom/whose, that,* and *which* as function words in essential and nonessential clauses.

Who/whom/whose is used in both essential and nonessential clauses.
That is used in essential clauses.
Which is generally used in nonessential clauses.

EXAMPLES

This is a 26-year-old male *who* cut his left index finger on a pocket knife.

The patients *whose* Pap smears are class II must be notified.

She twisted her left knee, *which* has an artificial prosthesis in it.

The recommendation *that* she undergo radiation therapy was rejected by the family.

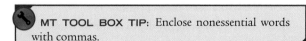

🔧 **MT TOOL BOX TIP:** Enclose nonessential words with commas.

RULE 3.1b Nonessential appositives are separated from the remainder of the sentence by commas.

Remember that appositives merely explain or describe other nouns or pronouns in a sentence.

EXAMPLES: *Appositive*

John Munor, *your patient,* was admitted to Center City Hospital today.

Laralyn Abbott, *the head nurse,* summoned me to the phone.

As with phrases and clauses, appositives may be essential to the complete meaning of the sentence, and then they must not be separated from the remainder of the sentence by commas. Remember that there are appositives that help identify a word by limiting or restricting its meaning, and so you must ask yourself whether you need to know *which one.*

EXAMPLE: *Essential appositive*

Your patient *Ralph Swansdown* died at 3:45 a.m.

To recap:

Specific term: Ralph Swansdon
General term: your patient

When the specific term *follows* the general term, you do not enclose the term in commas. When the general term *follows* the specific term, enclose that term in commas. Notice that if *Ralph Swansdown (the specific term)* is separated from the rest of the sentence with a pair of commas, it appears that the person being addressed by this remark had only one patient, the lately deceased Mr Swansdown. It is *essential* to know *which* patient. Likewise, one-word appositives do not require commas.

EXAMPLES

I *myself* will stay late and finish the report.

My cousin *Pat* just became a certified medical transcriptionist.

RULE 3.1c Use a comma, or pair of commas, to set off a short parenthetical expression from the remainder of the sentence

These expressions may begin, interrupt, or end a sentence and are always nonessential.

EXAMPLES

However, I want this report completed immediately.

I want this report completed immediately, *however.*

These comma pairs can also be used to draw emphasis to a nonessential expression. The rule is not superseded in this case, of course.

EXAMPLE

He is an excellent surgeon, *whether or not you care for my opinion,* and I feel that you must trust his judgment.

Recall that some of the words used as parenthetical expressions are *indeed, for example, I suppose, of course, after all, by the way, it seems, to be sure, therefore, however, furthermore, in my opinion, strictly speaking,* and so on. However, no word or expression in itself is parenthetical. When closely connected in meaning with other words in a sentence, they are not set off.

EXAMPLE

However upset she is, she will finish the report.

To restate these three similar rules: Set off nonessential words from the main body of thought; commas must be placed before and after such words, phrases, or clauses; if nonessential words occur at the beginning of a sentence, a single comma follows the expression. Your ability to recognize the difference between essential words, phrases, or clauses and those that are nonessential is important. Remember that an essential or a restrictive element identifies or further defines the meaning of the sentence and must *not* be separated from the sentence.

One final note: Many dictators give a vocal clue indicating whether something is nonessential by dropping their voices. The voice goes up when something is emphasized. Examine these two sentences by reading them aloud.

EXAMPLES

We were determined, nevertheless, to proceed with the surgery.

We were nevertheless determined to go ahead with the surgery.

Listen for these vocal hints and observe also the position of *nevertheless* in each sentence.

3-2 SELF-STUDY

DIRECTIONS: Using Rules 3.1a, 3.1b, and 3.1c, add a comma or comma pair to the following sentences where required. Be careful not to enclose essential sentence parts. In the space provided, briefly state why you did or did not punctuate the sentence. A simple test for a nonessential element is to read the sentence without it. If the missing element does not change the basic meaning of the sentence, it should be set off by commas.

EXAMPLE

She said *if my memory serves me right* that she had graduated from medical school in 1998.

The phrase *if my memory serves me right* is nonessential. It is also a parenthetical expression.

1. John Munro your patient was admitted to Center City Hospital today.

   _____

2. He is an excellent surgeon whether or not you care for my opinion and I feel that you must trust his judgment.

   _____

3. She required trifocal not bifocal lenses at this time.

   _____

4. Dr Mitchell having been in surgery since two this morning collapsed on the day bed.

   _____

5. The wound was closed with #3-0 silk sutures.

   _____

The answers to these Self-Study questions are in Appendix A, p. 430. Check your answers before you continue. Review the rules, if necessary.

3-3 SELF-STUDY

DIRECTIONS: Using the directions in Self-Study 3-2, complete the following problems. Notice that your attention is directed to words in italics in some of the sentences.

1. Please telephone my nurse *if you are agreeable to postponing the surgery.*

   _____

2. He has done well since the transurethral resection of his prostate *with the exception of one episode of postsurgical hemorrhage.*

   _____

3. Our daughter Pat *who is a senior this year* is studying for a degree in rehabilitation therapy.

_____

4. I want to examine all of the children *who have been exposed.*

_____

5. Bill Birch's father *Ralph Birch* is chief of staff at Mercy Hospital now.

_____

6. His decision *not to operate* was a bit hasty if you ask me.

_____

7. Only the second copy which is a photocopy should be mailed to the referring physician.

_____

8. I will contact the anesthesiologist *as soon as the operating room is free.*

_____

9. *Essentials of Medical History* my textbook is excellent.

_____

10. Nephritis *Bright disease* will be the topic of his presentation at our meeting.

_____

11. I had lunch with Alex St. Charles the new resident.

_____

12. I would like to thank all of those patients *who donated blood.*

_____

13. All patients wearing pacemakers should be told the good news.

_____

14. Medical staff members *who fail to attend the meeting* will lose their consulting privileges however.

_____

15. The emergency department dictation not the pathology department dictation was diverted to the per diem staff.

_____

16. Furthermore she is to be prepped before Dr Summers arrives.

_____

17. Your patient Ethel Clifford saw me in consultation.

_____

18. Ethel Clifford your patient saw me in consultation.

_____

19. It was of course essential for him to be admitted immediately.

_____

20. It was essential for him to be admitted immediately of course.

_____

The answers appear in Appendix A, p. 430.

RULE 3.2a Use a comma to set off an introductory dependent phrase or clause.

EXAMPLES

After you have an x-ray, I will examine you. *(Simple introductory clause)*

Dr Chriswell was having difficulty dictating; however, *after the equipment was adjusted,* she was able to finish her reports. *(Part of the second independent clause)*

Fully aware of his budget restrictions and with concern for the high cost of the equipment, Dr Jellison approved the purchase of speech recognition technology equipment. *(Compound introductory phrase)*

NOTE: The comma follows the second phrase.

To transcribe this accurately the first time is the main goal. *(This introductory phrase serves as the subject of the sentence and must not be separated from the rest of the sentence by a comma.)*

Recall that this introductory element can be thought of as being "out of place" in the sentence. Many of these introductory dependent phrases or clauses begin with words such as *since, because, after, about, during, by, if, when, while, although, unless, between, so, until, whenever, as,* and *before* and with verb forms such as *hoping, believing, allowing, helping,* and *working.*

RULE 3.2b Do *not* use a comma when the essential or restrictive clause appears in natural order: at the end of the sentence or at the end of the independent clause.

Essential clauses limit the meaning of the main clause.

EXAMPLES

I will examine you *after* you have an x-ray. *(Tells when the patient will be examined)*

She was able to finish her report *after* the equipment was adjusted.

EXAMPLE: *Introductory*

During the course of the procedure, a power failure occurred.

EXAMPLE: *Natural order*

A power failure occurred *during* the course of the procedure.

OPTIONAL: The comma may be omitted after a very brief introductory element if clarity is not sacrificed.

EXAMPLE

If possible schedule the thoracotomy to follow the bronchoscopy.

If possible, schedule the thoracotomy to follow the bronchoscopy. *(Also correct)*

The comma is also omitted after short introductory phrases that answer such questions as when, where, why, or how often.

EXAMPLE

This afternoon she needs to pick up her referral.

Sometimes I feel exhausted after such a long shift.

 3-4 SELF-STUDY

DIRECTIONS: Using the rules you have just learned, add a comma or comma pair where required. Be wary of separating the subject from the verb with a comma, which you might attempt to do when the subject is lengthy. Always check to be sure there is an intact independent clause. Please insert and circle optional commas.

EXAMPLE

After the surgery was completed, he dictated the operative report. *(Note the comma after the introductory phrase.)*

1. Although she had been in pain for some time she failed to seek medical attention.
2. That you have lost your promotion is not my concern.
3. If you are not feeling better by tomorrow take two aspirin and call Dr Meadows.
4. When initially seen the patient was in restraints lying in bed.
5. To transcribe and complete the insurance billing is her responsibility.
6. Our receptionist whom I hired yesterday failed to come in today.
7. Recently we reviewed all discharge summaries for the month of July.

You will find the answers in Appendix A, p. 431. Before you continue with your next Self-Study, be sure to check any errors you may have made by reviewing the comma rules.

3-5 SELF-STUDY

DIRECTIONS: Use the rules you have learned thus far and place commas, as needed, in the following problems. Then, briefly state the reason for the commas you have added. It is important to state why you have placed punctuation, because it will assist you in correcting a misunderstanding, if there is one, about a particular placement.

1. She will go immediately into the operating room as soon as it is free.

2. Whatever he said to her was misunderstood.

3. Dr Johnston the pathologist deserves the credit for that diagnosis.

4. The delivery of the baby a girl was uneventful.

5. Furthermore I will not be here to interview the new medical transcriptionist.

6. After successful general anesthesia padding was placed under the left buttock.

7. To be sure she was safe the nurse took her to the car in a wheelchair.

8. After lunch he must rest quietly.

9. Thinking he was at home the patient attempted to get out of bed.

10. Helping the visually impaired transcriptionist research a word is Janet's responsibility.

The answers are in Appendix A, p. 431. Check them carefully, and review when necessary.

RULE 3.3 Use a comma to set off a year date that is used to explain a preceding date of the month.

EXAMPLES

He was born on *March 3, 1933,* in Reading, Pennsylvania.

Make her an appointment for Wednesday, *July 6, 20XX.*

Omit commas when the complete date is not given.

EXAMPLES

We will see the patient again on *May 6.*

He had surgery in *April 20XX* in Tucson, Arizona.

Omit the comma with the military date sequence.

EXAMPLE

11 November 2006

RULE 3.4 Use a comma to set off the name of the state when the city precedes it.

EXAMPLE

The pacemaker was shipped to you from Syracuse, *New York,* by air express.

Use commas to separate all the elements of a complete address.

EXAMPLE

Please mail this to my home address: 132 Winston Street, Park Village, IL 60612.

NOTE: Do not place a comma between the state name and the ZIP code. The ZIP code is considered part of the state name.

RULE 3.5 Do not use a comma to set off *Inc.* and *Ltd.* after the name of a company unless the company prefers the usage.

EXAMPLES

I was employed by Thoracic Surgery Medical Group *Inc.,* in Encino, California, for five years.

Headquarters for The Reader's Digest Association, *Inc.,* is Pleasantville, New York.

RULE 3.6 Use a comma or pair of commas to set off titles and degrees after a person's name.

EXAMPLES

John A. Meadows, *MD,* saw the patient in consultation.

Ms Nancy Bishop, *risk manager,* gave him ten days to bring his incomplete charts up to date.

If there are multiple degrees or professional credentials after a person's name, place them in the order in which they were awarded and separate them with commas.

EXAMPLES

Mary Watkins, *BS, MS, JD*

Nancy Casales, *CMT, AHDI-F,* is the new president of AHDI, Mountain Meadows Chapter.

Frances Knight, *LLB, MD,* will be speaking about risk management.

NOTE: There is a trend to eliminate commas, particularly when meaning is not sacrificed. Some writers are not using commas to separate degrees and titles after a person's name. As always, follow the wishes of the bearer of the name.

Do not place a comma before roman numbers that indicate first, second, third, and so forth, or before *Jr* or *Sr* after a name unless the bearer of the name prefers that usage.

EXAMPLES

Kip I. Praycroft *Sr,* MD

Howard J. Matlock *III*

Carl A. Nichols *Jr* was admitted to Ward B.

RULE 3.7 Use a comma after each element or each pair of elements in a series of coordinate nouns, adjectives, verbs, or adverbs.

OPTIONAL: You *may* omit the comma before the conjunction if clarity is not sacrificed. However, many writers avoid this option, and it is recommended that you not take this option.

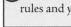 **MT TOOL BOX TIP:** Ignore "optional" forms of rules and you will always be safe.

EXAMPLES

Please copy the patient's operative report, pathology report, and consultation report for Dr Gifford.

The various hospital departments were decorated in green and yellow, blue and brown, and green and white.

There were papers to be filed, charts to be sorted, ledgers to be posted.

The patient underwent daily group, milieu, and individual psychotherapy.

Often medical dictators use several descriptive adjectives such as size, shape, age, color, and nationality to describe a patient. These descriptors may be thought of as a single unit and therefore not separated by commas.

EXAMPLE

The patient is a well-developed, well-nourished 35-year-old white female dispatch officer.

When you have a list such as this, be careful not to separate the adjective that forms a noun phrase with the noun it modifies. The noun phrase is *female dispatch officer,* and the adjective immediately preceding the noun phrase is *white.*

A test of whether commas are needed is to transpose the final two modifiers. For example, one would not say *female white dispatch officer.*

EXAMPLE

He is a 37-year-old Hispanic married ICU nurse.

One would not say *ICU married nurse.* Thus the noun phrase is *ICU nurse* and you would not use a comma in this phrase.

Additionally, no comma is used before the ampersand (&) in a series of names in a business.

EXAMPLE

The law firm is listed as Claborne, Franklin & Bowers.

NOTE: The abbreviation *etc* in a series has a comma both before and after it unless it occurs at the end of a sentence; then its period ends the sentence.

When the items in a series are connected by *and* or *nor,* do not use commas to separate the series.

EXAMPLES

Neither the interns nor the residents nor the medical students were invited to attend the lecture series.

RULE 3.8 Use a comma to separate two or more independent clauses when they are joined by the conjunction *and, or, nor, but, for, yet,* or *so.*

NOTE: The comma is placed in front of the conjunction.

EXAMPLES

She used a cane in her right *hand, but* now she cannot use a cane at all because of pain in her right shoulder.

Your appendix appears to be *inflamed, but* I do not believe that you need surgery at this time.

BUT: Your appendix appears to be inflamed but not acutely. *(Not two independent clauses)*

EXAMPLE

The diagnosis of urinary tract infection was *made, and* he was treated with Septra.

Do not identify a compound predicate in a simple sentence as two independent clauses.

EXAMPLES

The child weighed 7 pounds at birth *and* was the result of an uncomplicated pregnancy and delivery. *(Not two independent clauses; a compound predicate, no comma)*

She has no other current skin complaints and no history of skin cancer.

Examine the sentence this way: first, *She has* no other skin complaint; then, *she has* no history of skin cancer.

The simple subject goes with each predicate. No independent clause; no comma.

Two of the preceding examples do not contain two independent clauses, and it would be incorrect and misleading if you placed commas in front of the conjunctions. Be careful not to make this error. Check the sentence to see whether the clauses are independent by testing each clause to see whether it expresses a complete thought and could stand alone as a sentence, without the conjunction. When the second (or third) clause is *dependent,* the subject is usually missing. There must be a subject in the second clause to make it independent. Do not make the mistake of using a comma just because a conjunction is present. Know why you are punctuating, and when in doubt, leave it out!

> **MT TOOL BOX TIP:** When in doubt, leave it out (a punctuation mark, that is).

OPTIONAL: Some writers omit a comma between two short, closely related independent clauses if there is no chance of the meaning being confused. However, dictation editors are discouraged from using this option, and you may waste time trying to decide.

EXAMPLE

She came in just after noon *so* we invited her to lunch.

BUT: I kicked the ball, and John accidentally slipped reaching for it.

If you omit the comma after *ball,* it appears, at first glance, as if you also kicked John accidentally.

Please look at the example *The diagnosis of urinary tract infection was made, and he was treated with Septra.* Many experts would eliminate this comma because the sentence is rather brief and straightforward. Now you have another "option" to deal with! Make it easy and correct: ignore the option.

3-6 SELF-STUDY

DIRECTIONS: Using Rules 3.3 through 3.8, add a comma or commas where required. Briefly state why you inserted the comma or commas. Remember: This suggestion is important.

1. The patient was first seen in my office on Wednesday July 14 20XX.

   _____

2. Please send this to Natalie Jayne RN Chief of Nurses Glorietta Bay Hospital.

   _____

3. Carl A. Nichols Jr was admitted to Ward B.

   _____

4. The blood test included a white blood count red blood count hematocrit and differential.

   _____

5. There is a history of a mild head injury at age 10 and she was in a moderately severe motorcycle accident about 15 years ago.

   _____

6. The condition is now stationary and permanent and he should be able to resume his normal workload.

   _____

7. She was fully dilated at 2:30 a.m. but did not deliver the second twin until 2:55 a.m.

   _____

8. He denies any visual problem but he uses glasses.

   _____

See p. 432 in Appendix A for the answers to this Self-Study. If necessary, review carefully before you continue.

3-7 SELF-STUDY

DIRECTIONS: In the following sentences, fill in the missing punctuation, and in the space after each sentence, fill in the letter or letters of the rule or rules you used from the list given after Rule Review. Each rule may be used more than once, and it is not necessary to refer to the point in the chapter where the rule was introduced. Place a circle around any optional commas and write your reason for the option in the "rule" blank.

RULE REVIEW: Use a comma or pair of commas to

a. set off nonessential words from the remainder of the sentence

b. set off nonessential appositives

c. set off a parenthetical expression

d. set off an introductory phrase or clause

e. set off the parts of a date

f. set off *Inc.* or *Ltd.* in a company name only if the firm prefers this style

g. set off titles and degrees after a person's name

h. separate words in a series

i. separate two independent clauses

j. separate the name of the state from the name of the city

EXAMPLE

On auscultation, there are diffuse rhonchi and occasional rales heard.

Rule ___d___

1. He will be able to return to light work at any time but he should not be allowed to operate a jackhammer.

   Rule _____

2. His wounds are all healing well and he has had no further pain.

   Rule _____

3. In the preceding week he had had an automobile accident and was under the care of Dr Finish.

   Rule _____

4. The patient continued her labor and was closely monitored for fetal heart tones.

   Rule _____

5. I have consulted with the Radiation Therapy Department at University Hospital and they have suggested that radiation therapy would be the best approach to this problem.

   Rule _____

6. It is my understanding that you will do the history and physical examination for the hospital but not the consultation.

   Rule _____

7. Please contact Charles Rick MD in Nogales Arizona as soon as possible.

   Rule _____

8. He had surgery July 14 2006 for carcinoma of the prostate but is now free of disease.

   Rule _____

9. Dr Phillip is the newest member of St. Peter's Medical and Surgical Group Inc.

   Rule _____

10. On physical examination I found a well-developed well-nourished white woman in no acute distress.

    Rule _____

11. He noticed increasing dyspnea with effort extreme shortness of breath and night sweats.

    Rule _____

12. She is to be admitted with your concurrence on Wednesday July 1 20XX at 2 p.m.

    Rule _____

13. Before you call surgery to schedule this and before you telephone Mrs Jones will you report to me?

    Rule _____

14. As you know John Briggs MD my partner is retiring on July 31 this year.

    Rule _____

15. On March 26 20XX she had a left lower lobectomy and postoperatively had bronchopneumonia which required intravenous antibiotics.

    Rule _____

See p. 432 in Appendix A for a list of the rule or rules used in this exercise. After you have completed the assignment, you may consult this list to check yourself. If you chose the wrong rule, perhaps you have misplaced the comma!

RULE 3.9 Enclose names of persons used in direct address and the words *yes* and *no* in commas.

EXAMPLES

My thanks, *Paul*, for sending Mr Byron in for a consultation.

No, it is not our policy to give out that information.

Now is the time, *medical documentation specialists*, to make your voices heard.

RULE 3.10 Coordinate adjectives (two or more words that independently modify the same noun) are separated by a comma.

NOTE: Check to see whether the modifiers are coordinate by placing a mental *and* between them or see whether you can reverse their sequence.

EXAMPLES

She is a *tall, slender* woman.

It was a *wide, deep* wound.

BUT: She is an efficient medical scribe.

Do not place a comma after the last modifier in front of the noun. In the following sentence, we would not place a comma in front of *memo*.

We received a poorly punctuated, rude memo from your department.

RULE 3.11 Use a comma or a pair of commas to emphasize a word, to avoid misleading or confusing the reader, and to set off contrasts and omissions.

EXAMPLES

In *20XX, 461* babies were delivered in the new obstetrics wing.

It is one thing to be *assertive, another* to be rigid.

We are here to *work, not* visit.

Soon *after, he* got up and discharged himself from the hospital.

The day *before, I* had seen her in the emergency department.

She was caught in the trap called "last *hired, first* fired."

He *demanded, rather hastily, that* she be released from further care.

Diagnosis: *Fractures, 3rd* and *4th* ribs on right.

Operation performed: *Hemorrhoidectomy, radical.*

Impression: *Diverticulosis, moderate.*

RULE 3.12 Use a comma after the complimentary close when using "mixed punctuation" in a letter.

EXAMPLE

Sincerely yours,

RULE 3.13 Use commas to group large numbers in units of three.

EXAMPLE

platelets *250,000;* WBC *15,000*

NOTE: Addresses, year dates, ZIP codes, four-digit numbers, and some ID and technical numbers are traditionally not separated by commas, nor are commas used with decimals or the metric system.

EXAMPLES

1000 mL *(correct); 1,000* mL *(incorrect)*

My bill to Medicare was *$1250.*

CAUTION: Do not separate numbers that are parts of complete units.

EXAMPLE

She was in labor for *6 hours 40 minutes* before we decided to do a cesarean section.

NOT: 6 hours, 40 minutes

EXAMPLE

The infant weighed *4 pounds 15 ounces* on delivery.

NOT: 4 pounds, 15 ounces

EXAMPLE

He died *3 years 4 months 13 days* after the implant.

NOT: 3 years, 4 months, 13 days

RULE 3.14 Use a comma to separate the parts of a date in the date line of a letter.

EXAMPLE

November *11, 20XX*

BUT: 11 November 20XX

3-8 PRACTICE TEST

DIRECTIONS: Using your textbook and any other reference materials, properly punctuate the letter on p. 80. There are 13 commas missing. Other punctuation marks, including two commas, are provided for you, so your completed letter will contain 15 commas, including any optional commas. In the margin, number each comma you insert, and on a separate sheet of paper, give your reason for using each comma.

Please retype and punctuate this letter using letterhead paper of your choice.

Punctuate it on the page if there is a time problem or equipment is not available in the teaching laboratory.

The answer is on p. 433 in Appendix A.

September 16 20XX

Tellememer Insurance Company
25 Main Street, Suite R
Albuquerque NM 87122

Dear Sir or Madam

Re: Ron Emerson

I understand from Mr Emerson that the insurance company feels that the charges for my services on June 30 20XX are excessive.

Mr Emerson was seen on an early Sunday morning with a stab wound in his chest, which had penetrated his lung producing an air leak into his chest wall. In addition he had a laceration of his lung.

After consultation and review of his x-rays his laceration was repaired. He was observed in the hospital for 2 days to be sure that he did not have continuing hemorrhage or collapse of his lung.

I feel that the bill given to Mr Emerson is a fair one. We received on July 31 20XX a Tellememer Insurance Company check for $200; and I feel that your payment of $200 is unreasonable. It is doubtful that one could get a plumber to come out early Sunday morning to fix a leaky pipe for $200; and Mr Emerson's situation in my opinion was much more serious than would be encountered by a plumber.

We will bill Mr Emerson for the remainder of the $680 balance on his account but I want you to know that we feel that your payment is insufficient. If he feels that the bill is excessive we would be glad to submit to arbitration through the County Medical Society Fee Committee. If this fails I suggest we seek help through the New Mexico Insurance Commission.

Sincerely yours

William A. Berry MD

mlo

Enclosed: X-ray report; history and physical report

Copy: Mr Ron Emerson

3-9 REVIEW TEST

DIRECTIONS: Place a comma or commas where needed in the sentences that follow. Please circle any that may be optional.

1. In the meantime he was discharged to his home.

2. She is scheduled to be seen again on February 3 at 10:30 a.m.

3. Laralyn Abbott the trauma team nurse issued a code blue.

4. Your patient Salvador Rodriquez was readmitted to the hospital with a diagnosis of cholecystitis pancreatitis and mild gastritis.

5. As demonstrated earlier chemotherapy had little effect on the rate of tumor growth.

6. In 20XX 461 cases were reviewed by the Tumor Board.

7. Soon after he got up and discharged himself from the hospital.

8. Dr Powell not Dr Franklyn delivered the infant.

9. After three surgeries are not scheduled.

10. I would like her to be and she probably will be a candidate for heart surgery.

11. She is a spastic developmentally delayed child.

12. He had crystal clear urine.

13. It has been a pleasure Winton to help you take care of Mr Ibarra.

14. She required trifocal not bifocal lenses at this time.

15. Dr Chriswell was having difficulty dictating; however, after the equipment was adjusted she was able to finish her reports.

16. He was indeed concerned about her progress.

17. Even though he was experiencing difficulty breathing we decided not to perform a tracheotomy.

18. The patient was placed in four-point restraints and gastric lavage was carried out.

19. The surgery was completed in 2 hours 40 minutes.

20. The infant demonstrated normal reflexes of suck root and startle.

The voice of the dictator usually gives us clues such as voice inflection, pauses, tone, and word emphasis that help in understanding the meaning of what is being said. To convey this meaning to the person to whom the dictator is communicating, the vocal clues must be translated into written clues.

You have just completed your study of the most used written clue: the comma. Now you can tackle the remainder of the basic aids to understanding the written word. Again, special emphasis has been placed on the punctuation rules you will use most often in medical transcribing.

THE PERIOD AND DECIMAL POINT

NOTE: Some dictators indicate the end of a sentence by saying "period" or "full stop." Others drop their voice to indicate closure. You will need to learn the individual styles of your dictators.

RULE 3.15 Place a period at the end of a sentence and at the end of a request for action that is phrased as a question out of politeness. (You may use one or two spaces following the period. Find out if your site permits this choice; some sites do not allow two spaces as they perceive this to add unnecessary spaces in line counts.)

EXAMPLES

His chest was clear to percussion and *auscultation.*

You must be seen by a surgeon at *once.*

Will you please send a copy of the operative report to Dr *Blanche.*

NOTE: Use only one period at the end of a sentence, even if the sentence ends with a punctuated abbreviation.

EXAMPLE

The surgery is scheduled to begin at 7 *a.m.*

RULE 3.16 Place a period with the following:

▶ Single letter abbreviations

Joseph P. Myers

▶ The name of the genus when it is abbreviated and used with the species

E. coli   M. tuberculosis   E. histolytica

▶ Lowercase Latin abbreviations

a.m.   p.m.   e.g.   t.i.d.   p.o.

▶ After letters and numbers in alphanumeric outlines except those enclosed in parentheses

I. ....
   A. ....
   B. ....
     1. ....
     2. ....

Diagnoses
1. Bilateral external canal exostoses.
2. Deafness, left ear, unknown etiology.

The following are *not* punctuated:
▶ Metric and English units of measurement

wpm   mph   m   g   kg   mg   mL   L   cm   km

▶ Certification, registration, and licensure abbreviations

CMA-A   CMT   RN   RRA   ART   LPN

▶ Acronyms

CARE   Project HOPE   AIDS   MAST

▶ Most abbreviations typed in capital letters

UCLA   PKU   BUN   CBC   COPD   D&C
T&A   I&D   PERRLA

▶ Scientific abbreviations typed in a combination of capital and lowercase letters

Rx   Dx   ACh   Hb   IgG   mEq   mOsm
Rh   Na   K   pH

▶ Abbreviations that are brief forms of words

exam   phenobarb   sedrate   flu   Papsmear   chem

▶ Academic degrees and religious orders

BVE   DDS   MD   MS   PhD   RCSJ   SJ

Some individuals prefer that these abbreviations be punctuated with a period. It is not incorrect to do this.

▶ It is optional to place a period with abbreviated professional and personal abbreviated titles.

Mr.   Jr.   Dr.   Msgr.   Mr   Jr   Dr   Msgr

RULE 3.17 A period (decimal point) is used to separate a decimal fraction from whole numbers.

EXAMPLES

His temperature on admission was *99.8 degrees.*

The new surgical instrument cost *$64.85.*

Epinephrine dose: *0.3 mL.*

The wound measured *2.5 x 2.5 cm.*

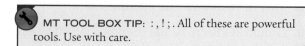 **MT TOOL BOX TIP:** : , ! ; . All of these are powerful tools. Use with care.

THE SEMICOLON

The semicolon is always used as a mark of separation. It is frequently equivalent to a period; in this situation, both sides of the semicolon must be independent clauses. Sometimes the semicolon replaces a comma and tells the reader, "Keep reading; the second part is related."

RULE 3.18 Use a semicolon to separate two or more closely related independent clauses when there is no conjunction such as *and, or, but,* or *nor.*

EXAMPLES

You have requested our *cooperation;* we have complied.

The nose is remarkable for loud congestive *breathing;* there is no discharge visible.

RULE 3.19 Use a semicolon to separate independent clauses if either one or both have already been punctuated with two or more commas and misreading might occur if a comma also separates the clauses.

EXAMPLES

Around the first of July, he developed pain in his chest, which he ignored for several *days;* and finally he saw me, at the request of his family doctor, on July 16.

There was no history of pneumonia, tuberculosis, chronic cough, or *hemoptysis;* and there was no exposure to substances at home, at work, or at school that may have contributed to this event.

RULE 3.20 Use a semicolon before a parenthetical expression and a comma after it when the expression is used as a transitional word between two independent clauses.

EXAMPLE

I attempted a labor induction with Pitocin, and contractions *occurred;* however, the patient failed to develop an effective labor pattern, and I discharged her after 8 hours.

However, when a conjunction is used along with a parenthetical expression in a compound sentence, it is separated by commas.

EXAMPLE

The phenobarbital keeps her in a drowsy state, so *consequently,* she is not able to think creatively or participate in sports activities.

NOTE: Parenthetical expressions are nonessential words or phrases that are used as independent comments that modify the entire sentence rather than any particular words in the sentence. Here are some commonly used parenthetical expressions: *accordingly, actually, apparently, as a matter of fact, as you know, by all means, certainly, clearly, consequently, fortunately, frankly, furthermore, happily, however, if possible, in my opinion, indeed, moreover, needless to say, nevertheless, obviously, personally, therefore, unfortunately.*

RULE 3.21 Use a semicolon between a series of phrases or clauses if any item in the series has internal commas. (This usage gives a clear indication of where one word group ends and another begins.)

EXAMPLES

Among those present at the Utilization Committee Meeting were Dr Frank Byron, *chief of staff;* Mrs Joan Armath, *administrator;* Ms Nancy Speeth, *medical records technician;* and Mr Ralph Johnson, director of nurses.

Medications: She will continue her 1800-calorie ADA diet and usual medicines, which include estradiol, micronized, 2 mg/d for 25 of 30 *days;* propoxyphene HCl 65 mg q.i.d., which is an increase from her current t.i.d. regimen; and flurazepam HCl 30 mg at bedtime.

THE COLON

Think of the colon as a pointer, drawing your attention to an important and concluding part. It is a mark of *anticipation.* It helps to couple separate elements that must be tied together but emphasized individually. Often, the material to the right of the colon means the same as the material to the left of the colon. In the past, a double space was always inserted after the colon in narrative copy. Today a single space is acceptable; whichever method you choose, be consistent.

RULE 3.22 Use a colon to introduce a *list* preceded by a *complete sentence.* These lists are often introduced by the following expressed or implied words: *as follows, such as, namely, the following.*

EXAMPLE

Please bring the following items with you to the *hospital:* robe, slippers, toilet articles, and two pairs of pajamas.

INCORRECT: The patient had: a history of chronic obstructive lung disease and congestive heart failure.

CORRECT: The patient had a history of chronic obstructive lung disease and congestive heart failure.

RULE 3.23 In business letter preparation, a colon is placed after the salutation (when mixed punctuation is used) and in the following other document components.

EXAMPLES

Gentlemen:

Dear Dr Berry:

Dear Bill: (or) Dear Bill,

To Whom It May Concern:

Dear Sir or Madam:

Re: Florence Gregg

CC: William Norris, MD

Attention: Bradley Wilhite

Enclosure: Pathology report

PS: Please note our new area code.

OPTIONAL: When the salutation is informal and the person is addressed by first name, you *may* use a comma (see the third example).

RULE 3.24 Use a colon with numbers in expressing ratios and dilute solutions and between the hours and minutes indicating the time. (There are no spaces on either side of the colon.)

EXAMPLES

The solution was diluted *1:100.*

The odds are *10:1.*

Her appointment is for *10:30* a.m.

NOTE: The colon is not used in expressions of military (24-hour) time.

EXAMPLE

Time of death was called at *1434 hours.*

See Rule 5.17 for a description of 24-hour time.

NOTE: The colon and double zeros are not used with the even time of day.

EXAMPLE

10 a.m.

RULE 3.25 Place a colon after the introductory word or words in preparing a written history and physical, in introducing a reference line, in listing the patient's vital signs, or with the introductory words in an outline.

EXAMPLES

Chief complaint: Hyperemesis.

Past history: Usual childhood diseases; no sequelae.

Allergy: Patient denies any drug or food sensitivity.

Re: Mrs Blanche Mitchell.

Reference: #306-A.

Subject: Stress test.

Vital Signs

 Temperature: 101 degrees.

 Pulse: 58.

 BP: 130/90.

 Respirations: 18.

Diagnoses: 1. Gastritis.

    2. Pancreatitis.

    3. Rule out cholecystitis.

NOTE: A colon is not required when the list begins on the line following. (See also *Vital Signs* above)

EXAMPLE

Diagnoses

1. Gastritis.

2. Pancreatitis.

3. Rule out cholecystitis.

NOTE: Close your listed items with a period.

RULE 3.26 Use a colon to introduce an example or a clarification of an idea.

NOTE: There is no coordinating conjunction, and the second clause explains or completes the first. Notice, for instance, that in the first two examples of the following, these words cannot be appositives because they are needed to complete the entire thought.

EXAMPLES

I see only one *alternative*: chemotherapy.

You have only one goal *here*: accuracy.

Now for some brighter *news*: We will be able to begin hiring again in a month.

NOTE: These examples are often introduced by the expressions *thus* or *that is*, or the expression could be supplied mentally.

Colons are generally used in sentences in which the second set of words amplifies or clarifies the first. A *capital letter* is used to begin the set of words after the colon if it is a formal statement.

EXAMPLE

This is how the equipment is stored: Leave the cord to the headset loose, and place it in the plastic bag provided.

3-10 SELF-STUDY

DIRECTIONS: Using Rules 3.15 through 3.26, add a semicolon, colon, or period where required.

1. Mr Clark E Rosamunde is scheduled to arrive at 4:30 pm

2. Josephine Tu, MD, will present six cases to the Oncology Review Board Dr Richland will be unable to attend

3. Would you please send this on to Ralph Desmond Jr

4. Please place the following warning on the door to Room 16 "Caution Radioactive materials in use"

5. The ambulance arrived at precisely 2110

6. The patient was treated for the following problems insomnia, malaise, depression

7. The consultation fee of $85 was not covered by insurance

8. General On examination the patient is awake, alert, and cooperative

9. Condition on Discharge Good

Check your answers in Appendix A, p. 433.

3-11 SELF-STUDY

DIRECTIONS: In the following exercises, fill in the missing punctuation, and in the blank after each exercise, fill in the letter of the rule you used from the list given after Rule Review. Each rule may be used more than once, and it is not necessary to refer to the point in the chapter where the rule was introduced.

RULE REVIEW: Use a period:

a. with single capitalized word abbreviations.

b. to separate decimal fractions.

Use a semicolon:

c. between two independent clauses that have internal punctuation.

d. between two independent clauses with a parenthetical expression acting as a conjunction.

e. between two independent clauses with no conjunction.

f. to simplify reading the sentence because of other punctuation marks.

Use a colon:

g. to introduce a series of items.

h. to clarify an idea.

i. with introductory words in an outline.

j. with a reference notation.

EXAMPLE
The child had a full-term gestation; his birth weight was 9 pounds 4 ounces.
Rule ____e____

1. She has not quite returned to full physical activity yet therefore, I will want to see her again in a month to reevaluate her status.

Rule _____

2. As you recall, Mr Scout is a 41-year-old man with severe angina, myocardial ischemia, and triple artery disease but he does have a well-functioning ventricle.

Rule _____

3. The procedures performed were as follows bronchoscopy, bronchography, scalene node biopsy, right pneumonectomy. The insurance reimbursement (welcome as it was) amounted to only $65075 [six hundred fifty dollars and seventy-five cents].

Rule _____

4. The panel members included the following staff Dr Mary A Jamison, chief resident Dr Peter R Douglas Jr, surgical director Mrs Nancy Culpepper, operating room supervisor and Jane Morris, RN, ICU supervisor.

Rule _____

5. One fact stands out in all this discussion about this young man he has a great element of fear about being anesthetized.

Rule _____

6. The patient was admitted with a temperature of 1012° [one hundred one and two tenths degrees], chills, and nausea she also complained of low back pain and cervical pain.

Rule _____

7. The operative site was injected with 05% [point five percent] Xylocaine and epinephrine.

   Rule _____

8. Her neurologic examination now, as in the past, has been completely normal and there has never been any evidence of cerebral injury as a result of the gunshot wound.

   Rule _____

9. According to Dr Kahn, the neurosurgeon, her neurologic examination is normal she has full rotation of her neck, with flexion and extension unlimited.

   Rule _____

10. Final clinical diagnosis Acute cervical sprain, resolved. Condition on discharge Improved.

   Rule _____

Answers are given in Appendix A, p. 434.

THE HYPHEN

RULE 3.27 Use a hyphen when two or more words have the force of a single modifier before a noun. These are *called compound adjectives* and the *set* together modifies the noun.

EXAMPLES

figure-of-eight sutures

seizure-inducing drug

end-to-end anastomosis

self-inflicted knife wound

well-known speaker

ill-defined tumor mass

large-for-dates fetus

non-English-speaking patient

new-car salesman

non-ski-related injury

end-of-dose deterioration

acid-base balance

C-reactive protein

AIDS-related complex

barrel-shaped thorax

behind-the-ear hearing aid

fat-soluble vitamins

The resident consulted the alcoholism counselors on his two *MAST-positive* patients.

That was an *ill-advised* remark written in the medical record.

(See also Rule 3.28.)

🔧 **MT TOOL BOX TIP:** Watch out for hyphenated words that have become a single word.

NOTE: Omit the hyphen when the compound follows the noun.

EXAMPLES

The patient is a *well-developed, well-nourished* black male.

HOWEVER: The patient is well developed.

This is a very *up-to-date* reference for drug names.

HOWEVER: This reference is up to date.

This *19-year-old* Mayview College student was injured in the accident.

HOWEVER: This Mayview College student is 19 years old.

During her pregnancy, she experienced a *45-pound* weight gain.

HOWEVER: She gained 45 pounds during her pregnancy.

NOTE: An adverb ending in "-ly" is not hyphenated before the adjective and noun.

EXAMPLES

She is a *moderately obese* waitress.

That was a *poorly dictated* report.

He is an *exceptionally gifted* diagnostician.

NOTE: *Common* compound expressions, as well as essential parts of disease descriptions, are not hyphenated. We quickly understand these words as a unit without the help of a hyphen.

EXAMPLES

word processing software

income tax refund

low cervical incision

normal sinus rhythm

pelvic inflammatory disease

congestive heart failure

right upper quadrant

chronic obstructive pulmonary disease

central nervous system

intensive care unit

Social Security check

civil rights issue

special delivery letter

deep tendon reflexes

ad hoc committee

in vitro testing

amino acid residue

rapid frozen section

atrial septal defect

low back pain

NOTE: The expression *status post* is not hyphenated.

Status post automobile accident

Status post hysterectomy

NOTE: Some compounds are permanent

EXAMPLES

on-site

long-term

state-of-the-art

RULE 3.28 Use a hyphen between conflicting terms of equal weight that occur both before or after the verb.

EXAMPLES

The waiting room was painted a sort of *yellow-orange.*

The results were *false-positive.*

The *false-positive* result

The lesions were *blue-black.*

Blue-black lesions

The patient's expression was *happy-sad.*

Her *happy-sad* expression

RULE 3.29 Use a suspending hyphen in a series of compound modifiers.

EXAMPLES

There were *small-* and large-sized cysts scattered throughout the parenchyma.

He has a *2-* or 3-month convalescence ahead of him.

A *1-* to 2-inch longitudinal incision will be made just above the umbilicus.

RULE 3.30 Use a hyphen when numbers are compounded with words and they have the force of a single modifier.

EXAMPLES

He is a *56-year-old* janitor in no acute distress.

We work a *35-hour* week.

She is a *3-day 6-hour-old* surviving twin.

Admitted with a *5-day* fever.

Four-vessel angiography showed a narrowing of the left carotid artery.

However, you do not use the hyphen with metric abbreviations

A *2 mm* drill bit was selected for the craniotomy.

The patient was seen in the ER with 9 *day-old* abrasions. *(How did the MT know this was not "9-day-old" abrasions? The context of the rest of the report helped.)*

RULE 3.31 Hyphenate compound numbers 21 through 99 when they are written out.

EXAMPLES

Fifty-five medical transcriptionists attended the meeting last night.

Ninety-nine percent of the time, I am confident of the diagnosis.

RULE 3.32 Use a hyphen when there is a prefix before a proper noun.

EXAMPLES

trans-Golgi reticulum

anti-American

pseudo-Christian

The estimated date of confinement is *mid-May.*

RULE 3.33 Use a hyphen after the prefixes *ex, self,* and *vice* and after other prefixes to avoid an awkward combination of letters, such as two or three identical vowels in a sequence.

EXAMPLES

ex-wife	self-medicating
ex-patriot	self-assured intern
self-inflicted	anti-immune
self-limited disease	ex-patient
self-retaining catheter	salpingo-oophorectomy
vice-president *(also written as two words: vice president)*	

BUT: coordinate   intraarterial

RULE 3.34 Use a hyphen after a prefix when the unhyphenated word would have a different meaning.

EXAMPLES

re-collect (collect again)

re-cover (cover again)

re-create (create again)

re-present (present again)

re-sign (sign again)

re-sort (sort again)

re-treat (treat again)

You should also hyphenate a word for ease of reading, comprehension, and pronunciation.

EXAMPLES

re-do

re-type

co-op

RULE 3.35   Do not use a hyphen with the prefixes *bi, tri, uni, co, extra, infra, inter, intra ,mid, mini, multi, pseudo, sub, super, supra, ultra, out, over, ante, anti, semi, un, non, pre, post, pro, trans,* and *re* unless there are identical letters in a sequence.

EXAMPLES

preoperative	antidepressant
antenatal	nondrinker
semiprone	intra-abdominal
semi-independent	midaxillary
postoperative	

BUT: non-Hodgkin (see Rule 3.32)
   transsacral
   microorganism
   posttraumatic

NOTE: Most words beginning with *pre* and *re* are not hyphenated even when identical letters are in a sequence.

preenroll	preexisting
preeclampsia	preelection
preemergent	preempt
preenzyme	preepiglottic
preeruptive	preextraction
reemploy	preevaluate
reenlist	reenact
reexamine	reenter

NOTE: Because hyphens are not generally used with prefixes, it is easiest to remember the few that are hyphenated: *ex, self,* and *vice,* along with the suffixes that take the hyphen: *odd, elect,* and *designate.*

EXAMPLES

ex-husband	president-elect
self-made	papal-designate
vice-chair	self-addressed envelope
twenty-odd	

When *mid* is used as an adjective meaning "the middle of," it may be written as a separate word.

EXAMPLES

We made an incision in the *mid finger*.

A *midfinger* incision was not possible in this case.

mid life

mid Atlantic

RULE 3.36   Use a hyphen with letters or words describing body chemicals, elements, or drugs except with subscripts or superscripts.

EXAMPLES

IL-1 (interleukin-1)

Glofil-125

5-AZA

M-protein

17-hydroxycorticosteroids

gallium-67 citrate (^{67}Ga)

uranium-235

BUT: ^{131}I ^{18}F

NOTE: If you are unable to use superscript, these must be transcribed on line as follows:
I 131 and F 18

RULE 3.37   Use a hyphen to take the place of the words *to* and *through* to identify numeric and alphabetical ranges unless the range is accompanied by a symbol.

EXAMPLES

Rounds were made in Wards *1-4*.

Check *V2 through V6* again.

Take 100 mg Tylenol *1-2* at bedtime.

NOTE: Avoid using the hyphen to describe blood type.

EXAMPLE

O-negative blood was in short supply. (Rather than *O-blood was in short supply.*)

Her blood type is AB negative. (Rather than *Her blood type is AB-*).

RULE 3.38   Use a hyphen after a single letter joined to a word that together form a coined word.

EXAMPLES

V-shaped	V-Y flap	x-ray	S-shape
Z-plasty	T-cell	T-shirt	U-bag
K-wires	T4 cell	T-8 suppressor	

BUT: 3M   T square

RULE 3.39 Place a hyphen between compound nouns and compound surnames.

EXAMPLES

Nonne-Milroy disease

Arnold-Chiari type II malformation

Legg-Calvé-Perthes disease

A *Davis-Crowe* mouth gag was used.

Mary *Smyth-Reynolds* was in today for her yearly Pap smear.

Antonia is the *secretary-treasurer* for our local chapter of the AHDI.

Refer to Chapter 8 for further discussion on use of the hyphen.

THE DASH

A dash is made on the keyboard with two hyphens. You may use your symbols menu and insert an em dash, which is about twice as long as the keyboard hyphen. Before you use the menu to insert a dash, be sure that your equipment is able to print the symbol. There is no space before, between, or after the two hyphens or the em dash. This chapter uses double hyphens in the examples. The dash indicates a sudden shift in thought and should be used very sparingly.

RULE 3.40 Use a dash as a forceful break for emphasis, for an abrupt change of thought, or to call attention to explanations not closely connected with the remainder of the sentence.

EXAMPLES

I want you *to--no,* I insist that *you--consult* a surgeon about the lump in your breast.

We may be so busy analyzing physical signs that we *miss--or dismiss--clues to* frame of mind.

For this patient, a polyp meant a fatal *malignancy--and* all the awful experiences that attend it.

I do the *transcription--you* do the editing.

RULE 3.41 Use a dash for summary.

NOTE: A dash is sometimes used instead of a colon. This practice works well if a list is in the middle of a sentence, because the second dash shows clearly where the list ends. Dashes are also helpful with appositives that are already punctuated with commas.

EXAMPLES

Red, white, and *blue--these* are my favorite colors.

She soon became bored with the nontranscription details of her job--*editing, printing, collating*--but finally realized they were part of the duties of the position.

NOTE: Never begin a new line with a dash. You must continue the last word before the dash to the following line along with the dash. Use the nonbreaking hyphen (in Microsoft Word, press Option + Hyphen or press Ctrl + Shift + Hyphen).

THE APOSTROPHE

RULE 3.42 Use an apostrophe to show singular or plural possession of nouns, pronouns, abbreviations, and eponyms.

▶ Singular nouns that do not end in *s*: add apostrophe *s ('s).*

EXAMPLES

the *transcriptionist's* responsibility

Bob's doctor

my fitness *coach's* exercise list

Dr *Farnsworth's* office

New *Year's* Eve

Father's Day

▶ Singular nouns of more than one syllable that end in *s* or an *s* sound: add an apostrophe after the *s (s')* if the addition of another *s* after the apostrophe would make it awkward or difficult to pronounce.

EXAMPLES

the *waitress'* table

Mr *Moses'* surgery

Los *Angeles'* traffic

Dr *Griffiths'* monograph

In reference to Dr Walters:

Dr *Walters'* point of view (*Not Dr* Walter's *point of view)*

▶ Singular nouns that end in an *s* sound or a *z* sound: add an apostrophe *s ('s).*

EXAMPLES

for *appearance's* sake

James *Rose's* appointment

▶ Singular one-syllable nouns that end in *s*: add an apostrophe *s ('s)* after the *s.*

EXAMPLES

Mr *Jones's* radiology report

Francine *Dees's* vacation

Marijane *Noonan-Moss's* employee badge

▶ Singular nouns that end in a silent *s*: add an apostrophe *s ('s)* after the *s.*

EXAMPLES

Arkansas's beauty

Jacques's appointment to the staff

▶ Plural nouns that end in *s* or an *s* sound: add an apostrophe at the end of the noun.

EXAMPLES

the *farmers'* crops (more than one farmer)

the *Joneses'* medical records (more than one member in the Jones family)

the *attorneys'* fees

proofreaders' marks

workers' compensation

HINT: With surnames, first make the name plural and then form the possessive.

Singular	Plural	Plural possessive
Otis	Otises	Otises'
Woods	Woodses	Woodses'
Gomez	Gomezes	Gomezes'
Rabinowitz	Rabinowitzes	Rabinowitzes'

Mr Sanchez's medical records (singular)

The Sanchezes' medical records (plural)

▸ Names in joint possession: add the possessive to the final name.

EXAMPLES

The Holloways and *Bryans's* summer cabin *(They own it together.)*

Those are my *brothers-in-law's* books.

Dr Pate and Dr *Frank's* office *(one office)*

Knight, Peachtree, and *Hoffman's* law office

John and *Sheila's* children

Mike, Ralph, and *Paul's* graduating class

▸ Names in separate possession: add the possessive to the name of each.

EXAMPLES

The *Shaw's* and *Tracy's* homes were on the tour.

We needed the *Keene's* and *Albright's* signatures.

Dr *Pate's* and Dr *Frank's* offices *(Two offices)*

Both *Pat's* and *Claire's* gardens are beautiful.

▸ Hyphenated and compound nouns and pronouns: add an apostrophe *s ('s)* on the final word.

EXAMPLES

my *brother-in-law's* book

my *brothers-in-law's* book (One book, two or more owners)

Mrs *Campbell-Munroe's* operative report

someone *else's* parking space

everyone *else's* opinion

▸ Double possessive: add the apostrophe *s ('s)* to each noun that should be possessive.

EXAMPLE

Dr *Thornton's associate's* diagnosis is the admitting diagnosis.

▸ Irregular plural nouns (that do not end in *s*): add apostrophe *s ('s)*.

Singular	Plural	Plural possessive
child	children	children's
man	men	men's
woman	women	women's
alumnus	alumni	alumni's

▸ Understood noun: use an appropriate possessive just before the understood word.

EXAMPLES

The stethoscope is *Dr Greenley's.* (Meaning *Dr Greenley's stethoscope*)

I consulted *Dorland's.* (Meaning *Dorland's dictionary*)

▸ Nonpersonal pronouns: add an apostrophe *s ('s)*.

EXAMPLES

nobody's fault

anyone's guess

somebody *else's* responsibility

▸ Personal pronouns *(its, hers, yours, his, theirs, whose, ours)* do not require an apostrophe.

EXAMPLES

The next appointment is *hers.*

The day shift is now officially *ours.*

I cannot tell if that is *his* or *hers.*

We never seem to be sure if *its* surface is smooth enough.

The dog injured *its* foot.

That dictionary is *yours.*

Notice this: That *Dorland's* is *yours.* (*The word* dictionary *is understood.*)

NOTE: Be very careful about *who's* (a contraction for *who is*); do not confuse it with *whose.*

Be careful about *it's* (a contraction for *it is*); do not confuse it with *its.*

EXAMPLE

The dog injured *it's* foot. (Incorrect)

This mistake is a very common one and very easily avoided. When using *it's,* speak the contraction out, *it is,* and see whether the sentence makes sense: "The dog injured *it is* foot."

 MT TOOL BOX TIP: Own *its* and *it's*—really own it.

▸ Abbreviations: add apostrophe *s ('s)*.

EXAMPLES

Proofreading is the *CMT's* responsibility.

We found the *EMT's* missing gurney.

It was our *HMO's* decision.

▶ Eponyms

Many eponyms (adjectives derived from a proper noun) are used in medical writing. Most of these are no longer written in the possessive case. However, some dictators prefer the older style and wish to have the possessive expressed. It would be nice (not to mention easier) if everyone would agree. You will often find both styles in reference books. When eponyms are used to describe parts of the anatomy, diseases, signs, or syndromes, they *may* be possessive. However, for names of places, patients, or surgical instruments, the possessive is not used, nor is it used in a compound eponym. This practice is often confusing—how do you recognize the name of a place or patient in contrast to that of a researcher or physician? In addition, if the eponym is preceded by the article *an, a,* or *the,* you can eliminate the possessive. In the meantime, follow the guidelines as best you can and consult your reference books. If you hear the possessive dictated, use it (and use it correctly). If it is not dictated, do not use it. Eventually the use of these particular possessive eponyms will most likely be eliminated.

EXAMPLES: *Where possessive is acceptable when dictated*

Signs and tests

Romberg's sign	or	Romberg sign
Hoffmann's reflex	or	Hoffmann reflex
Babinski's sign	or	Babinski sign
Ayer's test	or	Ayer test

Diseases and syndromes

Fallot's tetralogy	or	Fallot tetralogy
Tietze's syndrome	or	Tietze syndrome
Hirschsprung's disease	or	Hirschsprung disease

Anatomy

Bartholin's glands	or	Bartholin glands
Beale's ganglion	or	Beale ganglion
Mauthner's membrane	or	Mauthner membrane

Exceptions (always use the possessive)
Ringer's lactate
Taber's Cyclopedic Medical Dictionary

EXAMPLES: *No possessive used*

Use of the article
A Pfannenstiel incision   *The* Babinski sign

EXAMPLES: *Possessive never used*

Surgical instruments

Mayo scissors	Richard retractors
Foley catheter	Liston-Stille forceps

Names of places or patients
Christmas factor
Lyme disease
Chicago disease

Compounds
Stein-Leventhal syndrome
Adams-Stokes disease
Leser-Trélat sign
Bass-Watkins test
Gruber-Widal reaction

But this is not a compound
Blackberg and Wanger's test or
Blackberg and Wanger test

NOTE: Be careful to check the correct spelling of the name. Is it Water's view or Waters' view? (The second spelling is correct: Waters' view.)

NOTE: Do use the possessive when the possessive closes the sentence.

EXAMPLE

The infant shows early signs of Reye's. *("Reye's syndrome" is understood)*

RULE 3.43 Use an apostrophe in contractions of words or figures.

EXAMPLES

'94	won't	can't
she'll	o'clock	doesn't
couldn't	wouldn't	I'll

NOTE: *Avoid* the use of contractions of words or figures except for *o'clock* in formal medical documents and formal business letters. Contractions are acceptable in direct quotes. See examples in Rule 3.46.

EXAMPLES

You hear	You type
ought four	2004
won't	will not
she'll	she will
doesn't	does not
I'll	I will
nine o'clock	9 o'clock

RULE 3.44 Use an apostrophe in possessive expressions of time, distance, and value. Remember that nouns, not adjectives, can be possessive.

EXAMPLES

He should be able to return to work in a *month's* time.

You should have full range of motion in your elbow in 2 *months'* time. *(Notice the position of the apostrophe with this plural noun)*

The bullet came within a *hair's* breadth of the thoracic aorta.

I want the patient to feel that she got her *money's* worth. *(Notice that it is not "monies' worth.")*

Be careful to place your apostrophe appropriately for singular or plural possession.

EXAMPLES

He should be able to return to work in 3 *weeks'* time. *(Plural: use s apostrophe [s'])*

He should be able to return to work in 1 *month's* time. *(Singular: use apostrophe s ['s])*

NOTE: Sometimes it is confusing to decide whether certain word sets are possessive or not. Use the suggestion in the examples to determine whether you have chosen the possessive correctly.

After 6 *months'* convalescence, the patient was able to return to her usual and customary work. *(Correct)*

However, notice that there is no apostrophe in the following examples:

EXAMPLES

She is nearly *6 months* pregnant. *(Not 6 months' pregnant because she cannot be 6 months of pregnant)*

I believe that he is *2 hours* late. *(Not 2 hours' late because he cannot be 2 hours of late)*

RULE 3.45 Use an apostrophe to form the plural of the capital letters *A, I, O, M,* and *U* when used alone; the plural of all lowercase letters; and after a lowercase letter in an abbreviation.

NOTE: The reason for this rule is to avoid making what might appear to be a word with the combination of some letters and *s,* such as *Is, Ms, Us, is,* and *as.* It is not necessary to use the apostrophe to form the plural of numbers or capital letter abbreviations.

EXAMPLES

When you make an entry in a chart, be careful that your *2s* don't look like *z's.*

You used four *I's* in that first paragraph.

He has a note for three *Rx's* on his desk.

The *TMs* were intact.

QUOTATION MARKS

RULE 3.46 Use quotation marks to enclose the exact words of a speaker.

EXAMPLE

The patient said, *"There has been hurting in the pelvic bones."*

BUT: The patient says there has been some pain in the pelvic bones.

Be careful to enclose only direct quotations.

The patient said, *"she's always been told that her mother died of cancer." (Incorrect)*

The patient said, *"I've always been told that my mother died of cancer." (Correct)*

The patient said she has always been told that her mother died of cancer (Correct)

RULE 3.47 The titles of minor literary or artistic works are placed within quotation marks.

EXAMPLE

His photographic entry *"The Country Doctor"* won first place in the contest.

NOTE: Underline or use italics for the titles of published books, magazines, articles, and newspapers. Place in quotation marks the titles of chapters, papers, sections, and subdivisions of published work.

EXAMPLE

Your homework assignment is to read *"Causes of Disease"* in <u>*Diseases of the Human Body*</u>.

RULE 3.48 Use quotation marks to single out words or phrases for special attention.

EXAMPLES

I see no need for *"temper tantrums"* in the operating suite.

"Accommodate" is at the top of the list of *"most frequently misspelled words."*

The technical term for Lou Gehrig disease is *"amyotrophic lateral sclerosis."*

NOTE: If the expression *so-called* precedes the term in question, quotation marks are not needed.

EXAMPLE

These *so-called* seizure states occur once or twice a week. *(No quotation marks around seizure states)*

🔧 **MT TOOL BOX TIP:** *Accommodate* tops the list of misspelled words.

RULE 3.49 Use quotation marks to set off slang, coined, awkward, whimsical, or humorous words that might indicate ignorance on the part of the author if it is not known that the writer is aware of them.

EXAMPLE

See whether you can schedule a few *"well"* patients for a change.

NOTE: Punctuation with quotation marks in American English is as follows: periods and commas go *inside* the quotation mark; semicolons and colons go *outside* the quotation mark. Question marks and exclamation marks belong *inside* the quotation marks when they are part of the quoted material; they are placed *outside* the final quotation marks when they are part of the entire sentence.

EXAMPLES

The third chapter, *"Punctuation,"* is the most difficult for me. *(Notice the placement of the comma here)*

The patient related that she spoke with her hands *"like an Italian."*

The medical report answers my original question, *"What is the secondary diagnosis?"*

Notice the placement of the period and question mark in these examples.

PARENTHESES

Parentheses, commas, and dashes are used to set off incidental or nonessential elements in text. Which you choose will be determined either by the dictator/writer of the material or by the closeness of the relationship between the material enclosed and the remainder of the sentence. In general, commas are used to set slightly apart material that is closely related, and parentheses are used when commas have already been used within the nonessential element or when the material itself is neither grammatically nor logically essential to the main thought. The dash is a more forceful and abrupt division and draws attention to a statement; parentheses deemphasize. Material enclosed within parentheses can range from a single punctuation mark, such as "(!)," to several sentences. Again, the voice of the dictator may assist you in choosing to use parentheses, because the voice normally drops when the dictator utters strongly nonessential material.

RULE 3.50 Use parentheses to set off words or phrases that are clearly nonessential to the sentence. These are often definitions, comments, or explanations.

EXAMPLES

She felt that she had inhaled some sort of ornamental dust *(gold, silver, bronze, and so forth.)* while working in her flower shop.

Suzanne *(my coworker)* and I usually attend the conferences together. *(Note: In this instance, the appositive needs to be enclosed in the parentheses rather than commas to make clear that two, not three, of us attend the conferences together.)*

The administrative medical assistant *(receptionist, secretary, bookkeeper, insurance clerk, file clerk)* requires the same length of training as does the clinical medical assistant.

Please fax *(930-555-7231)* the transcript to me immediately.

RULE 3.51 Use parentheses around figures or letters that indicate divisions in narrative copy when the items are "run in."

EXAMPLE

It is my impression that she has *(1)* progressive dysmenorrhea, *(2)* uterine leiomyoma, and *(3)* weakness of the right inguinal ring.

NOTE: You may elect to use a period after figures or letters that indicate divisions as long as they do not occur within a sentence.

EXAMPLE

1. Sterile field
2. Suture materials
3. 4 × 4 sponges

THE SLASH (ALSO CALLED THE BAR, VIRGULE, OR DIAGONAL)

RULE 3.52 Use the slash when writing certain technical terms. The slash sometimes substitutes for the words *per, to,* and *over.*

EXAMPLES

She has *20/20* vision. *(Indication of visual acuity)*

His blood pressure is *120/80. (120 over 80)*

The dosage is *50 mg/d. (Milligrams per day)*

RULE 3.53 Use the slash to offer word choice.

EXAMPLES

and/or

his/hers

plus/minus

Mr/Mrs/Miss/Ms

she/he

RULE 3.54 Use the slash to write fractions or to create a symbol.

EXAMPLES

2/3

c/o

1-1/2

SPACING WITH PUNCTUATION

RULE 3.55   NO SPACE

before a colon, semicolon, apostrophe, period, comma, question mark, exclamation point

between a number and the degree symbol

after a period within an abbreviation

after a period used as a decimal point

between quotation marks and the quoted material

before or after a hyphen

before or after a slash

before or after an em dash (two hyphens)

between parentheses and the enclosed material

between any word and the punctuation after it

between the number and the colon in a dilute solution

before or after a comma used within numbers

before or after an ampersand in abbreviations (e.g., L&W)

on either side of the colon in expressions of ratios

on either side of the colon in expressions of the time of day

after the closing parenthesis if another mark of punctuation follows

EXAMPLE

If Mrs Ross is promoted *(to lead transcriptionist),* she will leave this department.

RULE 3.56   ONE SPACE

after a comma

after a semicolon

after a period that follows an initial

after a colon (optional: you may use two)

after a period at the end of a sentence (optional: you may use two)

on each side of the ampersand (&) in a series of names after the closing parenthesis

on each side of the "×" symbol in an expression of dimension

EXAMPLE

a 2 × 2 sponge

 MT TOOL BOX TIP: Use only one space after a comma, a semicolon, and a period.

 MT TOOL BOX TIP: Put a space on each side of an "×" when it is used to describe dimensions.

EXAMPLE

Use 8-1/2 × 11-inch paper.

RULE 3.57   TWO SPACES

after a question mark or exclamation point at the end of a sentence (optional: you may use one)

after a quotation mark at the end of a sentence (optional: you may use one)

after a colon used with topic words in a memo (for example, *TO:, FROM:, DATE:*)

after a period when it follows a number in an enumeration

after a colon or a period at the end of a sentence (optional, you may use one)

Do not be intimidated because there are so many rules to remember. You are probably already comfortable with a great many of them, so some of this instruction is just a review for you. Take a little time to reexamine those rules that cause you problems.

3-12 SELF-STUDY

DIRECTIONS: Using Rules 3.27 through 3.54, add a hyphen, dash, apostrophe, quotation mark, parentheses, or slash where required.

1. Her favorite response is weve always done it this way.

2. It was an ill defined tumor mass.

3. The diagnosis is grim I feel helpless.

4. Her temperature peaked at 106.5 degrees we were relieved when this occurred, and the seizures subsided.

5. There were no 4 × 4s left in the box.

6. Because of his condition emphysema and age 88, he is a poor risk for anesthesia at this time.

7. Eighty five of the patients were seen first in the outpatient department.

8. The patient with the self inflicted gunshot wound had a poorly applied bandage.

9. The blood pressure ranged from one hundred twenty over eighty to one hundred forty over eighty.

10. This is a very up to date drug reference.

The answers are in Appendix A, p. 434.

3-13 SELF-STUDY

DIRECTIONS: In the following exercises, fill in the missing punctuation and indicate which of the rules you used. (Refer to the brief Rule Review.) In the blank after the sentence, write the letter of the rule or rules used. Each rule may be used more than once.

RULE REVIEW: Use a hyphen
  a. when two or more words have the force of a single modifier.
  b. when figures or letters are mixed with a word.
  c. between compound names or words.
  d. between coordinate expressions.

Use an apostrophe

  e. to show possession.
  f. to show letters are missing.
  g. to form the plurals of lowercase letters.

Use quotation marks

  h. to show slang or awkward wording.

Use parentheses

  i. to set off a strongly nonessential phrase.

Use a slash

  j. to divide certain technical terms.

EXAMPLE
"Accommodation" is spelled with two c's, two m's, and three o's. Rule ____g____

1. Mrs Gail R. Smith Edwards was hospitalized this morning. She is the 47 year old woman Dr Blank admitted with a self inflicted knife wound. Her blood pressure was 60 40 [sixty over forty].

   Rule _____

2. Barbara Ness happy go lucky personality was missed when she was transferred from the medical records department.

   Rule _____

3. Glen Mathews, the well known trial lawyer, and the hospitals surgeon in chief, Dr Carlton Edwards, will appear together if you can believe that on TVs latest talk show tonight. Its the only subject on the hospitals gabfest.

   Rule _____

4. I want a stamped, self addressed envelope enclosed with this letter and sent out with todays mail.

   Rule _____

5. Dr Davis said his promotion was a good example of my being kicked upstairs. He obviously didnt want to leave his position in the x ray department.

   Rule _____

6. Havent you ever seen a Z fixation? Bobbi Jo will be happy to explain it to you.

   Rule _____

7. Were all going to the CCU at 4 oclock for instructions on mouth to mouth resuscitation.

   Rule _____

8. Right eye vision: 20 20.
   Left eye vision: 10 400.
   Right retinal examination: Normal.
   Left retinal examination: Inferior retinal detachment.

   Rule _____

9. You were seen on September 24 at which time you were having some stiffness at the shoulders which I felt was due to a periarthritis a stiffness of the shoulder capsule; however, xray of the shoulder was negative.

   Rule _____

10. After he completed the end to end anastomosis, he closed with #1 silk through and through, figure of eight sutures.

    Rule _____

11. Dr Chriswells diagnosis bears out the assumption that the red green blindness is the result of an X chromosome defect.

    Rule _____

12. After his myocardial infarction MI, his blood test showed high levels of C reactive protein.

    Rule _____

The answers are in Appendix A, p. 434.

3-14 SELF-STUDY

DIRECTIONS: In the following exercises, the marks of punctuation are missing, but the number of marks that are needed has been provided for each exercise. This number includes any optional marks and the periods needed at the end of a sentence. Some periods are indicated for you with an asterisk (*). Parentheses and quotation marks count as two marks. You may use your text or reference materials as your instructor directs. The exercise is to be retyped and double-spaced for proper placement.

1. Dr Younger couldnt find the curved on flat scissors therefore all heck broke loose* (Needs 8 marks)

2. The patients admission time is 330 [three-thirty] pm* When he comes in please call me for a face to face confrontation with him about his visitors* (Needs 8 marks)

3. This 68 year old right handed Caucasian retired female telephone operator was well until mid February* While sitting in a chair after dinner she had the following symptoms paralysis of her left arm and left leg paresthesia in the same distribution bilateral visual blurring and some facial numbness* (Needs 14 marks)

4. The patient was admitted to the ward at one oclock in the morning screaming Alls fair in love and lust the attending physician sedated him with Thorazine six hundred milligrams per day*) (Needs 7 marks)

5. The following describes a well prepared business letter neat accurate well placed correctly punctuated and mechanically perfect* The dictator expects to see an attractive letter with no obvious corrections smudges or unevenly inked letters* It is an insult in my opinion to place a letter that appears other than described on your employers desk for signature* (Needs 15 marks)

Answers are in Appendix A, p. 435.

3-15 REVIEW TEST

DIRECTIONS: Follow the directions provided in Self-Study 3-14. Use a double space on your computer between the following exercises.

1. She inadvertently sterilized the Smith Petersen nail instead of the V medullary* (Needs 3 marks)

2. She has had no further spells but she did have 2 episodes prior to this one several years ago* (Needs 4 marks)

3. The patient presents as a well developed asthenic elderly extremely bright and oriented Asian woman* She is fully alert and able to give an entirely reliable history however she is somewhat anxious and concerned over her present condition* (Needs 5 marks)

4. The patient has just moved to this community from Anchorage Alaska where he was engaged in the lumber industry* He had an emergency appendectomy performed at some remote outpost in January 1996* According to the patient he has always felt like somethings hung up in there* Roentgenograms taken July 17 200X failed to reveal anything unusual* (Needs 13 marks)

5. He is a 35 year old well developed well nourished Native American truck driver oriented to time place and person* (Needs 8 marks)

6. The X chromosome defect resulted in her ovarian aplasia undeveloped mandible webbed neck and small stature Morgagni Turner syndrome* (Needs 7 marks)

7. Vital signs Blood pressure 194 97 pulse 127 respirations 32 regular and gasping* General Healthy appearing male looking his stated age in moderately severe respiratory distress with slightly dusky colored lips* (Needs 12 marks)

8. His heart is in regular sinus rhythm without murmurs or thrills the distal pulses are all palpable and Phalens maneuver is negative* (Needs 4 marks)

9. I want to raise the charge for office calls to $125 this is long overdue and hospital calls to $180* Please explain this to all the patients including the new ones when they call for an appointment* (Needs 6 marks)

10. I took the samples of the powder to Dr Peterson White pathologist and he has not as yet made any report* As you can see from the initial report there is no evidence of powder in the biopsy specimen* (Needs 8 marks)

11. Really the prognosis is not too good but well hope that maybe shell defy the usual course of events* (Needs 5 marks)

12. I will restate the situation Mr Goodman has a right superior mediastinal widening that has proven to be secondary to some dilatation and lateral displacement of the superior vena cava* (Needs 2 marks)

13. It is anticipated that after completion of this radiation therapy and your recovery from it in a period of 4 to 6 weeks you should be able to return to your former employment without difficulty* (Needs 3 marks)

14. Dr Lopez advice was to transfer the patient* Please see that his x rays are sent with him to the Veterans Affairs Medical Center* (Needs 4 marks)

15. She is a spastic developmentally delayed child with bilateral hip bowing greater on the right than on the left whose mother is very very anxious for noninvasive correction* (Needs 5 marks)

16. Notice please There will be no further parking allowed in the staff lot without an up to date sticker vehicles in violation will be towed away at the owners expense* (Needs 6 marks)

17. According to the pathology report see enclosed there is no evidence of Mr Neibauer my patient having active pulmonary tuberculosis at this time* The debate concerning the approval of his attending the Contagious Disease Conference became heated we had to recess several times once for 40 minutes and we finally adjourned with no definite policy established* Ann Reynolds my administrative assistant will get in touch with Mr Neibauer to let him know* (Needs 14 marks)

DIRECTIONS: In the following questions, select only one, best answer and write the letter describing it in the blank.

18. Which of the following sentences contains a punctuation error? _____
    a. Joan is the "smilingest" nurse on the ward.
    b. He has a positive Kehr sign.
    c. I ordered a #7 Jackson bronchoscope.
    d. The infant suffered compression of the umbilical cord, which resulted in it's death.

19. Which of the following contains a punctuation error? _____
    a. Diagnosis: Fracture, right distal radius.
    b. Please send both of the Smithes' records to Dr Berry.
    c. I want to see this patient back in three week's time.
    d. It's a well-known fact that she's a respected physician.

20. Which of the following sentences is correct? _____
    a. This is my sister's-in-law's medical record.
    b. Those were Dr Brown's and Dr Brooks' diagnoses.
    c. This is Dan's and Mary's new transcription reference.
    d. This is the transcriptionists's test.

 3-16 REVIEW TEST

DIRECTIONS: Using your text and reference materials, punctuate the letter on page 99. Use mixed punctuation for the salutation and complimentary close. The letter is to be retyped, but you may proofread it by marking your text before you copy the letter.

William A. Berry, MD
3933 Navajo Road
GrandView, XX 87453
Telephone: 212.555.0124

August 13 20XX

John D. Mench MD
Applegate Suite 765
455 Main Street
Bethesda MD 20034

Dear Dr Mench

Re Debra Walters

This letter is to bring you up to date on Mrs Walters who was first seen in my office on March 2 20XX at which time she stated that her last menstrual period had started August 29 20XX. Examination revealed the uterus to be enlarged to a size consistent with an estimated date of confinement of June 5 20XX.

The pregnancy continued uneventfully until May 19 at which time the patients blood pressure was 130 90. Hygroton was prescribed and the patient was seen in one week. Her blood pressure at the next visit was 150 100 and additional therapy in the form of Lozol was prescribed in addition to other antitoxemic routines. Her blood pressure stabilized between 130 90 and 140 90.

The patient was admitted to the hospital on June 11 20XX with ruptured membranes mild preeclampsia and a few contractions of poor quality. Intravenous oxytocics were started and after 2 hours of stimulation there was no change in the cervix with that structure continuing to be long closed and posterior. The presenting part was at a -2 to a -3 station and the amniotic fluid had become brownish-green in color suggesting some degree of fetal distress.

Consultation was obtained and it was recommended that a low cervical cesarean section be performed. A female infant was delivered by cesarean section. It was noted at the time of delivery that the cord was snugly wrapped around the neck of the baby 3 times and this might have contributed to the evidence of fetal distress as evidenced by the color of the amniotic fluid.

The patients postoperative course was uneventful and she and the baby were discharged home on the fifth postpartum day.

Sincerely yours

William A Berry MD

mlo

Let's Have a Bit of Fun

1. In which sentence is Miss Hamlyn in trouble?
   a. Miss Hamlyn, the medical assistant failed to report for work.
   b. Miss Hamlyn, the medical assistant, failed to report for work.

2. Which shows a breach of ethics?
   a. Five nurses knew the diagnosis, all told.
   b. Five nurses knew the diagnosis; all told.

3. Which shows compassion?
   a. I left him, feeling he'd rather be alone.
   b. I left him feeling he'd rather be alone.

4. Which is harder for the interns?
   a. Down the hall came four interns carrying equipment and several doctors with their patients.
   b. Down the hall came four interns, carrying equipment, and several doctors with their patients.

5. Which is unflattering to the hostess?
   a. The party ended, happily.
   b. The party ended happily.

6. In which does the writer know about the private lives of her fellow workers?
   a. Every secretary, I know, has a secret ambition.
   b. Every secretary I know has a secret ambition.

7. Where would you prefer to work?
   a. The hospital employs a hundred odd men and women.
   b. The hospital employs a hundred-odd men and women.

8. Who is late?
   a. The receptionist said the nurse is late.
   b. The receptionist, said the nurse, is late.

9. Which is the worse problem?
   a. All my money, which was in my billfold, was stolen.
   b. All my money which was in my billfold was stolen.

10. Who filled up the emergency ward?
    a. All of the students who ate in the snack bar got food poisoning.
    b. All of the students, who ate in the snack bar, got food poisoning.

11. Who is the best leader?
    a. I intend to serve you fairly energetically and enthusiastically.
    b. I intend to serve you fairly, energetically, and enthusiastically.

The answers are given in Appendix A, p. 435.

PUNCTUATION RULE SYNOPSIS

PUNCTUATION	RULE	PAGE
Use a Comma or Pair of Commas		
To set off a nonessential word or words from the rest of the sentence	3.1a	69
To set off nonessential appositives	3.1b	70
To set off a parenthetical expression	3.1c	70
To set off an introductory phrase or clause (See also Rule 3.2b)	3.2a	73
To set off the year in a complete date	3.3	74
To set off the name of the state when the city precedes it	3.4	74
To set off *Inc.* or *Ltd.* in a company name	3.5	74
To set off titles and degrees after a person's name	3.6	74
To separate elements of words in a series	3.7	75
To separate two independent clauses	3.8	75
To set off the name of a person in a direct address	3.9	78
To separate certain modifiers	3.10	78
To avoid confusion	3.11	78
After the complimentary close	3.12	78
In certain long numbers	3.13	79
To separate the parts of a date in the date line of a letter	3.14	79
Use a Period		
At the end of a sentence	3.15	81
With single capitalized word abbreviations	3.16	82
When the genus is abbreviated	3.16	82
In certain lowercase Latin abbreviations	3.16	82
To separate a decimal fraction from whole numbers	3.17	82
Use a Semicolon		
Between two independent clauses when there is no conjunction	3.18	82
Between independent clauses if either or both are already punctuated	3.19	82
Before a parenthetical expression when it is used as a conjunction	3.20	83
Between a series of phrases or clauses when any item in the series has internal commas	3.21	83

PUNCTUATION	RULE	PAGE
Use a Colon		
To introduce a list or series of items	3.22	83
After the salutation in a business letter when "mixed" punctuation is used	3.23	83
Between the hours and minutes indicating the time	3.24	83
In ratios and dilutions	3.24	83
After the introductory word or words in a history and physical examination report	3.25	84
With the introductory words in an outline	3.25	84
To introduce an example or clarify an idea	3.26	84
Use a Hyphen		
When two or more words have the force of a single modifier	3.27	86
Between conflicting terms	3.28	87
In a series of modifiers	3.29	87
When numbers are compounded with words	3.30	87
Within compound numbers 21 to 99 when they are written out	3.31	87
Between a prefix and a proper noun	3.32	87
After prefixes *ex, self,* and *vice;* to avoid awkward combinations of letters	3.33	87
After a prefix when the unhyphenated word would have a different meaning (Exceptions, see Rule 3.35)	3.34	87
In certain chemical expressions	3.35	88
To take the place of the words *to* and *through*	3.36	88
	3.37	88
After a single letter joined to a word that together form a coined term	3.38	88
Between compound nouns and compound surnames	3.39	89
Use a Dash		
For a forceful break	3.40	89
For summary	3.41	89
Use an Apostrophe		
To show singular or plural possession	3.42	89
In contractions	3.43	91
In possessive expressions of time, distance, and value	3.44	91
To form the plural of some letters	3.45	92

PUNCTUATION	RULE	PAGE
Use Quotation Marks		
To enclose the exact words of a speaker	3.46	92
To enclose the titles of minor literary and artistic works	3.47	92
To single out words or phrases	3.48	92
To set off slang, coined, awkward, or whimsical words	3.49	92
Use Parentheses		
To set off clearly nonessential words or phrases	3.50	93

PUNCTUATION	RULE	PAGE
Around figures or letters that indicate divisions in narrative copy	3.51	93
Use a Slash		
In certain technical terms	3.52	93
To offer a word choice	3.53	93
To write fractions	3.54	93
Spacing with Punctuation Marks		
No space	3.55	94
One space	3.56	94
Two spaces	3.57	94

3

CHAPTER

CHAPTER 4

Capitalization

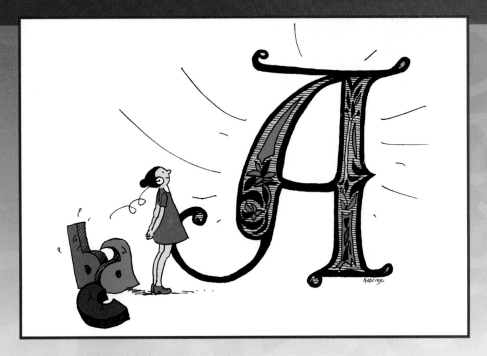

OBJECTIVES

After reading this chapter and completing the exercises, you should be able to

1. Demonstrate the ability to capitalize words accurately from copy prepared in lowercase letters.

2. Recognize when capital letters are required in ordinary business writing and in specific medical words and abbreviations.

3. Explain the special uses of capital letters in the preparation of medical reports and correspondence.

4. Use reference materials to check unfamiliar medical and business terms.

INTRODUCTION

This review of capitalization rules should be a pleasant interlude after your study of punctuation. Only a few capitalization rules may cause problems for transcriptionists, so this chapter reviews those and emphasizes where they most commonly occur in medical and business transcription.

The purpose of capitalizing a word is to give it emphasis, distinction, authority, or importance. Avoid unnecessary capitalization, and do not use all capital letters to highlight something unnecessarily, such as a person's name on a document. Words composed completely of capital letters often are more difficult to read because there is not as much "white space" around them.

EXAMPLE

Hazel Tank, CMT (Correct)

HAZEL TANK, CMT (Avoid)

Like rules regarding punctuation, rules regarding capitalization can differ. The current trend is toward less, rather than more capitalization. Consequently, as with a punctuation mark, be sure you have a reason for using a capital letter, and when in doubt, check your references.

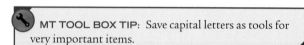 **MT TOOL BOX TIP:** Save capital letters as tools for very important items.

VOCABULARY

Capital Letter: Uppercase letter, also called "cap."

Small Letter: Lowercase letter, noncapital letter.

Eponym: An adjective derived from a proper noun.

EXAMPLES

Mayo scissors

Noone-Milroy disease

Amsler chart

Acronym: A word formed from the initial letters of other words.

EXAMPLES

NOW (National Organization for Women)

HOPE (Health Opportunities for People Everywhere)

WHO (World Health Organization)

CAD (coronary artery disease)

ECMO (extracorporeal membrane oxygenation)

AIDS (acquired immunodeficiency syndrome)

SOAP (subjective, objective, assessment, plan)

Lowercase letters are used when an acronym is commonly used in the language.

EXAMPLES

laser   radar   scuba

Proper Noun: The name of a specific person, place, or thing.

Some *common nouns* may be used to name a specific person, place, or thing but are often modified by *my, your, his, our, their, these, the, this, that,* or *those.*

EXAMPLE: *Common nouns*

my mother   the doctor   your patient   our president

NOTE: These refer to specific persons, yet they are not proper nouns.

EXAMPLES: *Proper nouns*

Secretary of State Lewis

Dr Smith

Mary Tunnell

President Lincoln

the Brooklyn Bridge

Aunt Margaret

RULES

The following five rules pertain to typing business letters.

RULE 4.1 Capitalize the first word of the salutation and the complimentary close.

EXAMPLES

Dear Sir or Madam:

Dear Dr Reynolds:

Sincerely yours,

Yours very truly,

RULE 4.2 Capitalize *boulevard, street, avenue, drive, way,* and so on, when used with a proper noun.

EXAMPLES

321 Westvillage *Drive*

One of the most attractive *streets* in Cuyamaca Woods is Grand View *Road.*

RULE 4.3 Capitalize a person's title in business correspondence when it appears in the inside address, typed signature line, or envelope address.

EXAMPLES

Ms Marilyn Alan, *President*

W. Peter Deal, MD, *Director*

ATTENTION: Ralph Cavanaugh, *Buyer*

Gene Ham, *Instructor*

RULE 4.4 Capitalize the first letter or all of the letters in the word *Attention* when it is part of an address; capitalize the first letter of each word or all the letters in *To Whom It May Concern*.

EXAMPLES

ATTENTION: Reservation Clerk

or

Attention: Paul Glenn, MD, Dean

TO WHOM IT MAY CONCERN:

or

To Whom It May Concern:

RULE 4.5 Capitalize both letters of the state abbreviation in the inside address and the envelope address. Follow the abbreviation with the ZIP code.

EXAMPLES

District Heights, *MD* 20028

San Diego, *CA* 92119

Appendix B contains a complete list of U.S. Postal Service abbreviations for state names. You should either remove this from your book and place it in your reference notebook or photocopy it for your reference book.

The next eight rules are often used in transcribing medical letters and reports.

RULE 4.6 Capitalize professional titles, political titles, family titles, and military ranks when they immediately *precede* the name.

EXAMPLES: *Military and professional titles*

Capt. Max Draper, USN Medical Corps, will be the guest speaker at the annual meeting of the AMA. *Dr* Smith, the president, plans to meet his plane. The *doctor* will leave for the airport at 4 o'clock. We will meet with *President* Austin at the university this evening. *Dean* Caldwell may not be able to join us, however.

EXAMPLES: *Professional and political titles*

Dr Randolph, the *president* of the medical society, was invited to speak at the joint meeting with the local bar association.

Rev. John Hughes will give the invocation.

Maxine Wong has just been approved as the new *quality assurance manager*.

Do *not* capitalize the names of medical or surgical specialties or the type of specialist.

NOTE: Only titles of high distinction are capitalized *after* a person's name except in the address and typed signature line. "High distinction" can be very subjective, depending on who is doing the writing. High distinction often refers to the persons of rank in one's own firm and to high government officials.

EXAMPLES

The internist referred him to a *thoracic surgeon*.

He is studying to be an *emergency room specialist*.

We asked for a second opinion from the *cardiologist*.

EXAMPLE

Parkland Community College

3261 Parkview Drive

Boise, ID 83702

ATTENTION: Ms P. Lombardo, *Administrator*

EXAMPLES: *Family titles*

My *father* is bringing *Aunt* Mary here this afternoon for her flu shot.

The patient's *mother* died of carcinoma of the breast at age 56, and his *father* is living and well.

EXCEPTION: A title is not capitalized when used with an appositive.

EXAMPLE

My *uncle*, William Paulls, moved here recently from Cleveland.

RULE 4.7 Capitalize names, proper nouns, well-known nicknames for proper nouns, and eponyms.

MT TOOL BOX TIP: Eponyms are always capitalized.

EXAMPLES: *Proper names*

Pieter von der Mehden

Be careful with the spelling, spacing, hyphenation, punctuation, and capitalization of people's names. If there is *any* doubt, check with someone who can verify

---

the correct form.* Be alert for particles such as *Mc, Mac, de, de la, del, van, von, y, von der, O',* and so on.

You already are aware of the various spellings that even common names can take, so watch out for the variety of ways that names are further expressed:

Mary Jane, Marijane, Mari Jayne, Mary-Jane, Merry Jane

Fitz Hugh, Fitzhugh, Fitz-Hugh

Sanjuan, San Juan

Santa Rosa, Santarosa

Mc Clain, McClain, Mac Lain, Mc Lean, Mac Lean

St. George, Saint George, San George

Alicia Morales y Gonzales

Frank de la Vera

Reina de Saint Luc

Ai-Mei Sung

Antony Smith-Haynes

Rosario Sanchez Martinez (Family name with no hyphen: *Sanchez Martinez*)

Get the sequence correct:

Robert Joyce or Joyce Robert

A further problem:

Robertson Jayne (The family name is *Jayne*)

Check for the proper version:

Jean/Gene Leslie/Lesley Adrienne/Adrian Laverne/Lavern/LaVern

EXAMPLES: *Proper nouns*

Dr Watson was a fictional hero in *Sherlock Holmes's* classics.

I couldn't remember whether he joined the *Air Force* or the *Navy*.

Do you realize that *Mother* will have to be placed in a nursing facility if she is unable to care for herself?

COMPARE WITH: Our *mother* will have to be placed in a nursing home.

EXAMPLES: *Proper nouns and well-known nicknames for proper nouns*

Josephine Holman just moved here from the *Rockies* and is looking for a job as a human resources specialist.

We learned that valley fever is endemic to *Imperial Valley, San Joaquin Valley,* and the *Sonoran* deserts.

She moved to the *Bay Area* after winning the *Nobel Prize*.

Ellen wanted to return to the *Deep South* after working in *California* for just a few years.

EXAMPLES: *Eponyms*

We need a #15 *Foley* catheter.

The diagnosis was *non-Hodgkin* lymphoma.

It is interesting that *Christmas* disease was named for a family with a particular type of hereditary condition.

The procedure was performed through a *McBurney* incision.

The patient was placed in the *Trendelenburg* position and prepped for surgery.

Some interesting names from mythology are used to describe parts of the anatomy, such as "*Achilles* tendon," or conditions, such as "*Oedipus* complex."

Newcomers to medicine often misspell *Burow* solution and think that the *Sippy* diet is one you sip!

NOTE: Words *derived* from eponyms are not capitalized, nor are those that have acquired independent common meaning. (When in doubt, check the dictionary.)

EXAMPLES: *Nouns derived from eponyms*

Parkinson disease but *parkinsonism*

Cushing syndrome but *cushingoid* facies

Gram stain but *gram-positive* results

Addison disease but *addisonian* crisis

EXAMPLES: *Common nouns and adjectives formed from proper nouns*

arabic number	klieg light
atlas	kocherize
braille symbol	koebnerization
brussels sprouts	manila folder
cesarean section	mendelian genetics
chinese blue	mullerian duct
curie unit	paris green
epsom salt	pasteurized milk
eustachian tube	petri dish
french fries	plaster of paris
freudian slip	politzerize
graafian follicle	portland cement
haversian system	roentgen unit
hippocratic clubbing	roman numeral
india ink	watt
joule	

EXCEPTION: Americanization

RULE 4.8 Capitalize the names of ethnic groups, religions, and languages.

EXAMPLE

He is a well-developed, well-nourished *Asian* businessman in no acute distress.

*Hint for name verification: Contact whoever has a social document sheet (name, address, phone number, place of employment, and so on) from the patient. This document could be with the referring physician, the primary care physician, clinic, nursing home, insurance company, workers' compensation carrier, emergency department, medical records, the unit where the patient is confined, and so on. See Appendix C on Evolve for a hospital admission document.

EXAMPLE

She is a *Catholic*, but they decided to be married in the *Jewish* temple.

EXAMPLE

We are taking an evening course in medical *Spanish* because we have many *Hispanic* patients who do not speak *English*.

NOTE: Designations based on skin color are not capitalized.

EXAMPLES

She is a well-developed, well-nourished *black* female student.

This 43-year-old *white* farm worker fell from the back of a truck at 3:55 a.m.

RULE 4.9 Capitalize the name of the genus when used in the singular form (with or without the species name), but do not capitalize the name of the species that follows it. When the genus name is used alone, it implies the genus as a whole.

EXAMPLES

The patient was admitted by the ophthalmologist with *Onchocerca volvulus* infection.

Ralph saw the doctor because he had a bad reaction to *Cannabis sativa*.

NOTE: The genus may be referred to by its first initial only; this is capitalized with a period and followed by the species name. You may eliminate the period after the genus name with site approval. This is becoming the acceptable format. The examples will show it both ways.

EXAMPLES

E. coli (Escherichia coli)

M. tuberculosis (Mycobacterium tuberculosis)

H influenzae (Haemophilus influenzae)

NOTE: Spell out, do not abbreviate, the genus the first time it is dictated in a report. Subsequent to that, it may be abbreviated. Use the abbreviated form when dictated.

🔧 MT TOOL BOX TIP: The genus is capitalized; the species is not.

▶ Remember not to capitalize the plural or adjectival form of a genus name.

EXAMPLES

Giardia lamblia but giardiasis

Diplococcus but diplococci and diplococcal

Streptococcus but streptococci and streptococcal

Infections caused by chlamydiae are increasing.

▶ Bacterial names applied to laboratory media are lowercase.

EXAMPLES

brucella agar

bacteroides bile

esculin agar

Refer to Appendix B for a list of some of the most frequently used genus and species names.

RULE 4.10 Capitalize trade names and brand names of drugs, other trademarked materials, and commercial products.

NOTE: It is often difficult for the beginning medical transcriptionist to recognize a brand name (capitalized) in contrast to a generic name (lowercase). Until you become familiar with these and various suture materials and instruments, it is necessary to use reference materials.

After completing Chapter 8, you will have more competence in determining which terms for drugs are capitalized.

EXAMPLES: *Generic names of drugs and suture materials*

nitroglycerin	analgesic	hydrocortisone	alcohol
ether	silk	catgut	cotton

EXAMPLES: *Trade names of drugs, suture materials, and other commercial products*

Cortisporin	Darvon	pHisoHex	Theokin
Dermalon	Gelfoam	HydroDiuril	Ser-Ap-Es
Ace bandage	ChapStick	Dacron	Dictaphone
Q-tips	Band-Aid	Motrin	RhoGAM
Surgicel	ibuprofen		

It is not necessary to follow the idiosyncratic capitalization of some drug names unless your employer prefers it.

EXAMPLES

HydroDiuril   Hydrodiuril

Exceptions are chemotherapy protocols and investigative agents.

EXAMPLES

ProMACE   CaT   IfoVP   CyADIC

NOTE: See Rule 4.22.

▶ Be alert to the internal capital letters and spacing in these commercial products:

PowerPoint	StairMaster	Wii
DuraSoft lenses	NeXT	WordPerfect
iMac	Post-it notes	iPad

RULE 4.11 Capitalize the names of *specific* departments or sections in the hospital.

EXCEPTION: Some teaching hospitals and military hospitals prefer capitalization for individual departments within their facility. Many large hospitals today have a variety of named outbuildings: The Eye Center, Imaging, The Women's Center, Rehabilitation, and so on. The entire entity is often referred to as "the campus."

EXAMPLES

Please see that the records are sent to St. Joseph's Hospital *Admitting Department.*

The *admitting department* was overwhelmed with 45 new admissions yesterday.

Albertson City Hospital *Pathology Department* received an award from the Greater Albertson County Industrial Council.

The specimen was sent to the *pathology lab.*

All *pathology departments* should have this notice posted.

The *Emergency Department* at Westside General Hospital has just received a new hyperbaric unit.

Some *emergency departments* are sending patients to *acute care centers* after triage.

The baby was born in the hallway somewhere between the *hospital pharmacy* and *The Women's Center.*

The patient was admitted to 4-North for observation; he is scheduled for an appointment at 1 p.m. in the *Advanced-Imaging Center.*

NOTE: Capitalize the names of departments when they are referred to as the people who represent them.

EXAMPLES

I asked *Pathology* to send the report to me STAT.

He reported that *Oncology* called again about the change in their schedule.

RULE 4.12 Capitalize specific designations used with numbers.

EXAMPLES

You have a reservation on *Flight* 707.

We ordered a *Model* 14 Medtronic pacemaker.

Kennedy *Class II*

We found a deficiency in *Complex I.*

NOTE: The following common nouns are not capitalized when used with numbers.

case	chapter	chromosome	column
fraction	grade	grant	group
lead	line	method	note
page	paragraph	part	patient
phase	section	series	size
stage	type	sentence	volume
wave	experiment	factor	

There is an error in your copy on *page 27, paragraph 2, line 3.*

The *stage III* tumor had invaded the chest wall and the nodes in the supraclavicular area.

RULE 4.13 Capitalize the first word of each line in an outline or subheading of a report and the entire main heading of a formal report.

EXAMPLE: *Diagnoses*

1. *Stress* incontinence of urine.
2. *Monilial* vaginitis.

EXAMPLE

HEENT

HEAD: Normal.

EYES: Pupils round and equal, react to L&A.

EARS: Hearing normal, TMs intact, canals patent.

EXAMPLE

PHYSICAL EXAMINATION
  HEENT
    Head: Normal.
    Eyes: Pupils round and equal, react to L&A.
    Ears: Hearing normal, TMs intact, canals patent.
    Nose: Canals patent.
    Throat: Trachea in the midline.

EXAMPLE

OPERATIVE REPORT

PREOPERATIVE DIAGNOSIS: Glaucoma, chronic, simple, bilateral.

POSTOPERATIVE DIAGNOSIS: Glaucoma, chronic, simple, bilateral.

OPERATION PERFORMED: Iridencleisis, right eye.

NOTE: When direct reference is made within a document to specific parts of a report, capitalize the heading or subheading used within the report.

EXAMPLES

Please refer to Past History in the June 9, 20XX, report.

There is nothing in her past history to alarm us at this time.

The next eight rules are used in all kinds of writing.

RULE 4.14 Capitalize the first word of a sentence, the first word of a complete direct quotation, and the first word after a colon if that word begins a complete thought.

EXAMPLES

The instructor said, "*Strive* for mailable copy even when you are practice-typing."

These are your directions: *Begin* typing as soon as you hear the signal and stop when the timer rings.

RULE 4.15 Capitalize the first and last words and all other words in the titles of articles, books, and periodicals with the exception of conjunctions, prepositions, and articles of three or fewer letters.

NOTE: Remember that book titles are also underlined or italicized.

EXAMPLES

I just purchased the latest edition of the Pharmaceutical Word Book by Drake & Drake; it is now available on CD-ROM as well.

The last online issue of *Perspectives on the Medical Transcription Profession* has an excellent article about job satisfaction written by Sidney Moormeister, PhD.

RULE 4.16 Capitalize the names of the days of the week, the months of the year, holidays, historic events, and religious festivals.

EXAMPLES

There will be no class on *Friday, November* 11, because it is *Veterans' Day*.

Do we get an *Easter* holiday or *Passover* vacation? Neither. It's called "*Spring Vacation.*"

BUT: I am taking an advanced transcription class in the *spring* semester; I wish I had taken it this *fall.*

RULE 4.17 Capitalize both the noun and the adjective when they make reference to a specific geographic location with real or imaginative names.

EXAMPLES

The patient was born and raised in the *Southwest;* he has lived in the *Big Apple* only a short while.

We plan to stay at a resort by the *Atlantic Ocean* when we go *east* for the medical meeting this fall.

The Great Lakes
Cape of Good Hope
Apache Reservation
Statue of Liberty
Down East
Silicon Valley

EXCEPTION: Some parts of the names of places are not capitalized when they appear *before* the names of a specific place or are general directions.

EXAMPLES

New York State but the state of New York

It's south of Atlantic City.

RULE 4.18 Capitalize abbreviations when the words they represent are proper nouns. Capitalize most abbreviations of English words; capitalize each letter in an acronym.

> 🔧 MT TOOL BOX TIP: Most abbreviation tools are capitalized.

EXAMPLES

ECG is the preferred abbreviation for "electrocardiogram."

Ronda A. Vasquez, *MD,* graduated from *UCSD.*

Dr Bowman is working with Project *HOPE* and *UNICEF.*

Our patient *JB* has progressed from being *HIV*-positive and now has *AIDS.*

Dr Ashamed is scheduled to assist with the *T&A.*

The *DTRs* are intact.

We changed from a *PC-DOS* operating system.

NOTE: Metric and English forms of measurement or Latin abbreviations are not capitalized.

EXAMPLES

t.i.d.	cm	mph	mg
p.o.	q.4 h.	mL	kg g

> 🔧 MT TOOL BOX TIP: Latin and foreign abbreviations are not capitalized.

RULE 4.19 Capitalize the abbreviations of academic degrees and religious orders.

EXAMPLES

MD PhD	DDS	MS	SJ	BVE
DPM	LLB	AS	OCSO	OSB

Please refer to Chapter 5 for a complete review of the use of abbreviations and to Chapter 3 for the use of punctuation with abbreviations.

RULE 4.20 When transcribing an organizations' minutes, bylaws, or rules, capitalize the names of all organizations, institutions, business firms, government agencies, and conferences, as well as the names of their departments, divisions, and titles of officers.

NOTE: The word *the* is not capitalized when it immediately precedes the name of the organization unless it is an official part of the name.

EXAMPLES

Then the *Secretary* read the minutes, and they were approved as read.

Dr Sanderson has recently retired from *the Navy*.

Utilization Committee

Mortality and Morbidity Conference

Tumor Board

International Clinical Congress

American College of Internal Medicine

the Internet

America Online

Knights of Columbus

NOTE: Do not confuse a general term for a formal name.

U.S. Postal Service but the post office

Beta tests but beta cells

Eastridge Clinic but the clinic

Gram stain but gram-negative culture.

RULE 4.21 Capitalize the names of specific academic courses.

BUT: Academic subject areas are not capitalized unless they contain a proper noun.

EXAMPLE

I am enrolled in *Medical Transcription Skill Building* 103; I am also taking keyboarding and *business* English.

These last five rules are frequently used in medical writing.

RULE 4.22 Capitalize each letter in the name of a drug, use bold print, or do both when reporting drug allergies in a *chart note* or in a patient's *history*. Some institutions request capitalization of other codes, such as *DO NOT RESUSCITATE* and *COMFORT CARE ONLY*, so that they will stand out on the record.

EXAMPLES

Allergies: Patient is allergic to PHENOBARBITAL and CODEINE.

Allergies: The patient reports a sensitivity to **SULFA**.

RULE 4.23 Capitalize the names of diseases that contain proper nouns, eponyms, or genus names. The common names of diseases and viruses are not capitalized.

EXAMPLES

The patient tested positive for *Rocky Mountain* spotted fever. (Proper noun)

She was given the final series of *diphtheria, pertussis,* and *tetanus* vaccine. (Common diseases)

She is now suffering from *postpoliomyelitis syndrome* and is unable to breathe without the use of her respirator. (Virus name)

Frequently, *Toxocara* infections are acquired from household pets. (Genus)

We have had the usual problems with *rubella, rubeola,* and *chickenpox* in the kindergarten population. (Common diseases)

He is showing early signs of *Lou Gehrig* disease. (Eponym)

RULE 4.24 Capitalize cardiologic symbols and abbreviations that are used to express electrocardiographic results.

EXAMPLES

The *P* waves are slightly prominent in *V1* to *V3*. (Or *V1-V3* or *V1-V3*)

It is not clear whether it contains a *U* wave.

The *QRS* complexes are normal, as are the *ST* segments.

There are *T*-wave inversions in *L1, aVL,* and *V1-V4*.

RULE 4.25 Capitalize the initial letter symbol for chemical elements; second letters are not capitalized.

EXAMPLES

Co (cobalt)   Ba (barium)   K (potassium)   I (iodine)
N (nitrogen)   O (oxygen: capital "O," not a zero)

Written-out chemical compounds are not capitalized

EXAMPLES

sodium   hydrogen   oxygen

RULE 4.26 Capitalize the first letter in the abbreviation for immunoglobulins (Ig) and follow it with a capital letter designation of one of the 5 class designations.

EXAMPLES

IgG   IgA   IgM   IgD   IgE

MT TOOL BOX TIP: Accept that policies, rules and procedures keep your tools in perfect working order.

4-1 SELF-STUDY

DIRECTIONS: Draw a single line under each letter that should be capitalized. You may refer to your reference materials. Refer to **Saunders Pharmaceutical Word Book**, or similar reference if that is not available, for help with some of the drug terms.

1. after i finish medical transcription 214, i will take a class in medical insurance billing. i want to get a job with goodwin-macy medical group.

2. all the patients were reminded that the office would be closed on labor day, monday, september 7.

3. dr albert k. shaw's address is one west seventh avenue, detroit, michigan.

4. two of the commonly sexually transmitted pathogens are chlamydia trachomatis and neisseria gonorrhoeae.

5. it was mr geoffry r. leslie, vice president of medical products inc., who returned your call.

6. the university hospital rotation schedule has been posted, and i am assigned to the emergency department and you report to cardiology.

7. patsy, who works in the valley view medical center, is studying to become a certified medical transcriptionist.

8. the dorcus travel bureau arranged dr berry's itinerary through new england last fall.

9. keep this in mind: accuracy is more important than speed.

10. the following are my recommendations:
    1. continuing treatment through the spinal defects clinic.
    2. evaluations at 2-month intervals during the first year of life.
    3. physical therapy reevaluation at 6 months of age.

11. the patient has four siblings, all living and well; his mother died of heart disease at age 45 and his father in an automobile accident when he was 24; there is no history of familial disease.

12. we expect judge willard frick to arrive from his home on the pacific coast for the memorial day weekend.

13. i find current medical terminology by vera pyle, cmt, to be an excellent reference book for the transcribing station in the department of internal medicine.

14. my uncle, sam, is a thoracic surgeon in houston.

15. mr billingsgate wrote to say that he had moved to 138 old highway eight, space 14.

16. we are waiting for confirmation of the diagnosis from the centers for disease control and prevention; it could be four corners virus.

17. whenever she takes perocet, she develops psychosis and was actually committed to a psych ward after taking it.

18. there is a recent study demonstrating increased benefit of adding bevacizumab (avastin) monoclonal antibody to the carboplatin and taxol regimen.

Answers are in Appendix A, p. 436.

4-2 SELF-STUDY

DIRECTIONS: Draw a single line under the letters that should be capitalized in the sentences below. Again, choose a good drug reference book for help (see Chapter 8).

1. the right rev. michael t. squires led the invocation at the graduation ceremony for greenlee county's first paramedic class.

2. nanci holloway, a 38-year-old caucasian female, is scheduled for a cesarean section tomorrow.

3. the internist wanted him to have meprobamate, so he wrote a prescription for miltown.

4. johnny temple had chickenpox, red measles, and german measles his first year in school.

5. i understand that bob, our p.m. shift mt, is proficient in american sign language.

6. the pathology report showed a class IV malignancy on the pap smear.

7. some patients have been very sick with kaposi sarcoma, the rare and usually mild skin cancer that seems to turn fierce with aids victims.

8. the mustard procedure is often used to reroute venous return in the atria.

9. the young man was an alert, asthenic, indochinese male who was well oriented to time and place.

10. the gynecologist wrote a prescription for flagyl for the patient with trichomonas vaginalis.

11. he was stationed at the naval training center before deployment to the gulf.

12. dr collier recommended a combination of benzathine penicillin g such as bicillin, for our patient with endocarditis.

13. barbara, our lpn, is the new membership chairman for the local now chapter; she asked me to join.

14. the od victim was taken to the riverview urgent care center by his roommate.

15. her right achilles tendon reflex is +1 compared to the left.

16. she is to begin her first glac chemotherapy on june the first.

17. he received an injectiion of crofab in the ed after being bitten by a rattlesnake.

18. the incision was dressed with adaptic, dry gauze, sterile webril, and a modified jones dressing.

19. we will hold the propranolol, lisinopril, and hydrochlorothiazide, as the patient is on a cardizem lyo-ject.

20. pain management: tylenol 650 mg p.o. q6 h p.r.n. pain.

The answers to these problems are on p. 436 in Appendix A. Do not be concerned with your progress if you had trouble with some of the abbreviations; Chapter 5 provides an in-depth study.

4-3 SELF-STUDY

DIRECTIONS: Retype the following letter, inserting capital letters and punctuation where necessary. You may use your reference materials. Use the U.S. Postal Service abbreviations for the state name in the address. After you have retyped the letter, check your answer in Appendix A, p. 437.

FAX: 212.555.1247   Telephone: 212.555.0124

William A. Berry, MD
3933 Navajo Road
GrandView, XX 87453

1   may 17, 20XX

2   barbara h. baker md
3   624 south polk drive
4   boothbay harbor, me 04538

5   dear dr baker:

6   re: mrs brenda woodman

7   at the request of dr thomas brothwell, i saw his patient in the office today.
8   he, apparently, felt that her thyroid was enlarged.

9   she stated that she is on dyflex g 1/2 tablet q.i.d., sski drops 10 t.i.d., brethine
10   2.5 mg b.i.d. and prednisone 10 mg. she has had asthma for 12 years and,
11   other than a t&a in childhood, has never been hospitalized.

12   on physical examination her thyroid was 2+ enlarged, especially in the lower
13   lobes, and smooth. the heart was in regular sinus rhythm of 110, and she had
14   findings of moderate bronchial asthma at this time. on pelvic examination, she
15   had a virginal introitus and a moderate senile vaginitis. she had heberden
16   nodes on the fingers and vibration sense was decreased by about 25
17   seconds.

18   the laboratory tests, a copy of which is enclosed, showed a normal thyroid
19   function. the urinalysis was negative; and the electrocardiogram, a copy of
20   which is enclosed also, showed some nonspecific st- and t-wave changes
21   and some positional change, suggestive of pulmonary disease.

22   in summary: i do not feel that the lady has hyperthyroidism but simply an
23   enlarged thyroid due to the prolonged iodide intake.

24   it was my pleasure to see your sister in the office, and i hope that the above
25   findings will reassure her family in the northeast.

26   sincerely,

27   william a. berry, md

28   ir

29   enclosures

30   cc: thomas b. brothwell, md

4-4 REVIEW TEST

DIRECTIONS: Retype the following letter, inserting capital letters and punctuation where necessary. Use the correct U.S. Postal Service abbreviations for the state name in the address.

John B. Scott, MD
8730 Engineer Road
Winnetka, Illinois 60141
463-4400

march 3, 20XX

state compensation insurance fund
p.o. box 2970
winnetka, illinois 60140

dear sir or madam:

re: james r. gorman, account number 6754

the above referenced patient was seen today for presurgical examination in the office. he has an acute upper respiratory infection with a red left ear and inflamed tonsils. therefore his surgery was cancelled and he was placed on keflex 250 mg every 6 hours.

mr gormans surgery was rescheduled for march 15 at mercy hospital. he will be rechecked in the office on march 14.

very truly yours,

john b. scott, md

efr

4-5 REVIEW TEST

DIRECTIONS: Retype the following letter, inserting capital letters and punctuation where necessary. Use the correct U.S. Postal Service abbreviations for the state name in the address.

FAX 213.555.2347   **Telephone 213.555.0124**

**William A. Berry, MD
3933 Navajo Road
GrandView, XX 00983**

may 6 20XX

mrs adrianne r shannon
316 rowan road
clearwater florida 33516

dear mrs shannon:

dr berry asked me to write to you and cancel your appointment for friday may 15.

we hope this will not inconvenience you but dr berry has made plans to attend the american college of chest physicians meeting in kansas city at that time. i have tentatively rescheduled your appointment for monday may 18 at 10:15 am

by the way you might be interested to know that dr berry has been asked to read the paper that he wrote, entitled "the ins and outs of emphysema." i believe that you asked him for a copy of this article the last time you were in the office

sincerely yours

laverne shay
secretary

CAPITALIZATION RULE SYNOPSIS

CAPITALIZE	RULE	PAGE
Abbreviations	4.18	109
Abbreviations for state names	4.5	105
Academic courses	4.21	110
Academic degrees	4.19	109
Acronyms	4.18	109
Allergies	4.22	110
Article titles	4.15	109
Attention lines	4.4	105
Avenue in addresses	4.2	104
Book titles	4.15	109
Boulevard in addresses	4.2	104
Brand names for drugs	4.10	107
Brand names for products	4.10	107
Capitals with colons	4.14	109
Cardiologic abbreviations	4.24	110
Cardiologic symbols	4.24	110
Chemical elements	4.25	110
Colons with capital letters	4.14	109
Complimentary closes	4.1	104
Days of the week	4.16	109
Degrees	4.19	109
Departments in the hospital	4.11	108
Direct quotations	4.14	109
Diseases	4.23	110
Drugs	4.10, 4.22	107, 110
Eponyms	4.7, 4.23	105, 110
Family titles	4.6	105
Genus names	4.9, 4.23	107, 110
Geographic locations	4.17	109
Headings	4.13	108
Historic events	4.16	109
Holidays	4.16	109
Immunoglobins	4.26	110
Languages	4.8	106
Military ranks	4.6	105
Months of the year	4.16	109
Names	4.7, 4.23	105, 110
Names for courses	4.21	110

CAPITALIZE	RULE	PAGE
Nicknames	4.7	105
Nouns	4.7	105
Nouns used as adjectives	4.7	105
Nouns with numbers	4.12	108
Numbers with words	4.12	108
Officers' titles	4.20	109
Organizations' names	4.20	109
Outlines	4.13	108
People	4.8	106
People's titles	4.3	105
Periodical titles	4.15	109
Place names	4.17	109
Political titles	4.6	105
Professional titles	4.6	105
Proper nouns	4.7, 4.23	105, 110
Quotations	4.14	109
Races	4.8	106
Religions	4.8	106
Religious festivals	4.16	109
Religious orders	4.19	109
Salutations	4.1	104
Sentences	4.14	109
Signature lines	4.3	105
Species	4.9	107
Specific departments	4.11	108
State abbreviations	4.5	105
Street name in addresses	4.2	104
Title in addresses	4.3	105
Title of articles	4.15	109
Title of books	4.15	109
Title on envelopes	4.3	105
Title of officers	4.20	109
Title of periodicals	4.15	109
Title with signatures	4.3	105
Titles	4.6	105
Titles for people	4.3	105
To Whom It May Concern lines	4.4	105
Trade names	4.10	107
Viruses	4.23	110

4-6 FINAL REVIEW

DIRECTIONS: In the blank, write the letter identifying the sentence with a capitalization error.

1. _____
   a. Some body-cavity-based lymphomas can occur independently of Kaposi Sarcoma in patients with AIDS.
   b. He was sent to be examined by the chairman of the Department of Neurology at Chantel General Hospital in Delaney.
   c. The pathogen is a susceptible gram-negative bacillus such as P. aeruginosa, though some resistance has appeared in this species.
   d. She is a 27-year-old woman from the French West Indies, with a history of seizures since childhood, who was brought to the emergency department because of a sharp left anterior pleuritic chest pain.

2. _____
   a. We placed a Cloward instrumentation and removed the disk contents, which were degenerated.
   b. He was seen and tested in the Neuro-Otology Laboratory in Orlando, Florida, where the Dix-Hallpike Test demonstrated a right-beating nystagmus, the left ear being normal.
   c. The diagnosis of Down syndrome was promptly confirmed, and the infant was sent to the Level III Neonatal Unit.
   d. Persistent hypotension or hemodynamic instability may necessitate hemodynamic monitoring via Swan-Ganz catheterization.

3. _____
   a. A Pfannenstiel abdominal entry and transverse lower uterine segment incision were easily performed with the patient under epidural anesthesia.
   b. I give antibiotic prophylaxis for endocardial or valvular lesions, history of endocarditis, and patent ductus arteriosus.
   c. It should be well known that Coccidioides immitis is a saprophytic, dimorphic fungus endemic to the southwestern United States and a portion of Central and South America.
   d. This 75-year-old black man has had a biopsy-proved bullous pemphigoid for more than a year, which has steadily improved.

4. _____
   a. This 35-year-old Hispanic man was referred to the Dermatology Service for evaluation of refractory rosacea.
   b. A 2-year-old from French Guiana was referred with a strange erosive tinea capitis of the crown that fluoresced under Wood light examination.
   c. A culture of sputum yielded a moderate growth of Streptococcus pneumoniae and Branhamella catarrhalis.
   d. The patient was brought to the Emergency Room with a flaccid right arm, weak right leg, and positive Babinski sign.

5. _____
   a. She was returned to the care of her primary physician with advice to obtain a telephone connection to Lifeline, an emergency assistance service.
   b. Those living in crowded groups should consider vaccination for influenza, varicella, measles-mumps-rubella (MMR), and Hepatitis A.
   c. Cytologic evaluation was conducted according to the Bethesda system from among the largely Latino population.
   d. Testing for human papillomavirus (HPV) was not performed.

6. _____
   a. A routine PAP test is recommended for patients on a yearly basis.
   b. The decrease in serum potassium is usually transient, not necessitating supplementation.
   c. His work in medical jurisprudence took place after his graduation from law school and his medical residence program in forensic medicine.
   d. Before anyone can be enrolled in a clinical trial, the study must receive approval by an ethics committee.

CHAPTER 5

Transcribing Numbers, Figures, and Abbreviations

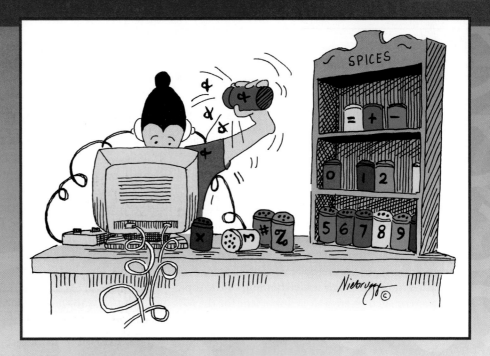

OBJECTIVES

After reading this chapter and completing the exercises, you should be able to

1. Explain when a number should be typed as a figure, typed in spelled-out form, or typed as a Roman numeral.
2. Type medical and business symbols as abbreviations only when appropriate.
3. Demonstrate your ability to prepare accurately typed material containing numbers, symbols, and abbreviations commonly found in medical writing.
4. Recognize and correctly use metric abbreviations.
5. State the reasons for spelling out abbreviations.
6. Demonstrate the proper use of metric system abbreviations in medical records.

INTRODUCTION

This chapter continues the discussion of the various typing techniques peculiar to medical and scientific reports, also known as *style*. We are working with rules, and they, like those introduced previously, are not sacred; however, they are sound and practical. When you master the techniques presented in this chapter, you will have the mechanical skills necessary to type medical and scientific papers with confidence.

> 🔧 **MT TOOL BOX TIP:** Accept that policies, rules, and procedures keep your tools in perfect working order.

One of the most difficult tasks in studying machine transcription is learning the technical and mechanical manner of writing used by those already working in the field. Therefore, even a mastery of medical terminology may not give you the confidence that you are transcribing in exactly the way it should be done.

Furthermore, absence of basic mechanical skill results in copy that lacks refinement or accuracy. Unfortunately, errors can occur because the medical transcriptionist (MT) "thought" he or she heard a certain word and then typed a senseless remark or a fragment of material. A more thorough understanding of the topic helps prevent such an error. It is important for the MT to be both grammatically and technically proficient.

If you want to avoid mistakes in your work, you must learn correct terms and practices and, at the same time, keep current by reading medical reports, papers, and journals. You do not have to understand the complete technical content of an article, but you must read to become familiar with how the copy is prepared. Some formats used in journal writing (for example, the use of italics for foreign words) are not generally used in medical transcription unless something is being transcribed for publication. In this case, the transcriptionist must be sure to follow all the stylistic rules used by that journal or publication.

You will find that there may be several ways of doing something—not several ways of doing something "right," just several ways of doing something. Some of the ways are preferred, although other methods might be acceptable. Sometimes MTs are not able to do what they know is technically correct because the software or hardware does not support it. In this case, MTs carry out the function the "best" way under the circumstances. For instance, it is correct to write "the patient's temperature is 102°," but if you know the printer cannot print a degree symbol, you input *102 degrees*.

You might hear a veteran MT say, "I have always done it this way," with a tone of voice indicating that the declaration therefore makes the practice correct. However, the MT's way might not always be correct. Many people learn by copying the work of other people whom they trust and admire. However, others might have just "invented" a format, setup, or method of transcription. Years of doing something incorrectly does not make it correct. Rules do change, too, and there may be a better way of completing certain tasks. Learn now which references and role models are trustworthy. Learn to question practices that do not look or sound right. Know why something is done one way and not another.

Before you start working with numbers in general, take a quick look at the metric system and how it is used in medical records.

USE OF THE METRIC SYSTEM IN MEDICAL RECORDS

This section focuses on just the metric units and abbreviations that are commonly used, and is not a comprehensive discussion of the entire metric (SI) system. Notice that all the abbreviations are written in lowercase letters except for *liter*, for which you use a capital *L*. (Note also *mL*.)

Units That You Need To Know

UNIT	SYMBOL	MEASURES	REPLACES
meter	m	length, distance, thickness	*inch, foot, yard, mile*
gram	g	mass (weight)	*ounce, pound*
liter	L	volume	*cup, pint, quart, gallon, fluid ounce*
Celsius	C	temperature	*Fahrenheit, although Fahrenheit may also be used*

Prefixes Commonly Used for More than One of a Unit

PREFIX	SYMBOL	RELATION TO UNIT	EXAMPLE
kilo-	k	1000 of them	1 kg, 1000 g

Prefixes Commonly Used for Less than One of a Unit

PREFIX	SYMBOL	RELATION TO UNIT	EXAMPLE
centi-	c	1/100 of a unit	1 cm
milli-	m	1/1000 of a unit	1 mL

There is more than one way of expressing a metric measurement. Usually, the least complex expression is chosen. For example, 1.5 meters (1.5 m) is also expressed as 150 centimeters (150 cm) or 1500 millimeters (1500 mm). We use the 1.5 m measurement as the least complex of the three.

Rules to Follow in Typing Metric Measurements

▶ Symbols are abbreviated when used with numeric values. They are written out when they are not used with numeric values.

EXAMPLES

There was a bruise more than a centimeter long over the bridge of her nose. *(Correct)*

There was a bruise more than a cm long over the bridge of her nose. *(Incorrect)*

There was a bruise more than 1 cm long over the bridge of her nose. *(Incorrect. This was not dictated.)*

▶ Symbols are not followed by a period or other marks of punctuation unless they occur at the end of a sentence or a series of values.

EXAMPLES

25 cm	115 kg	1000 mL *(Correct)*
25 cm.	115 kg.	1000 mL. *(Incorrect)*

▶ A zero is placed in front of the decimal point for numbers less than 1.

EXAMPLES

0.5 mL	0.1 cm	0.75 mg *(Correct)*
.5 mL	.1 cm	.75 cm *(Incorrect)*

EXCEPTION: Metric description of firearms does not use the zero.

EXAMPLE

A .22-caliber slug was lodged in the wound.

▶ A space is placed between the number and the symbol.

EXAMPLES

25 mg	1 m	*(Correct)*
25mg	1m	*(Incorrect)*

▶ Symbols are not made plural, no matter how many units are described.

EXAMPLES

6 m	75 mg	3 L *(Correct)*
6 ms	75 mgs	3 liters *(Incorrect)*

▶ Zeros after the decimal point are not placed after a whole number unless dictated.

EXAMPLES

Dictated: The wound was three centimeters at its widest point.

The wound was 3.0 cm at its widest point. *(Incorrect)*

The wound was 3 cm at its widest point. *(Correct)*

Dictated: The wound was three point zero centimeters at its widest point.

The wound was 3.0 cm at its widest point. *(Correct for this dictation)*

EXCEPTIONS

▶ Specific gravity is expressed with four digits with a decimal point between the first and second digit.

NOTE: Specific gravity of urine is a measurement of volume of urine at a specific temperature and compared with the same volume of water at the same temperature. The normal range for specific gravity is just slightly above 1. For example, H_2O pH = 1.000.

▶ When the pH of a substance is given, use two numerals. If only one numeral is dictated, place a zero after the decimal point.

EXAMPLES

Dictated: Specific gravity is ten twenty.

Transcribed: Specific gravity is 1.020.

Dictated: The "pee h" was seven.

Transcribed: The pH was 7.0

▶ Common fractions are not used with the metric system.

EXAMPLES

1/2 cm	3/4 liter *(Incorrect)*
0.5 cm	0.75 L *(Correct)*

▶ The derived unit for volume *cubic centimeters* and its abbreviation (cc) are not used. The abbreviation for milliliters (mL) is the proper abbreviation for this unit of measurement.

▶ The degree symbol (°) is used with the abbreviation for Celsius (C). The word *degrees* is written out with the word *Celsius*.

EXAMPLES

Her temperature on admission was 38°C. *(Correct)*

Her temperature on admission was 38 degrees Celsius. *(Correct)*

Her temperature on admission was 38 degrees C. *(Incorrect)*

TYPING NUMBERS

Let's begin now with a general overview of numbers so that when we start working with them, the rules will fall into place quickly.

There are several ways of expressing numbers: *written out as words, Arabic figures,* and *Roman numerals.* Of the written-out types, there are two: One set is called *ordinals:* these are such words as *first, second, third,* and so on. The other written-out words are just the words *one, two, three,* and so on. There are certain times when we use these word forms. Most of the time in medical writing, we use figures (*1, 2, 3,* and so on) because the figures have technical significance, serve as measurements, or deserve special emphasis. This practice makes things a lot easier. Figures are quick and easy to understand, quick and easy to type. Finally, we have the unusual use of Roman numerals: *I, II, III,* and so on. They are reserved for certain sorts of expressions, usually when the range of numbers is not expected to go very high.

An interesting issue is how to express the time of day. This task seems simple enough, but you can either write out the time or use figures. This is an easy rule to remember: When the time of day is all by itself (come at *three,* the party was over at *two* in the morning), you write it out. If it is expressed with *a.m., p.m., o'clock, noon,* or with minutes as well as hours (*3:30*), use figures. One exception: You also can write out the time when it is used with *o'clock.* It is a little formal, but some people like it that way. The military uses a 24-hour clock, so use a set of four figures to write the military time of day (*1400, 0900*).

Now you can begin with a more formal introduction to the vocabulary of numbers:

▸ *Numeral* and *Arabic numeral* mean 0, 1, 2, 3, 4, 5, 6, 7, 8, and 9 and their combinations.
▸ *Numeric term* refers to written-out numbers.
▸ *Roman numerals* refer to the use of certain letters of the alphabet: Most frequently, certain capital letters and combinations of the letters I, V, and X.
▸ *Cardinal numbers* refer to the quantity of objects in the same class. A cardinal number may be a whole number, a fraction, or a combination: 3 days, $15, and so forth.
▸ *Ordinal numbers* express position, sequence, or order of items in the same class. They can be spelled out or written as a figure plus a word part: first, 1st, third, eleventh, 14th, and so forth.

The following rules are separated into these different groups: Some numbers are expressed in more than one way.

Some style guides suggest that all numbers in medical documents be expressed in numerals. This practice certainly makes it easier to use numbers. These variations are shown in the examples. You will use more written-out numbers in formal documents, such as letters; therefore, be prepared to use each style appropriately and consistently according to the situation. Finally, you will type numbers in the style preferred by the dictator and supported by technology.

Ordinal Numbers: First, Second, Third, and So On

RULE 5.1 Spell out ordinal numbers (*first* through *ninth*) when they are used to indicate a time sequence. Use figures for ordinals when the ordinals are part of a series that includes a higher ordinal (10th and above) and when the number indicates any technical term. Ordinals are meant to express rank rather than quantity.

EXAMPLES: *Spelled-out, nontechnical numbers*

This is her *second* visit to the clinic. (*2nd*)

The patient was discharged to his home on the *fifth* postoperative day. (*5th*)

The *first* stage of the disease went by relatively unobserved. (*1st*)

Most spontaneous abortions occur during the *first* or *second* week of pregnancy, just after the *first* menstrual cycle is missed.

She has a *first*-degree relative with breast cancer. (*1st*)

EXAMPLES: *Figures for technical ordinals*

The *7th* cranial nerve was involved in his facial paralysis.

The clinic was for children in the *1st* through *12th* grades. (*First through twelfth*)

The *4th, 5th,* and *6th* ribs were fractured.

The injury was between the *1st* and *2nd* cervical vertebrae.

It occurred sometime between the *14th* and *30th* weeks of pregnancy.

Change the mailing address from PO Box 254 to 1335 *11th* Street.

Give the patient an appointment for the *6th* of August. (Or *August 6,* not *August 6th*)

NOTE: As with all numbers, use a spelled-out ordinal number to begin a sentence, or recast the sentence to avoid beginning with a number. See Rule 5.2.

EXAMPLE

Twelfth-grade students in the honor programs are simultaneously enrolled in community college classes.

Numbers Spelled Out or Written as Words: One, Two, Three, and So On

RULE 5.2 Spell out numbers at the beginning of a sentence.

🔧 MT TOOL BOX TIP: Spell out a number when it begins the sentence.

EXAMPLE

Fourteen patients were studied at the request of the staff, *four* were studied at the request of their physicians, and *eleven* were studied as interesting problems for discussion.

NOTE: When several related numbers are used in a sentence, be consistent; type all numbers in figures or write them all out. Normally, it is easier to type all of them in figures. If the number beginning the sentence is large (more than two words), it may be necessary to rewrite the sentence so that the number can be used as a figure elsewhere in the sentence. However, *if you must begin a sentence with a numeric term, you are not obligated to write out the other large numbers in the sentence.*

EXAMPLES

Seventy-one percent responded to the questionnaire; *33%* were positive, *21%* were negative, and *17%* gave a "no opinion" response.

Or recast the sentence:

Of the *71%* who responded…

NOTE: Be sure to spell out an abbreviation or symbol used with a number if the number has to be spelled out for some reason, such as the word *percent* in the first example.

RULE 5.3 Spell out all whole numbers *one* through and including *ten* in medical reports when they do *not* refer to technical terms or when they are used as pronouns.

EXAMPLES

I think that *one* should give him the benefit of the doubt. (Pronoun)

They will need *one* another's help in the crisis.

The first *three* documents were out of order.

They plan to open *six* more urgent care centers here within the next *two* years.

The address for our risk management team is *One* East Wacker Drive, Chicago, IL 60601.

She said she would be very upset if she made that mistake *one* more time.

He is serving his *first* week of a *two*-month volunteer program.

RULE 5.4 Spell out numbers used for indefinite expressions or made to appear as indefinite.

EXAMPLES

I received *thirty-odd* applications.

He had diphtheria in his late *forties*.

Hundreds thronged to see my "celebrity" patient.

She said she had a *hundred* reasons for avoiding surgery.

RULE 5.5 Spell out fractions when they appear without a whole number or are *not* used as a compound modifier.

EXAMPLES

He smoked a *half*-pack of cigarettes a day.

He smoked *one-half* pack of cigarettes a day. *(1/2)*

BUT: He smoked *1-1/2* packs of cigarettes a day.

A *1/2*-inch incision was made in the thenar eminence. (Use of modifier)

There was damage to *one fourth* of the distal phalanx. (No use of modifier)

NOTE: Figures in the last example may read better: *1/4th* of the distal phalanx

NOTE: Make all fractions on the keyboard by using the whole number, the slash, and the second whole number, with no spacing *(1/3)*. Mixed fractions are made with a space between the whole number and the first number of the fraction. Place a hyphen between the whole number and the first number of the fraction in medical reports *(2-1/2)*. Some software converts fractions to reduced-sized figures *(1½)*. Do not mix these reduced-sized fractions with those you construct. Some software does not support these automated fractions, so avoid using them.

EXAMPLE: *1-1/2 inch*

NOT: *1 and 1/2 inch*, which the dictator might say.

RULE 5.6 Spell out the first number and use a figure for the second number when two numbers are used together to modify the same noun.

EXAMPLES

six 3-bed wards

two 1-liter solutions or *two* 1 L solutions

fifty 3-gallon tanks or 50 *three-gallon* tanks (When the first number is large)

NOTE: Remember Rule 3.30 and use a hyphen when words are compounded with figures.

RULE 5.7 Spell out the *even time of day* when written without *o'clock* or without *a.m.* or *p.m.*

EXAMPLES

The staff meeting is scheduled to begin at *three*.

He is due at *nine* this evening.

Give her an appointment for *half-past two*.

NOTE: Figures are used for all other expressions of time. See Rule 5.9. The phrases *in the morning, in the afternoon,* and *at night* are written with *o'clock* and not with *a.m.* or *p.m.* Do not use *o'clock* with *a.m.* or *p.m.* or when both hour and minutes are expressed.

EXAMPLES

I met her in the emergency room at *3* o'clock in the morning.

She is expected at *3* o'clock p.m. (Incorrect)

She is expected at *3* o'clock. (Correct)

She is expected at 3 p.m. (Correct)

She is expected at *3:30* o'clock. (Incorrect)

She is expected at *3:30* p.m. (Correct)

NOTE: It is also acceptable to write out an even time of day with the expression *o'clock*. This style is more formal.

EXAMPLES

The award ceremony is planned for three o'clock. (Correct)

Please ask her to come at *3* o'clock. (Correct)

RULE 5.8 Spell out large round numbers that do not refer to technical quantities and are more or less indefinite. Figures give such numbers an undesired emphasis.

EXAMPLES

There are more than a *million* people living in Pitman County now.

There were *eighteen hundred* physicians present at the symposium.

NOT: There were one thousand, eight hundred present. (Nor *1800* present)

HOWEVER: He was given *600,000* units of penicillin. (Technical)

 MT TOOL BOX TIP: Indefinite numbers (e.g., several *hundred*) are spelled out.

Numbers as Figures: 1, 2, 3, and So On

These are also called *cardinal figures* or *Arabic figures*.

RULE 5.9 Use figures to express the time of day with *a.m.* or *p.m.* and the time of day when both hours and minutes are expressed alone.

 MT TOOL BOX TIP: The time of day is usually written in figures.

NOTE: Even times of day are written without the colon and zeroes.

EXAMPLES

He arrived promptly at *2:30*.

Office hours are from *10:00 a.m.* to noon. (Incorrect)

Office hours are from *10 a.m.* to noon. (Correct)

NOTE: Do not use *a.m.* or *p.m.* with 12. You may use the figure 12 with the word *noon* or *midnight* or use the words alone without the figure 12.

EXAMPLES

We close the office at *12 noon*. (Or simply *noon*)

My shift is over at *midnight*.

My shift is over at 12 p.m. (incorrect)

 MT TOOL BOX TIP: When using 12:00 as the time of day, use noon or midnight for that time of day.

RULE 5.10 Use figures to write numbers larger than ten.

Use a comma to punctuate large numbers when five or more digits are represented. Addresses, year dates, ZIP codes, fax numbers, four-digit numbers, and some ID and technical numbers are traditionally not separated by commas, nor are commas used with decimals or the metric system.

 MT TOOL BOX TIP: Technical numbers are written using figures.

EXAMPLES

The piece of equipment is valued at *$12,300*.

Piedmont Hospital Association serves a population of *150,500*.

Please send this to Union Annex Box *87543*.

All of the ZIP codes changed in our area; please note that the new one is *06431*.

Platelet count was 350,000.

NOTE: The last example is often dictated as *platelet count was three fifty*. Since a platelet count is correctly indicated with six numerals, you need to expand the *three fifty* to 350,000; and a dictated *two twenty five* expands to 225,000.

Some very large numbers are written by using scientific notation. See example below. (See p. 128 for the use of subscript.)

EXAMPLE

2.5×10^8 (Not *250,000,000*)

RULE 5.11 Use figures to write numbers less than ten when they occur with a larger number on the same subject.

EXAMPLE

There are *3* beds available on the maternity wing, *14* on the surgery wing, and *12* on the medical floor.

RULE 5.12 Use figures to write numbers with the expression *o'clock* when designating areas on a circular surface.

NOTE: Only whole numbers are used, and the word *area* or *position* is added to the expression.

EXAMPLES

The sclera was incised at about the *3 o'clock* area.

The cyst was in the left breast, just below the nipple about half way between the
5 o'clock and *6 o'clock* positions.

HOWEVER: Omit the *o'clock* term if the following clock-face figures are used.

EXAMPLE

The cyst was in the left breast at about the 5:30 position just below the nipple.

RULE 5.13 Use figures to write dollar amounts.

NOTE: Even amounts are written without the period and zeroes.

EXAMPLE

The initial consultation is *$185*. (Not *$185.00*)

RULE 5.14 Use figures in writing vital statistics such as age, weight, height, blood pressure, pulse, respiration, dosage, size, temperature, and so on.

EXAMPLE

You hear: he is a sixteen year old well developed well nourished white male height is seventy two inches weight is one hundred forty five pounds blood pressure is one hundred twenty over eighty pulse is seventy two and respirations are eighteen.

You type: He is a *16-year-old*, well-developed, well-nourished white male. Height: *74 inches*. Weight: *145 pounds*. Blood pressure: *120/80*. Pulse: *72*. Respirations: *18*.

NOTE: In the preceding example, the transcriptionist eliminated the verbs *is* and *are* and substituted the colon when the vital statistics were given. Each set of vital statistics is closed off with a period (a semicolon would also be correct).

You may also type: Height is 74 inches, weight is 145 pounds, blood pressure is 120/80, pulse is 72, and respirations are 18.

EXAMPLES

Height: *72 inches*. (Correct)

Height is *72 inches*. (Correct)

Height: is *72 inches*. (Incorrect)

He was described as a *2-year 3-month-old* boy.

You hear: this is a three day old black female infant with a rectal temperature of one hundred two degrees weighing seven pounds and nine ounces and measuring twenty-one inches in length.

You type: This is a *3-day-old* black female infant with a rectal temperature of *102°*, weighing *7* pounds *9* ounces, and measuring *21* inches in length.

NOTE: You would write out the word *degrees* when the degree symbol is unavailable.

You hear: he is to take tofranil ten milligrams per day for three days to be increased to twenty-five to fifty milligrams per day if there is no response.

You type: He is to take Tofranil *10* mg/day for *3* days, to be increased to *15-50* mg/day if there is no response.

NOTE: When a whole number is dictated, do not add a decimal point and a zero. 6 mg (correct) not 6.0 mg (incorrect) This latter could have fatal consequences if misread. Use a trailing zero only when it is dictated as part of a measurement.

You hear: We removed a three point oh by three point five millimeter cyst from the right ovary.

You type: We removed a 3.0 x 3.5 mm cyst from the right ovary.

You hear: the patient has twenty forty vision in the right eye and twenty one hundred in the left eye.

You type: The patient has *20/40* vision in the right eye and *20/100* in the left eye.

RULE 5.15 Use figures when numbers are used *directly* with symbols, words, or abbreviations.

There *is* a space between the number and the words or the abbreviation; there is *no space* between the symbol and the number.

EXAMPLES: *Number and abbreviation*

15 mmHg (It is spoken *millimeters of mercury* and pertains to barometric reading)

1 q.i.d.

400 mOsm of solute

6 mL

8 pounds *3* ounces

5 feet *6* inches

3 a.m.

1.5 cm

q.4 h. (Notice the space between the *4* and the abbreviation for hour)

EXAMPLES: *Number and degree symbol*

There is no space between the degree symbol (°) and the abbreviations C or F nor between the number and the degree symbol.

36°C

When angles are referred to, there is no space between the degree symbol and the number

Abduction was limited to 10°.

There was a 15-degree angle achieved at this time. (also 15° angle)

If the word degree is not dictated, do not use either symbol or word.

EXAMPLES: *Numbers and other symbols*

1+ protein

at a *−2* station

+2.50

120/80

Rh−

Rh+

2%

$10 (Not $10.00)

#14 Foley

#3-0

1:100

20/40

EXCEPTION: *3 × 5* (Spaces are used because the symbol × crowds the figures.) Use the lower case *x*.

 MT TOOL BOX TIP: The symbol # may often be substituted for *number* or *No.*

NOTE: Do not use symbols and hyphens together.

EXAMPLES

a *2 L* bottle (Correct)

a *3-inch* incision (Correct)

a *3″-incision* (Incorrect)

O-negative blood (Correct)

O-blood (Incorrect)

You Hear	*You Type*
one plus protein	*1+* protein
fifteen millimeters of mercury	*15* mmHg
two percent	*2%*
two by three centimeters	*2 × 3 cm*
seventy five milliliters per kilogram per twenty four hours	*75 mL/kg/24 hours*

You Hear	*You Type*
Strength is five out of five in all extremities.	Strength is *5/5* in all extremities.
one "cue eye dee"	*1* q.i.d.
ten milligrams "tee eye dee"	*10* mg t.i.d.
the "bee you en" is forty five milligrams percent	the BUN is *45* mg%
ninety nine degrees fahrenheit	*99*°F (also *99 degrees* Fahrenheit)
a ten day history	a *10*-day history
ten dollars	*$10* (not $10.00)
sixty three cents	*63* cents (not $.63)
number fourteen foley	*#14* Foley (also *No. 14* Foley)
thirty to thirty five milliequivalents	*30-35* mEq (also *30 to 35* mEq)
four hundred milliosmoles of solute	*400* mOsm of solute
oh-ess equals plus two point five oh plus oh point seven five	OS = *+2.50 + 0.75**
times one	*×1* (not *times 1* or *× one*)
right eye was a minus zero point fifty plus one point zero zero axis one thirteen	OD: *−0.50 + 1.00* axis *113**

 MT TOOL BOX TIP: Illegal abbreviations are simply not used in medical documents.

RULE 5.16   Use figures for the day of the month and the year; write out the month when used in narrative text and in the date line of a letter. Use figures separated by slashes or hyphens in other formats.

EXAMPLES: *Date line for letter or report*

November 3, *20XX*

3 November *20XX* (Military and foreign style; not used in text format)

EXAMPLES: *Text use*

The patient was first seen in the emergency department on *March 3, 20XX.* (Correct)

The patient was first seen in the emergency department on *3/3/00.* (Incorrect)

The patient was first seen in the emergency department on *3 March 20XX.* (Correct in military documents)

The patient was first seen in the emergency department on *March 3* last year. (Incorrect. Find out the correct year and insert it.)

*Right eye (OD) and left eye (OS) abbreviations are used here because it is obvious what they mean and they will not be misunderstood. See Table 5-1.

TABLE 5-1 Illegal Abbreviations (see www.ismp.org)

ABBREVIATION	INTENDED MEANING	USE INSTEAD
AS, AD, AU	left ear, right ear, each ear	right ear, left ear, each ear
OD, OS, OU	right eye, left eye, both eyes	right eye, left eye, both eyes
BT	bedtime	bedtime
cc	cubic centimeters	mL (for *milliliters,* the correct term)
DC	discharge or discontinue	discharge or discontinue
HS	half-strength	half-strength
hs	bedtime	bedtime
IU	international units	units
od	once daily	daily
QD or q.d.	every day	daily
sub q or SQ	subcutaneously	subcutaneously
U	unit	unit
×3 d	for 3 days	for 3 days
> and <	greater than/less than	use *greater than* and *less than*

If one of these terms is dictated and the dictator and dictation is clear, a determination must be made by the facility concerning the transcription of the abbreviation. The MT should not be responsible for translating the dictation into its "presumed meaning."

NOTE: The date is spelled out in text of the body of the report because the primary purpose is ease of communication of information, and the risk for misunderstanding is increased if numerals are used in text. However, for specific information in the header/footer information, numerals are preferred for ease in filing and comparison of dates. This is a facility preference.

EXAMPLES: *In reports*

Office visit: *3-3-XX* or *3/3/XX*

Office visit: *03/03/0X* (Double-digit method also acceptable)

DOB (date of birth): *3-3-93* or *3/3/1993 or 03/03/1993*

D (date of dictation): *11/3/XX*

T (date of transcription): *11/4/XX*

EXAMPLES: *The double-digit dating system*

D: 11-03-XX

T: 11-04-XX

Also

D: 11/03/20XX

T: 11/04/20XX

 MT TOOL BOX TIP: Double-digit dating is often required in medical documents (e.g., 03/07/2010).

RULE 5.17 Use figures when writing the military time of day (24-hour clock time).

You Hear	You Type
oh three fifteen (3:15 a.m.)	0315 hours
twelve hundred hours (noon)	1200 hours
fourteen hundred hours (2 p.m.)	1400 hours
sixteen thirty (4:30 p.m.)	1630 hours

EXAMPLES

Time of death was called at *16:34.* (Incorrect)

Time of death was called at *1634 p.m.* (Incorrect)

Time of death was called at *1634 hours.* (Correct)

NOTE: Military (or 24-hour) time is not used with *a.m., p.m.,* or *o'clock.* It is frequently used to state birth and death times, as well as time of day in autopsy protocols. It is customary to write the word *hours* after the figures.

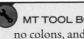 **MT TOOL BOX TIP:** 24-hour clock time uses 4 digits, no colons, and no *a.m.* or *p.m.* (e.g., 1450 hours).

RULE 5.18 Use figures in describing sutures and materials.

NOTE: When the dictator says *two oh* or *double oh* in referring to suture materials, you type *2-0.* For reading ease, use only the number, hyphen, and the zero (0) from 1-0 to 11-0. It is not necessary to insert the # symbol unless dictated.

EXAMPLES

Dictated: The incision was closed with number six oh fine silk sutures.

The incision was closed with *#6-0* fine silk sutures. (Correct)

The incision was closed with *#000000* fine silk sutures. (Incorrect)

The incision was closed with *#60* fine silk sutures. (Incorrect)

She used *2-0* chromic catgut for suture material. (Correct)

RULE 5.19 Use figures and symbols when writing dimensions. Leave a space on each side of the ×. Place a zero in front of a decimal fraction when there is no whole number before it, whether dictated or not.

You Hear	You Type
eight point five by five by four	*8.5 × 5 × 4*
three point five by three	*3.5 × 3*
point five by point seventy five	*0.5 × 0.75* (Correct)
	0.5 × .75 (Incorrect)
point two seven five	*0.275* (Correct)
	.275 (Incorrect)

Use a trailing zero only when it is dictated as part of a measurement.

You hear: We removed a three point oh by three point five millimeter cyst from the right ovary.

You type: We removed a 3.0 x 3.5 mm cyst from the right ovary.

SUBSCRIPT AND SUPERSCRIPT

At one time, many numbers were typed in subscript or superscript (slightly below or above the line). With the advent of software formatting features, this technique has become somewhat easier, but it can still be time consuming to locate the proper formatting. Some MTs make macros for commonly used formats, such as ^{131}I, pO_2, CO_2, B_{12}, and ° (the degree symbol). However, some printers do not support this format, and therefore it has become acceptable to execute *most* subscript and superscript symbols on the line or spelled out, as in the case of the word "*degree.*" Numbers are more easily read when typed on the line, because most reports are single-spaced. Again, some dictators or authors may insist on traditional formatting; therefore, be alert to this possibility. Preparation of documents for publication incorporates these styles, as well as superscript footnote symbols.

EXAMPLES

H_2O (The symbol for water)

A_2 is greater than P_2 (The aortic second sound is greater than the pulmonic second sound)

The L_4 area was bruised (Reference to the fourth lumbar vertebra)

Subsequently ^{131}I was given (Reference to radioactive iodine)

You might want to learn this technique. It is shown in the examples, along with numbers typed on the line. An exception to the general rule of avoiding subscripts and superscripts is in the case of numbers given to the *power of 10;* for example, urine culture grew out 10^5 colonies of *E. coli*. It is obvious that in this case to write the superscript on the same line would change the value of the number. However, in some situations, this exponent will not print or upload, and your only option would be to type *10 exp 5* or *10 to the 5th* (or whatever number is dictated). It is important for you to understand printing and technological parameters for the healthcare provider.

RULE 5.20 Use figures with capital letters to refer to the vertebral (spinal) column, vertebral spaces, and disks.

NOTE: *C* is used for the cervical vertebrae 1 through 7.

T (or *D*) is used for the thoracic (or dorsal) vertebrae 1 through 12.

L is used for the lumbar vertebrae 1 through 5.

S is used for the sacral vertebrae 1 through 5.

C2-3 is the intervertebral disk space between the second and third vertebrae.

Normally the physician would not say *thoracic six* but *tee six.* You would type *T6* or T_6.

You hear: he has a herniated disk at el four five.

You type: He has a herniated disk at *L4-5* (also L_{4-5}).

You hear: the patient has respiratory paralysis due to injury of spinal nerves see three through see five.

You type: The patient has respiratory paralysis due to injury of spinal nerves *C3* through *C5*. (Do not use the hyphen, as in *C3-C5*, because you need to use the word *through* to indicate the unspoken C4.)

You hear: there was an injury to the spine between see seven and tee one.

You type: There was an injury to the spine between *C7* and *T1* (Also C_7 and T_1 or *C7-T1*).

NOTE: Reference to the spinal nerves is made in the same manner. There is a *C8* spinal nerve.

RULE 5.21 Use figures when writing electrocardiographic *chest* leads. These leads are V_1 through V_6 and aV_L, aV_R, and aV_F.

▶ Leads for recording electrocardiographic tracings are designated by numbers and letters. The standard leads are indicated by Roman numerals; the central terminal lead is designated by *V* and a letter for right or left arm or foot.

EXAMPLES

lead *I*

lead *III*

VR or V_R

aVR or aV_R

aVF or aV_F

▶ Chest leads are indicated with a *V* for the central terminal and an Arabic number for the chest electrode and a Roman numeral for intercostal space positions.

EXAMPLES

lead *V1* or V_1

lead *VR1* or V_{R1}

lead *3V3* or $3V_3$

You hear: lead vee-r-two

You type: lead *VR2* or V_{R2}

You hear: lead-three vee-three

You type: lead *3V3*

You hear: there is es tee elevation in leads vee two and vee six.

You type: There is ST elevation in leads *V2* and *V6.* (Also V_2 and V_6)

You hear: the leads one, two, a vee el, and a vee ef are missing in this sequence.

You type: The leads *I, II, aV_L* (*aVL* also correct), and aV_F (*aVF* also correct) are missing in this sequence.

NOTE: Roman numerals are used with standard bipolar ECG and EKG leads. See p. 132.

Sequential leads should be typed as follows:

You hear: lead vee one through vee five.

You type: lead *V1 through V5* or V_1 *through* V_5 (not *V1-V5* nor *V1-5.*)

RULE 5.22 Use figures in writing technical ratios and ranges.

You hear: the solution was diluted one to one hundred.
You type: The solution was diluted *1:100.*

You hear: there is a fifty-fifty chance of recovery.
You type: There is a *50-50* chance of recovery.

NOTE: A *ratio* expresses the elements of a proportion and expresses the number of times the first contains the second.[*] A *range* is the linking of a sequence of values or numbered items by expressing only the first and last items in the sequence or the difference between the smallest and the largest varieties in a statistical distribution.

▶ Ratios composed of words are expressed with a slash, a hyphen, or the word *to.*

EXAMPLES

The odds are *ten to one.*
the *female/male* ratio (also *female-male* ratio)

▶ Ratios composed of numbers are expressed with a colon.

EXAMPLES

The odds are *10:1.*
The solution was diluted *1:100,000.*

▶ Symbolic ratios are written with a slash.

EXAMPLE

The *a/b* ratio

▶ The word *to* or a hyphen may be used in expressions of range. When in doubt, use the word *to.*

EXAMPLES

The projected salary increases are *$2.75 to $3.00* per hour.
The projected salary increases are *$2.75-$3.00* per hour.

---

*An example in making lemonade might be the following: ratio of water : lemon juice : sugar is 10:1:2 tablespoons.

We scanned all the medical records from *2002-2010 to* the EMR system.

There is a waiting period of *3-6* months.

NOTE: Do not use the hyphen when the range includes a plus and/or a minus sign.

EXAMPLES

The expected weight change was anywhere from *−6.5 kg to 10.5 kg.*

The presenting part was at a *−2 to a −3* station.

▶ The symbol or abbreviation is used with each of the figures in the range; the hyphen is not used.

EXAMPLES

The survival rate was consistent at *20% to 25%.*

The temperature fluctuated daily between *100° and 103°.*

EXCEPTION: It was *2 to 3* cm long. (*2-3 cm long* is also correct.)

NOTE: Use words rather than a hyphen when symbols are part of the range. Repeat the percent symbol (%) with each number in a range.

You hear: Quality assurance reported accuracy from ninety four to one hundred percent.
You type: Quality assurance reported accuracy from *94% to 100%.*

You hear: Leads vee one through vee five were rechecked
You type: Leads V1-V5 were rechecked. (correct)
You type: Leads V_1 through V_5 were rechecked. (correct)
You type: Leads V_{1}-$_{V5}$ were rechecked (not correct)

You hear: Blood pressure ranged from sixty-five over one hundred forty to ninety over one hundred sixty.
You type: Blood pressure ranged from *65/140* to *90/160.*

RULE 5.23 Use figures and symbols when writing plus or minus with a number.

You hear: one to two plus
You type: 1 to 2+

You hear: pulses were two plus
You type: pulses were 2+

You hear: the presenting part was at a minus two station
You type: The presenting part was at a *−2* station.

You hear: the refractive error in the left eye was a minus zero point fifty plus one point zero zero axis 113
You type: The refractive error in the left eye was a *−0.50 + 1.00 axis 113.*

You hear: visual acuity with correction was increased to twenty two hundred by plus eight point fifty lens
You type: Visual acuity with correction was increased to *20/200 by +8.50* lens.

NOTE: Someone unfamiliar with this last expression might interpret the first part to read *22 hundred* because that is how it sounds when it is spoken. Visual acuity is expressed with the figure *20* in front of the slash: *20/20, 20/40, 20/100, 20/200, 20/400,* and so on. A distance vision chart is read at 20 feet, and the basic expression describes the patient's ability to read the chart at this distance. A person with poor vision would have a visual acuity of 20/200, whereas perfect vision would be 20/20. A speech recognition document could show this transcribed as 2200 because that is what is heard by the speech engine. You would edit that to 20/200.

Mixed Numbers

RULE 5.24 Use figures to write both technical and non-technical mixed numbers (whole numbers with a fraction).

> **NOTE:** Fractions are not used with the metric system or with the percent (%) sign. Decimals are used with the metric system to describe portions of whole numbers.

EXAMPLE

You hear: three-fourths percent

You type: 0.75% (Not *3/4%*)

EXAMPLES

The patient moved to this community *2-1/2* years ago. (Mixed number)

You hear: one and one half years ago

You type: *1-1/2* years ago

You hear: one and a half centimeters

You type: *1.5* cm (Not *1-1/2* cm)

> **NOTE:** To type fractions, type the numerator, the slash, and the denominator. Place a hyphen between the whole number and the numerator of the fraction: for example, *2-1/4.* If your computer converts these fractions to reduced-sized figures, then there is no space or hyphen in 2¼. Remember to make sure that your printer recognizes these figures.

RULE 5.25 Use figures in writing numbers containing decimal fractions.

EXAMPLE

You hear: the incision site was injected with point five percent xylocaine.

You type: The incision site was injected with *0.5%* Xylocaine. (Not *1/2%*)

> **NOTE:** A zero is placed before a decimal that does not contain a whole number so that it will not be read as a whole number. Be very careful with the placement of the

zero and decimal. Incorrect placement could result in a 10- or 100-fold error, or worse.

A zero is not placed in front of or after other numbers unless dictated.

EXCEPTION: Specific gravity is expressed with 3 numbers after the decimal point, dictated or not.

EXAMPLE

You hear: **Specific gravity is one twelve.**

You type: **Specific gravity is 1.012**

Kirshner wires (K-wires) are also transcribed with 4 digits, a zero in front of the decimal point and 3 digits after the decimal point.

EXAMPLE

You hear: **The bones were held in alignment with a point six two inch kay wire.**

You type: **The bones were held in alignment with a 0.062-inch K-wire.**

EXCEPTION: By convention, a zero is not used in front of the decimal point of the measure of the bore of a firearm.

EXAMPLE

He used a *.22*-caliber rifle.

Unrelated Numbers and Other Combinations

RULE 5.26 Unrelated numbers in the same sentence follow the rules governing the use of each number.

EXAMPLE

He has *three* offices and employs *21* medical assistants and *2* transcriptionists. (Rule 5.3 and Rule 5.11)

RULE 5.27 Round numbers in millions and billions are expressed in a combination of figures and words.

EXAMPLE

Do you know that Keane Insurance sold over *$3-1/2 billion* of medical insurance last year? (*$3.5 billion* is also correct. *$3.5 billion dollars* is not correct.)

Note the placement of the dollar sign ($).

Spacing

The symbols ' (called *prime*), +, −, %, #, $, °, and / are typed directly in front of or directly after the number to which they refer, with no spaces. There is a space on each side of the times symbol (×) in expressing dimensions.

5-1 SELF-STUDY

DIRECTIONS: Here are phrases you might hear. Quotation marks define a *phonetic* expression for you. Please use double spacing and *transcribe* the correct version of what you have heard; use the proper format. Be careful with all numbers, symbols, abbreviations, punctuation, and capitalization. There is a synopsis of rules on p. 143 to help you locate the rules quickly.

EXAMPLE

You hear: the patient was seen in the emergency room at eighteen hundred on eleven august two thousand and ten.
You type: The patient was seen in the emergency room at 1800 hours on August 11, 2010.

1. the wound was closed in layers with "two oh" and "three oh" black silk sutures
2. the three month premature infant was delivered by cesarean section
3. he is a twenty four year old black male with an admitting blood pressure of one hundred eighty over one hundred
4. paresis is noted in four fifths of the left leg
5. it was then suture ligated with chromic number one catgut sutures
6. there were multiple subserous fibroids ranging in size from point five to two point five centimeters in diameter
7. there are a thousand reasons why i wanted to be a doctor but at three "ay em" after i have been awakened from a deep sleep it is hard to think of any
8. my charge for the procedure is seven hundred and fifty dollars and the median fee in the community is eight hundred dollars
9. the patient received four units of blood
10. the bullet travelled through the pelvic plexus into the spinal cord shattering "es" two "es" three and "es" four

After you have completed this exercise, check Appendix A, p. 438, to see whether you completed it properly. *Retype* any problems that you missed so that you get the "feel" of producing them correctly and another chance to see them written accurately.

5-2 PRACTICE TEST

DIRECTIONS: Follow the directions given in Self-Study 5-1. This test is just a bit more difficult; therefore, be sure that you understand any errors you made in Self-Study 5-1.

1. on september twenty six two thousand and ten she had a left lower lobectomy
2. two sutures of triple oh cotton were placed so as to obliterate the posterior cul de sac
3. he smoked one and one half packs of cigarettes a day
4. there was a small splinter of glass recovered from just to the right of the iris in the four o'clock area
5. the resting blood pressure is seventy six over forty
6. please mail this to doctor ralph lavton at ten dublin street bowling green ohio four three four oh two
7. we had seven admissions saturday twenty four sunday and three this ay-em
8. in the accident the spine was severed between see four and five
9. the child was first seen by me in the esther levy imaging center on the evening of eleven may two thousand and six.
10. i recommend a course of cobalt sixty radiation therapy

After you check your answers, retype any questions you missed so that you have the opportunity to produce the sentences correctly. Check your answers in Appendix A, p. 438.

MT TOOL BOX TIP: Taking frequent breaks when you are studying or working is a tool for health.

Roman Numerals

Roman numerals are generally used as noncounting numbers. There are many medical phrases *traditionally* expressed with capital Roman numerals. These are made on the keyboard with the capital letters *I, V,* and *X.* Lowercase Roman numerals are used in the preparation of prescriptions and are made with the lowercase *i, v,* and *x;* however, they are seldom required in transcription. Capitalize a proper noun occurring with a Roman numeral and a noun occurring with a Roman numeral at the beginning of a sentence. Because the use of Roman numerals is based only on tradition, some professionals prefer the use of Arabic numbers. Always follow the desires or customs of your employer. The examples that follow show the use of the Roman numerals along with similar expressions in which the Arabic figure is preferred.

 MT TOOL BOX TIP: Roman numerals are unusual; use them only when required.

RULE 5.28 Use Roman numerals for numbers with the following expressions.

NOTE: The examples include some Arabic numbers that are exceptions to or a second way to use the expression.

Expressions	*Examples*
Axis	axis *I-V*
Cranial leads (EEG)	lead *I* reading
Limb lead (ECG)	leads *I-III* readings
Cranial nerves	cranial nerves *II-XII* intact (also cranial nerves *2-12*)
Phase	phase *II* clinical trials
	phase *III* drug trial
	phase *3* study
Type	type *1* hyperlipoproteinemia
	type *2* diabetes
	Alzheimer type *II*
	type *1B* comminuted fracture
Fracture	Salter *III* fracture
	LeFort fracture *I*
Factor (blood)	missing factor *VII*
	antithrombin *III*
	clotting factors I-V
	factor *VIII*: Ag
	factor *XI* deficiency
	factor *V* Leiden mutation
	plasma coagulation factor *I*
	platelet factor *2*
Step	Step *I* diet

Expressions	*Examples*
Level	level *I* trauma center
	level *III* lymph node
	amnesia levels *I-VIII*
	cognitive function scale *I-VIII*
	Clark level *III* melanoma
Class	class *III* antigens
	cardiac status: class *IV*
	class *III* malocclusion
	class I-V Pap test
	class *II* malignancy*
Technique	Coffey technique *III*
	Bruce *II* protocol
Stage	stage *I* coma
	lues *II* (secondary syphilis)
	Billroth *I* (first stage of an operation)
	Tanner *IV*
	decubitus ulcer stage *IV*
	Binet stage C (anemia and thrombocytopenia)
Cancer stages	stage *I-IV**
Grade	grade *IV* astrocytoma
	grade *II* hip dysplasia
	cognitive scale rating *I-VIII*
Histological grades	grade *1*
Heart murmurs	grade *2* systolic murmur (also expressed in a sort of fraction fashion: grade *3/6* [grade three over six])
	TIMI grade *3*
Miscellaneous	Schedule *II* drugs
	Chiari *II* syndrome
	Axis *I-V* (psychiatric diagnoses) *(Note: See page 353 for a description of the 5 axis expressions)*
	Sensolog *III* pacemaker
	Natural-Knee *II* systems prosthesis
	DSM-*IV* (fourth edition of handbook)
	GP *IIb/IIIa* (drug)
	alpha *II*†

Pregnancy and delivery are expressed by using the words *gravida* for the number of pregnancies and *para* to indicate the number of deliveries. On occasion, the dictator will also specify the number of abortions. Again, follow the preference of the author of the material in using these traditional expressions. These may be written in the following manner:

gravida 2 para 2

gravida 2 para 2 abortus 0

Some dictators abbreviate the three main topics with *GPA* after the topic "obstetrics."

---

*Cancer stages and classes are Roman; cancer grades are Arabic.
†The symbols for Greek letters cannot be made on a standard keyboard so the names are written out. The most commonly used letters are lowercase *alpha, beta, gamma, delta, lambda,* and *theta.*

EXAMPLE

OB: G3 P3 A0

Another method for representing a patient's obstetric history is the use of a set of four numbers to indicate the number of pregnancies resulting in term deliveries, the number of deliveries of premature infants, the number of abortions, and the number of living children. These are separated with a hyphen.

EXAMPLE

OB: Gravida 5 para 4-1-0-5

This expression indicates that the patient who has been pregnant (gravida) five times; has delivered four infants at term, one prematurely; had no abortions; and has five living children. This is called TPAL terminology. It is easily found on the Internet by entering *TPAL*.

 5-3 SELF-STUDY

DIRECTIONS: Imagine that you hear the following phonetic words, phrases, or sentences. On a separate sheet of paper, retype the sentences properly. Watch for the proper use of capitalization and punctuation.

1. unfortunately the last biopsy revealed that his carcinoma has changed from a class one to a class three malignancy
2. bleeding was controlled with "two oh" ties
3. there are well healed incisions beneath each areolar border from three through nine oclock.
4. the doctor's callback time is every day at four oh clock
5. i was called to the "ee are" at three in the morning where i performed an emergency tracheotomy on a four day old male infant. i remained in attendance for two hours to be sure he was out of danger
6. he came in for a class three flight physical
7. he has passed the five year mark without any evidence of a recurrence
8. he has a grade two hip dysplasia
9. the patient had respiratory paralysis due to injury of spinal nerves "see three through see five"
10. this is her fourth admittance this year

After you have checked your answers, retype any questions you missed so that you have the opportunity to produce the sentences correctly. Check your answers in Appendix A, p. 438.

 5-4 PRACTICE TEST

DIRECTIONS: Follow the directions given in Self-Study 5-3.

1. we must watch mrs olsen carefully because she has two stage three decubitus ulcers on her dorsal spine and one stage two on her right heel
2. she was gravida six para four one one four and denied venereal disease but gave a history of vaginal discharge
3. i can see only fifteen to twenty patients a day
4. please order twelve two gauge needles
5. use only one eighth teaspoonful
6. the dorsalis pedis pulses were two plus and equal bilaterally
7. the ear was injected with two percent xylocaine and one to six thousand adrenalin
8. please check the reading in "vee four" again
9. at precisely "oh seven thirty" she delivered a "thirty four hundred gram" infant with apgar scores of nine at one minute and nine at five minutes
10. please recheck those "e-see-gee" limb lead readings from lead one and lead two

After you have checked your answers, retype any questions you missed so that you have the opportunity to produce the sentences correctly. Check your answers in Appendix A, p. 438.

USE OF SYMBOLS

You will notice many symbols printed in medical journals and texts, but the only symbols this book considers are those generally used in medical transcription. However, there are many symbols on the "hidden keyboard" of computers. The MT needs to be able to find these symbols and use them when appropriate. For example, some MTs avoid using the degree symbol because it is not represented on the standard keyboard. This practice may be unacceptable to some dictators, and so you must learn how to access this symbol on your computer.

Symbols are substitutes for words and may be useful and desirable to speed up reading and comprehension.

SYMBOL	MEANS	EXPLANATION
&	and	symbol is called an *ampersand*
°C	degree Celsius	degree symbol
°F	degree Fahrenheit	degree symbol
=	equals	on the keyboard
-	minus *or* to	made with the hyphen
#	number	on the keyboard
/	per *or* over	made with the slash
:	ratio	made with the colon
%	percent	on the keyboard
+	plus	on the keyboard
×	times *or* by	the lowercase x

NOTE: Some printers and/or electronic record system applications cannot recognize the *&, °C, °F,* bold, superscript, or subscript; be sure of this restriction before you use any of these symbols.

RULE 5.29 Use symbols *only* when they occur in immediate association with a number written as a figure.

EXAMPLES

You Hear	You Type
eight by three	*8 × 3*
four to five	*4 to 5 or 4-5*
number three oh	*#3-0*
pulses are two plus	pulses are *2+* (not *two +*)
vision is twenty twenty	vision is *20/20*
times two	*×2*
six per day	*6 per day*
diluted one to ten	diluted *1:10*
at a minus two	at a *−2*
sixty over forty	*60/40*
grade four over five grade	*4/5*
patient had nocturia times two	patient had nocturia *×2* (not *nocturia × two*)
performed a tee and a	performed a *T&A*
25 millimeters per hour	*25 mm/h or 25 mm per hour*

You Hear	You Type
extension limited by forty-five percent	extension limited by *45%*
thirty degrees celsius	*30°C or 30 degrees Celsius*
seventy five to eighty percent	*75% to 80%* (repeat the % percent symbol)

NOTE: You may spell out *degrees Celsius* or *degrees Fahrenheit,* but do not use the word *degrees* with the abbreviation *C* or *F.* It is also correct to simply type the temperature with or without the symbol or the word *degree* if it is dictated that way.

EXAMPLES

The patient's admitting temperature was 99. (This is correct if it was dictated this way.)

99 degrees, 99°F, and 99 degrees Fahrenheit are also correct expressions.

The patient's admitting temperature was 99 degrees F. (Incorrect)

The patient's admitting temperature was 99° Fahrenheit. (Incorrect)

NOTE: The *percent symbol (%)* is used only with a specific number; write out *percent* or *percentage* when referring in general to an amount stated as a percentage.

EXAMPLE

What *percentage* of the class earned an A on that last test?

Be consistent when you have a choice. Further illustration of symbol usage is combined with the discussion of abbreviations.

USE OF ABBREVIATIONS, ACRONYMS, INITIALISMS, AND BRIEF FORMS

Acronyms are words that are formed from the letters of the abbreviations. Sometimes they spell actual words (*AIDS, HOPE, CAT*), and other times a combination is pronounced as if it were a word (*CABG, cabbage; ARC, ark; ECMO; PERLA*).

An *initialism* is an abbreviation in which each letter of the abbreviation is pronounced: *CBC, T&A, CHF, b.i.d., DNA.*

Some abbreviations are said as a word but are always typed as an abbreviation: *milligrams* becomes *mg; doctor* as a title becomes *Dr; mister* as a title becomes *Mr.* An *abbreviation* is the term used to describe all these handy and troublemaking symbols of whole words and expressions.

Finally, there are brief forms or short forms of words. Some of these (such as *Pap smear*) include the shortened form or abbreviated form of a word (*Papanicolaou*) with the noun (*smear* or *test*). In others (such as *C-section*), a capital letter (in this case, *C*) is used to stand for a term *(caesarean)*. Other examples include *afib,* which is short for *atrial fibrillation,* and *T max,* which is the patient's maximum temperature.

The most difficult of these to deal with are acronyms, because when we hear a familiar word, we do not know whether we are, in fact, dealing with an abbreviation or a word. Look at these examples of what you might hear:

The patient was given a *cage* screen. (This is a *CAGE* screen. *CAGE* is an acronym for questions about drinking alcohol: *cutting, annoyance, guilt, eye-opener.*)

We need to consider using a *tens* unit. (This is a *TENS* unit. *TENS* is an acronym for *transcutaneous electrical nerve stimulation.*)

For reconstruction we plan to use a *tram* flap. (A *TRAM* flap is used for reconstruction after a mastectomy. *TRAM* is an acronym for *transverse rectus abdominis myocutaneous.*)

He was given an *ace* inhibitor for his hypertension. (By now, you have figured out that must be an *ACE inhibitor.*)

Sometimes the construction of the sentence will help alert you to the possibility of an acronym, or the word simply makes no sense as it is. Of importance is that you can be alert for these.

Medicine, like other technical fields, involves the use of many abbreviations and symbols that are particularly familiar to the medical writer and reader; this section is a guide to the proper use of these shortened forms.

It is difficult for the beginning MT to know exactly how abbreviations should be typed. In addition, some abbreviations are typed with all capital letters, some in lowercase, and some in a combination of the two. They are written with or without periods. Chapter 3 contains a punctuation rule for the use of periods with abbreviations; that rule is repeated in this chapter, and so you need not turn back for review.

Symbols and abbreviations can save time, space, and energy and can prevent the needless duplication of repetitious words. The overuse of abbreviations is to be avoided, however; only standard abbreviations should appear in the patient's record where permitted.

Hospitals and other medical facilities often have lists of abbreviations that are acceptable for use in their facilities. The MT transcribing chart notes for the medical office or emergency department has far greater latitude in using abbreviations than do hospital MTs, dictation editors, or those employed by transcription services. However, medical office, emergency department, and hospital "shortcuts" and hieroglyphics should be confined to memos and telephone messages.

Furthermore, abbreviations of any type should never be used when there is a chance of misinterpretation. To add to the problem, some references may be inconsistent with regard to both the capitalization and the punctuation of abbreviations. When in doubt (and you know the meaning of the abbreviation), spell it out. Do not abbreviate expressions that were not dictated as abbreviations; for example, do not type *t.i.d.* if the dictator said *three times a day.*

Neil M. Davis offers this warning in his book *Medical Abbreviations:*

> *"Abbreviations are a convenience, a time saver, a space saver, and a way of avoiding the possibility of misspelling words. However, a price can be paid for their use. Abbreviations are sometimes not understood. They can be misread, or are interpreted incorrectly. Their use lengthens the time needed to train individuals in the health fields, wastes the time of healthcare workers in tracking down their meaning, at times delays the patient's care, and occasionally results in patient harm."*

(From Davis NM: *Medical abbreviations: 30,000 conveniences at the expense of communication and safety,* ed 14, Warminster, Pa., 2008, Neil M Davis Associates.)

RULE 5.30 Do *not* abbreviate the names of drugs or medications. Do *not* use abbreviations in the following parts of the patient's medical record: admission and discharge diagnoses, preoperative and postoperative diagnoses, names of surgical procedures, the names of diseases or syndromes, and orders for nursing care.

EXAMPLES

Discharge diagnosis: *PID* (Incorrect)

Discharge diagnosis: *Pelvic inflammatory disease* (Correct)

Postoperative diagnosis: *OMChS* (Incorrect)

Postoperative diagnosis: *Otitis media, chronic, suppurating* (Correct)

Operation performed: *T&A* (Incorrect)

Operation performed: *Tonsillectomy and adenoidectomy* (Correct)

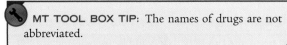

MT TOOL BOX TIP: The names of drugs are not abbreviated.

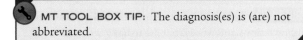

MT TOOL BOX TIP: The diagnosis(es) is (are) not abbreviated.

RULE 5.31 Use symbols and abbreviations in the medical record only when they have been approved by the medical staff and there is an explanatory legend available (to authorized users) to make entries in the medical record and to those who must interpret the entries. (See Table 5-1 for a list of illegal abbreviations that should not be used.)

> **NOTE:** These lists vary, of course, among institutions. Obtain lists from the institutions for which you work and refer to the lists carefully.

RULE 5.32 Spell out an abbreviation when you realize there could be a misinterpretation of the definition. You must be certain, of course, that *your* interpretation is correct; otherwise leave it alone or flag the transcript for the dictator to interpret. Be particularly careful with medicolegal documents.

EXAMPLE

The patient had a history of CVRD. (This could mean *cardiovascular renal disease* or *cardiovascular respiratory disease*. The MT should not expand it, but flag it if the meaning is unclear from context.)

 MT TOOL BOX TIP: Expand ambiguous abbreviations for a work-smart tool.

RULE 5.33 Use an abbreviation to refer to a test, committee, drug, procedure, and so on in a report or paper *after* the term has been used once in its completely spelled-out form.

EXAMPLE

All newborns are routinely tested for *phenylketonuria (PKU)*. As a result, the incidence of *PKU* as a cause of infant…

RULE 5.34 Check any unfamiliar abbreviations or those that seem inappropriate with your reference lists. Initialisms can sound alike.

EXAMPLE

I performed an *IND*… (It could be interpreted as *I&D, IMD, IMB, IMP,* or *IME* and so on. This list could go on and on.)

RULE 5.35 Type as abbreviations the familiar, common abbreviations and words that are usually seen as abbreviations.

EXAMPLES

Mr	Dr	Mrs	a.m.	p.m.	CBC	C-section
DNA	ER	pH	Rh	ED	ICU	

Appendix B contains a brief list of some abbreviations, acronyms, and short forms that are commonly used in office chart notes and hospital records. You might want to remove it from the book or photocopy it and place it in your standard-size, three-ring binder for a quick reference. Later, you can add new abbreviations that you discover along with the institution-approved list. You also could add a few pronunciation hints from time to time. Be alert to unusual abbreviations and record them for future reference; for example, *CAMP factor* but *cAMP receptor*, *rDNA* (recombinant DNA), *F2N test* (finger to nose), *FOOSH* injury (fell on outstretched hand), *5′ SeeNT* (five prime nucleotidase), and *C1q* (assay).

RULE 5.36 Use abbreviations for all metric measurements used *with* numbers.

 MT TOOL BOX TIP: Metric units are abbreviated when used with numbers.

 MT TOOL BOX TIP: Metric abbreviations are not punctuated.

EXAMPLES

You Hear	*You Type*
five by six centimeters	5 × 6 *cm*
one millimeter	1 *mm*
five grams	5 *g*
two liters	2 *L*
two and a half meters	2.5 *m* (not 2-1/2)
ten centimeters	10 *cm*
point five millimeters	0.5 *mm*
seven milliliters	7 *mL*
twenty kilograms	20 *kg* (not *kilos*)
thirty seven degrees celsius	37°C
six milligrams	6 *mg*

NOTE: There was only *a centimeter* difference between the two. (No abbreviation)

NOTE: Do not separate the figure from the abbreviation that follows it. If the figure occurs at the end of a line, carry to the next line so it will appear with the abbreviation.

EXAMPLES

Correct:

. . . . .There was *1400 mL* of serosanguineous fluid.

or

.... There was
1400 mL of serosanguineous fluid.

Incorrect:

.... There was *1400
mL* of serosanguineous fluid.

For example, you can keep this set together by using the nonbreaking space provided in your software program. In some Microsoft Word programs, you can press Option + Spacebar to carry the entire expression to the next line. You can do the same for the hyphen. When you have *x-ray* at the end of the line and do not want it to separate, carry out the same function so the expression will be intact on the next line: press Option + Hyphen. Other programs require that you press Ctrl + Shift + Hyphen or Ctrl + Shift + Space.

RULE 5.37 Periods are used with some single capitalized words and single-letter abbreviations.

EXAMPLES

Inc.   Ltd.
Joseph P. Myers   *E. coli*

▶ Punctuate the name of the genus when it is abbreviated and used with the species name.

E. coli   M. tuberculosis   E. histolytica

NOTE: Some professionals are omitting the period after the genus abbreviation.

▶ Brief forms are not punctuated.

Sed rate   exam   phenobarb
Pap smear   flu   lab

▶ Lowercase abbreviations made up of single letters.
a.m.   p.m.   e.g.   t.i.d.

▶ Units of measurement are *not* punctuated.

wpm   mph   mg   mL   mm
L   cm   km   g

▶ Certification, registration, and licensure abbreviations are *not* punctuated.

CMA-A   CMT   RN   RRA   ART   LVN

▶ Acronyms are *not* punctuated.

CARE   Project HOPE   AIDS   ELISA   PET

▶ Most abbreviations typed in full capital letters are *not* punctuated.

UCLA	PKU	BUN	CBC	WBC	COPD
D&C	T&A	I&D	P&A	NBC	FICA
KEZL	TV	FM	AM	PM	

MT TOOL BOX TIP: Capital letter abbreviations are not punctuated.

▶ Scientific abbreviations written in a combination of capital and lowercase letters are *not* punctuated.

Rx   Dx   ACh   Ba   Hb   IgG   mEq   NaCl
mOsm   Rh   pH

▶ Academic degrees and religious orders are now *generally* not punctuated.

MD   PhD   DDS   BVE   MS   SJ

(This is also Rule 3.16.)

RULE 5.38 Chemical and mathematical abbreviations are written in a combination of both uppercase and lowercase letters without periods. These abbreviations are not substituted for the spoken word; for example, if *potassium* is dictated, do not use *K*.

EXAMPLES

Abbreviation	Meaning
CO_2 (CO2)	carbon dioxide
Hb	hemoglobin
Hg	mercury
Na	sodium
T_4 (T4)	thyroxine
O_2 (O2)	oxygen
Ca	calcium ion
NaCl	sodium chloride
DNA	deoxyribonucleic acid
HCl	hydrochloric acid
10^4	ten to the fourth
K	potassium
pH	hydrogen ion concentration

NOTE: The *pH* of a substance is a measure of its acidity or alkalinity (ranging from 0 to 14). It is indicated with a whole number or a whole number and a decimal fraction. If there is no following fraction, this is indicated with a zero (0).

Dictated: the patient had a pee h of five point two.
Transcribed: The patient had a *pH* of *5.2*.

Dictated: pee h was seven.
Transcribed: The *pH was 7.0*.

Since no following number was dictated, the zero is added. We do not expand the abbreviation to its meaning: *hydrogen ion concentration*.

Dictated: The dee en a is unavailable for further study.
Transcribed: The DNA is unavailable for further study.

Dictated: stat report shows sodium one hundred thirty eight milliequivalents per liter potassium three point three milliequivalents per liter chloride ninety seven milliequivalents per liter and a total see oh two of five milliequivalents per liter blood glucose is seven hundred milligrams percent.

Transcribed: STAT report shows sodium 138 mEq/L, potassium 3.3 mEq/L, chloride 97 mEq/L, and a total CO_2 of 5 mEq/L. Blood glucose is 700 mg%. (Not mg percent or milligrams percent)

NOTE: You may use a slash to express *per* in technical expressions when at least one element is a number: for example, Respirations: *60/min.*

RULE 5.39 Latin abbreviations are typed in lowercase letters, with periods.

MT TOOL BOX TIP: Latin abbreviations are punctuated.

EXAMPLES

Abbreviation	Meaning
t.i.d.	three times a day
q.i.d.	four times a day
a.m.	antemeridian (before noon)
p.m.	postmeridian (after noon)
p.c.	after meals
a.c.	before meals

EXCEPTION: *A.D.* (in the year of Our Lord)

NOTE: It has become acceptable to write *a.m.* and *p.m.* in capital letters. This form is not punctuated: *AM* and *PM.*

RULE 5.40 Do *not* abbreviate proper names unless the name is abbreviated in the correspondent's letterhead. Shortened forms of a person's name, such as nicknames, are allowed in the salutation.

EXAMPLE

Steven J. Clayborn and *Dear Steve:*

NOTE: Do not use *Geo.* or *Chas.* with a last name unless thus abbreviated in the letterhead.

NOTE: Some nicknames might not be a shortened form but rather the entire name.

EXAMPLES

Ray	Gene	Will	Al	Alex
Ben	Ed	Fred	Sam	Pat
Beth	Hugh	Betty	Rob	Dan

Do *not* abbreviate in these other cases:

▶ Titles other than *Dr, Mr, Mrs,* and *Ms,* unless a first name or initial accompanies the last name.

EXAMPLES

Maj. Ralph Emery but Major Emery

Hon. John Wilson but Honorable Wilson

Rt. Rev. Donald Turnbridge but Right Reverend Turnbridge

MT TOOL BOX TIP: Titles no longer require punctuation when abbreviated; it is an option (e.g., Mr, Dr, Ms).

▶ The words *street, road, avenue, boulevard, north, south, east,* and *west* in an inside address. However, *Southwest (SW), Northwest (NW),* and so on, are abbreviated *after* the street name.

EXAMPLES

936 *North* Branch *Street*

1876 Washington *Boulevard NW*

▶ Days of the week and months of the year. To avoid confusion, numbers should not be substituted for the names of the months in correspondence; however, they are acceptable in other records and reports.

EXAMPLE

January 11, 20XX (Narrative copy)

NOT: Jan 11, 20XX *or* 1-11-0X *or* 1/11/XX *or* 01-11-XX

Typing Drugs

As a review of some of the rules, these are some hints for typing drug information into documents when numbers and symbols are used.

▶ Metric units of measure are used in abbreviated form with numerals. They are not made plural.

25 mg   0.50 mg   150 mL   2 cm

▶ Dosage instructions are preferably written in lowercase letters with periods separating the initials.

p.o.   t.i.d.   q.i.d.   b.i.d.   p.r.n.   q.4 h.

▶ Do not separate the number at the end of the line from the symbols that may follow.

25 mg (Correct)
. 25
mg (Incorrect)

▶ Do not use either the lowercase or capital letter *o* on the keyboard for zero; use the zero symbol.

50 mg (Correct)
5O mg (Incorrect)
5o mg (Incorrect)

▶ Brand or trade name drugs and methods of administration are capitalized; generic and chemical names are not.

Dalmane (brand name)

Gris-PEG (brand name)

Humalog KwikPen (brand name drug and trademarked packaging form)

captopril (generic name)

▶ It is not necessary to follow an unusual capital letter–small letter combination or all capital letter spelling given by the drug company unless you or your employer wishes it. However, someone might like to keep a name like *pHisoHex* intact, but it is not necessary. Use a capital letter after a hyphen in a brand-name drug.

Di-Delamine (Correct)

HydroDIURIL (*Hydrodiuril* also correct)

Neggram (NegGram), Rhogam (RhoGAM), Tace (TACE)

▶ Drugs in a simple narration, especially without dosages given, are separated by commas.

The patient was discharged home on *Lanoxin, Calan, and Solu-Medrol.*

▶ In a more complex combination, when commas are needed within a string of information concerning a single drug, the units are separated by semicolons.

MEDICATIONS: She will continue her 1800-calorie ADA diet and usual medicines, which include the following: estradiol, micronized, 2 mg/d for 25 of 30 days; propoxyphene HCl 65 mg q.i.d., which is an increase from her current t.i.d. regimen; flurazepam HCl 30 mg at bedtime; hydrocodone bitartrate 5 mg; ibuprofen 600 mg q.i.d.

▶ A complex string is easier to read in stacked-list format:

MEDICATIONS

1. Continue her 1800-calorie ADA diet.
2. Estradiol (micronized) 2 mg/d for 25 of 30 days.

3. Flurazepam HCl 30 mg at bedtime.
4. Hydrocodone bitartrate 5 mg b.i.d.
5. Acetaminophen 500 mg b.i.d.
6. Ibuprofen 600 mg q.i.d.
7. Levothyroxine sodium 25 mg/d.
8. Metoprolol tartrate 25 mg/d.
9. Prednisone 5 mg/d.
10. Propoxyphene HCl 65 mg q.i.d. (which is an increase from her current t.i.d. regimen).

Periods are included at the end of each medication to alert the reader that the item is complete.

ABBREVIATION REFERENCE

See Appendix B for a list of some abbreviations commonly used in the completion of medical office and hospital reports of all types. This list is not comprehensive, but it will be helpful to you when you complete the exercises. The list will serve as a reference for your exercises and as an illustration of the variety of ways that many common abbreviations are typed: all capital letters, combination of capital letters and lowercase letters, and all lowercase letters. The italics indicate how acronyms are pronounced. Furthermore, you should know that abbreviations, symbols, and contractions are used far more freely in chart notes (progress notes) and in history and physical examination reports than they are in a discharge summary, an operative report, a legal report, or formal correspondence. For example, you would type *The GU tract was clear* in the patient's medical office record, but you would type *The genitourinary tract was clear* in a report to an insurance examiner. The medical office record might note that *the pt had an appy on 7-1-XX* and *she's waiting for the results of a cysto.* The letter to another physician would report that *the patient had an appendectomy on July 1, 20XX;* likewise, *she is waiting for the results of a cystoscopy.*

Also in Appendix B is a list of short forms (brief forms) and medical slang. Some words, such as *C-section* and *Pap smear,* do not fall in a set category.

 5-5 PRACTICE TEST

DIRECTIONS: Study the Abbreviation Reference and type the answers to the questions on a separate sheet of paper.

1. You hear: "eye gee gee."

   You type: _____

2. You hear: "fifteen millimeters of mercury."

   You type: _____

3. You hear: "ten to the fourth."

   You type: _____

4. You hear: "blood is are-h negative."

   You type: _____

5. You hear: "clear to pee-en a."

   You type: _____

6. You hear: "h double e en tee."

   You type: _____

7. You hear: "take one bee eye dee pee are en for pain."

   You type: _____

8. You hear: "h en pee."

   You type: _____

9. You hear: "pee oh two."

   You type: _____

10. You hear: "acetylcholine."

   You type: _____

5-6 SELF-STUDY

DIRECTIONS: Imagine that you hear the following phonetic phrases or sentences. On a separate sheet of paper, retype the sentences and phrases properly. Watch for proper use of symbols, numbers, abbreviations, punctuation, and capitalization.

EXAMPLE

You hear: the "pee-h" was seven neutrality just between alkalinity and acidity

You type: The *pH* was 7.0: neutrality; just between alkalinity and acidity.

1. flexion was limited to fifteen degrees extension to ten degrees adduction to ten degrees and abduction to twenty degrees

2. by use of a half inch osteotome one centimeter of the proximal end of the proximal phalanx was removed

3. "dee tee arz" are one to two plus

4. range of motion of the neck is limited to approximately seventy percent of normal

5. the date on the cholecystogram was september one two thousand and nine

6. estimated blood loss was one hundred milliliters; none was replaced

7. at two "ay-em" the patients temperature was thirty eight point nine degrees celsius

8. the "pee-ay" and right lateral roentgenograms show a fracture of the right third and fourth ribs

9. lenses were prescribed resulting in improvement of his visual acuity to twenty thirty in the right eye and twenty forty five in the left eye. the visual field examination was normal and the tension is seventeen millimeters of mercury of schiotz with a five point five gram weight

10. she has one sister who is "ellen w"

11. i removed six hundred milliliters of serosanguineous fluid from the abdomen

12. we need to use thirty five millimeter film for this process

After you have checked your answers, retype any questions you missed so that you have the opportunity to produce the sentences correctly. Check your answers in Appendix A, p. 439.

 ## 5-7 PRACTICE TEST

DIRECTIONS: Follow the instructions given in Self-Study 5-6.

1. hemoglobin on seven twenty seven was eleven point two grams hematocrit was thirty seven

2. did you know that the postal rates were twenty five cents for the first ounce and twenty cents for each additional ounce to mail something first class in nineteen eighty nine

3. the protein was sixty five milligrams percent

4. electromyography shows a three plus sparsity in the orbicularis oris

5. an estimated point two milliliters of viscid fluid was removed from the middle ear cavity

6. he entered the "e-are" at four "ay-em" with a temperature of ninety nine

7. there was a reduction of the angle to within a two degree difference

8. take fifty milligrams per day

9. i then placed two four by four sponges over the wound

10. the "tee-bee" skin test was diluted one to one hundred

11. drainage amounts to several "see-sees" a day

12. he is to take flurazepam "h-see-el" s thirty milligrams " h-ess "

After your answers have been checked, retype any questions that you missed so that you have the opportunity of producing the sentences correctly. Check your answers in Appendix A, p. 439.

 ## 5-8 SELF-STUDY

DIRECTIONS: Follow the instructions given in Self-Study 5-6.

1. the urine was negative for sugar, "pee-h" was seven and specific gravity was one point zero one two

2. the "bee-you-en" is forty five milligrams percent, one plus protein

3. i excised a small well circumscribed tumor two millimeters in diameter

4. use a three "em" vi-drape to cover the operative site

5. she received her second dose of "five-ef-you"

6. the culture grew one hundred thousand colonies of e coli per cubic centimeter

7. the surgeon asked for a number seven jackson bronchoscope

8. there were high serum titers of "gee" immunoglobulin antibodies

9. the phenotype "a-two-b" was found consistently in the family blood history

10. respirations sixteen per minute

After you have checked your answers, retype any questions you missed so that you have the opportunity to produce the sentences correctly. Check your answers in Appendix A, p. 440.

5-9 REVIEW TEST

DIRECTIONS: Follow the instructions given in Self-Study 5-6.

1. the patient has a "pee-h" of six point ninety six "pee oh two" of twelve and "pee see oh two" of fifty four

2. there is a one point zero by point five centimeter area of avulsed tissue and a three centimeter gaping deep laceration of the chin

3. lungs clear to "pee and a" heart not enlarged "ay-to" is greater than "pee-to" there was a grade one over six decrescendo early diastolic high frequency murmur

4. cycloplegic refraction "oh-dee" equal plus three point two five plus oh point seven five times one hundred twenty five equals twenty thirty minus one

5. the patient received a six thousand gamma roentgen dose

6. iodipamide sodium "eye" one hundred thirty one was used

7. we used a concentration of five times ten to the fifth per milliliter

8. a dilute solution of one to one was used

9. he was scheduled for a "tee three" uptake

10. aqueous procaine penicillin "gee," four point eight million units intramuscularly with one gram of probenecid orally, is still recommended for uncomplicated gonorrhea

11. she returned today for her vitamin "bee-twelve"

12. my plan was to give her six hundred thousand units of penicillin on the first day and give her half that on the second

13. he denied symptoms of dysuria hematuria and urgency but did report nocturia times two

14. she is to take her medication "cue-four-h" with an additional one half dose "a-see"

15. i have an appointment for the eleventh of june and i need to change it to the first of july

16. six case histories were presented at the tumor board meeting today for a total of ninety seven this year

17. we expect that thousands of students will be able to participate in this surgery through the use of closed circuit "tee vee"

18. he has been a two pack a day cigarette smoker for the last forty years

19. please order six twenty gauge catheters

20. wbc count twenty nine point seven hemoglobin thirteen platelet count three hundred eighty

21. i feel that my fee of twelve hundred dollars is fair

22. the jury awarded one point two million dollars in damages to the parents of the child

23. i removed a forty five slug from the left lower liver margin

24. how many centimeters long was that tear in her thumb

25. the hemoglobin was eight point eight, hematocrit twenty six point five white blood cells eight thousand one hundred with eighty segs and eighteen lymphs

26. you will notice that the standard leads one, two, "a vee el" and "a vee ef" are missing in the "ee-see-gee" lead-sequencing formats

27. then five milliliters of one percent lidocaine was injected into the right breast at the four oclock and eight oclock areas

28. we will check a "pee ess ay" and "kem seven" today

29. the six by seven millimeter nodule was treated with shave biopsy and "ee-dee-en-see" in three layers

30. a twenty-four french foley with a thirty "see-see" balloon two way was advanced up the urethra

POSTSCRIPT

Some of the phrases and expressions discussed in this chapter occur frequently in dictation and are worthy of mention one more time. Be sure that you are able to use them correctly.

You Hear	*Properly Transcribed*
it was her fifth admission.	It was her *fifth* admission. (Also *5th*)
will be admitted at four pee em	will be admitted at *4 p.m.* (*PM*)
came to see me at four o clock	came to see me at *4 o'clock* (or *four* o'clock)
ay two is greater than pee two	*A2* is greater than *P2* (or A_2 and P_2)
vision is twenty twenty	vision is *20/20*
a twenty nine year old	a *29-year-old*
taken tee i dee for three days	taken *t.i.d.* for *3 days*
ninety nine degrees	*99°* (*99 degrees*)
diluted one to ten	diluted *1:10*
sixty-five milligrams percent	*65 mg%*
bee pee is one hundred over eighty	*BP is 100/80*
forty five degree angle	*45°* angle (also *45-degree* angle)
ten percent weight loss	*10%* weight loss
twenty-one gauge needle	*21-gauge* needle
sutured with three oh chromic	sutured with *3-0* chromic
injected with point five percent	injected with *0.5%*
used three four by fours	used *three 4 × 4s*
nocturia times two	nocturia *×2*
one plus protein	*1+* protein
drink seven hundred fifty milliliters per twelve hour period	drink *750 mL/12-hour period* (also *750 mL per 12-hour period*)
herniated disk at tee three four	herniated disk at *T3-4* (or T_{3-4})
dorsalis pedis pulses were two plus	dorsalis pedis pulses were *2+*
class two infection	class *II* infection
cranial nerves two through twelve	cranial nerves *II-XII* (also *2-12*)
cut was ten centimeters long	cut was *10 cm* long
fifteen millimeters of mercury	*15 mmHg*
the pee h was seven	the *pH* was *7.0*
he takes two pee see	he takes *2 p.c.*
seen on four twenty-one	seen on *April 21*
platelet count three hundred forty	platelet count *340,000*

SYMBOL AND NUMBER RULE SYNOPSIS

ELEMENT	RULE	PAGE
General		
Abbreviations and numbers	5.15	125
Date	5.1, 5.16	122, 126
Decimals	5.24, 5.25	130
Dimensions	5.19	127
Fractions	5.5, 5.24	123, 130
Indefinite expressions	5.4	123
Large numbers	5.8, 5.10, 5.27	124, 130
Metric numbers		121
Money	5.13	125
Multiple use of numbers	5.2, 5.6, 5.11, 5.24, 5.26	122, 123, 124, 130
Numbers in the address	5.1	122
Ordinal numbers (first, second)	5.1	122
Spelled-out numbers	5.2 to 5.8	122 to 124
Time of day	5.7, 5.9, 5.17	123, 124, 127
Unrelated numbers	5.26	130
Written-out numbers	5.2 to 5.8	122 to 124
Technical		
Abbreviations	5.30 to 5.40	135 to 138
Capitalization of abbreviations	5.37	137
Chemical abbreviations	5.38	137
Dilute solutions	5.22	129
Electrocardiographic leads	5.21, 5.28	128, 132
Figures with plus or minus	5.23	129
Foreign abbreviations	5.39	138
Greek letters	5.28	132
Metric abbreviations	5.36	136
Military time	5.17	127
Subscript and superscript	5.10	124
Suture materials	5.18	127
Symbols	5.15, 5.29	125, 134
Units of measurement	5.14, 5.19, 5.22	125, 127, 129
Vital statistics	5.14	125
When not to abbreviate	5.30 to 5.32, 5.40	135-136, 138
Miscellaneous		
O'clock area	5.12	125
Punctuation with abbreviations	5.37	137
Ranges	5.22	129
Ratios	5.22	129
Roman numerals	5.28	132
Spacing with symbols	5.15	125
Spinal column and nerves	5.20	128

5
CHAPTER

5-10 METRIC REVIEW TEST

DIRECTIONS: Select the set that is incorrectly expressed in the groups that follow. Place the answer in the blank provided.

1. _____

    a. meter - basic word for distance
    b. liter - basic word for volume
    c. gram - basic word for liquid
    d. Celsius - basic word for temperature

2. _____

    a. g is the abbreviation for gram
    b. mL is the abbreviation for milliliter
    c. cm is the abbreviation for centimeter
    d. kilo is the abbreviation for kilogram

3. _____

    a. 25 mg
    b. 0.25 mg
    c. 25 mg.
    d. 0.025 mg

4. _____

    a. 3.5 L
    b. 3 Ls
    c. 3000 mL
    d. 3 L

5. _____

    a. degree Celsius
    b. °C
    c. °Celsius
    d. degrees C

6. _____

    a. 2-1/2 km
    b. 0.25 km
    c. 25 km
    d. 2.5 km

INSTRUCTOR'S REVIEW TEST

In this multiple-choice test, you will review some of the things you learned in this chapter and in previous chapters. Be alert to punctuation, capitalization, numbers, abbreviations, and medical records.

DIRECTIONS: Select the best answer and write the corresponding letter on the line provided.

1. What is "mmHg" an abbreviation for, other than millimeters of mercury? _____
    a. specific gravity
    b. urinalysis
    c. barometric reading
    d. acid-base

2. Select the word group that is correctly expressed. _____
   a. S-1, S-2 fracture
   b. self-administration
   c. mid-line incision
   d. three fold error

3. Select the sentence that is the preferred expression. _____
   a. Her next clinical appointment is for July 15, 20XX, for further tests.
   b. Her next clinical appointment is for July 15, 20XX for further tests.
   c. Her next clinical appointment is for July 15 20XX for further tests.
   d. Her next clinical appointment is for 7-15-XX for further tests.

4. Please select the correct sentence in the following: _____
   a. Neither of my sister-in-laws' health records was faxed to the office.
   b. Neither of my sisters-in-law's health records was faxed to the office.
   c. Neither of my sisters'-in-laws health records was faxed to the office.
   d. Neither of my sisters-in-laws' health records was faxed to the office.

5. What is the Latin abbreviation for "that is"? _____
   a. etc.
   b. e.g.
   c. i.e.
   d. ibid.

6. In addition to the period, which other punctuation mark is always placed inside the closing quotes? _____
   a. question mark
   b. comma
   c. exclamation point
   d. semicolon

7. What is the correct way to transcribe "one-half centimeter"? _____
   a. one-half cm
   b. .5 cm
   c. 1/2 cm
   d. 0.5 cm

8. Which of the following sentences is *correctly* punctuated? _____
   a. The patient had an acute cellulitis; and he was admitted to the hospital.
   b. The patient had an acute cellulitis, and he was admitted to the hospital.
   c. The patient had an acute cellulitis, he was admitted to the hospital.
   d. The patient had an acute cellulitis and, he was admitted to the hospital.

9. The primary reason for a medical record is _____
   a. to assist in treatment and diagnosis of a patient.
   b. for defense in a possible law suit.
   c. for research and diagnostic analysis.
   d. to comply with the law.

10. A semicolon is used _____
    a. to separate two independent clauses with a conjunction.
    b. to separate two independent clauses without a conjunction.
    c. to introduce a list.
    d. with a salutation in a business letter.

11. Which sentence is correct? _____
    a. Several physicians' opinions' were considered.
    b. Several physician's opinions were considered.
    c. Several physicians opinion's were considered.
    d. Several physicians' opinions were considered.

12. Which of the following *unpunctuated* sentences contains a nonrestrictive (also called *nonessential*) clause or phrase? _____
    a. The medical records that require signatures are placed near the dictating station.
    b. Assignment One which I found interesting was supposed to be typed.
    c. The chart was forwarded before I received your instructions.
    d. The patients may be placed in the examination rooms as soon as Dr Hamlyn arrives.

13. Which of the following sentences is *incorrectly* punctuated? _____
    a. Little Brenda is the "perkiest" baby on the pediatric ward.
    b. He has a positive Kehr sign.
    c. I ordered a #7 Jackson bronchoscope.
    d. The infant suffered a compression of the umbilical cord, which resulted in it's death.

14. Select the incorrect expression. _____
    a. the baby was just 3-months-old
    b. the 52-year-old retired secretary
    c. at her 6-month followup visit
    d. a self-inflicted knife wound

15. When can the transcriptionist make a change to a medical report? _____
    a. under no circumstances
    b. only after the dictator sees it
    c. with the risk manager's direction
    d. before it is signed

16. Which of the following sentences is *incorrectly* transcribed? _____
    a. The patient is a 45-year-old male.
    b. The patient is a 45 year old male.
    c. This male patient is 45 years old.
    d. The patient's age is 45 years.

17. Who owns the *information* in the medical record? _____
    a. The patient
    b. The medical records director
    c. The physician who dictated it
    d. The healthcare institution

18. Which of the following parts of speech modifies a verb? _____
    a. adverb
    b. adjective
    c. noun
    d. another verb

19. Which of the following sentences is *incorrectly* punctuated? _____
    a. It is our policy to accept applications from all who offer them.
    b. Please send Mr Smith's records to the VA Hospital.
    c. I want to see this patient back in three week's time.
    d. It's a well-known fact that she's a respected physician.

20. Which of the following is a compound modifier? _____
    a. self-administered
    b. ex-governor
    c. 3-years-old
    d. baby-sit

CHAPTER 6

Letter Transcription

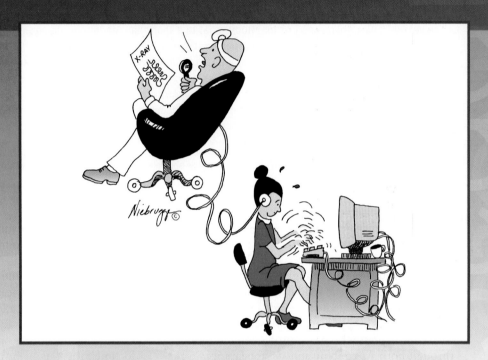

OBJECTIVES

After reading this chapter and completing the exercises, you should be able to

1. Appraise the value of an attractive letter to a business.
2. Assess how the business letter reflects the public image of a medical practice.
3. Describe the specific qualities that make a letter mailable.
4. Demonstrate the three basic mechanical formats of letter preparation.
5. Demonstrate the ability to paragraph properly and to place a letter attractively on a page.
6. Use a specific letter format when preparing a letter from a draft copy that was typed as a single paragraph.
7. Prepare a two-page letter by following the rules for multiple-page letters.
8. Identify the unique format for "To Whom It May Concern" documents.
9. Recognize the use of displayed extract text.

Note from the Author

Correspondence was my first experience with medical transcription, and I was not as good at it as I thought I would be. I knew the proper letter mechanics and had good English grammar skills, so I thought it was going to be easy. It was not. The fact that I could not spell medical words (or understand them, for that matter) in addition to the fact that some English words that I thought I could spell I did not spell correctly, prompted me to go to night school. No, I did not receive any training in medical transcription—it was another 10 years or so before those books and classes became available. I worked on spelling, homonyms, and obscure grammar rules.

I acquired that initial job because I could take shorthand, but it was no time at all before I "talked" my employers into purchasing dictation/transcription equipment. I thought that this step surely would make me a good "medical secretary."* Alas, there was just too much more to it than that: learning to paragraph; putting punctuation marks exactly where they belonged; using numbers and symbols correctly; and making sure the finished document was perfect. ("Perfect" was not a word to be taken lightly, inasmuch as the overall appearance was very important too.) However, I became proficient at doing chart notes and began to enjoy my new skills. When one of the physicians started training me to prepare operative reports, diagnostic studies, history/physical examinations reports, and discharge summaries, I learned that the complexities of doing this job well were very interesting and rewarding. Soon I learned to transcribe and format those difficult letters too. Good luck!

Medical transcriptionist was not a term anyone used in those days. It was many years later, in fact, before the term came into use. No one would have referred to me as a "medical language specialist" either, unless they were part of a stand-up comedy routine.

INTRODUCTION

Letter preparation is unique in many ways and has several special attributes that can make it challenging to plan. These include the following:

▶ The overall appearance; unlike documents that are meant only for the medical record, a letter must be attractive. It is the personal representative of the writer and expresses his or her professional standing through both its content and its appearance. You control its appearance, and you may in part control how it reads; thus, it also represents you. The placement of the letter on the page must be considered, with top and bottom white areas taken into account and with even and equal margins maintained.

▶ Formats are important; traditionally, they are followed exactly.

 MT TOOL BOX TIP: Proper formats for letters are important tools.

▶ Paragraphing is important: the beginner must learn to recognize when shifts to new subject matter occur.
▶ Correct punctuation, although important in all documents, can be a particular challenge in letters.
▶ Shifts of emphasis and format can be confusing. For example, the dictator may decide to place an abbreviated version of the patient's physical examination within the body of the letter. In this situation, the MT cannot expect to provide a strictly traditional document and must know how to handle variations in paragraphing.

▶ Lengthy lists of enclosures and/or courtesy copies can make it difficult to maintain an attractive overall appearance.
▶ Confusing opening and closing remarks can be bewildering to the novice. For example, the dictator may give both a street address and a post office box address, dictate a lengthy reference line that is not in the proper sequence, address the recipient of the document by a name other than the one previously dictated (this may be a mistake or a nickname), close the letter with unusual, nontraditional greetings or salutations (e.g., "Shalom!", "Happy New Year!", or "Kindest personal regards"), or sign off with just a first name instead of the usual full name.

This chapter discusses all of the standard letter transcription practices and introduces some common variations so that you can be confident that you are setting up a document in the best possible way. You are the key factor in turning out this product: the letter.

It is important that the letter be perfect in every way, beginning with "eye appeal" and with great attention to detail. Your success depends on your ability to produce a mailable letter. Therefore, in learning to identify the specific qualities that make a letter mailable, you should also be able to recognize errors in form, grammar, punctuation, typing, and spelling.

 MT TOOL BOX TIP: A tool for formal letter formatting is to provide "eye appeal."

Vocabulary

Open punctuation: Style of letter punctuation in which no punctuation mark is used after the salutation or complimentary close (Figure 6-1, *B*).

Mixed punctuation: Style of letter punctuation in which a colon or a comma (only when a first name is dictated) is used after the salutation and a comma is used after the complimentary close (see Figure 6-1, *A*).

Letter format: The mechanical setup of a letter, which dictates placement of the various letter parts (Figure 6-2).

Continuation sheets: The sheets of paper used to type a second page and subsequent pages of a letter. These are often called *second sheets*.

Full block: The name of a particular letter format (see Figure 6-1, *A*).

Modified block: The name of a particular letter format (see Figure 6-1, *B*).

QUALITIES OF A MAILABLE LETTER

1. *Placement.* The following are important aspects:
   - The content should be attractively placed on the page with the right margin fairly even. Because the right margin is not justified on medical documents, ragged right margins often occur. A maximum of five characters in variation is ideal, but sometimes this is not possible.
   - The letter should have "eye appeal," with the letterhead taken into consideration when format is chosen.
   - The letter should have picture-frame symmetry if possible.
2. *Form.* The following should be taken into consideration:
   - Correct format (such as *full block* or *modified block*).
   - Double spacing between paragraphs.
   - Consistent punctuation (*open* or *mixed*).
   - Correct use of enclosure and copy notations.
3. *Typing techniques.* There should be no keyboarding, formatting, or printout errors, such as improper word wrapping to the next line, incorrect spacing, transposition of words, typographical errors, omitted material, or words divided incorrectly at the end of a line.
4. *Proper mechanics.* You should show proper knowledge of technical writing techniques (e.g., abbreviations, numbers, and symbols). (See Chapter 5.)
5. *Grammar.* The words in the letter should be used correctly in accordance with their meaning (e.g., *all ready/already*).
   - Homonyms should be used correctly (e.g., *their/there, site/sight/cite*).
   - Contractions should be avoided whenever possible.
6. *Spelling.* There must be no doubt about the correct spelling of a word, and references must be consulted without hesitation. (See Chapter 8.)
7. *Overall appearance.* Be sure to check the following:
   - The printout is clear and sharp with no smudges.
   - Page startup and page breaks are correct.
   - Letterhead is not in conflict with printout.
8. *Content.* Be sure of the following:
   - The material is accurate as dictated.
   - No material is omitted.
   - No material is changed to alter the meaning of the letter.

LETTER FORMATS

Secretarial manuals illustrate and name many different formats in which letters may be prepared. The names given to these arrangements vary, but the formats are standard.

The following formats have been named to match closely the names you might already have learned and, at the same time, to describe as nearly as possible the appearance of the letter:

Full block (see Figure 6-1, *A*). The full-block format is the most frequently used format. Notice that the date line, address, salutation, reference line, all lines of the body of the letter, complimentary close, and typed signature line are flush with the left margin. This is a popular format because no tab stops are needed. As long as it is compatible with the letterhead and the wishes of the dictator, you may use it.

Modified block (see Figure 6-1, *B*). In the modified block format, the date line, reference line, complimentary close, and typed signature line are typed to begin just to the right of the middle of the page. This format has a little more "personality" and is compatible with most letterheads. Most dictators are comfortable with the signature area.

Notice that placement of the date line sets your format. If you place the date at the left margin, you must continue with full-block format. If you place your date at the center point, you must follow through with this format, making sure that

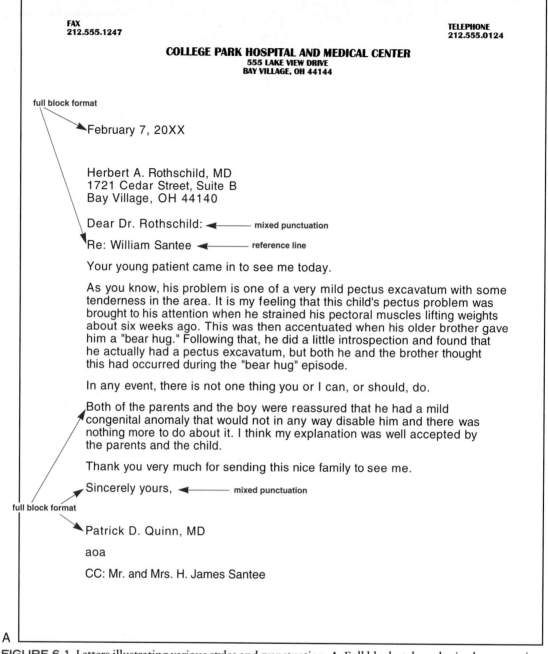

FIGURE 6-1 Letters illustrating various styles and punctuation. **A,** Full block style and mixed punctuation.

the complimentary close and typed signature line are lined up with it.

Modified block with indented paragraphs (see Figure 6-1, *C*). The third and final format is not as popular as the first two because of the tab stops necessary for beginning each paragraph. It is a traditional format and might be preferred by the dictator. Additional formats you may have learned in business typing classes are not used for medical letters because the formats are too informal.

Many general business offices have one letter format that is used by all the transcriptionists in the company, but you might find that there are few formal rules about letter styles for medical dictation.

In the following items, I examine a business letter and discuss its components. Each item refers to a corresponding number in Figure 6-2; refer to this figure as I examine a business letter and discuss its components.

Also, refer to Figure 6-1, *D,* to see how to handle spacing between sections. Note the placement of the

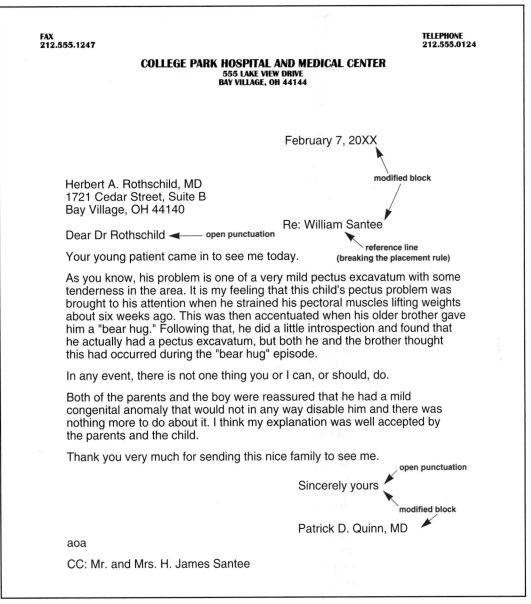

FAX
212.555.1247

TELEPHONE
212.555.0124

COLLEGE PARK HOSPITAL AND MEDICAL CENTER
555 LAKE VIEW DRIVE
BAY VILLAGE, OH 44144

February 7, 20XX

modified block

Herbert A. Rothschild, MD
1721 Cedar Street, Suite B
Bay Village, OH 44140

Re: William Santee

Dear Dr Rothschild ◄──── *open punctuation*

*reference line
(breaking the placement rule)*

Your young patient came in to see me today.

As you know, his problem is one of a very mild pectus excavatum with some tenderness in the area. It is my feeling that this child's pectus problem was brought to his attention when he strained his pectoral muscles lifting weights about six weeks ago. This was then accentuated when his older brother gave him a "bear hug." Following that, he did a little introspection and found that he actually had a pectus excavatum, but both he and the brother thought this had occurred during the "bear hug" episode.

In any event, there is not one thing you or I can, or should, do.

Both of the parents and the boy were reassured that he had a mild congenital anomaly that would not in any way disable him and there was nothing more to do about it. I think my explanation was well accepted by the parents and the child.

Thank you very much for sending this nice family to see me.

open punctuation

Sincerely yours

modified block

Patrick D. Quinn, MD

aoa

CC: Mr. and Mrs. H. James Santee

B

FIGURE 6-1, cont'd B, Modified block style and open punctuation. Illustrates reference line that breaks the placement rule.

reference line in particular, because it was typed in accordance with the "break-the-rule" placement.

> **MT TOOL BOX TIP:** Save and name a new document as soon as you create it.

Item 1: Paper

Standard 8½ × 11-inch, 25% cotton content bond paper is most often used. The paper is usually white, although off-white or eggshell colors may be preferred. Be sure that the paper is compatible with the printer and is inserted properly.

Item 2: Letterhead

The letterhead must be appropriate and current. The physician, clinic, or hospital will use stationery with his or her name (or the corporate name or institution name) and address printed on it. Other information, such as the telephone number, fax number, medical specialty, or board membership, is often included. The letterhead should be confined to the top 2 inches of the page. Avoid a letterhead that is continued to the bottom of the page because it makes placement difficult and the style is unnecessary. Printed borders on the paper are equally distracting.

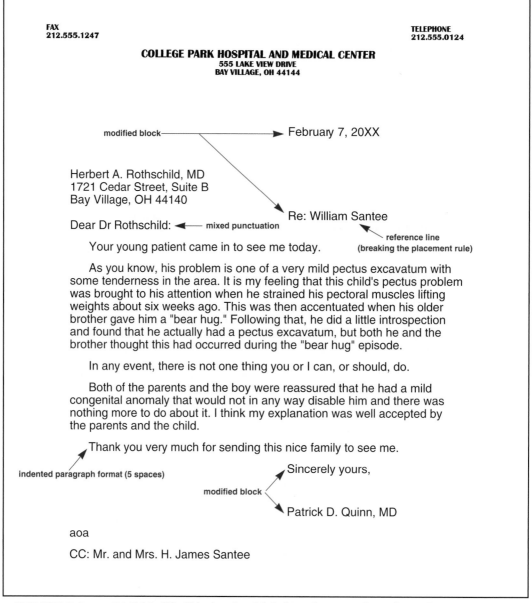

FIGURE 6-1, cont'd C, Modified block style with indented paragraphs and mixed punctuation.

Many physicians choose to have steel-die engraved letterhead. Engraving establishes the finest quality letterhead; it looks professional and further enhances the appearance of the correspondence.

Embossing and color art, which are very popular on business letters, were seldom seen on physicians' letterheads until recently. However, these are gaining in popularity. Be sure to obtain the approval of your employer before you change the letterhead, the type of printing, or the quality of the paper you have been using.

Continuation sheets do not have a letterhead but are of the same color and quality as the first sheet. When using continuation sheets, be careful to print out on the face (front) of the paper. You can tell the face from the back by holding the paper to the light. The watermark (a faint symbol that is part of the paper) is visible and can be read from the face. If you print out on the back, the paper may appear to be of a different color and texture and will not match your letterhead paper. Be sure to insert the proper number of continuation sheets into the printer (and remove any spare sheets later). It is incorrect to print the second and subsequent pages on paper that happens to be in the paper tray.

Number 10 (4⅛ × 9½-inch) envelopes should match the paper in color and quality. The return address is engraved or printed to match the letterhead. Because

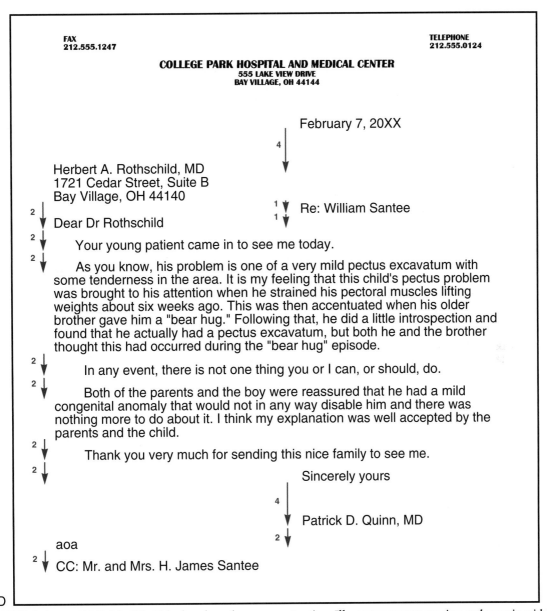

FAX
212.555.1247

TELEPHONE
212.555.0124

COLLEGE PARK HOSPITAL AND MEDICAL CENTER
555 LAKE VIEW DRIVE
BAY VILLAGE, OH 44144

February 7, 20XX

4

Herbert A. Rothschild, MD
1721 Cedar Street, Suite B
Bay Village, OH 44140

2

1   Re: William Santee
1

Dear Dr Rothschild

2   Your young patient came in to see me today.

2   As you know, his problem is one of a very mild pectus excavatum with some tenderness in the area. It is my feeling that this child's pectus problem was brought to his attention when he strained his pectoral muscles lifting weights about six weeks ago. This was then accentuated when his older brother gave him a "bear hug." Following that, he did a little introspection and found that he actually had a pectus excavatum, but both he and the brother thought this had occurred during the "bear hug" episode.

2   In any event, there is not one thing you or I can, or should, do.

2   Both of the parents and the boy were reassured that he had a mild congenital anomaly that would not in any way disable him and there was nothing more to do about it. I think my explanation was well accepted by the parents and the child.

2   Thank you very much for sending this nice family to see me.

2   Sincerely yours

4   Patrick D. Quinn, MD

2

aoa
2   CC: Mr. and Mrs. H. James Santee

D

FIGURE 6-1, cont'd D, Modified block style and open punctuation. Illustrates proper spacing and margin width.

6

CHAPTER

the envelope makes the first impression on a correspondent, deliberate care must be taken in its preparation.

A variety of typefaces and setup styles are available (Figure 6-3). You might be asked to create an appropriate letterhead when a change is made. A reputable printer will provide you with a list of available typefaces and will help design an attractive letterhead.

Item 3: Date

The date is in keeping with the format of the letter and is placed in line with the complimentary close and typed signature line. It is typed approximately three or four lines below the letterhead (no closer, but you may drop it farther down for a brief letter). The date used is the day on which the material was dictated and *not* the day on which it was transcribed. This point is very important because comments made in the document could reflect this date. Spell out the date in full in either the traditional or the military style. Note the use of the comma in the traditional style.

EXAMPLES

December 22, 20XX (traditional style)

22 December 20XX (British and military style)

NOT: 12-22-XX or 12/11/XX

Item 1 — Paper

KARL ROBRECHT, MD
INTERNAL MEDICINE

Gulf Medical Group

A PROFESSIONAL CORPORATION
800 GULF SHORE BOULEVARD
NAPLES, FLORIDA 33940
TELEPHONE 262-9976

ROBERT T. SACHS, MD
PHYSICIAN AND SURGEON

2 — Letterhead

Approximately 3
blank lines
below letterhead

_____ 3 — Date

Fifth line below
date line

_____ 4 — Inside address
_____ 5 — Street address
_____ 6 — City and state
_____ Reference

Double space after
last line of address

_____ : 7 — Salutation

_____
_____
_____
_____ . 8 — Body

Single spaced with
double space
between paragraphs

_____
_____
_____
_____ .

Double space after
last line typed

_____ , 9 — Complimentary
close

Signature area

3 blank lines

_____ 10 — Typed
signature line

_____ Title

Double space — 11 — Reference
initials

Double space — 12 — Enclosure
notation

Double space — 13 — Distribution
notation

FIGURE 6-2 Business letter setup mechanics, showing modified block format and mixed punctuation. (See the text for a description of each item illustrated.)

FIGURE 6-3 Letterhead styles and typefaces.

Item 4: Inside Address

The inside address is typed flush with the left margin and is begun on approximately the fifth line below the date (it may be moved up or down a line or two, depending on the length of the letter). The name of the person or firm is copied exactly as printed on the person's or firm's letterhead or as printed in the medical society directory or the telephone book. A courtesy title is added to a name whenever possible. If you do not know whether the person is a man or woman, omit the courtesy title. The title "Ms" is used when you do not have a title for a woman; it is also used as a substitute for "Miss" or "Mrs" because many women prefer this usage. The degree is preferred over a title in the case of a physician, and in no case should a title and a degree be used together. Use the middle initial when it is known. (You will recall that punctuation rules permit dropping the period from titles, such as Dr., Mrs., Mr., and so on. However, if you want to punctuate these titles, it would not be incorrect to do so.)

EXAMPLES

Ms Mary T. Jordan

Professor Otis R. Laban

Drs Reilly, Lombardo, and Hamstead

Dora F. Hodge, MD

Captain Denis K. Night, Jr.

Glenn M. Stempien, DDS

Franklyn Battencourt, Esq.

Neal J. Kaufman, MD, FACCP

Rabbi Bernice Gold

Paul Kip Barton, MD, MAJ, USN

NOT: Dr Clifford F. Adolph, MD
　　　 Dr Bertrum L. Storey, PhD
　　　 Ms Janet Holloway, DO

When "doctor" is dictated and you have no way of finding out if the person being addressed is a medical doctor, an osteopath, a podiatrist, a dentist, or another professional with a doctoral degree, use the title format.

EXAMPLES

Dr Phillip R. Wood

Dr Suzanne P. Markson

If a business title accompanies the name, it may follow the name on the same line or, if lengthy, it may appear on the next line. (Note the punctuation in the examples.)

EXAMPLES

F.E. Stru, MD, Medical Director

Ms Sheila O. Wendall
Purchasing Agent

William Peter Sloan-Wilson, MD
Captain, USN, USCG

Adrian N. Abott, MD
Chief-of-Surgery
Sinai-Lebanon Hospital

Item 5: Street Address

After the name of the person or firm is the street or post office box address. (If both are given, use the post office box address. The street address has been provided for persons visiting the firm and provides a site for express-mail deliveries. The firm may not even have the facilities for receiving regular mail on site. If the post office box is given, the person or firm has indicated that delivery to the post office box is preferred.) Abbreviations are permitted *after* the street name only; they include NW, NE, SW, and so on. Avoid abbreviating North, South, East, West, Road, Street, Avenue, or Boulevard. "Apartment" is abbreviated only if the line is unusually long. The apartment, suite, or space number is typed on the same line with the street address, separated by a comma.

EXAMPLES

321 Madison Avenue

1731 North Branch Road, Suite B

845 Medford Circle, Apartment 54

8895 Business Park NW

PO Box 966

If all of the delivery address line information cannot be typed in a single line above the city, state, and ZIP code, then place the secondary address information (e.g., suite, apartment, building, room, space numbers) on the line immediately *above* the delivery address line. This placement may seem awkward, but it is correct. The envelope address is a copy of the inside address, and post office personnel and scanning equipment read only the last two lines of the address, so these lines must contain the street address, city, state, and ZIP codes. The mail carrier is the only one interested in the suite, apartment, or space number. When you do not know whether a suite or apartment is indicated, use the pound sign (#) and the number.

> 🔧 **MT TOOL BOX TIP:** The envelope address matches the letter address.

EXAMPLES: *Entire address*

Mrs Lila Hadley
Apartment 21
1951 52nd Street
Tucson, AZ 85718

Mrs Marijane Simmons
8840 Marshall Place, #5
Jamestown, NY 14701

James Woo
Wildflower Estates
325 Park Drive
Lakewood, CO 80215

Item 6: City and State

The name of the city is spelled out and separated from the state name with a comma. The state name may be spelled out or abbreviated and is separated from the ZIP code by one letter space and no punctuation. The United States Postal Service state abbreviations are not used without the ZIP code. (See Appendix B for these state abbreviations.)

EXAMPLE

Honolulu, Hawaii 96918 *or* Honolulu, HI 96918

NOT: Honolulu, HI *or* Honolulu, Hi

Item 7: Salutation

The salutation is typed two line spaces below the last line of the address, as follows:

▶ Open punctuation format: no mark of punctuation used.
▶ Mixed punctuation format (formal): followed by a colon.
▶ Mixed punctuation format (informal—first name used): followed by a comma or a colon.

EXAMPLES

Open: Dear Mr Walsh

Mixed (formal): Dear Mr Walsh:

Mixed (informal): Dear Don: or Dear Don,

See Figure 6-1, *A* and *C*, for examples of mixed punctuation and Figure 6-1, *B* and *D*, for examples of open punctuation.

EXAMPLES: *Salutations used for men, showing mixed punctuation*

Gentlemen:

Dear Mr Sutherland:

Dear Dr Hon:

Dear Dr Blake and Dr Fortuna:

Dear Mr Tony Lamb and Mr Peter Lamb:

Dear Rabbi Ruderman: (likewise, Father, Bishop, Reverend, Monsignor, Cardinal, Brother, Deacon, Chaplain, Dean, and so on)

EXAMPLES: *Salutations used for women, showing mixed punctuation*

Ladies:

Mesdames:

Dear Dr Martin:

Dear Mrs Clayborne:

Dear Ms Robinson:

Dear Judge Peterson: (likewise Reverend, Rabbi, Chaplain, Dean, Deacon, Bishop, Captain, Professor, and so on)

Dear Sister Rose Anthony:

Dear Miss Thomas and Mrs Farintino:

EXAMPLES: *Salutations used for addressing men and women together*

Dear Sir or Madam:

Ladies and Gentlemen:

Dear Doctors:

Dear Mr and Mrs Knight:

Dear Dr and Mrs Wong:

Dear Professor Holloway and Mr Blake:

Dear Dr Lois Candelaria and Dr Fred Candelaria:

Dear Mr Clayborne and Mrs Steen-Clayborne:

Dear Dr Petroski and Mr Petroski:

Dear Captain and Mrs Philips:

Dear Dr Mitchelson et al.: (used for addressing large groups of men and/or women)

Item 8: Body

The body of the letter is begun a double space below the salutation or the reference line (when used here) and is single-spaced. Even very brief letters are single-spaced.

The first and subsequent lines are flush with the left margin unless indented paragraphs are used; in that case, the first line of each paragraph is indented one tab stop. There is always a double space between paragraphs.

Make use of displayed extract text when it is appropriate. This practice adds emphasis to the material, makes the letter easier to read, and supplies visual interest. This part of the letter is indented at least five letter spaces (one tab stop on left margin) from *both* left and right margins. Figures 6-4 and 6-5 illustrate two examples of appropriate use of displayed extract text. Be sure to double-space before and after this feature.

When the author decides to include an outline for the proposed plan for the care of the patient, an abbreviated version of the patient's history or current status, or a brief physical examination, prepare it in the form as illustrated. Be sure you carry the block indentation to continuing pages when necessary, and remember to return to the established margin when this material is complete.

Item 9: Complimentary Close

The complimentary close is lined up with the date and is typed a double space below the last typed line. Only the first word is capitalized. A comma is used after the close if a colon appears with the salutation (mixed punctuation). No punctuation mark is used with the open format. If the author of the document dictates some other greeting at the end of the letter, such as "Kindest personal regards," "Merry Christmas to Janet and the children," "Regards in the holiday season," "Happy New Year!" and so on, type it as a final paragraph, and use the complimentary close as usual.

EXAMPLES: *Mixed punctuation*

Sincerely,

Yours very truly,

EXAMPLES: *Open punctuation*

Sincerely

Yours very truly

See Figure 6-1, *A* to *D*, for examples of mixed and open punctuation.

Item 10: Typed Signature Line

The dictator's or writer's name is typed exactly as it appears in the letterhead, with three blank lines inserted after the complimentary close. Press the return/enter key four times after you type the complimentary close. Then type the name, lined up with the complimentary close. If an official title accompanies the name, it may appear on the same line, preceded by a comma, or on

---

Kwei-Hay Wong, MD
1654 Piikea Street
Honolulu, Hawaii 96818
Telephone 555-534-0922
Fax 555-534-9512

Diplomate, American Board
Of Otolaryngology

Ear, Nose, Throat
Head and Neck Surgery

March 27, 20XX

Roy V. Zimmer, MD
6280 Jackson Drive
San Antonio, TX 78288   Re: Mrs Florida Sanchez

Dear Roy:

Thank you for referring this pleasant young lady to my office. She was first seen on February 17, 20XX.

Her past history is of no great significance and will not be reiterated at this time.

Physical examination revealed the following:

Thyroid: Normal to palpation, with no cervical adenopathy.

Breasts: No masses, tenderness or axillary adenopathy.

Abdomen: Flat. Liver, kidneys, and spleen not felt. There is a well-healed McBurney scar present. No masses, tenderness, or...

FIGURE 6-4 Part of a letter illustrating the use of displayed extract text set off from the rest of the letter for emphasis.

GULF MEDICAL GROUP

A PROFESSIONAL MEDICAL CORPORATION
800 GULF SHORE BOULEVARD
NAPLES, FLORIDA 33940
865-262-9976
FAX 865-893-4353

KARL ROBRECHT, MD
INTERNAL MEDICINE

CELESTYN SACHS, MD
PHYSICIAN AND SURGEON

March 27, 20XX

PERSONAL

Mrs Lila Hadley
Apartment 21
1951 52nd Street
Naples, FL 33941

Dear Mrs Hadley:

This is in reply to your letter concerning the results of your tests that were done here and by Dr. Galloway.

1. Intestinal symptoms, secondary to a lactase deficiency.

2. Generalized arteriosclerosis.

3. Mitral stenosis and insufficiency.

4. History of venous aneurysm.

You were seen on February 2, at which time you were having some stiffness at the shoulders, which I felt was likely to be due to a periarthritis. (This is a stiffness of the shoulder capsule.)

FIGURE 6-5 Part of a letter illustrating the use of displayed extract text set off from the rest of the letter for emphasis.

the line directly below the signature line without a comma. If the dictator signs off with just a first name, type his or her complete name (and title, if there is one).

EXAMPLE

Sincerely,

Samuel R. Wong, MD
Chief-of-Surgery

EXAMPLE

Yours very truly,

Kathryn B. Black, MD, Medical Director

Note the punctuation.

NOTE: An office employee using the letterhead stationery always identifies his or her position in the firm and provides a courtesy title. The title enables the correspondent to have a title to use in writing or telephoning. The title is enclosed in parentheses, or the title may accompany the name when it is signed.

EXAMPLES

(Ms) Lynmarie Myhre, CMT

(Mrs) Mai Chang
Receptionist

(Miss) Paula de la Vera, CMA-A
Office Manager

NOTE: *Signature:* The typed signature line indicates where the originator of the document will sign and also spells out the signature to be sure it is understood. Be sure that all documents are signed by the author of the document before it leaves your facility.

Item 11: Reference Initials

The transcriptionist's initials are typed using lowercase letters two line spaces below the typed signature, flush with the left margin. Only two or three of the transcriptionist's initials are used, and humorous or confusing combinations are avoided. Do not type your initials when you type a letter for your own signature.

EXAMPLES

crc (rather than *cc*)

db (rather than *dmb*)

dg (rather than *dog*)

NOTE: If the author wants his or her initials used, they precede the initials of the transcriptionist, or if the author differs from the person who signs the document, the author's, the signer's, and the transcriptionist's initials are used.

EXAMPLES

lrc/wpd or lrc:wpd

RF:BJT:wpd

Item 12: Enclosure Notation

If the author is enclosing one or more items with the letter, attention is called to the item or items with a notation. The notation is typed flush with the left margin, and the number of enclosures should be noted if there is more than one. A variety of styles is acceptable. The single word *Enclosure* is the most commonly used.

> 🔧 **MT TOOL BOX TIP:** Use an enclosure notation when appropriate.

EXAMPLES

Enc.	**Enclosure**	**Check enclosed**
Enc. 2	**2 Enc.**	**2 enclosures**
Enclosures		
Enclosures: 2		
Enclosed:	1. Operative report	
	2. Pathology report	
	3. History and physical	

NOTE: This last notation can help you ensure that all items are enclosed before the letter is sealed. The recipient's secretary should also check the enclosure line when the letter is opened, to ensure that he or she has all of the mentioned items before the envelope is discarded.

Item 13: Distribution Notation

It is understood that a file copy is made of every item prepared by the transcriptionist. If a copy of the correspondence is sent to someone else, this fact is noted on the original version. The notation is typed flush with the left margin and is two line spaces below the reference initials or last notation made. In other words, it is the last entry on the page, unless there is a postscript. Various styles are used, and all are followed by the complete name of the recipient. A colon is used with the notation. Copies mailed out are photocopies of the original document, or the document may be printed out again and mailed. Use the abbreviation *cc* or simply *C* in capital or lowercase letters and identify the recipient of a copy of the document. The abbreviation *cc* remains correct and popular. It used to mean "carbon copy" and now means "courtesy copy."

EXAMPLES

cc: Frank L. Naruse, MD

c: Ruth Chriswell, Business Manager

C: Hodge W. Lloyd

Copy: Carla P. Ralph, Buyer

Copies: Kristen A. Temple
　　　　Anthony R. McClintock

NOTE: *Never* type a copy notation without a name following it.

Second and subsequent copy notations are lined up under the first notation. In general, the names are ranked in alphabetical order. If you have a very lengthy list of copy notations, consider making a two- or three-column list rather than a long string that could affect another page.

EXAMPLES

CC: Claire Duennes, MD   Norman Szold, MD
    Sharon Kirkwood, MD   James Tanaka, MD
    Amrum Lambert, MD   Robert Wozniak, MD
    Clifford Storey, MD   Vell Yaldua, MD

OTHER LETTER MECHANICS

Blind Copy

If the sender wants a copy of the correspondence to be sent to a third party and does not want the recipient of the original version to know that this was done, he or she will direct that a "blind copy" be mailed. Do *not* make a copy notation on the original but do make a notation on the file copy with the name of the recipient after the notation. Print out the original, and then add the *bcc* notation with the recipient's name to the master and print two copies: one to mail and one to file.

> **EXAMPLE:** *Typed on file copy and Taylor's copy*
>
> bcc: Ms Penelope R. Taylor

Postscript

The postscript is typed a double space below the last reference notation and is flush with the left margin. The abbreviation *PS* followed by a colon usually introduces the item. It is no longer punctuated.

> **NOTE:** The postscript can be an afterthought or a statement deliberately withheld from the body of the letter for emphasis or a restatement of an important thought (e.g., a telephone number in a letter of application). A handwritten afterthought, added by the dictator, does not need to be introduced with PS.

> **EXAMPLE:** *An afterthought*
>
> PS: Thanks for your offer to borrow your mountain cabin. I'll telephone you when I see I have a weekend off.

> **EXAMPLE:** *Emphasis*
>
> PS: Please do not hesitate to call on me if I can help you in any way.

If the postscript is longer than one line, indent any subsequent lines to align with the first word of the message.

If the postscript is simply something forgotten from the body of the letter such as "By the way, I will return the x-rays to your office after I see Mrs Theobald next week," you may insert the statement in the body of the letter where the x-rays were last mentioned and then eliminate the postscript. This maneuver is easy to accomplish with the "cut and paste" feature of word processing software.

Attention Line

The attention line is no longer used in business correspondence because of the software feature that enables you to copy the inside address to the envelope. Type the recipient's name and title, if necessary, above the name of the business. The word *Attention* is no longer used unless you want to use it or unless you are using a title for an unknown recipient.

EXAMPLES

Josephine Simmons, PhD, Administrator
Altamont Springs Community Hospital
321 Fifth Avenue
Altamont Springs, FL 32716

Attention: Administrator
Altamont Springs Community Hospital
321 Fifth Avenue
Altamont Springs, FL 32716

To Whom It May Concern

The phrase *To Whom It May Concern* is used when you have no person or place to send a document. It is typed in full capitals, or the first letter of each word is capitalized. It may be typed flush with the left margin or centered on the page. Open or mixed punctuation is used with it. In general, the complimentary close is not used with this format.

> MT TOOL BOX TIP: Use TO WHOM IT MAY CONCERN when you don't know to whom a letter is intended.

When a reference line is used with this document, it is typed a double space below the To Whom It May Concern line.

EXAMPLE:

TO WHOM IT MAY CONCERN:

RE: Rudy Carpenter, SS # 576-39-9654

EXAMPLE

THORACIC SURGERY MEDICAL GROUP, INC.
ROBERT B. STEINWAY, MD
STEPHEN R. CLAWSON, MD
CHRISTIAN M. LOW, MD
MARY SUE LOW, MD

504 WARFORD DRIVE
SYRACUSE, NY 13223
TELEPHONE 555.567.2342

19098 CHATHAM ROAD
SYRACUSE, NY 13203
TELEPHONE 555.562.4290

August 18, 20XX

TO WHOM IT MAY CONCERN

RE: Capt. R. J. Reynolds, USMC

The above-named individual has been under my care for chronic obstructive pulmonary disease since March 2010. He has seen some improvement of his symptomology . . .

Reference Line

Reference lines are commonly used in medical correspondence and medicolegal reports.

A patient's name is always placed in a reference line. Using recent guidelines, some dictators avoid using the name elsewhere in the document, so that the patient is identified only in this initial entry. Exact placement is determined by the letter style chosen. In some documents, a reference line may also include file numbers, name of employer, name of insurance carrier, or date of accident or injury. Examine the following examples closely.

FULL-BLOCK PLACEMENT
(SEE FIGURE 6-1, *A*)

▸ Flush with the left margin
▸ Two line spaces after the salutation
▸ Use *RE:* or *Re:* to introduce the patient's full name

EXAMPLES

Matthew R. Bates, MD

7832 Johnson Avenue

Denver, CO 80241

Dear Dr Bates

RE: Leah Hamlyn

MODIFIED BLOCK PLACEMENT

▸ Use when the reference line is long or contains more than one entry
▸ Flush with the left margin

▸ Two line spaces after the salutation
▸ Use *RE:* or *Re:* to introduce the patient's full name

EXAMPLE

Matthew R. Bates, MD

7832 Johnson Avenue

Denver, CO 80241

Dear Dr Bates

Re: Leah Hamlyn, Accident report E 14-78-9865

EXAMPLE

Matthew R. Bates, MD

7832 Johnson Avenue

Denver, CO 80241

Dear Dr Bates

RE: Leah Hamlyn
    Colorado Workers' Compensation Company
    Date of Injury: October 1, 20XX

MODIFIED BLOCK PLACEMENT
(SEE FIGURE 6-1, *B*)

▸ Breaking the placement rule
▸ Lined up with the date
▸ A single line space after the last line of the address
▸ Use *RE:* or *Re:* to introduce the patient's full name
▸ A single line space between *Re:* and salutation

EXAMPLE

October 14, 20XX

Matthew R. Bates, MD

7832 Johnson Avenue

Denver, CO 80241

RE: Leah Hamlyn

Dear Dr Bates

However, the reference line is *misplaced* so often that transcriptionists who place it correctly not only are in the minority but also begin to think that they are in error. There is no arbitrary rule about this line. It is considered a part of the body of the letter. The problem with misplacement began when custom dictated that the "rule could be broken" when modified block format was used and the reference line was very brief. The second part of the problem occurred when dictators, unconcerned with style or format, gave information for the reference line before pronouncing the salutation. Finally, instead of inserting a single line space and then inserting the reference followed by another single line space, some transcriptionists inserted two line spaces both before and after the reference in the breaking-the-placement-rule format. Take care to place this line correctly, and begin by looking closely at and studying the following examples, which show incorrect placements. The correct versions are given in the preceding examples.

EXAMPLE: *Incorrect placement of reference line (out of place)*

Matthew R. Bates, MD

7832 Johnson Avenue

Denver, CO 80241

RE: Leah Hamlyn

Dear Dr Bates:

EXAMPLE: *Another incorrect placement of reference line (too much space)*

Matthew R. Bates, MD

7832 Johnson Avenue

Denver, CO 80241

RE: Leah Hamlyn

Dear Dr Bates:

PERSONAL OR CONFIDENTIAL NOTATION

Personal or confidential notations are typed on the second line below the date, starting at the same point as the date. Type the notation in capital letters. Follow with the inside address on the fourth line down, depending on the length of the letter (see Figure 6-5, p. 158).

EXAMPLE: *Full-block format*

October 23, 20XX

PERSONAL

TWO-PAGE LETTERS

If a letter is too long for one page, it must be appropriately continued on a second page or subsequent pages. The following rules apply:

1. Continue to the second page at the end of a paragraph whenever possible.
2. If a paragraph must be divided between pages, carry at least two lines of the paragraph to the second page.
3. Leave at least two lines of a paragraph on the first page.
4. Type no closer than 1 inch from the bottom of the page.
5. Do not divide the last word on the page.
6. Place headings no less than 1 inch from the top of the page.
7. Leave two blank lines between the last line of the heading and the first line of the continuation of the letter. To do this, press the return or enter key three times at the end of the typed data in the heading.
8. To prevent the first line of a new paragraph from appearing as the last line on the page or to prevent the final line of a paragraph from printing on a new page, use the widow/orphan control feature of your word processing software. (An "orphan" is a single short line or the last few words of a paragraph left on the bottom of a page. A "widow" is a short line ending a paragraph that is positioned at the top of a page.)

The second sheet or continuation sheets are plain paper the same color, size, and quality as the letterhead paper. Headings are placed on the second sheet to identify it as belonging to the first sheet. There are two styles for page headings.

EXAMPLE: *Horizontal form*

RE: Leah Hamlyn   2   October 3, 20XX
(patient's name)   *(page number)*   *(date)*

EXAMPLE: *Vertical form*

RE: Leah Hamlyn

Page 2

October 3, 20XX

NOTE: The page number is centered in the horizontal form. In a nonmedical letter, the name of the correspondent is listed in place of the patient's name.

Always do a print preview to ensure the page markings appear where they are intended, and take care to number each sheet in the series properly. It is an insult to ask the document author to sign a letter in which new page markings are on the bottom of the page or a few lines into a paragraph on page 2. If documents are printed off site and you do not have the opportunity to review the final printed document, be sure that someone on site checks them and the printer setup for you.

COPIES

The transcriptionist makes a copy (paper copy or electronic copy) of every item transcribed. Great care must be taken to ensure that a copy is made of every corrected original before the original is mailed. A document may need to be rushed to the mail after it is signed; therefore, make it a habit to photocopy the letter *before* the signature is added. If corrections or additions are needed, make another copy and shred the first photocopy. Be sure that good-quality paper is used for copies that are mailed out of the office. You might consider printing a duplicate of your original for the copy to be mailed out. The office copy becomes part of the patient's permanent record and is filed in his or her medical chart.

FILE NOTATION

You already have experience in naming your individual files. You might also need to code the document itself with your unique file name. This way transcribed documents can be retrieved easily and quickly when needed. You might be able to use your own file name conventions; however, the dictator or organization may prefer that you use specified codes. If you can use your own codes, here are some hints for making it simple:

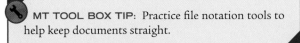

MT TOOL BOX TIP: Practice file notation tools to help keep documents straight.

▸ Use minimal data: ID number for the dictator, patient name, and date.
▸ Use letters and numbers for dates: use just the last digit of the year and then use 1 to 9 for the first nine months and O, N, and D for October, November, and December.
▸ Use a period for a separation mark.

▸ Place the file name as the last entry on the page.
▸ Decrease the font size to 8 or 9 point.
▸ Use the identical code as your saved file name.

EXAMPLES: *D.P.D: doctor.patient.date*

(using Figure 6-1)
(Your ID number for Dr Quinn is Q1)
Q1.Santee.27X

Uncoded: Dr Quinn dictated a letter about patient Santee on February 7, 20XX.

(using Figure 6-4)
(Your ID number for Dr Wong is W3)
W3.Sanchez.327X

Uncoded: Dr Wong dictated a letter about patient Sanchez on March 27, 20XX.

NOTE: Be sure that you back up your document files on a daily basis.

PLACEMENT

Placement should have picture-frame symmetry and balance of the three blank margins and the letterhead. A good rule to follow for margins is to use 2-inch margins with short letters (fewer than 100 words), $1^{1}/_{2}$-inch margins with medium-length letters (100 to 200 words), and 1-inch margins with long letters (200 words).

To achieve symmetry and to squeeze a letter onto one page, you can adjust the spacing at the end of the letter (beginning with the typed signature line). Leave two, rather than three, line spaces for the signature and a single line space between the typed signature line, the reference initials, and other notations. If you are using the modified block format, you can type the reference initials on the same line as the typed signature line to save more space. If you still find that you cannot fit the letter on one page, then reformat, widen the margins, and type the final paragraph on a second page.

The visual appeal of the letter is very important. Try to keep the right margin as even as possible, and try not to vary the line length by more than five characters.

To make a very short letter appear attractive on the page, widen the margins and increase the space between the date line and the letterhead; increase the space between the date line and the inside address.

6-1 TYPING ASSIGNMENT

DIRECTIONS:
▶ Retype the following material into letter form. Paragraph beginnings are indicated by the symbol ¶.
▶ Make a letterhead by using a computer macro to match the name of the author and inventing an appropriate address, or use any prepared letterhead paper as your instructor directs.
▶ Use full-block format, open punctuation, a reference line, and the current date. Refer to the vocabulary list at the beginning of the chapter if necessary. Pay close attention to placement and mechanics.
▶ Remember to use the proper state abbreviations that you learned in Chapter 4. (See Appendix B.)
▶ Prepare a file maintenance notation and insert it on the bottom of your document.

Save this letter after your instructor has checked it because you will need it for Self-Study 6-3.

The letter is from Laurel R. Denison, MD; is to Gregory O. Theopolis, MD, 4509 Roessler Road, Detroit, Michigan 48224; and is in reference to Bobby West.

Dear Dr Theopolis ¶ This one-month-old baby was seen in my office yesterday for evaluation of difficulty with the right foot. ¶ The mother reports that this is the third sibling in the family. The older two siblings have no difficulty with the feet. When this baby was born, there was obvious deformity of the right foot, which has not corrected itself. ¶ Physical examination reveals that the hips are normal. There is internal tibial torsion. There is pes equinus; there is hindfoot supination and forefoot adduction. It is obvious that this baby has a congenital talipes equinovarus in the right foot. ¶ He was casted in the office yesterday. ¶ We do not know the prognosis yet since this is the first experience with the child. Prognosis depends on the congenital factors that caused the deformity, in the first place, and the elasticity of the tissues, in the second place. We will follow the child at weekly intervals. ¶ Thank you for the opportunity of seeing this baby. Sincerely

6-2 TYPING ASSIGNMENT

DIRECTIONS:
▶ Retype the following material into letter form. Paragraph beginnings are indicated by the symbol ¶.
▶ Make a letterhead by using a computer macro to match the name of the author and inventing an appropriate address, or use any prepared letterhead paper as your instructor directs.
▶ Use modified block format, mixed punctuation, a reference line that breaks the placement rule, and the current date. Pay close attention to placement and mechanics. (See Figure 6-2.)
▶ Remember to use the proper state abbreviations learned in Chapter 4. (See Appendix B.)
▶ Prepare a file maintenance notation and insert it on the bottom of your document.

This letter is from Emery R. Stuart, MD, to Walter W. von der Meyer, MD, 6754 Sunrise Circle, Ft. Lauderdale, Florida 33312. Copies should be sent to Dr Barney P. Haber and Dr Herbert W. Delft. (It is not necessary to make these copies; make just the notation.) The patient is Mrs Nora George.

Dear Walter. ¶ This is a final follow-up letter on your patient, who, you will recall, was admitted to Sunrise View Hospital in February 20XX for aortic valve replacement with a diagnosis of aortic stenosis. ¶ Nora has done well; she is in normal sinus rhythm, and she is well controlled on her Coumadin. She, at times, has some swelling of her hands and feet and has gained considerable weight since surgery. She needs continued close medical observation of her prothrombin level, which should be maintained at about 20% of normal, indefinitely. She should also be maintained on Lanoxin and may possibly require diuretics intermittently. ¶ We will not follow Nora any further for her heart disease. She has had an uneventful postoperative course and can continue her medical follow-up through your office or that of Dr Herbert Delft, whichever you decide. ¶ Thank you very much for letting us see this patient with you and perform her surgery. We will be glad to see her at any time if there are any questions regarding her valve function or clinical course. Sincerely yours.

Save this letter after your instructor has checked it.

PARAGRAPHING

Paragraphs give the letter shape. The subject is divided into topics, and these topics constitute paragraphs. Paragraphs aid the reader by signaling a *new* idea with each division.

The paragraphing will contribute to the visual appeal of the letter and should be well balanced. Therefore, the first and last paragraphs are usually brief, and the middle paragraphs are longer. Nevertheless, a paragraph may be of any length, and you should not hesitate to make one sentence a paragraph when it is appropriate. A series of brief paragraphs in a row, however, can be distracting to the reader. On the other hand, in a brief letter, a long paragraph may appear uninviting, and you may have to break the paragraph up to provide visual appeal.

Most authors do not directly indicate the beginning (or end) of a paragraph, but they may give indirect clues with voice inflections or other subtle voice changes. Each new paragraph is begun with a sentence that suggests the topic or further explains it in a different way.

Correct paragraphing is not difficult with most medical letters because the letters generally follow a well-established pattern. The knowledge of this pattern will help you determine the paragraph breaks with or without vocal hints.

Physicians' letters dealing with patient care are usually narrative reports to workers' compensation carriers, consultation reports, letters of referral, followup notes, or discharge summaries.

The first paragraph is normally a brief introduction or explanation for the letter. In patient-related letters, the patient and his or her chief complaint are introduced in the initial brief paragraph. The next paragraph may contain the history of the complaint, along with a general description of any contributing problems in the patient's history. This material is followed in the third or fourth paragraph with the findings on examination of the patient. (At times, these remarks may be so brief that they constitute only one sentence.)

The next-to-last paragraph is confined to a medical opinion, prognosis, diagnosis, recommendation, report of tests, results of surgical procedures, detailed outlines for proposed care or treatment, evaluation of return-to-normal status, or summary. The subject is then closed in the final paragraph. At this point, the author may thank a referring physician, indicate what will take place next with the patient, or request some action on the patient's behalf.

6-3 SELF-STUDY

DIRECTIONS: Refer to your copy of Typing Assignment 6-1. Notice the paragraph breaks. Answer the following questions here or on a separate sheet of paper as your instructor directs.

1. Notice that paragraph 1 is only one sentence long. What does the dictator do with this sentence?

   _____

2. Notice that paragraph 2 is three sentences long. Could the first of these sentences have been placed in the first paragraph? _____

   Why or why not? _____

3. What is the author *doing* in paragraph 2? _____

4. Could any part of paragraph 3 logically be part of the second or fourth paragraph? _____

   Why or why not? _____

5. What is the author *doing* in paragraph 3? _____

6. Again, we have one sentence in paragraph 4. Could the transcriptionist have joined this sentence to paragraph 3? _____

7. What did the author *do* in this paragraph? _____

8. What is the subject of paragraph 5? _____ Could this paragraph be joined to paragraph 4?

   _____

   Why or why not? _____

9. Notice the last line of paragraph 5. Could this have been a paragraph on its own? _____

   Why or why not? _____

   Could you make it a part of the last paragraph? _____

   Why or why not? _____

10. What is the dictator doing in the final paragraph, number 6? _____ Do you think it is appropriate to have this single sentence standing as an entire paragraph? _____

    Why or why not? _____

    Turn to p. 440 in Appendix A for the answers to these questions.

 6-4 SELF-STUDY

DIRECTIONS: Refer to your copy of Typing Assignment 6-2. Notice the paragraph breaks. Answer the following questions here or on a separate sheet of paper as your instructor directs.

1. Paragraph 1 tells you the type of document this is. What is it?

   _____

2. Paragraph 1: What is the subject(s) of this paragraph? _____

3. Paragraph 2: What is the author *doing* in this paragraph? _____

   Could the last two sentences of this paragraph be used to form a new paragraph? _____

   Why or why not? _____

4. Paragraph 3: What is the dictator saying in this paragraph?_____

Could this paragraph have been combined with the last two sentences of paragraph two?_____

Why or why not? _____

5. Paragraph 4: What is the subject of this paragraph? _____

Should this be arranged as two short paragraphs? _____

Turn to p. 440 in Appendix A for the answers to these questions.

 6-5 TYPING ASSIGNMENT

DIRECTIONS:
- Retype the following material into letter form.
- Use full-block format, mixed punctuation, and the current date.
- Watch for proper paragraphing, placement, and mechanics.
- Use letterhead paper.
- Carefully mark your book where you think the paragraph breaks should be. Ask yourself whether they follow the pattern you have just learned. If they do not, consider some different breaks. Remember that there is sometimes more than one choice for a new paragraph break.
- On your final draft, write a number by each paragraph break.
- On a separate sheet of paper, type an explanation for that paragraph break, and turn it in with your letter.

The letter is from Steven A. Flores, MD, and is to another physician, Willard R. Beets, at 7895 West Sherman Street, San Diego, California 92111.

Dear Dr Beets. I saw Mr Tim Molton, your patient, in my office yesterday afternoon. As you will recall, Mr Molton is a 49-year-old professional gardener who came to see you with a chronic cough and a history of expectoration of a whitish material. He brought the x-rays from your office with him, and I noted a fossa on the superficial surface of his lung. He was afebrile today and stated that he had been so since the onset of his symptoms. He did not complain of pain but did experience some dyspnea on exertion and some shortness of breath. I did not carry out a physical examination, but I did skin test him for both tuberculosis and coccidioidomycosis. I did not give him a prescription for any medication and will wait until we get the results of his skin tests. It seems to me that your diagnosis of his problem is correct, so we will proceed with that in mind. As you probably know, valley fever is endemic to San Diego; and since Mr Molton was born and raised in New York State, he could be very susceptible. You may tell his employer that if he does have valley fever, he will have to convalesce for a month to six weeks, after which time he should be fully able to return to his normal duties. I will keep you posted on the results of his tests. Thank you very much for letting me help you with Mr Molton's problem. Sincerely.

NOTE: Please notice how many times the patient's name was used in this document. There is a trend toward using the patient's name only in the reference line. That style would be difficult for this dictator. You cannot change this pattern unless asked to do so. Always transcribe what is dictated.

6-6 TYPING PRACTICE TEST

DIRECTIONS:
▶ Retype this material in letter form. Use full block format open punctuation, and a reference line.
▶ Use letterhead paper.
▶ You will have to supply proper punctuation, capitalization, paragraphing, and mechanics. Good luck!

may 1 20XX ian r wing m d 2261 arizona avenue suite b milwaukee wisconsin 53207 dear dr wing i saw your patient mrs elvira martinez in consultation in my office today. she brought the x-rays from your office with her. she was afebrile today but on questioning admitted a low grade fever over the past few days i removed the fluid as seen on your film of april 30 from the right lower lung field and she felt considerably more comfortable. on thoracentesis there was 50 mL of straw colored fluid her history is well known to you so i will not repeat it. on physical examination i found a well developed well nourished white female with minimal dyspnea there was no lymphadenopathy breath sounds were diminished somewhat on the right there was dullness at the right base the left lung was clear to percussion and auscultation. the remainder of the examination was negative. because of her history of chronic asthma i suggested she might consider bronchoscopy if this fluid reaccumulates. because she is a heavy smoker i insisted she stop smoking completely. if she does not she will not enjoy continuing good health although i have no idea of the actual prognosis. your patient has been returned to you for her continuing care i will be glad to see her again at any time you think it necessary thank you for letting me see this pleasant lady with you sincerely yours jon l mikosan m d ps i am enclosing a copy of the pathology report on the fluid as you can see it is negative

This letter, prepared properly, is in Appendix A, p. 441. Do not refer to it until your document is complete and printed.

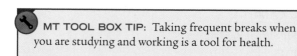

MT TOOL BOX TIP: Taking frequent breaks when you are studying and working is a tool for health.

ENVELOPE PREPARATION

A No. 10 (4⅛ × 9½ inch) envelope, printed to match your letterhead stationery, is always used with your 8½ × 11 inch paper. The traditional style for addressing envelopes by using both uppercase and lowercase letters can now be read by the optical character readers used by the United States Postal Service. The proper formatting style that you have learned in this chapter conforms to Postal Service regulations: Single-spaced; blocked each line to the left; capitalized first letter of every word in the address; city, state, and ZIP code on the last line; street address on the line above the city, state, and ZIP code. (If the apartment, suite, space, room, building, or development name or number cannot fit on the line with the street name and address, it is placed on the line above the street address.)

To print an envelope, do the following:

1. Select the default placement specifications for your printer with the proper-sized envelope. (This step ensures that the address falls within the optical character readers' read zone.)
2. Verify that you have properly prepared the inside address.
3. Highlight the inside address on your letter.
4. Select the envelope feature of your word processing program.
5. Insert your envelope into the printer and select print. The address will be printed on the envelope.

If notations such as "Confidential," "Personal," or "Special Delivery" need to be typed on the envelope, do not type them below or alongside the address, the so-called read zone.

EXAMPLE

Attention: Sales Director
National Paper Company
Franklin-Pratt Building
1492 Columbus Avenue North
Syracuse, NY 13224

EXAMPLE: *Poorly arranged format*

Victory R. Langworthy, MD
Medical Director
West View Community Hospital and Inland
Medical Center, Inc.
321 Roseview Drive
St. Louis, MO 63139

EXAMPLE: *Better arrangement*

Victory R. Langworthy, MD, Medical Director
West View Community Hospital and
Inland Medical Center, Inc.
321 Roseview Drive
St. Louis, MO 63139

EXAMPLE: *Poorly arranged format*

Miss Josie M. Brooks
1879 Westchester Boulevard, Apartment 170 B
Normal Heights, SD 57701

EXAMPLE: *Better arrangement*

Miss Josie M. Brooks
Apartment 170 B
1879 Westchester Boulevard
Normal Heights, SD 57701

If you are unable to print an envelope with your computer, prepare the envelope exactly as you did the inside address. Begin typing 2 inches down from the top of the envelope and 4 inches from the left edge, so that your address will appear in the proper read zone.

Mail addressed to a foreign country should have the name of that country as the last line of the address block. Place the name two line spaces below line that has the city, state or province, and postal code. Coding varies from country to country. Type the name of the country in full capital letters.

EXAMPLE

Prof. Wolfgang Hinz
Art Director, Rhineland Institute
Schulstrasse 21
Siegelbach, Pfalz 6751

GERMANY

EXAMPLE

Ms Marijane N. Woods
Manager, Abbott Realty
1804 31st Avenue SW
Calgary, AB T2T 1S7

CANADA

NOTE: There is one letter space between the city name and the two-letter abbreviation for the province or territory, followed by two letter spaces and the six-character postal code.

Mail addressed to members of the military who have Army Post Office (APO) or Fleet Post Office (FPO) addresses is set up as follows:

EXAMPLE

Warrant Officer John R. Meadows, USAF

Company R

5th Infantry Regiment

APO New York, NY 09801

If your mail is addressed to a private mailbox (rented from a private company), insert the private mail box number (PMB) above the delivery address.

EXAMPLE

Mr Steven R. Madruga

PMB 9982

115 South Olive Street

Philadelphia, PA 10101

 6-7 TYPING PRACTICE TEST

DIRECTIONS: Prepare envelopes for the letters you typed in Typing Assignments 6-1 and 6-2. Do not be concerned about the names (if any) in the return address block.

SIGNING AND MAILING

When the letter is ready for signature, use a paper clip to attach the envelope (and any enclosures) to the top of the letter, with the flap over the letterhead. Until you present the letter for signature, keep it in a folder to keep it clean and out of the view of any passerby. After the letter is signed and before you place it in its envelope, make sure that there are no smudges and that all enclosures are attached.

Fold the letter by bringing the bottom of the page one third up the page and then creasing. Next, fold the upper third down to within $1/2$ inch of the first crease and make the second crease. Insert the letter into the envelope so that when it is removed, it will open right side up. Figure 6-6 illustrates the proper way to fold a letter.

On occasion, the dictator is unavailable to sign the mail but requests that it be sent out rather than delayed for his or her signature. You should handle this situation as directed, by signing his or her name and then adding your initials, by typing below the signature area "Dictated but not signed" and adding your initials, or by simply signing his or her name. Be particularly careful that the letter is completely error-free in every way. Keep the copy available for the dictator's return rather than filing it immediately.

> 🔧 **MT TOOL BOX TIP:** Your initials on your product show your pride in your use of tools.

No. 10 Envelope (9-1/2 x 4-1/8 Inches)

Fold the letter by bringing the bottom of the page one third up the page and crease. Fold down the upper third within 1/2 inch of the first fold and crease. Insert the last creased edge into the envelope first.

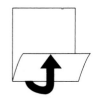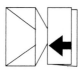

FIGURE 6-6. Proper way to fold a letter for insertion into a No. 10 envelope. (From Diehl MO: *Medical Transcription Guide: Do's and Don'ts*, ed 3, St Louis, Saunders, 2004.)

A FINAL NOTE

Letterhead stationery in addition to the standard $8\frac{1}{2} \times 11$-inch type is often kept for brief letters or secretarial correspondence. There are two standard sizes: Monarch ($7\frac{1}{2} \times 10\frac{1}{2}$ inches) and Baronial ($5\frac{1}{2} \times 8\frac{1}{2}$ inches). Envelopes are printed to match these two sizes, and papers and envelopes should *not* be mixed. Follow the same general guidelines in preparing the envelopes, except that you should begin the address $2\frac{1}{2}$ inches from the left edge of the envelope, rather than 4 inches.

6-8 TYPING REVIEW TEST

Instruction Sheet for Retyping the Following Material into Letter Form

1. Paper: Use letterhead, size 8½ × 11
2. Envelope: Use No. 10
3. Copies: Single
4. Equipment: Computer
5. Format: Modified block, open punctuation
6. Date: May 16 plus current year
7. Mechanical needs: Proper paragraphing, placement on page, *some* internal punctuation, other mechanics as may be required
8. Placement on page: Proper alignment for attractiveness and "eye appeal"
9. Patient's name: LeeAnn Jensen
10. Dictator: Dr Randolph R. Bever
11. Addressed to: Dr Norman C. Kisbey Jr, at Post Office Box 1734, Washington, DC 20034

Dear Dr Kisbey. Today I have seen your patient in neurosurgical consultation at your request. As you know, she is a very pleasant 40-year-old, right-handed lady who comes in with a history of seizure-like episodes beginning in January of 20XX. These seizures consist of a sense of unreality and a feeling as though she were observing herself as an actress on a stage. Prior to the onset of, or associated with, these seizure-like episodes, she has noted a smell of heavy fragrant flowers. She describes the smell of the flowers as slightly unpleasant, almost funereal. Each of these so-called seizure states lasts only a few seconds and is followed by a tremendous feeling of unreality. This is also associated with a great fear that she won't be able to move and she always gets up and walks around afterward to make sure she is not paralyzed. During the episode there is no loss of cognitive ability and she is able to converse with her husband and she has virtually total recall for the entire episode. She had episodes, as described, in January and February of 20XX, four in March and five in April. There is no family history of seizures. There is a story of a mild head injury at age ten and apparently she was in a moderately severe motorcycle accident about fifteen years ago which resulted in a broken mandible. The neurological examination at this time is essentially normal. The extraocular movements and fundi show no abnormalities. The visual fields and confrontation testing are intact. There is no Babinski sign. The only abnormality that I could detect in the entire examination was a stiffened right shoulder which she tells me came on after a lengthy game of tennis. I could palpate no masses over the head and there were no audible bruits over the head or over either carotid bifurcation. She has been on a dose of 30 mg of phenobarbital b.i.d. and did not care to add any Dilantin. The phenobarbital keeps her in a drowsy state consequently she is not able to think creatively or participate in sports activities. She brought with her the skull x-rays and brain scan taken at University Hospital and I have reviewed them. In my opinion, they are within normal limits. In addition, she brought with her several EEG records which I have gone over. The neurologist's summary is enclosed. I thought there was a slight abnormality present in the right temporal area. At this time, I do not believe there is evidence of intracranial mass lesion or of focal neurologic deficit. A number of features argue against interpreting her spells as true psychomotor seizures: Firstly, the fact that the aura is unusual, and secondly the fact that she has total recall for the entire episode. Thirdly, there is the fact that she has no postictal abnormality. My tendency at this time would be to gradually switch her over to Dilantin 30 mg t.i.d. and, in addition, place her on Diamox 125 mg each morning. I suggest the Diamox because she tells me that the "seizure" episodes tend to come on within a few days of her menstrual periods. We have agreed that if she is not markedly improved within a period of one month on this regimen she would come into the hospital for 4-vessel angiography. Thank you for the privilege of seeing this interesting patient and for thinking of me in connection with her problems. Yours sincerely. Randolph R. Bever, MD Professor of Neurosurgery, Weeks Medical School.

FOOD FOR THOUGHT

Imagine for a few minutes that you have just received the preceding letter in the mail. Try to read it with the assumption that it is to you personally. What is your reaction to the letter? How many errors can you find? Briefly express your opinion on a separate sheet of paper or as your instructor directs.

If nothing else, you have formed a definite opinion about this company that is based entirely on the written representation of them. It is doubtful that you would consider asking them for any information about their tours. Nor would you give them further thought other than to wonder how they stay in business.

Certainly, you would not feel they could be trusted to handle a tour because they are unable to handle their correspondence.

The recipients of your office correspondence will be equally affected by the preparation and thought that go into the letters they receive from your office. It is inconsistent to ignore the fact that careless preparation could affect their opinion of *your* employer.

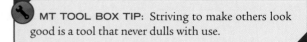

MT TOOL BOX TIP: Striving to make others look good is a tool that never dulls with use.

EXAMPLE

B L O T C H E T T   T O U R S

8888 Malarky Drive
Fun Valley, UT 99999

1   4/1/XX

2   Ms. Glendora Kirsch
3   211 Elm Ave. Apt a
4   Losangeles, Cal. 99999

5   Dear Miss Kirsch,

6   It seems that each year about this time we sent you a
7   letter inquiring about your plans for this sumer. Each
8   year for the passed three years now we have had no answer.

9   According to our records, you wrote Blotchett Tours inquiring
10 about some information concerning different tours. We sent you our price lists,
11 departure date list, special off season excursions, etc. Wouldn't it be nice if you
12 could plan to travel this summer. Why not reserve
13 a place for yourself in one of our package deals..

14   Enclosed herewith please find an application blank for
15 you to fill out. Just return it in the business reply
16 envelope with your small check for only $35 and your Place will be assured.
17 Naturally your deposit will aply toward the full purchase of your tour. We are
18 guaranteed and bonded.

19 We will will be looking for your response soon.

20 Very Truly Yours,

21 Hank Behn, Sales rep.

CHAPTER 7

Proofreading, Making Corrections, and Quality Assurance

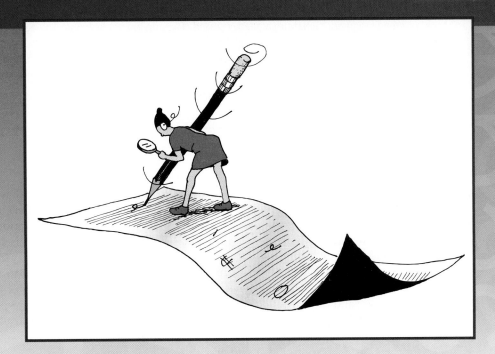

OBJECTIVES

After reading this chapter and working the exercises, you should be able to

1. Explain where errors could occur in your transcript.
2. Define critical, major, and minor errors.
3. Illustrate how important it is to check your transcript very carefully for possible errors.
4. Demonstrate the ability to use and recognize proofreader's symbols.
5. Demonstrate the ability to proofread and correct your transcripts.
6. Recognize the word hazards and printout problems associated with electronic shortcuts.
7. Identify and correct errors after editing phrases, sentences, and documents.
8. Demonstrate the ability to proofread and correct documents transcribed by others.
9. Explain the importance of submitting your work for quality assurance and evaluation.
10. Recognize transcription practices to avoid in order to produce quality documents.

Note from the Author

Of course I believed in quality assurance. What I did not believe in was the form it took.

I read and reread the documents that I transcribed in the very beginning—I thought with great care. I was mistaken. One of my dictators took a heavy black ink pen and carefully drew a circle around any misspelled word or any punctuation mark that he did not like. First, I was very upset to see the mistakes, and then I was twice as upset when I had to completely retype the document on a typewriter. After a while, I was resigned to the fact that I could not see these mistakes myself, so I very tactfully approached the dictator and asked him if he would not mark the document with the ink pen. I told him that I was becoming very clever at putting the paper back in the correcting typewriter and lifting the offending letter or punctuation mark right off the page, but I could not do that if the page was marked. He not only readily agreed; he happily agreed. I smiled. The grin did not last long. The next "batch" was given to me the following day. No mistakes! I was delighted. I commented on the fact. He replied, "Oh, no, there are mistakes indeed. On the first one, two misspelled words, the second has three punctuation mark errors, and the third has a misspelled word." "Well, where are they?" I implored. His ominous reply: "You told me not to mark them so that you could fix them. I presume that now you will go about finding them and correcting them."

Aren't you lucky?

INTRODUCTION

You have been typing copy and practicing transcribing by now, or you are starting to prepare to transcribe. Here are a few hints for transcribing.

▶ Listen all the way through a dictation from a new dictator, even several times, to get the general feel of the dictator's voice and the document itself.

▶ Play the dictation when you are alone in the room to hear how it sounds.

▶ Listen for the same expressions being said over and over again.

▶ Use your own small reference book to record names of drugs, instruments, and so on that a particular dictator uses.

▶ Notice the context of the document. When you know the context, it is easier to fit the troublesome words into a meaningful group. For example, a history and physical examination has a context quite different from that of an operative report. A radiology report does not resemble a pathology report.

▶ Look at the various documents in Appendix C on Evolve and notice the context and groups of words that are repeated.

As you begin to produce good medical transcripts, it is important that you also learn sound proofreading skills. The largest medical vocabulary, the fastest fingers, and the latest equipment mean nothing if the final document does not reflect the professional quality for which you strive. Proper proofreading skills can give you this quality, and the lack of it can cause embarrassment and possibly harm. You need these skills now because you will have to check your work carefully to earn high marks on the version you submit for grading. Later, you will want to have excellent skills when you begin your career as a medical transcriptionist (MT) or medical dictation editor. Because accurate written communication is so important, the abilities to proofread your own work and to work without supervision will give you an advantage. If you work for an organization that does quality assurance checks, your work must be able to pass scrutiny. If you are an independent MT, you must be secure about your own work standards.

A great deal of self-discipline is required of the MT who wants to turn out perfect documents. No matter how accurate a speller you are and no matter how well honed your punctuation, capitalization, and mechanical skills, errors can and do occur, and it is necessary to approach every document you prepare with the attitude that errors may be present. A systematic search for errors is then begun. Generally, mistakes are not made from ignorance or carelessness but rather from the inability to "see" the mistake (to recognize it) or because you have become too familiar with the material or because you are dealing with unfamiliar material. If you have never heard of something, you might not consider questioning it. Many errors are of this type. You could also commit errors of interpretation, or you could inadvertently leave out a word.

Because you have progressed this far, you know where many mistakes can be found. It is unlikely that you will make errors in format; if you learned your punctuation, capitalization, and mechanical rules well, these areas should not bother you. If you are careful to stop and check spelling, remembering not to depend on your spellchecker, each time you have a doubt about accuracy, where will you look for errors?

WHERE ERRORS OCCUR

Differences of opinion exist among teachers, students, and your prospective employers as to what an error is and how important different errors are. For example, transposed letters in the name of a drug could be very serious, whereas the incorrect use of a capital letter, although upsetting to a fastidious instructor, would hardly be grounds for dismay on the part of an employer. In addition, many other kinds of errors are value judgments on the part of the student, teacher, or quality assurance manager (QA).

In fact, some kinds of errors are "permissible" and with them the document is still usable; most errors are easily corrected. The important thing is to *find* our mistakes before they become part of the medical record.

 MT TOOL BOX TIP: A flaw in your work is a chance to learn.

On the other hand, you do not want to work so slowly to avoid making errors that your production drops or you become nervous about the errors you "could" be making. Instead, try to keep your errors to a minimum, learn to find those you do make, and learn to correct them quickly and easily.

When transcribing from equipment (in contrast to copy typing or transcribing from notes), you can look at your work while keyboarding; therefore, you can see most mistakes and correct them as they occur.

On-screen proofreading itself is not as easy as proofreading hard copy (the printed page) because you could overlook some errors (e.g., punctuation marks, letters that tend to blend together). You must train your eyes to spot the smallest of errors. In the classroom, always proofread your work on screen until you feel it is perfect. One trick is to increase the font size to 14 points. Most of the letters that tend to blur and blend (*e, o*) will show up. Return the document to the proper font size, print it out, and proofread it, and notice what, if anything, has slipped past your previous efforts. Keep track of the errors you make so that you can be particularly careful in this area in the future. Keep a running score of how many documents were actually print ready. Your skills will improve in time, and proofreading is easier and less time consuming than redoing your work. Listen ahead to avoid grammar problems. Make your goal perfect on-screen editing. In real life, you won't have the luxury of printing to paper. Arrive quickly at the goal of not relying on needing to have a print copy.

A beginning student is often concerned with whether he or she should stop and research unfamiliar material as it occurs or should continue with the work and thoroughly proofread the document later, making corrections and insertions. One point in favor of continuing to work is that some "mystery words" are no longer mysteries when seen in the overall context; also, the dictator could use the word again, and you are now able to understand it. Becoming accustomed to a dictator's voice as you progress into a document clears up misunderstood words. If you decide to try this approach, highlight the area to which you must return and carefully leave clues for yourself about the missing material. Certainly it is wise to completely punctuate a sentence when you have the sentence in front of you. Clues such as drops and inflections of the voice help with the punctuation as you progress, but it is usually necessary to review the material later for final punctuation. Once again, never rely on a spellchecker to correct the overall document; but stop as you go along and check any words about which you are in doubt. It is not a good idea to research these later because you could overlook them and the spellchecker may not find them.

MT TOOL BOX TIP: Computer spellchecking—tool with hazards. Use carefully.

ACCURACY

Medical records must be as accurate as you can possibly type them. Achieving this goal requires accuracy on the part of *both* dictator and MT. The problem with accuracy sometimes is the meaning of the word "accuracy." Who determines what is accurate? For example, you have just learned some basic letter formats, and yet the dictator may ask that the reference line be placed at the top right edge of the page, which cancels the professional appearance of the letter. You know this placement is incorrect, and you know that those who receive the document will also question your skills, but you must do as the dictator directs. To him or her, that is accuracy.

Likewise, you have just completed a thorough study of punctuation, capitalization, and abbreviations. An employer may insist that all drug names be typed in full capitals, all abbreviations be punctuated, or inappropriate dashes be used. When you comply with these directions, you are being accurate. In certain circumstances, you might consider discussing these and any similar problems with the dictator, always remembering that the employer's version of accuracy must be followed.

Additionally, a hospital or its governing body can have rules already in place. The physician may dictate an abbreviation in the final diagnosis that you know is incorrect. However, both you and the dictator *must* comply with these rules; therefore, accuracy demands that you spell out these abbreviations and that you check with the dictator to be sure you have the correct words if you have any doubts.

Often the issue is not whether the document has been transcribed accurately but the definition of accuracy itself according to the dictator and/or the end user. Some dictators want the document to reflect the *meaning* of the dictation, requiring that gaps be filled in, grammar edited, style and formatting carried out according to the facility requirements; others want the transcribed report to reflect *exactly* what was dictated.

As an MT, you need to develop a trust relationship with the dictator, and when you become aware of inappropriate, incomplete, or inconsistent use of grammar, abbreviations, and so on, inform the dictator or supervisor and discuss the situation with him or her. If possible, discuss these possible problem areas when you are hired so that you will know what you should do.

Editing is like housecleaning; if you have done it well, no one will notice the work you put into it. However, if the work has not been done, you look careless.

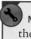 **MT TOOL BOX TIP:** Accuracy is a tool for which there is no substitute—keep it sharp.

QUALITY ASSURANCE

The quality of medical transcription is vital because of patient safety. The healthcare document also affects healthcare costs, because inefficient work can result in revenue loss and increased exposure to malpractice. As you learned in Chapter 1, the MT is the first line of defense in risk management. Good quality assurance provides for the standardization of style and format. Documentation must be of the highest quality and must be completed on a timely basis. The MT shares responsibility with the dictator to complete a high-quality transcript but should not be penalized for the failure of the dictator to be clear. The quality assurance manager is supportive of your efforts, and the process is meant to be educational, not critical, so that your performance will improve. You perform the evaluation most effectively while listening to your transcript and reading it. At this point, it would be a good idea for you to practice being the QA editor on one of your own documents or to share documents and dictation with a fellow student to get the feel of an evaluation.

 MT TOOL BOX TIP: Quality assurance—a reassurance tool.

TYPES OF ERRORS

The elimination of errors is paramount to the safety of the patient and to the completeness of the medical record. Elimination begins with the prevention of possible errors and close examination of the places where they could occur. (See overview of errors, Figure 7-1)

Critical Errors

Critical errors are so named because they have direct effect on patient safety. These errors may occur in the following manner:

▶ Patient identification: This area includes the correct spelling of the patient's name, social data, the record number, hospital number, x-ray number, pathology specimen number, Social Security number, and so on.

▶ Medical word misuse or inappropriate expansion of an abbreviation: For example, the abbreviation *MR* meant by the dictator to expand to "mitral regurgitation" instead reads "mental retardation."

▶ Template error: The dictator says "use my normal," and the normal template says "heart and lungs are clear." This *normal* is entered in the record. Later the dictator says, "There is a 2/6 systolic murmur." Either the dictator indicated the wrong template or the MT used the wrong template. The MT does not flag the conflict, resulting in an additional error.

▶ Incorrect drug names or dosage: For example, dictation of "point five milligrams" is transcribed 5 mg.

▶ Incorrect lab values: A wrong lab value could result in a patient not receiving proper treatment or followup testing.

▶ Incorrect test names.

▶ Inventive transcription: The transcriptionist makes up words or phrases that "appear to fit" when the actual dictation is not clear.

▶ Wrong disease names or diagnosis: Incorrect treatment and medical decisions could be the result along with inaccurate billing for medical care. It could take years for the patient's medical record to be corrected after an incorrect diagnosis has become part of that record.

▶ Dictation omitted: This error could be dictated material of a critical nature that was carelessly left out or deliberately omitted by the transcriptionist because he or she did not understand what was said. It could be a word or an entire sentence. For example, The dictator says "there is no pedal edema," and it is transcribed "There is pedal edema."

Even the normal lack of symptoms is important. There is also the temptation to just leave out something that is not easily understood. What is left out could be more important than what is left in.

Abbreviated Error Value Table Quality control				
Error level	Error type	Value/ volume method	Value/ 100 method	Pass/fail method
Critical	• Medical word misuse • Omitted dictation • Patient ID error • Upgrade of major due to patient impact	4	8	Fails with 1 critical error or more
Major	• Misspelled word • Incorrect verbiage usage • Minor error upgrade due to patient impact • Critical error downgrade – minimal impact	1.5	3	Fails with 3 major errors or more
	• Failure to flag for QA • Abuse of flagging • Protocol failure	1	2	
Minor	• Grammar/formatting error • Other miscellaneous errors	0.5	1	Fails with 9 minor errors or more
	• Critical or major error downgrade for minimal impact on patient safety	0.25	.5	
	• Punctuation • Dictator effect error	0	0	

FIGURE 7-1 Brief overview of three major types of errors.

▶ Incorrect unique medical record number: This error could be downgraded if it does not have the potential to directly compromise patient safety.

Major Errors

Major errors are ones that have an impact on document integrity. In some instances, a major error could become a critical error, depending on where it appears in the record.

▶ Abuse of flagging or leaving blanks when a term could easily have been looked up and found: This error is followed by the document being released to the site in this manner.

▶ Misspelled medical words: This error could be a typo or the substitution of a sound-alike word. This "misspelling" could actually result in a critical error if it affects the patient's safety.

▶ Misspelled English words: This error could be a word that changes the meaning of the sentence so that the reader must stop and think about what is read. The flow of understanding is halted. Such as, "The patient is not *aloud* to ambulate."

▶ Incorrect verbiage: The MT overuses editing and overrides the dictator's style, which is lost. The dictator could notice this error and say, "I would not have said that!" Or the MT transcribes exactly what was heard, paying no attention to the inappropriate

words left in the transcript. For instance, the dictator says, "The patient will be started on outpatient physical therapy … I'm sorry …outpatient occupational therapy." That sentence is transcribed exactly, *not* omitting the incorrect part and apology.

▶ Failure to flag and alert that something is omitted: For example, the section "allergies" was not dictated.

▶ Protocol failure: The MT did not use the preferred or standard format designated by the institution.

▶ Inappropriate or inaccurate use of abbreviations and symbols.

▶ Not choosing the correct account, so the report is misfiled.

Minor Errors

Minor errors do not compromise document integrity or affect patient safety. A minor error could be an error in grammar, punctuation, capitalization (did not capitalize a brand name of a drug) or a simple typo. It could be a dictation error that the MT did not correct.

RULES FOR RECOGNIZING AND AVOIDING ERRORS

CRITICAL ERROR RULE 7.1   Double-check any vital materials you transcribe.

Errors occur when numbers, dates, times, names, positions, and types and kinds of procedures and treatments are changed slightly or transposed with other similar material.

Verify demographic data, including correct spelling of the patient's name, record number, hospital number, x-ray number, pathology specimen number, Social Security number, and so on. Verify that the name dictated is the full and correct legal name of the patient, and confirm unusual names, a nickname that might be an actual given name, foreign names, names that could be easily transposed (e.g., James Scott vs. Scott James). Naming conventions vary from one culture to another, and shortened forms of names may cause confusion along with the changes of names due to marriage and divorce. Be sure to verify the correct and complete names of the attending physicians and all others involved in patient care. Confirm the accuracy of all dates, including dates of admission, discharge, and procedures. Be alert to problems and conditions, admissions and discharges, procedures, and so on that were described as having taken place *last year, two days ago, last month,* and so on. Research records to find out when exactly *yesterday* was when it was dictated and insert the correct date. You may use inexact dates, such as *the day after surgery* or *the day before he came into the emergency department,* if those dates appear in the report (e.g., the day of the surgery or the day he came into the emergency department).

CRITICAL ERROR RULE 7.2   Check closely to see that the result of your word expansion is appropriate.

Abbreviation expanders are wonderful time-savers because they enable you to type in an abbreviation that, with a cue, becomes a complete word or series of words. You need to complete the process carefully, or bizarre expansions result. Seasoned MTs have collections of these slipups. The slipups could be funny unless *you* are the responsible party. They are never funny to the person in whose medical record they occur.

EXAMPLES

Memphis, Tenderness (TN, *the abbreviation for* Tennessee, *is also the cue for* tenderness.)

San Ramon, Carcinoma (or condyloma acuminatum) (CA, *the abbreviation for* California, *is also the cue for these expressions.*)

Patients' names have carelessly been printed as follows:

Iron deficiency anemia Robinson (The patient's first name was Ida.)

Rectal examination Morris (The patient's first name was Rex.)

Diagnoses have been printed as follows:

Diagnosis: Struck with a pancreas (*a* pan)

Diagnosis: Sterile saline solution (*instead of* sick sinus syndrome)

CRITICAL ERROR RULE 7.3   Recognize that macro and template insertions are a potential source for problems, and recheck not only the insertion point but also the context.

A dictator may provide you with a list of predictated paragraphs, which you could then store in your software program. (See "macros" Figures C-46, C-47, and C-48 in Appendix C on Evolve.) You insert the paragraphs where appropriate in the dictation. However, you must check to be sure that they are accurate. A simple change of a number by the dictator or MT could place a paragraph pertaining to the closure of an abdominal incision into a transcription about the closure of an eye incision. Do not assume that the dictator is incapable of making a mistake about the accuracy of these directions.

CRITICAL ERROR RULE 7.4   Use reliable reference books to confirm spelling and correct dosage of drugs.

Because most drug manuals do not provide the phonetic pronunciation of a drug, it is possible for a variety of drug names to be substituted for the name dictated. Do not depend on the drug name that the spellchecker provides. Instead, check your drug reference for additional information about the drug to be sure that you have made the proper selection. Some dictators carefully spell drug names (or medical words they think you may have trouble locating). It is important to double-check any orally spelled words.

Look at this brief list of drug names that are frequently confused:

Accupril: quinapril (for hypertension)
Accutane: isotretinoin (for severe acne)

Ambien: zolpidem (for insomnia)
Amen: medroxyprogesterone (to prevent pregnancy)

amiloride: Midamor (for hypertension)
amlodipine: Norvasc (for chest pain and hypertension)

Celebrex: celecoxib (for arthritis)
Celexa: citalopram (for depression)

Clinoril: sulindac (for pain and inflammation)
Clozaril: clozapine (for schizophrenia)

clonidine: Catapres (for hypertension)
Klonopin: clonazepam (for anxiety)

Coumadin: warfarin (to thin the blood)
Compazine: prochlorperazine (for psychosis)

Flumadine: rimantadine (for influenza)
flutamide: Eulexin (for prostate cancer)

Fosamax: alendronate (for osteoporosis)
Flomax: tamsulosin (for enlarged prostate)

Lodine: etodolac (for pain and inflammation)
iodine (for skin infections)

Lotensin: benazepril (for hypertension)
Loniten: minoxidil (for hypertension)

Nicoderm: nicotine (to quit smoking)
Nitro-Derm: nitroglycerin (for angina)

Norvasc: amlodipine (for chest pain and hypertension)
Navane: thiothixene (for psychosis)

Paxil: paroxetine (for depression)
paclitaxel: Taxol (for ovarian cancer)

Pravachol: pravastatin (for high cholesterol)
propranolol: Inderal (for hypertension)

Premarin: conjugated estrogens (for osteoporosis)
Primaxin: imipenem and cilastatin (for various infections)

Prinivil: lisinopril (for hypertension)
Proventil: albuterol (for asthma)

Prozac: fluoxetine (for depression)
Proscar: finasteride (for enlarged prostate)

rimantadine: Flumadine (for influenza)
ranitidine: Zantac (for heartburn and ulcers)

Xanax: alprazolam (for anxiety)
Zantac: ranitidine (for heartburn and ulcers)

Zyrtec: cetirizine (for allergies)
Zantac: ranitidine (for heartburn and ulcers)
Zyprexa: olanzapine (for psychosis)

CRITICAL ERROR RULE 7.5 Verify that the patient's unique medical record and other demographic information (account number and/or visit episode) are correct.

In large facilities using electronic records, the dictator enters the demographic information (account number and/or visit episode number) directly into the dictation system either manually or by scanning. The MT *must* verify these numbers or the document could be entered into the wrong electronic record. Caregivers could unknowingly make treatment decision based on incomplete or inaccurate data, posing a serious risk to patient safety. This part of the record must be treated with the same critical eye toward potential errors as the body of the report.

CRITICAL ERROR RULE 7.6 Flag any area of the transcript that you cannot understand rather than inventing something that appears to fit. By the same token, do not omit a word, phrase, or sentence that you simply cannot understand.

 MT TOOL BOX TIP: A flag is a tool asking for help.

MAJOR ERROR RULE 7.7 Always consult a reference when you have the slightest doubt about the spelling of any word.

Whether a word is misspelled or just mistyped, the result is the same: a spelling error that can mislead or distract the reader. A misspelling can be the result of a dropped letter, an added letter, transposed letters, wrong letters, substituted letters, or a homonym used in place of the word dictated. For simplicity's sake, we just refer to the word as "misspelled."

Most computer software programs have built-in English spellchecking capabilities. You also can install medical dictionaries and medical spellchecking systems. There is no excuse today for a misspelled word in your documents, and there is no excuse for failing to use the spellchecking feature. Whether you stop and check as you go along or check when you finish a document is your preference. If necessary, you must clarify any questionable word with a dictionary to be sure you select the correct word. If the spellchecking feature has no words to suggest, you must thoroughly research.

Also, it is imprudent to have a correctly spelled word that sounds like the word you want but makes no sense in the context of the sentence. Spellchecking systems give a false sense of security by indicating that the word is correct, whereas actually they signify that "this is a word and this word is spelled correctly." They do not indicate "this is the correct word." This characteristic can create a particular hazard for drug names that sound alike. Homonyms (words that sound alike or look alike) are not recognized by spellcheckers as misspelled words. Also, the spellchecker will not recognize a wrong word substitute or other grammatical errors.

Homonyms require the most careful scrutiny in proofreading. You need to be aware of the many English homonyms in use and be alert for the sound-alike medical word as well. Homonyms are dictated correctly but the MT perceives the word incorrectly or is unaware of the existence of another word that sounds like or is similar to what was dictated. In Chapter 10, you will study homonyms in depth. Also, Appendix B lists them for you.

MAJOR ERROR RULE 7.8   Never leave a blank unless you have exhausted research possibilities.

However, typing a word that you *think* matches the word you need is never appropriate. Never type in nonsense words that cannot possibly be correct even though the word sounds right. Every word that you use must be appropriate to the text. Dictionary research is required when there is any doubt. You need to have good judgment in contrast to good guessing. Students and MTs alike could say, "That is just what it sounded like" or "That is just what was said." Do not be guilty of repeating these phrases in defense of errors in your work.

EXAMPLES

Mucous membranes were intact. (*Correct* use of the adjective form)

Mucus membranes were intact. (*Incorrect* use of the noun form)

After delivery of the placenta, the *perineal* tear was suture ligated. (*Correct*)

After delivery of the placenta, the *peroneal* tear was suture ligated. (*Incorrect* because *peroneal* pertains to the fibula, a bone in the lower leg)

A *culdocentesis* was performed, which revealed pooling of blood. (*Correct*)

A *colpocentesis* was performed, which revealed pooling of blood. (*Incorrect* because *colpocentesis* is not a word but sounds logical because *colpo* has to do with the vagina and the dictation concerns a gynecologic problem.)

Therefore, blanks may be left inappropriately when the MT could have found the word or words with proper research and diligence. Consider the previous example. The MT could have decided that *colpocentesis* was not correct but did not know what word would be correct and so left a blank with a note indicating that the word sounded like *colpocentesis*. (Research skills are discussed in Chapter 8.) It could be easy to renege on responsibility, to give up quickly and go forward, if the MT knows that someone else can probably insert the proper word. You can easily understand why an excessive number of blanks is considered a major error. Remember that a blank must always be left rather than have erroneous information in a report when the MT feels that a significant error is in the dictation.

MINOR ERROR RULE 7.9   If you must divide a word, divide it only at the proper point when you are transcribing documents such as printed reports or letters. (Do not divide a word when transcribing documents for uploading into an electronic record. An MT also has to be careful about using hard returns in the wrong places because those hard returns "split" lines and uploading messes up the lines.)

With the word-wrap feature of word processing software, you seldom must concern yourself with word division. Only when a right margin is very ragged should you consider breaking a word in two. Also, avoid dividing words because unhyphenated words are easier to read; hyphenation slows down production and can require checking with reference materials. Words can be divided only between syllables or word parts. There are preferred places to divide a word, and every effort must be made to divide at these points. Dividing a word incorrectly is the same as misspelling it. Newspapers and magazines divide words in places that do not necessarily conform to spelling rules, so do not use journalistic material for a reference. Here are a few hints:

▶ Divide a solid compound word between the elements of the compound.

   time/table   gall/bladder   child/birth

▶ Divide a date between the day and the year, not between the month and the day.

   September 1,/2010 not September/1, 2010

▶ Divide a word with a prefix between the prefix and the root word.

   ante/natal   post/operative   trans/sacral

▶ Divide a word between the root and the suffix.

   gono/coccus   trache/ostomy   cyst/itis

▶ Divide a street address between the name of the street and the words *street, avenue, circle,* and so on.

   3821 Ocean/Street or

   821 East Hazard/Road or

   821 East/Hazard Road

Furthermore, do not divide the last line on a page, one-syllable words (e.g., *weight, thought, strength*), proper names, abbreviations, or word sets.

page 421	**8 pounds 3 ounces**	**gravida 1 para 1**
x-ray	**5 feet 6 inches tall**	**2 cm**

MINOR ERROR RULE 7.10   Always check printouts to be sure they conform to proper placement protocol.

Rules concerning the spacing after certain punctuation marks, abbreviations, and symbols should be carefully followed. Spacing problems often occur with word processing and computer printouts that automatically take material to another line (or page) when you did not intend to do so. Use the widow/orphan control feature of your software program so that lines are not left alone on the bottom or top of a page. Always check your printout to be sure that the headers appear where they were intended. If documents are to be printed off site and you do not have an opportunity to review the printed copy, be sure that someone on site checks the documents and the printer setup for you.

When you type or make changes to something you have entered into the computer, it is possible to create a new error in the process. Double-check your correction! The cut-and-paste feature can cause misplacement of material above or below the cut or pasted material. Reread both areas carefully to check that no misplacement has occurred. Another common "newly created" error is to repeat a word on the line after the word, such as "and and." Spellcheckers do alert you to this "double-word" entry, so remember to make a final spellcheck to catch this type of error.

MINOR ERROR RULE 7.11 Always know why you are placing a punctuation mark.

Placing punctuation marks where they do not belong and omitting others that should be included are obvious problems. A comma fault (e.g., one comma missing from a comma pair, a comma separating a dependent clause, or commas enclosing essential elements) is a common error. The improper use and substitution of marks (e.g., a colon for a semicolon or a comma for a semicolon) are examples of other errors. Punctuation errors are often made because the MT has not listened far enough ahead in the material to grasp the sense of the sentence or has forgotten to look at the entire sentence and to return to insert or delete marks.

MINOR ERROR RULE 7.12 Always know why you are using a capital letter.

Most capitalization errors are caused by a failure to capitalize. However, you should be careful not to capitalize unless there is a reason for the capital letter.

MINOR ERROR RULE 7.13 Know the technical symbols for your specialty area and use them correctly.

Errors with numbers and symbols are usually caused by writing out numbers rather than using numerals. Remember to express age, drug dosage, time of day, and other technical terms in numerals (see Chapter 5). Omission of a symbol is certainly a minor error and usually occurs because the transcriptionist is unaware of the symbol or abbreviation.

On occasion, symbols and abbreviations may be used incorrectly. For example, sometimes a symbol is avoided and the word is spelled out because it is

difficult to stop and make that symbol. However, this maneuver is not an error if the dictator approves of this substitution. The improper use of symbols and abbreviations, rather than the failure to use them, is usually what causes errors. Additionally, the use of some symbols is never acceptable in some situations, (e.g. the &, %, ° symbols), because the symbols do not upload properly. Be sure that you know your client's preferences for symbol use and the use of bold and underlining.

EXAMPLES

Postoperative diagnosis: *PID (Incorrect use of abbreviation)*

Postoperative diagnosis: *Pelvic inflammatory disease (Correct)*

a *3-cm.* incision was carried along the… *(Incorrect: a period is not used; the hyphen is incorrect)*

a *3 cm* incision was carried along the… *(Correct)*

We used a dilute solution of *ten to one. (Incorrect number use)*

We used a dilute solution of *10:1. (Correct)*

MINOR ERROR RULE 7.14 Proofread carefully, correct all typographical errors, and use all electronic shortcuts with caution. Carefully check the on-screen document before you indicate "send" or "print."

Many computer programs have the capability to convert certain codes or symbols that are typed within the text to complete words, phrases, sentences, or paragraphs by the use of abbreviation expanders. Codes or "boilerplates" are also used by some programs to indicate a certain style, setup, or format. The inadvertent use or mistyping of these symbols results in a printout containing an incorrect format (e.g., setup, underlining, spacing, centering, indenting) or an inappropriate word, phrase, or even an entire paragraph or two.

EXAMPLE

Conclusion:

Relatively

severe

L4–5

spinal

stenosis.

(Somehow a code was given to the computer to print this stacked format.)

Users of voice recognition systems enjoy knowing that the transcribed material generally has no spelling errors. However, other errors can appear, and sometimes they are a bit tricky to correct because they can slip by unnoticed.

EXAMPLES

When lifting a patient from *bad* to *share* with a coworker… *(bed to chair)* which *dies* not seem to aggravate her back pain. … *(does)*

She is able to bend forward at the *waste*. …*(waist)* *(homonyms are very common)*

He is able to perform toe raises with both the right *hand* left lower extremities … *(and)*

We saw your patient today who is still under our *car* for physical therapy. *(care)*

Thank you for permitting me to participate in this *patient' scare. (patient's care)*

Juan, Jon, one, won, and *yawn* often turn up in interesting places.

Editing

The area being discussed in your transcript has been material you have produced. Now look at the words themselves and see what, if any, control you have over the "sound" of the transcript. To a certain extent, the MT must edit the transcription. The term "editing" means making minor corrections in certain areas of the transcript *while preserving the exact meaning, style, and personality* of the author or dictator. Now examine where these problems lie. Editing is always inappropriate when it alters information or tampers with the author's style, or when there is uncertainty about what was actually said, second-guessing the dictator.

Grammar

Skilled MTs change, delete, and clean up work, often unaware that they are doing so. They would not consider such activity to be an integral part of their job, but it is. Dictators for whom they work consider them invaluable or, often, are unaware that MTs have carried out this function. There is no argument about correcting improper grammar; never leave in a grammatical error with the misguided notion that you are transcribing "exactly what was said." Grammar rules are thoroughly reviewed in Chapter 10. Some additional areas in which alert and careful proofreading is required include word usage, singular and plural nouns, position of modifiers, and verb tense.

One can "get away with" many bad habits in our spoken language that are not correct in written form. For example, in writing, avoid using contractions.

Nouns and adjectives must be used correctly (see Chapter 9).

EXAMPLES

He was scheduled for replacement of his *aorta* valve. *(aortic)*

She had a *vesicle* fistula to her vagina. *(vesical)*

The proper use of singular or plural nouns is discussed in Chapter 9 as well.

EXAMPLE

The *conjunctiva* were bilaterally inflamed. *(conjunctivae)*

Take care to position modifiers correctly.

EXAMPLES

The patient had a hysterectomy leaving one tube and ovary in Jacksonville. *(Incorrect)*

The patient had a hysterectomy in Jacksonville, leaving one tube and ovary. *(Correct)*

She was given ampicillin and gentamicin because of her heart murmur every 6 hours. *(Incorrect)*

She was given ampicillin and gentamicin every 6 hours because of her heart murmur. *(Correct)*

Sometimes the errors in positioning may lighten up our day.

EXAMPLES

The baby was delivered, the cord clamped and cut, and handed to the pediatrician, who breathed and cried immediately.

I saw the patient in the emergency room while you were on vacation for dysfunctional bleeding.

Finally, be careful to use the proper tense and not to shift it inappropriately. Past tense is used in the *history* part of a report, in discharge summaries, and in discussion about a patient who has died. Present tense is used in the current illness or disease and in the history and physical examination.

EXAMPLES

The patient *has had* left sciatica for the past two years; this *is* now exacerbated. *(Correct combination of history of problem and current problem)*

The conjunctivae *are* bilaterally inflamed. *(Correct for current examination)*

The conjunctivae *were* bilaterally inflamed. *(Correct for discussion of history of eye problem)*

Inconsistencies, Redundancies, and Technical Errors

Physicians do not dictate in the same manner that they would write out material, often editing as they go along. John Dirckx, MD, expressed it well in the Summer 1990 issue of *Perspectives on the Medical Transcription Profession:*

> By choosing to dictate a document rather than write it out, the dictator not only sidesteps many of the mechanical tasks associated with composition but implicitly delegates these tasks to the transcriptionist. No dictators have such perfect powers of concentration that they never accidentally repeat themselves, never inadvertently substitute one word for another, never leave a sentence unfinished. Sooner or later, the most alert and cautious dictator makes each of these mistakes, and others besides. Clearly, these normal human lapses ought not to be reproduced

in the transcript; and just as clearly, the duty of identifying and correcting them devolves on the transcriptionist.

Careful editing is necessary for good risk management, and dictators appreciate the time and trouble taken to retain accuracy and grammar.

Editing for medical accuracy often requires skill that even some experienced MTs have not acquired. The physician could be discussing a tendon in the hand and use the term for a tendon found in the foot. The MT who is alert to this either has an excellent knowledge of terms or, in researching the proper spelling for the tendon, sees that the incorrect term was used. Either way, the desired result is achieved. The researching MT uses the *lack* of knowledge to obtain more knowledge, and the beginner must focus on making research another learning tool. Another example is when, through a slip of the tongue, the dictator says "hypotension" when "hypertension" has been the subject of the report and the meaning for hypertension is implied; the MT notes and corrects this mistake immediately. Attendance at medical lectures helps the MT not only to acquire knowledge about new medical materials, techniques, and procedures but also to reinforce anatomy and physiology skills. An educated MT is prepared to recognize potential errors because of an increased understanding of medicine.

However, do not get on the wrong track about some errors. Ellen Drake, CMT, AHDI-F, reference book author, feels strongly about editing:

> *Too many people confuse style with correctness. Clear, unambiguous, medically correct communication should be the goal. I do not believe Q/A* staff or proofreaders should spend their time correcting what are essentially style errors. While quality is most important, turnaround time is important too. A report that does not get on the patient's chart in a timely manner because it was held up in Q/A is far more hazardous in terms of patient care than an omitted comma or the capitalization of a generic drug.*

MINOR ERROR RULE 7.15 Adjust or rephrase inconsistencies.

EXAMPLE

The patient drinks several beers per day, occasional cigars and cigarettes. *(Incorrect)*

The patient drinks several beers per day and occasionally smokes cigars and cigarettes. *(Correct)*

MINOR ERROR RULE 7.16 Delete redundancies.

EXAMPLE

The patient has no sisters and no siblings. *(Incorrect)*

The patient has no siblings. *(Correct)*

*Quality assurance

When you become more proficient at transcription, you will be able to recognize that there are other medical inconsistencies that you have the ability to correct. At this point, you probably will recognize them but you might not know what to do. You do have the obligation to ask when in doubt.

MINOR ERROR RULE 7.17 Spell out slang, jargon, and short-form expressions.

Unlike abbreviations, in which letters take the place of whole words, slang or short-form expressions are abbreviated forms of complete words. Slang expressions are used to avoid the real word (substitutes for *death* are very common) or because the dictator is comfortable with a colloquial expression and does not notice its use.

EXAMPLES

After repeated attempts at resuscitation, the patient *was flat line* and was *pronounced.* (Substitute *died* and finish the sentence with *pronounced dead* and the time of day.)

After three hours of labor, this *primip's* contractions *fizzled out,* and she was sent home. (Change to *primipara's* and consider the use of *stopped* or *diminished.*)

She was sent to the mental health unit for a *psych eval.* (Insert *psychiatric evaluation.*)

The pain did not *bug* her much. (Insert *bother.*)

Check the list of short forms or slang expressions in Appendix B and see which of these are acceptable in transcription. Expressions that may be allowable in an office chart note or emergency department note are not always acceptable in a letter or consultation report.

NOTE: Some unusual words used in medicine can appear strange the first time you hear them. Physicians use such words as *peanuts, fat* towels, *Dandy* scissors, and *cigarette* drains during surgery. Neurologists may make note of *gull-wing* signs and *dolls' eye* movements. See Appendix B for a list of many unusual medical terms.

MINOR ERROR RULE 7.18 Correct technical errors.

EXAMPLES

A *2 mm* incision was closed above the left eyebrow. *(Too small)*

A *2 cm* incision was closed.

The baby weighed *3-1/2* kg. *(Incorrect use of fraction with a metric unit of measure)*

The baby weighed *3.5* kg.

There was a *2 × 2 × 2* ovarian tumor.

There was a *2 × 2 × 2 cm* ovarian tumor. *(This information is confirmed by the pathology report, operative report, or dictating physician.)*

We removed *1800 mg* of serosanguinous fluid. *(Wrong unit of measurement)*

We removed *1800 mL* of serosanguinous fluid.

NOTE: Chapter 5 includes a complete review of the metric system to help you with these measurements.

EXAMPLES

The *suture* was closed with #6-0 silk sutures. *(Incorrect)*

The *wound* was closed with #6-0 silk sutures. *(Correct)*

NOTE: When you are working and errors like the preceding occur, you have to ask your supervisor or the dictator for the correct word unless you are *positive* you know what word was intended but not dictated.

EXAMPLES

The tonsils were removed by blunt and sharp *diagnosis.* *(Dissection)*

The patient is edentulous with carious teeth. *(Incorrect)* *(Either he has no teeth or many carious teeth or even some carious teeth and some missing teeth.)*

Most physicians depend on the MT to discover dictation errors, and they appreciate being alerted to possible errors or inconsistencies so that they can make appropriate corrections if necessary. Consider these sentences:

> This 33-year-old woman had her gallbladder removed in 1965.
>
> The patient presented with diffuse infiltrate in the *left* lower lung fields, and bronchography confirmed her lower lobe bronchiectasis; therefore, a *right* thoracotomy and *right* lower lobectomy were performed the following day.

If you have access to the patient's medical record, you can determine the correct age of the woman or the correct date of her cholecystectomy. Examination of the actual x-ray films or the medical record should help you clarify the right-left problem in the second sentence. If not, you must check these with the dictator. Other mistakes dictators make are *he/she* substitutions or substitution of the referring physician's name for the patient's name. Prefix mixups are common: *hyper/ hypo, hemi/semi, pre/post,* and so on.

If the physician dictates "the chest x-ray 'was negative'" or "the physical examination findings were 'within normal limits,'" flag the report so that these are expanded. For instance, the expanded version could say that "the chest film was reviewed and there were no abnormalities." You cannot make this editorial change, but you can flag it for those who can and should.

Computers provide wonderful editing features: you can change and rearrange words, insert and remove punctuation, manipulate and rearrange entire sentences or paragraphs, increase or decrease the size of the margins, add or delete tab stops, and so on.

However, while you are busy with these tasks, you could change a sentence so that there is no longer a subject, the verb is missing or is in a singular form instead of a plural form, a paragraph appears in the wrong place, a duplicate paragraph is added instead of an electronic cut-and-paste item, the headers appear other than where they were intended, and so on. A nightmare can be created. Particular care must be taken whenever you perform these procedures.

Abbreviations

Take particular care with abbreviations and use them only when appropriate. Remember that the letters *d, p, g, t,* and *e* sound very much alike, and *n* sounds like *and* or *in,* and vice versa.

Misunderstandings

One problem that even the most experienced MT confronts is that of not quite hearing, or not being able to understand, a word or phrase that is dictated. Because you can back up the dictation over and over again, the word or words could eventually "come to you." It helps to listen ahead; sometimes the word is used again and said more clearly, or the meaning of the word becomes obvious because of other words or other parts of the document. Many transcribing units have controls that permit the operator to increase and decrease the speed of playback. The use of this option can facilitate the understanding of a word. Here are some simple examples of such words or phrases:

EXAMPLES

There was a large grey "whirling tuna." *(whorling tumor)*

He had one "slight" dyspnea. *(flight)*

There were no rales or "bronchi." *(rhonchi)*

You would have difficulty transcribing these sentences because you cannot make the connection with the word needed. You should not transcribe sentences that do not make sense to you. Such problems become increasingly difficult as words or phrases become more complex.

Dictators for whom English is not a first language, speaking according to the grammatical rules governing their own language, know what they want to say but sometimes make odd English word choices. These expressions indicate a language barrier, not poor patient care. It is your responsibility to determine what the dictator intended to say and type the material that way, again taking care to preserve the integrity of the meaning of the sentence.

EXAMPLES

The incision was *prolonged.*

The incision was *extended.*

The patient's *painful feets had disappeared.*
The patient's *foot pain* had disappeared.

Many missing teeth *present.*
Many missing teeth. or Many teeth missing.

Mother *has* a history of bronchitis when she was *old.*
Mother *had* a history of bronchitis when she was *elderly.*

This goal is easier to accomplish if you are working in a setting in which you have regular conversation with a dictator whose first language is not English. Then you become used to the nuances of his or her English translation problems. Each language is structured in a particular way; when you know or understand that structure, it is easier to work with such problems as omitting the past tense participle, making all words plural by adding an *s* to the singular, transposing words, or choosing the incorrect synonym. Many foreign-born physicians have extensive English vocabularies and speak perfect English; however, a heavy accent or the inability to pronounce certain sounds in English makes it difficult to understand them until you have "tuned in your ears." You have the obligation to assist the dictator and make him or her sound good. Actually, the dictator trusts that you will make his or her dictation appear as correct and professional as possible.

Flagging

As you learned earlier, leaving an inappropriate blank is a major error. Carry out proper research for missing data before you decide you must leave a blank and flag it.

Again, do not type material that does not make sense to you. If you cannot understand a word and the dictator is unavailable, ask your supervisor or another MT for help. If they cannot help, then it is time to leave a flag. Marking a document with a flag is also called carding or tagging. Repositionable adhesive notes make the best flags. They have just enough adhesive on the back to hold them firmly in place until removed. You can also staple or paperclip your flag. When you flag a document, you leave an underlined blank space in your material that is long enough to allow you to insert the correct word later without disturbing the format (usually 10 spaces are enough to call attention to the blank), and then you attach a *flag* to the material. A flag should include the patient's name, the page number, the paragraph, and the line of the missing word. If you are in a large organization, add your name. It helps the editor if you put the missing word in context; that is, include a few words that come before and after it. Give a hint, if you can, of the sound of the word even if the sound seems pretty silly to you.

The QA can frequently fill in the missing word with these simple clues. The QA inserts the correct word with the guidance of your page and line number notes. Be sure to remember to follow up on your flag to learn how it was resolved so that you can resolve a similar issue in the future on your own. It is really the QA's responsibility to do this, but make it your responsibility to see that it is carried out to your satisfaction.

EXAMPLE

Williams, Maribeth #18-74-78. Under PX, Respiratory (page 2, line 8) "respirations present." Sounds like "chain smokes." Judy, 5-17-XX

The reply to this will read "*Cheyne-Stokes* respirations present." You should remember to also follow this format on your practice transcripts. See Figure 7-2 for an example of a preprinted note that can be attached to your transcript.

You may encounter a unique electronic flagging system that has a built in code so that when an indistinguishable word or phrase is dictated, the MT can depress a preset code key and a symbol (e.g., <...........>) is inserted into the document. With another preset code, a pop-up screen or window appears. The MT types the difficult word or phrase phonetically in this special flag screen. With the tap of another code key, the original document returns to the main screen and transcription continues. These "markers" prevent the document from going to the client; it is sent directly to QA personnel for completion. Later, the MT receives a printed copy of the document to learn what the mystery word was.

In a regular transcript you should not type in a series of periods, asterisks, or question marks; do leave an obvious underlined blank space. Do not type something about the missing word; this information must be put on the attached or electronic flag. If your material is printed off site and you are not able to flag or tag it, then you must leave an electronic flag with the transcript. Some MTs have a phobia about leaving blanks. Vera Pyle, CMT, a founding member of the American Association for Medical Transcription (now known as AHDI) and author of *Current Medical Terminology,* had this to say about blanks:

> To me a blank is an honorable thing; it means you don't know. If you have tried everything you can try to fill in that blank and can't, leaving a blank is preferable to guessing. Guessing is bluffing and to me it is more honest to admit, "I don't know; I couldn't hear." It is filled in in a doctor's handwriting in ink and is entirely legal and entirely acceptable.

Some MTs use a full sheet of paper for a flag, forcing the signer of the document to lift it from the signature area to sign, in the hope that it will be noticed. Do whatever works.

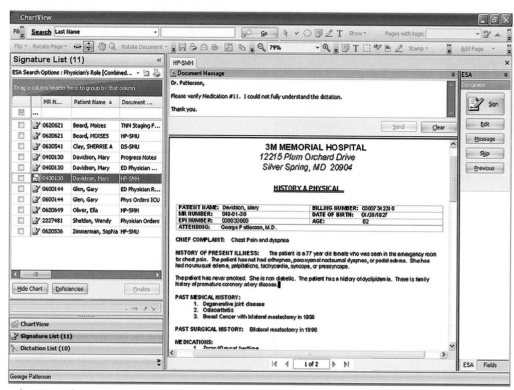

Screen shot showing a flag query for a problem in the dictation. (Courtesy of 3M Health Information Systems, Inc. © 3M. All rights reserved.)

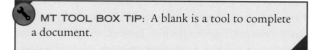

MT TOOL BOX TIP: A blank is a tool to complete a document.

Slang, Vulgar, and Inflammatory Remarks

When you are employed in the word processing department of a large clinic or hospital, your supervisor can assist you in handling questionable material. MTs working for a service with policies demanding verbatim transcription can likewise ask a supervisor or director for help. In a private medical office, you may, of course, approach the dictator directly for help.

Very few physicians make derogatory or inflammatory remarks, but it can happen. For example, they may be speaking in this manner because they are frustrated with the care of the patient. A surgeon may have just lost his or her patient to disease or accident and tears through the hospital, leaving a path of destruction behind. The *stupid physician* referred to in the dictation the surgeon leaves behind in your department reflects the frustration of not being able to help or loss of control of a situation. That remark, obviously, is not meant to appear in print.

Questionable remarks can reflect on you and your judgement, the physician, the hospital, and the patient.

What if the dictator refers to patients, patients' families, or other members of the healthcare team as *stupid, crocks, dumb, lousy surgeons, quacks, too dumb to know any better,* and so on? The dictator will usually have forgotten the irritation that precipitated the problem in the first place by the time you transcribe the dictation. Some institutions provide written policies on how to deal with inappropriate or inflammatory remarks written or dictated into the record. MTs must discover whether there are any written directions or rules for handling these kinds of remarks and follow these directives. Because most physicians are not legal experts, they can put themselves, and the institution, and you at risk if they are unaware of unprofessional language in the dictation.

In addition to inappropriate comments about the patient, statements referring to hospital personnel, other physicians, comments made regarding injury to the patient during a procedure, and comments made about complications or aborted procedures need to come to the attention of risk management personnel. Risk management personnel must be involved in any decision about what should or should not be written into the records. If procedures are enumerated and one of them was not dictated in the report, the MT must flag to alert either the dictator or QA. If you are uncomfortable with the dictation or the language used, you must ask for help.

Dear Doctor _____ :

RE: Patient name _____

Report name _____

Date dictated _____

☐ Please see blank on page ___ , paragraph ____ of this report. It sounded like _____

☐ Dictate more slowly and distinctly.

☐ Spell proper names.

☐ Spell unusual words in address.

☐ Spell patient names.

☐ Spell new and unusual surgical instruments.

☐ Spell new drug names.

☐ Spell new laboratory tests.

☐ Indicate unusual punctuation.

☐ Indicate closing salutation.

☐ Indicate your title.

☐ Indicate end of letter.

☐ Give dates of reports.

☐ Speak louder.

☐ Give patient's hospital number.

☐ Please read the area of this report indicated by the penciled checkmark for accuracy.

☐ Your dictation was cut off. Please fill in the rest of the report or redictate.

Thank you. Please return this note with corrections to:

Transcriptionist _____

Telephone No. _____ Date _____

FIGURE 7-2 Example of a flagging or tagging note to be attached to a medical manuscript for solving problem dictation. This form can be copied and then attached to the problem transcription. (From Diehl MO: *Medical Transcription Guide: Do's and Don'ts,* ed 3, St Louis, Saunders, 2004.)

Do you transcribe it? Consider these alternatives:

▶ Check with your supervisor before transcribing it.

▶ Contact the dictator, and diplomatically and tactfully ask about it.

▶ Make two transcripts, flag the problem, and ask the dictator to make a choice, destroying the original and copies of the rejected transcript (this method is costly and time consuming).

▶ Leave a blank with a flag that says, "I'm sorry, but I couldn't quite make out the first three words in paragraph 2."

It is better to leave a blank than to type a questionable remark. How you handle the problem depends on your work situation and your personal contact, if you have one, with the dictator.

EXAMPLE

This patient's condition would never have deteriorated to this extent if the nitwit charge nurse on four had brought it to my attention instead of taking it upon herself to practice medicine without a license.

Inflammatory remarks have no place in a medical record and could place innocent people in jeopardy. You were not there when the incident occurred, and you have no idea what precipitated this remark, and so it would not be your responsibility to edit or delete it. Your responsibility *is* to bring it to the attention of the dictator, supervisor, or risk manager *before* it becomes a permanent part of the patient's legal medical record. The risk manager is responsible for reporting, analyzing, and tracking any atypical occurrence in a hospital or other facility.

Sometimes the questionable remark is slang, overuse of contractions, or simply poor word choice.

EXAMPLES

Mom and *dad* were very accepting of the special care needed. (*A change to* The patient's parents were… *might be the choice of the QA.*)

The patient's scar has remained *pretty* much unchanged essentially. (*Pretty is generally a poor word choice, and in this case, combined with* scar, *it invites a simple edit:* The patient's scar has remained essentially unchanged.)

The sigmoidoscopy showed *tics*. (diverticula)

We DC'd the prednisone. (discontinued)

Hypospadias *doesn't look too bad. (Ask for help)*

Simple Editing

Your ability to analyze, polish, and proofread effectively and accurately will reflect your professional development. Remember: follow the protocol available, master the intricacies of English, and become familiar with trustworthy websites and reference materials and how to use them. Keep current; expand your vocabulary daily.

You must remember that medical records are legal documents, and although they are vital in the care of the patient, they are also vital historically and could be the major protection for the physician in the case of a misunderstanding or a professional liability lawsuit. It is imperative that they be current, accurate, legible, unaltered, and clear.

"Distance" Errors

Errors that typically (or usually) do not occur when transcribing local dictation with familiar names of places, businesses, hospitals, clinics, health groups, and so on can occur in "distance" transcription in which the names of people and places in health care are not in the MT's database. Doctor's names, place names, pharmacy names, and so on become a real problem. The unusual are bad enough, but even the ordinary place name can be a challenge if you have never heard it before. It could be mispronounced, you haven't a clue for an Internet search, and, of course, the dictator does not spell it for you or cannot spell it either. Every language has been borrowed from to name places, buildings, and landmarks. There can be no guessing. Leave clues and prepare to leave a blank and your flag.

Dr. Dirckx's comment in the Summer 1990 issue of *Perspectives on the Medical Transcription Profession* is an apt conclusion to the art of making corrections:

A permanent medical document dictated by one professional and transcribed by another is expected to conform to certain norms of precision, clarity, coherence, and taste. Most transcriptionists perform this operation so deftly and unobtrusively that the majority of dictators never even suspect that their dictation has undergone revision (or that it needed it).

Scoring Methods (Figures 7-3 and 7-4)

Scorers must do the following
1. Correctly identify the error.
2. Assign a predetermined value to the error.
   a. Critical errors affecting patient safety (3 points).
   b. Major errors affecting document integrity (1 to 2 points).
   c. Minor errors (0.25 to 0.5 points).
3. Determine the total score by using one of these criteria.
   a. Error values relative to total line counts.
   b. Scoring values subtracted from 100 regardless of size of the document.
   c. Pass/fail based on the number of major and minor errors.

Error scores can be upgraded from one category to another if they have the potential to compromise patient safety. Likewise, they can be downgraded if the impact to document integrity is minor or if there is minimal impact on the record. The main goal of correcting a minor error is instructional.

A defect in the document caused by poor dictation, inaccurate information provided by the dictator, failure of equipment, and so on, which add to the difficulties in producing an accurate document, is taken into consideration when a document is scored. QA standards apply to the originator of the document as well; however, if the document is returned from the originator as unacceptable, that is a problem.

These scores must be used to see the patterns of strengths and weaknesses so suggestions for improvement can be made. QA editors can assist MTs to do a better job, improve the quality of the output, and increase production.

The quality of the document produced by the MT directly affects the patient by influencing medical decisions and contributing to the continuity of care. Patient safety is paramount, but the data affect provider reimbursement as well. Additionally, healthcare compliance agencies inspect records for quality control. The goal of scoring is to eliminate errors, not to just achieve a good score. If errors are tracked and identified, the MT can concentrate on directed training to improve skills in that area (e.g., failure to recognize homonyms). The use of mentors for a time really positively affects the learning curve.

Quality Assurance Summary

Name: _____ MT ID#: _____

Date: _____ QA Staff: _____

Report Review Information

Job number(s)	Lines	QA score	Copy/feedback
1.			
2.			
3.			
4.			
5.			
6.			
7.			
Total			

Error	Qty	Value	Deduction
Critical errors affecting patient safety			
Medical word misuse		3.0	
Omitted dictation		3.0	
Patient identification error		3.0	
Upgrade of major or minor error due to patient safety impact		3.0	
Major errors affecting document integrity			
Abuse of flagging/blanks		2.0	
Medical word misspelling		1.5	
English word misspelling		1.5	
Incorrect verbiage		1.5	
Failure to flag		1.0	
Protocol failure		1.0	
Upgrade of minor error due to document integrity impact		1.5	
Downgrade of critical error due to less than critical impact		1.5	
Minor errors			
Grammar/formatting		0.5	
Miscellaneous/other		0.5	
Downgrade of error due to minimal critical or document integrity impact		0.25	
Punctuation/typo		0	
Dictation effects impacting documentation			
Critical dictator effect		0	
Major dictator effect		0	
Minor dictator effect		0	

Notes:

FIGURE 7-3 Quality Assurance Summary showing three major error types.

QUALITY ANALYSIS REPORT

Employee:

Evaluator:

Date Performed:

Document ID:
Date transcribed:
Voice ID:
Total Pages:
Total Lines:

TYPE OF ERROR	POINT VALUE		TICK MARKS	NUMBER OF ERRORS		TOTAL ERROR POINTS
Medical error	1	x			=	
Missing dictation or omitted text	1	x			=	
Wrong word	1	x			=	
Wrong numeric value	1	x			=	
Major missing or incorrect patient identifying data	1	x			=	
Minor missing or incorrect patient identifying data	.50	x			=	
Spelling, medical word	.75	x			=	
Spelling, nonmedical word	.50	x			=	
Punctuation, no change in meaning	.25	x			=	
Punctuation, change in meaning	.50	x			=	
Grammar	.50	x			=	
Syntax	.50	x			=	
Typographical (transposition)	.25	x			=	
Inappropriate editing	.50	x			=	
Format error	.25	x			=	
Proofreading	.50	x			=	
Word expander	.50	x			=	
Made up or nonsense term or phrase	.75	x			=	
Guessing	.75	x			=	
Wrong presentation	.25	x			=	
Wrong word or phrase	.50	x			=	
Careless blank	.50	x			=	

Comments: _____

Follow-up action:
☐ None required, information only
☐ None required, corrections already made
☐ Make corrections as noted STAT

Total number of error points: _____ ÷
Total number of lines in report: _____ =
Error quotient: _____ .
1.00 minus error quotient: _____ ×
100 = _____ % accuracy.

FIGURE 7-4 Quality Analysis Report for evaluating a transcript and grading the transcriptionist.

7-1 SELF-STUDY

DIRECTIONS: In the following sentences, locate and underline any error, and then write the correct word or words in the blank provided. If the sentence is correct, write *C* after it. It could be necessary to rewrite an entire sentence to correct some errors. Remember that all these sentences made it through a spellcheck program.

EXAMPLE

Her work restrictions at this time <u>or</u> no different than they had been.

Answer: change the *or* to *are*.

1. I have not seen him sense that time.

   _____

2. He has been taking naprosyn 4 his shoulder and elbow symptoms.

   _____

3. Dr. Thomas, a Thoracic Surgeon, has been setting in the reception room for over 1 hour waiting.

   _____

4. He was transported by the Paramedics to Brookview hospital.

   _____

5. She underwent a mastectomy back in 2008.

   _____

6. The patient was first seen in November of last year.

   _____

7. The patients hobbies are knitting, painting, and to read in her spare time.

   _____

8. The X-rays were red as normal.

   _____

9. He does not have and ability of the knee.

   _____

10. Examination of the eyes reveals that the extra ocular movements are normal.

    _____

11. The patient was mad as hell because of the delay in being seen.

    _____

12. She has the option, does she not, of still going ahead with the surgery?

    _____

13. She hurt her shoulder when lifting heavy packages out the warehouse.

    _____

14. She claims no radiation of pain down her right lady.

    _____

15. He has been absent from alcohol for the last 18 months.

_____

16. The patient is experiencing difficulty swallowing tires easily.

_____

17. The restrictions of disability are on changed.

_____

18. She was admitted for appendicitis.

_____

19. She experienced numb and swollen in her left leg.

_____

20. The sputum grew out H. flu.

_____

21. The examination had to be terminated because of a glossoepiglottic episode.

_____

22. Patient has chest pain if she lies on her left side for over a year.

_____

23. The patient is edentulous, and the teeth are in poor repair.

_____

24. She is a 36-year-old primip whose supposed to deliver twins.

_____

25. Sings warned that this was a biohazard area.

_____

26. He was seen on November 7 and is doing quite well.

_____

27. 4-0 plain chromic catgut was used to secure and reapproximate the skin edges of both incisions.

_____

28. The cranial nerves are in tact.

_____

29. The specimen was removed and sent to pathology in total.

_____

30. When three weeks old, his mother first noticed he was not responding to loud noises.

_____

See Appendix A, p. 442 for the answers to some of these problems. Some of these editing problems are discussed further in Chapter 10, so you will have more chances to perfect your skills.

HOW TO PROOFREAD

Computers have greatly changed how MTs proofread. Many practices (such as spellchecking) are so much easier that you could become careless. Because many MTs work in situations in which their final output is printed at a distance (in another room, another building, across town, across the state, in another country) or not printed at all as they become part of an electronic medical record, extra care must be taken to edit text very carefully on screen. In some settings, documents are selected from a day's or week's output, are proofread while listening to the voice file, and are scored. Figures 7-3 and 7-4 depict examples of QA worksheets and score sheets. Notice the scoring weight given to each item. Take a look at some of your scored transcripts and score yourself. Can you meet the expected standard?

Establish good proofreading habits now, and follow these general rules:

1. Always proofread as you transcribe or edit. Proofreading as you work is easy to do, unlike text typing, because you are able to look at your work as you transcribe. A production MT could have little time for complex editing, and thus give little thought to errors until reaching the end of the document. Precious time can be lost.
2. Do not proofread too fast. Read aloud, if you can, because this practice keeps you from skimming over material.
3. Read everything on the screen before you submit the document or print it. When you are learning and the equipment is available, print out a fast, low-quality copy. Check for typographical errors, mechanical errors, style, spelling, grammar, and meaning. Increase the font size when you read the material on screen. Enlarged letters expose errors. Do not forget to return the document to the normal font size before sending or printing it.
4. On long, complicated material, replay the dictation and check your work as you listen again.
5. After a "cooling off" period, when you are not as familiar with the material, read it again. "Cold" errors are easier to spot.
6. Always read everything before the final submission or printing. Check carefully for placement, appearance, and format.
7. Practice quality assurance on your own documents from time to time, and proofread while playing back the dictation. This practice is very time consuming, and you cannot do it daily, but do set aside a specific time to carry out this function on a document and score your document.

When you proofread your material, you do not mark it unless it is a rough draft. Rough-draft material is double-spaced, which leaves room for corrections and comments.

Most professionals have their own set of marks indicating their revisions. When your employer asks you to prepare a rough draft for revision before a document is typed in final form, informal marks and symbols are generally used. If, however, your employer is writing for publication, it will be necessary for you to recognize and use the more formal symbols.

Proofreader's Marks

When text is prepared for printing, it is corrected and marked with correction symbols placed either in the margin or between the lines to indicate the changes to be made.

In proofreading your own document, you may be more informal, using marginal notes when there is no room on the single-spaced copy to indicate the change.

While you are a student, your instructor will proofread your work and mark the document and use marginal notes in a variety of ways. Therefore, this section examines the proofreader's marks as they are used formally and shows you how to modify them for your own use. Your instructor might add other marking symbols as well.

The following examples will introduce you to the formal proofreader's marks (Figure 7-5) and will show you how the document is marked.

In addition, you will learn how you can use some of the symbols in a less formal way to mark your own copy.

> 🔧 **MT TOOL BOX TIP:** Correction and proofreading marks are little tools to explain changes.

SPACING
The proofreader's symbol ⧣ in the margin of the document indicates that spacing is to be increased. A slash (/) is made in the text to indicate where the correction is to be made. The mark ⌒ indicates that there is too much space and that the text should be closed up.

DELETE
The margin symbol to take out a word, a line, or a punctuation mark looks something like this: ℐ. A line ending in a "tail" is drawn through the text to be deleted.

INSERT BOTTOM PUNCTUATION
The symbol ∧ is drawn in the margin with the correct punctuation mark to be inserted within it.
    Comma: ⟨,⟩
    Colon: ⟨:⟩
    Semicolon: ⟨;⟩

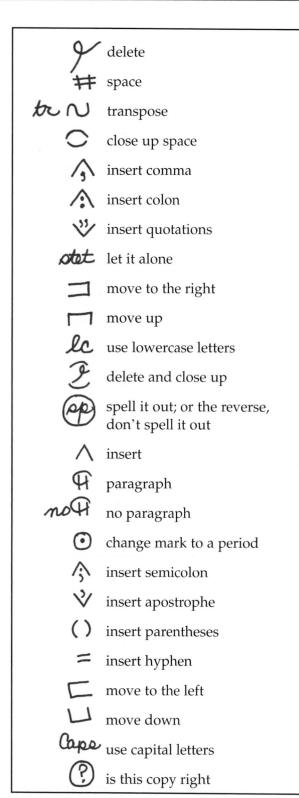

ℽ	delete
♯	space
tr ∿	transpose
◡	close up space
⋏	insert comma
⋏	insert colon
⋎	insert quotations
stet	let it alone
⊐	move to the right
⊓	move up
lc	use lowercase letters
ℯ	delete and close up
(sp)	spell it out; or the reverse, don't spell it out
∧	insert
¶	paragraph
no¶	no paragraph
⊙	change mark to a period
⋏	insert semicolon
⋎	insert apostrophe
( )	insert parentheses
=	insert hyphen
⊏	move to the left
⊔	move down
Caps	use capital letters
(?)	is this copy right

FIGURE 7-5 Proofreader's marks.

NOTE: Often one punctuation mark is deleted and another is added. When two or more margin notes are used in one line of text, they are separated by a slash (/).

INSERT TOP PUNCTUATION
The symbol ∨ is drawn in the margin with the correct punctuation mark to be inserted within it. Notice how this symbol for the margin differs from the three you just examined.

Apostrophe: ⋎
Quotation marks: ⋎

INSERT A PERIOD
A circle is drawn around a period in the margin (⊙) and is drawn around the punctuation mark in the text that is to be changed to a period.

INSERT A HYPHEN
The symbol = in the margin indicates a hyphen is to be inserted in the text.

INSERT A WORD
When you want to insert a word that is missing from a single-spaced document, the missing word is written in the margin, and a line is drawn to the place where it is to be inserted. When the document is double-spaced, it is fairly easy to insert the word above the text with the symbol ∧ showing where it belongs.

TRANSPOSE
The symbol ∿ is placed around the letters, words, or other marks to be transposed, and tr is written in the margin.

LET IT STAND
After a correction is made, the proofreader occasionally changes his or her mind. To undo the correction, the proofreader places dots under the material that was originally marked and writes the word *stet* (let it stand) in the margin.

USE CAPITAL LETTERS
Three lines are drawn under the lowercase letters that should be capitalized, and *Caps* is written in the margin.

USE SMALL (LOWERCASE) LETTERS
A slash (/) is drawn through the capital letter, and the letters *lc* are written in the margin.

SPELLING
Misspelled words, symbols that should be expressed as words, words that should be expressed as symbols, numbers that should be spelled out, and spelled-out numbers that should have been written as figures are circled. The margin notation is *sp*. If the editor is not

Proofing Symbol	Meaning	First Draft	Final Copy
#	insert space	Mr Jones is here.	Mr Jones is here.
◡	close up space	Too much sp ace here.	Too much space here.
ℰ	delete	There are too many waiting.	There are many waiting.
		Dictate the summary, but not the formal report.	Dictate the summary but not the formal report.
⋏	insert comma	Jean Bradley, your patient, was seen in the office.	Jean Bradley, your patient, was seen in the office.
⋏	insert semicolon	He agreed to the surgery, I scheduled it.	He agreed to the surgery; I scheduled it.
ℰ ⋏	remove one mark; insert another	I wanted to remove the the tumor, however, he refused	I wanted to remove the tumor; however, he refused.
⋏	insert colon	Gentlemen:	Gentlemen:
⋁	insert apostrophe	The patients incision ...	The patient's incision...
⋎⋎	insert quotes	She had these seizures frequently	She had these "seizures" frequently.
⊙	insert a period	Joaquin R Navarro, MD	Joaquin R. Navarro, MD
=	insert a hyphen	She is well developed, well nourished...	She is well-developed, well-nourished...
⋁	insert a word	The blood pressure on admission was 160/90.	The blood pressure on on admission was 160/90.
tr ∿	transpose	A new medication was prescribed and she...	A new medication was prescribed, and she...
⟶	move copy	She was, however, seen as an outpatient.	She was seen as an outpatient, however.
stet ⋯	let it alone	He should have cobalt-65 radiation therapy.	He should have cobalt-65 radiation therapy.
≡	caps	College park hospital	College Park Hospital
(cap word)	caps	College park Hospital	College Park Hospital

FIGURE 7-6 Illustration of proofreader's marks, how they are used, and the resulting corrected text.

Proofing Symbol	Meaning	First Draft	Final Copy
lc	lowercase	The patient's Mother died of heart disease.	The patient's mother died of heart disease.
circle word	spell out	She was placed in the (ICU.)	She was placed in the intensive care unit.
circle word	spelling error	(Ther) was no evidence of	There was no evidence of...
circle word	correct this	(3) of the most serious problems we have...	Three of the most serious problems we have...
circle word	correct this	The patient's temperature was (ninety-nine)	The patient's temperature was 99.
¶	insert paragraph	Her history is well known to you, so I will not repeat it. ¶On physical examination, I found....	Her history is well known to to you, so I will not repeat it. On physical examination, I ...
5]	move the copy to the right.	5]On physical examination,	On physical examination,
circle word	spell it out	On (PX) I	On physical examination, I
[5	move the copy to the left	On physical examination[5 I found a well-developed...	On physical examination I found a well-developed...

FIGURE 7-6, cont'd

sure what the writer meant with the circled word in question, a circled question mark (?) is written in the margin.

PARAGRAPHING

The symbol ¶ is used in the margin, and the document is also marked to indicate where a new paragraph should begin. If the paragraph beginning is incorrect, the symbol *no*¶ is used at the beginning of the paragraph to indicate the marked paragraph should be a continuation of the preceding paragraph.

MOVE THE TEXT

The following symbols indicate that text is to be moved as indicated: to the right ⊐, to the left ⊏, up ⊓, or down ⊔. Figure 7-6 shows how these symbols are used.

sp / = / = / sp   This (sixty-five) year old white widowed female was (begin) admitted

sp / sp   for the (1st) time. Her blood pressure was 120 (over) 80 supine.

lc / sp / sp   She Weighed 98 (lbs.) Height (fifty seven) (in.) she was   sp / ⊙ / caps

(?) / sp / lc   taking (quinadine) 324 (mgs) T.I.D.

This 65-year-old white widowed female was being admitted for the first time. Her blood pressure was 120/80 supine. She weighed 98 pounds. Height 57 inches. She was taking quinidine 324 mg t.i.d.

7-2 SELF-STUDY

DIRECTIONS: Now try to interpret these symbols yourself. Retype this paragraph on a separate piece of paper and use single-spacing. Next, compare it with the corrected text on p. 442 in Appendix A.

5 At cystoscopy, (their) were multiple urethral polyps, small in caliber, and an irritated bladder neck; the (urethra) orifices were normal, and the remainder of the bladder wall was (no) remarkable. I will have to presume that the bleeding is coming from the urethral polyps. I (don't) think this accounts for all this woman's symptoms, however. I am returning her to your care, and will follow her along for a while to see what we can do about the hematuria.

MT TOOL BOX TIP: Taking frequent breaks when you are studying and working is a tool for good health.

7-3 SELF-STUDY

DIRECTIONS: Retype the letter on p. 200, correctly following the proofreader's symbols. You will notice that the symbols used are a combination of formal and informal markings, just as your instructor or employer could use. Use letterhead paper and your own initials, but please be careful not to create any new mistakes! Check p. 443 in Appendix A to see the corrected text and compare it with your work.

PATRICK D. QUINN, MD
FAMILY PRACTICE
555 LAKE VIEW DRIVE
BAY VILLAGE, OHIO 44140
(216) 871-4701

July 17, 20XX

T.J. Thompson, Insurance Analyst
Northern Ohio Gas & Electric Co.
Post Office Box 1831
Bay Village, OH 44140

Re: Richard Wright

Dear Sir:

Mr Richard Right was seen in my office on July 9, 20XX. He was still having considerable pain in the right shoulder area, but there was full range of passive motion, and he felt like he was gradually improving, although he was not nearly as pain-free as before the recent surgery. The surgical wound was well healed on inspection. Their continued to be considerable tenderness to palpation in the depths of the surgical incision sight. There was not swelling or increased heat or redness and, as noted above there was a full range of passive motion of the right shoulder.

Because of the continuing rather excessive pain symptoms more x rays were obtained, and the findings were thought to be completely within normal limits.

I continue to have no real good explanation for the patients continuing rt. shoulder symptoms, particularly in there present degree of severity. It would seem to me that the would be much improved over he was prior too his recent surgery.

I have asked him to use the part as much as possible and to return in two weeks. Hopefully at that time some consideration can be given to a return-to-work date. Further reports will be forwarded as indicated. Thank you for the pleasure of caring for this patient.

Very Truly Yours,

Patrick D. Quinn, MD

ref

7-4 TYPING PRACTICE TEST

DIRECTIONS: Identify all errors in the following letter by marking them in red, using the proofreader's marks. (You do not have to make margin markings.) The letter should have been typed in full-block format, with a reference line and mixed punctuation. After you have proofread it, retype it properly. See the corrected version in Appendix A, p. 444.

Kwei-Hay Wong, MD

1654 Piikea Streeet
Honolulu, Hawaii 96818
Telephone 555-534-0922
Fax 555-534-9512

Diplomate, American Board   Ear, Nose, Throat,
   of Otolaryngology   Head and Neck Surgery

Sept. 15, 20XX

Dr. Carroll W. Noyes M.D.
2113 4th Ave. Suite 171
Houston, Tex. 77408

Dear Dr. Noyes;

I first saw Erma Hanlyn your patient on 7/18/XX with a history of a thyroid nodule since March of this year. This thirty five year old woman had it diagnosed at Alvarado Hospital where they urged her to have surgery I guess.

She gave a history that the nodule was quite tender when she was seen there and that she was on thyroid when they took her scan. However when I saw her the tenderness was gone. I couldnt feel any nodule.

     We have had her stay off of the thyroid so that we could get an accurate reading and on Sept. 8, 20XX we had another scintigram done at Piikea General hospital which revealed a symmetrical thyroid it was free of any demonstrable nodules.

All of the tenderness is gone and she feels well. She is elated over the fact that she has avoided surgery.

In my opinion, Mrs. Hannlynn probably had a thyroiditis when she was seen at Alvarado and the radioactive iodine that she was given for the test is responsible for the cure.

Thank you very much for letting me see her with you and I will be happy to see her again at any time you or she feel its necessary.

Sincerely

Kwei-Hay Wong, MD

wm

cc

Certainly, your letters will not look like those in the previous exercises, and you will be able to correct any errors while your document is still on the screen or being processed by the computer. You will mark your document only when it has been printed out.

In the beginning, you will want to transcribe letters and other documents in rough form. However, even in the beginning, try to make your rough version look as much as possible like the finished product as far as placement and spacing go. It is much easier to work with double-spaced material, but you lose your placement advantage when you type a document this way. Also, if you are trying to save paper and begin to type on the first inch of paper, another opportunity to achieve proper placement is lost. As you prepare your document, use letterhead paper or a letterhead macro, place the date, space properly, and work from there.

However, when the dictator or writer asks for a rough draft, double-space so that there will be plenty of room for editing.

An accomplished transcriptionist learns to make rough drafts mentally by learning how far ahead to listen. One day you will find that what started out as a rough version was actually polished as you typed. However, do not be dismayed if you never acquire this skill. The dictation of some employers is so disjointed that it is always necessary to type the document first in rough draft and then revise and edit. The use of a computer makes the job of revision an easy task.

Every transcriptionist or proofreader sees and hears a variety of interesting remarks that never (hopefully) find their way into print exactly as spoken or written. Hazel Tank, CMT, in San Diego, California, collected the following:

The child had a fever tugging at his right ear.
Return to the ED if worse or better.
I was beginning to lose patients with the patient.
The patient had her front end bent.
DX: Multiparous female who desires fertility.
She stepped wrong on her right hip.
The patient has Multi orgasm disease.
The baby was in the bass net all day.
The patient has trouble lying flat, particularly on his left side.
The patient was sleeping on my initial evaluation.
The end is almost in site.
The staff residence were called.

7-5 SELF-STUDY

DIRECTIONS: Each of the following sentences has an error. Please find and correct the error by placing the correct word or words in the blank provided. In the first part of the exercise, the error has been italicized because you might not have had an idea of where to look for a problem. Often the error is a homonym of the correct word.

1. The patient sustained a left distal radial ulnar *buccal* fracture. _____
2. Genitourinary: Normal testes, cords, *epididymus,* and penis. _____
3. I believe that he has a *mild dysplastic* anemia. _____
4. The specimen was removed *in block* and sent to pathology. _____
5. The tear was a half a centimeter above the end of her right eyebrow. _____
6. There was a *perfusion* of serous fluid in the abdomen. _____
7. He was given the *cage* screen as part of his initial workup. _____
8. There was a *sluffing* of skin about the right forearm just inside the elbow. _____
9. A portable scanner was brought to ED where a *plane* film of the abdomen was done. _____
10. It was necessary to use a jeweler's *loop* attached to my glasses during the surgical procedure on the eye. _____
11. I think the only problem he had was an old battery in his hearing *aide*! _____
12. The biopsy came back *basil* cell carcinoma. _____
13. The infant's cranium is round with a regular hair whirl. _____

14. The ligament was identified and released at the femoral head attachment and through _____
the phobia.

15. The patient had a tram flap reconstruction after mastectomy. _____

16. 2+ mitral regurgitation was note. _____

17. A urine CNS was ordered. _____

18. This has lead to significant orthostatic changes. _____

19. Ears: Purely white tympanic membranes bilaterally. _____

20. The patient is four and five-twelfths years old. _____

The answers are in Appendix A, p. 444.

7-6 PRACTICE TEST

PROOFREADING AND EDITING: Correct the word or words in the following phrases so that they properly reflect what the physician dictated or how the dictation should have been transcribed. You will need a medical dictionary to research any unfamiliar words.

EXAMPLE

normal post-operative coarse   postoperative course _____

1. used a number zero catgut suture _____

2. She uses oxygen binasal prongs. _____

3. The neck is subtle. _____

4. He had a mild cardial infarction. _____

5. sutured along the buckle sulcus _____

6. Dx: Hypertension, ideology unknown. _____

7. Palette and tongue are normal. _____

8. by manual examination of the uterus _____

9. no change in gate or stance _____

10. unable to breath _____

11. pressure at the sight of the bleeding _____

12. one sinkable episode _____

13. bleeding of the amniotic fluid _____

14. the right plural space _____

15. receptive aphagia for verbal commands _____

16. Planter reflex is negative. _____

17. Deep tendon refluxes are in tact. _____

18. There was some venus distention. _____

19. Retinal exam revealed papal edema. _____

20. He had 3 female sisters alive and well. _____

7-7 FINAL REVIEW

In this multiple-choice test, you will review some of the things you have learned in this chapter.

DIRECTIONS: Select the best answer and write the letter describing that answer on the line provided.

1. Which of the following is referred to as a critical error? _____
   a. using a capital letter incorrectly
   b. transposing letters
   c. misspelling a patient's name
   d. using faulty punctuation

2. Which of the following is referred to as a critical error? _____
   a. incorrect format
   b. omitted word
   c. improper paragraphing
   d. misspelled word

3. "Editing" the record does not mean which of the following? _____
   a. correcting grammar
   b. removing redundancies
   c. flagging blanks
   d. fixing the dictator's style

4. What do you do if the physician dictates an abbreviation in the final diagnosis? _____
   a. report it to the risk manager
   b. flag the document
   c. substitute the proper word
   d. contact the dictator

5. When you hear a number and "see see" dictated, what do you transcribe? _____
   a. cc
   b. cubic centimeter
   c. mL
   d. milliliter

6. Quality assurance is mainly a format for which of the following? _____
   a. setting pay scales
   b. providing education
   c. dispensing discipline
   d. training new hires

CHAPTER 8

Using Reference Books: Learn How to Get Help from the Experts

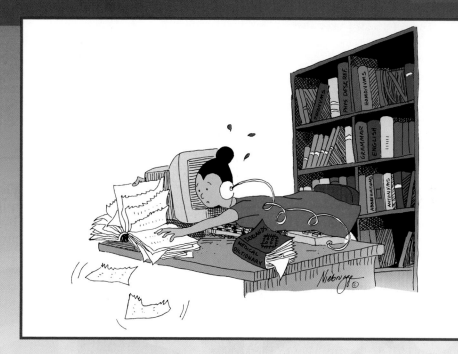

OBJECTIVES

After reading this chapter and completing the exercises, you should be able to

1. Locate the spelling of medical terms by using a medical dictionary.
2. Use cross-references to find medical terms.
3. Enhance your research skills by using books and websites used to locate medical words.
4. List the limitations of computer software spellcheckers as a final reference.
5. Name resources for locating newly coined medical terms.
6. Analyze ranges in standard laboratory tests.
7. Select the proper word form that could be written as one word, two words, or a hyphenated word.
8. Identify French and other unusual medical terms.
9. Use drug reference books to determine the correct spelling of drug names, to identify generic and brand-name drugs, and to verify dictated dosages.
10. Research and verify the accuracy of websites useful to MTs.
11. Develop critical thinking skills to determine an unknown word or words by using other words in the context of the document.

Note from the Author

When I started transcribing, the only reference books available to me were the physicians' copies of the previous year's drug reference book and the medical dictionary (which I am sure the senior physician had taken with him to medical school many years earlier). No one else had anything else to consult either, and so we MTs did a lot of networking. The librarian at the medical society was soon able to recognize my voice, I am sure. (Did you know that the library of the medical society in your area probably has a librarian who will help you with word research?) I did not call the medical society unless I had exhausted all other sources. The librarian would ask about the medical specialty and sometimes the words that surround the mystery word if the librarian had to do some research.

Today I am amazed by the books available, and it would be easy to develop the idea that one must have a copy of every reference book. That idea is simply incorrect. Today my former students, employed MTs in every field, are the ones who tell me what the really good reference books are for the classroom. It is nice when the classroom can provide many different books so that you can make some choices for your own library when you are employed. Yes, you do need reference books—good ones, too. Which ones? The books you need are pretty much determined by those for whom you transcribe and where you transcribe. The really important part is to be on familiar terms with the words you are using; if you do not understand the words you are transcribing, it makes no difference which reference books you consult. You cannot know that the word or words you select from any reference material are correct unless you spend some time learning the definition of the word you have just selected.

INTRODUCTION

If you are working through these chapters in order, you might have noticed that there have been many recommendations for you to "check with a reference." In this chapter, you can see what is available for references and how to use them efficiently. There is expert advice from specialists in the English language and from specialists in all the nuances of medicine.

As discussed in previous chapters, word processing programs include the capability to check the spelling of individual words and entire documents, as well as to allow the user to add words to an electronic dictionary. Many medical word books or spellers are available in computer-software format that allows the user to search for a word onscreen while working in a document. However, these devices are of little use if you do not have any idea of how to try to spell a word. Electronic spellcheck systems cannot find an unknown word for you; they can only make certain that the word you select is spelled correctly. Sometimes, a spellcheck system provides a noun when an adjective is needed, so you must learn good research and word selection skills. It is important that you recognize both noun and adjective forms. Remember that any spellchecker only alerts you to misspelled words; users must refer to dictionaries and other reference books to ensure that the proper word is selected and that the word makes sense. If you do not have a medical spellcheck system, then your word research and spelling skills for both medical terms and drug words must be excellent.

This chapter is designed to introduce you to the most common and helpful references for MTs, especially the medical dictionary, medical word books, drug reference books, and websites.

Remember how hard it is to find the correct spelling of a word in the dictionary if you cannot spell the word to begin with? Appendix B contains a Sound and Word Finder table. This table provides some phonetic clues to help you locate words more easily in your references. When you cannot find a word, look up the sound in the Sound and Word Finder table, and it will guide you to some possible letters or letter combinations with the same sound.

EXAMPLE

The physician has dictated "kon-DRO-ma." Refer to the Sound and Word Finder table and look under *K*. Notice the clues given are *cho, co,* and *con.* Using a medical dictionary helps you locate the correct spelling: *chondroma.*

An MT has no single or primary reference. In fact, it can take two reference checks to prove a word accurate. In the previous chapter, you learned that you often need a dictionary to be sure that the word selected by your program is the correct word for your document. Of course, you could also have an electronic dictionary installed on your computer. But for now, examine the hard copy of your dictionary and find out how to use it.

 MT TOOL BOX TIP: Reference books = huge tools.

THE ENGLISH DICTIONARY

Were you expected to know how to use a dictionary when you were a schoolchild? You asked for help with a word (spelling or meaning) and were told to "go look that up in a dictionary." I guess it is assumed that if you speak English, you can use an English dictionary. English speakers, however, are well aware of the various pronunciations and variances in the language. Spelling is not an easy proposition, and finding words when you first begin is not an easy task. The dictionary is not just a single reference book either; there is so much more information available in this multireference.

First, you must choose a good English dictionary. The dictionary should be a current edition (no more than 5 years old) and comprehensive. *Merriam-Webster's Collegiate Dictionary* was selected for the exercises in this chapter. You do not need a book with every word in it. In fact, avoid books that are so huge that you have difficulty storing and lifting them. On the other hand, you do not want a vastly condensed version. Collegiate-style dictionaries incorporate words at the level you will encounter. As with all reference books, the first thing you need to do with a dictionary is to open it and read the initial pages to see how it is set up and how to use the various pieces of information that are provided with each entry. The first time you examine your dictionary should not be when you first need to look for a word.

Many people find the phonetic diacritic marks tricky, and it is a good idea to see how these marks are used before you try to pronounce a new and difficult word. These aids are not to be overlooked, because they often help you choose between words that are spelled exactly the same but are pronounced differently and have entirely different meanings. You will have to select the meaning on the basis of the phonetics; consider, for example, *minute* (a 60-second period of time) and *minute* (a very small object), and *tear* (a rip) and *tear* (a product from your lacrimal gland). You will need to be able to discriminate between two words that sound identical but are spelled differently, have different meanings, and are different parts of speech; for example, *mucous*, an adjective relating to the secretion from the mucous membranes or mucosa, and *mucus*, a noun that names the secretion itself. Silent letters are also described and explained.

With the word entry itself, you have the following information in addition to the correct spelling (along with secondary variations or just variations, such as *disc* and *disk*) and current meaning of the word: the part of speech; the language of origin; homonym (sound-alike word); synonym (another word with the same meaning); antonym (a word with the opposite meaning); cross-reference; capitalization; usage; written open, closed, or hyphenated; end-of-line division of words; plural forms of nouns; rules of grammar; principal parts of verbs; and comparative and superlative forms of adjectives and adverbs (e.g., *good, better, best*). This material makes up the main body of the dictionary.

In general, you will find the secondary references located at the back. These may include the following: abbreviations; foreign words and phrases (foreign words and phrases that are generally used in English are included in the main body of the book); biographical names (famous persons); geographic names (this one is very important when you encounter patients who were born abroad or have been travelling abroad); signs and symbols; chemical elements; Roman numerals; time zones; weights and measures; punctuation and capitalization rules; and forms of address (useful if you have been directed to write a letter to a cleric, diplomat, or government or military official).

Along with your computer spellchecker, you now have an English-language reference book. The spellchecker makes a suggestion: you "check it out."

THE MEDICAL DICTIONARY

No matter how expert you become, you will always need a medical dictionary. Therefore, it is important to obtain the most comprehensive and recent edition (no more than 5 years old); or if you are working with software, to periodically upgrade it. A good medical dictionary can contain 100,000 words, but medical vocabulary contains 215,000 words. Among the many words not included in medical dictionaries are drugs, eponyms, instrument names, acronyms, and so on; therefore, additional reference books are vital. Thousands of new terms are coined each year by researchers, scientists, geneticists, and others; consequently, the usefulness of a medical dictionary as a reference diminishes with time. A beginning MT must spend time becoming familiar with the arrangement of the medical dictionary, because that knowledge will be an important asset in ensuring accuracy.

The best medical dictionaries usually include word origins, phonetics, abbreviations, and anatomical illustrations for each medical term. Please study Figure 8-1. Numerous words are not spelled exactly as they sound, and so you must learn to check the phonetic spelling to determine the correct word to use. This chapter refers to *Dorland's Illustrated Medical Dictionary*. All answers to Self-Study exercises, Practice Tests, and Review Tests are based on the 31st edition. If you have another medical dictionary, and because there are some variations in medical dictionaries, follow these explanations as closely as you can.

Check the index for the tables and plates (illustrations) so that you will have a better idea of what anatomical pictures and lists are present. Look through and review the pertinent information in the tables themselves. If you have not had a formal course in medical terminology, check your medical dictionary for a listing of prefixes, suffixes, combining forms, and roots (e.g., "Fundamentals of Medical Etymology" at the beginning of *Dorland's*) and become familiar with them.

Proper nouns are entered twice, once under the proper name and then as an eponym subtopic under a key entry. Use of the possessive form reflects the ongoing change, and even though the use of the nonpossessive form is increasingly common, it is not universal. The variation in forms is a reflection of change and not a prescription for the use of possessive and nonpossessive forms.

Some medical dictionaries also have a listing of muscles, nerves, and arteries grouped together in one place. In *Dorland's*, tables in the appendixes list the common name and three or more descriptive features of arteries, bones, muscles, nerves, and veins. These tables are helpful for quickly referencing anatomical parts. Remember that you have these lists readily

available when you have a mystery term in any of the categories. It is much easier to locate a word in a list than to find it hidden in the depths of the medical dictionary.

There are thousands of full color and line-drawing illustrations placed throughout the medical dictionary. The drawings are particularly helpful for research when you know the body part discussed but do not know the spelling of some area of the part. The illustrations are clearly labeled (Figure 8-2).

CROSS-REFERENCE

Often a physician will dictate a word or combination of words that you cannot find when you consult your dictionaries. An example is *biferious pulse*. Because *biferious* is difficult to spell, it may be hard for you to find under *B*; therefore, the first step is to look under *pulse*,

PRONUNCIATION   PLURAL FORM

THE WORD ⟶ **ar·thri·tis** (ahr-thri′tis) pl. *arthrit′ides* [Gr. *arthron* joint + -*itis*]⎤── ORIGIN (Greek, Latin, French, Old English)
inflammation of joints; see also *rheumatism.*

acute a., arthritis marked by pain, heat, redness, and swelling, due to inflammation, infection, or trauma.
acute gouty a., acute arthritis associated with gout.
acute rheumatic a., rheumatic fever.
acute suppurative a., inflammation of a joint by pus-forming organisms.
bacterial a., infectious arthritis, usually acute, characterized by inflammation of synovial membranes with purulent effusion into a joint(s), most often due to *Staphylococcus aureus, Streptococcus pyogenes, Streptococcus pneumoniae,* and *Neisseria gonorrhoeae,* but other bacteria may be involved, and usually caused by hematogenous spread from a primary site of infection although joints may also become infected by direct inoculation or local extension. Called also *pyoarthritis, septic a.,* and *suppurative a.*
Bekhterev's a., ankylosing spondylitis.
chronic inflammatory a., inflammation of joints in chronic disorders such as rheumatoid arthritis.
chronic villous a., a form of rheumatoid arthritis due to villous outgrowths from the synovial membranes, which cause impairment of function and crepitation; called also *dry joint.*
climactic a., menopausal a.
cricoarytenoid a., inflammation of the cricoarytenoid joint in rheumatoid arthritis; it may cause laryngeal dysfunction and rarely stridor.
Descriptive words with ── **crystal-induced a.,** that due to the deposition of inorganic crystalline material within the joints; see *gout* and *calcium pyrophosphate deposition disease.*
definitions of different   **a. defor′mans,** severe destruction of joints, seen in disorders such as rheumatoid arthritis.
types of diseases or   **degenerative a.,** osteoarthritis.
illnesses related to   **exudative a.,** arthritis with exudate into or about the joint.
the key medical term.   **fungal a., a. fungo′sa,** mycotic a.
gonococcal a., gonorrheal a., bacterial arthritis occurring secondary to gonorrhea, often characterized by migratory polyarthritis that usually involves one and sometimes two joints, and commonly associated with erythematous skin lesions and tenosynovitis.
gouty a., arthritis due to gout; called also *uratic a.*
hemophilic a., bleeding into the joint cavities.
hypertrophic a., osteoarthritis.
infectious a., arthritis caused by bacteria, rickettsiae, mycoplasmas, viruses, fungi, or parasites.
Jaccoud's a., see under *syndrome.*
juvenile a., juvenile chronic a., juvenile rheumatoid a.
Lyme a., see under *disease.*

FIGURE 8-1 A typical word entry from *Dorland's Illustrated Medical Dictionary,* 31st edition. (From *Dorland's illustrated medical dictionary,* ed 31, Philadelphia, Saunders, 2009.)

which is easy to spell. You will find that a subentry for *biferious* is listed alphabetically under the *pulse* heading. In other words, this term is located under the *noun* rather than the adjective. Many other medical terms can be found in a similar manner. This knowledge is very helpful because the noun is often much easier to spell than the adjective, and the adjective spelling probably brought you to the dictionary in the first place. Of note, however, in some medical phrases, the adjective is not necessarily the first word, as in *biferious pulse*. In

Latin terms it is usually the second (e.g., *pulsus bisferiens*) (Figure 8-3).

Some physicians use complete Latin terms to designate muscles and nerves. In these instances, consult the table of muscles or the table of nerves to obtain the correct spelling.

The following is a list of some frequently used nouns for which descriptive adjectives are listed alphabetically under the nouns in the dictionary.

Have your dictionary in hand now and look up *syndrome*. How many adjectives did you find as sublistings of this word?

NOTE: The same entity may be referred to as a disease or a syndrome (e.g., *Fabry disease–Fabry syndrome*) or as a sign or a phenomenon (e.g., *Gowers sign–Gowers phenomenon*). In some instances, the physician could have dictated a noun that does not list the adjective modifier you need. In this case, you will need to know the synonym for another choice. Here are some synonyms:

test (sign)	syndrome (disease)
phenomenon (sign)	procedure (operation)
test (reaction)	method (operation)
palsy (paralysis)	disorder (disease)
reflex (sign)	canal (duct)

It would be a good idea to copy the following list and place it in your full-size reference binder. For now, just briefly study these words so you can develop a feel for the type of words they are.

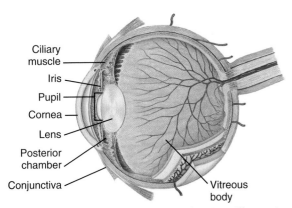

FIGURE 8-2 Example of a line-drawing illustration, one of many thousands found throughout the dictionary. (From Seidel HM, et al: *Mosby's guide to physical examination*, ed 5, St Louis, Mosby, 2003; shown in *Dorland's illustrated medical dictionary*, ed 31, Philadelphia, Saunders, 2009.)

Labels: Ciliary muscle, Iris, Pupil, Cornea, Lens, Posterior chamber, Conjunctiva, Vitreous body

aberration	capsule	disease (try *syndrome*)	ganglion	maneuver
abortion	carcinoma	disorder (try *syndrome*)	gland	margin
abscess	cartilage	duct (try *canal*)	gout	membrane
acid	cataract	ductus	graft	method (try *operation*)
acne	cavity	dysplasia	granule	microscope
agglutination	cell	dystrophy	groove	movement
alcohol	center	edema	group	muscle
alopecia	circulation	effect	heart	nerve
anastomosis	cirrhosis	embolism	hemorrhage	node
anemia	clamp	enzyme	hernia	nucleus
anesthesia	classification	erythema	hormone	oil
aneurysm	condyle	facies	immunity	operation (try *procedure* or *method*)
artery	conjunctivitis	factor	incision	
atrophy	corpus	fascia	index	os
bacillus	crisis	fever	inflammation	pain
bacterium	culture	fiber	jaundice	palsy
bandage	cycle	fissure	joint	paralysis (try *palsy*)
block	cyst	fistula	keratitis	pars
body	deafness	fold	lamina	pericarditis
bone	degeneration	formula	law	phenomenon (try *sign*)
bougie	dermatitis	fossa	layer	
bursa	diabetes	fracture	lesion	plane
canal (try *duct* or *tube*)	diarrhea		ligament	
	diet		line	

plate	rule	stage	theory	tunica
plexus	sac	stimulant	therapy	tunnel
pneumonia	scale	stomatitis	tic	typhus
point	score	strain	tissue	ulcer
position	serum	study	tongue	unit
pressure	shelf	substance	tooth	urine
procedure (try	shock	sulcus	tourniquet	vaccine
operation)	sickness	surgery	tract	valve
process	sign (try test)	suture	treatment	vas
pulse	sinus	symptom	tremor	vein
ramus	sodium	syndrome (try	triangle	vena
rate	solution	disease)	tube (try canal	vertebra
ratio	space	system	or duct)	vessel
reaction	speculum	tendon	tubercle	virus
reflex (try sign)	spine	test (try sign,	tuberculosis	wave
region	splint	reflex, or	tuberculum	wax
respiration	sprain	phenomenon)	tumor	zone

pulse (puls) [L. *pulsus* stroke] 1. the rhythmic expansion of an artery, palpable with the finger. See also *pulse rate*, under *rate*, and *beat*. 2. any rhythmic expansion, such as a venous pulse. 3. a brief surge, as of current or voltage.
abdominal p. the pulse over the abdominal aorta.
abrupt p. quick p. (def. 1).
allorhythmic p. irregular p.
alternating p. pulsus alternans.
anacrotic p. one in which the ascending limb of the tracing shows a transient drop in amplitude, or a notch.
anadicrotic p. one in which the ascending limb of the tracing has two waveforms separated by a notch, signifying a transient drop in amplitude.
anatricrotic p. one in which the ascending limb of the tracing shows three small additional waves or notches.
apical p. the pulse over the apex of the heart, as heard through a stethoscope or palpated.
arterial pressure p. pressure p.
atrial liver p. a presystolic pulse corresponding to the atrial venous pulse, sometimes occurring in tricuspid stenosis.
atrial venous p., atriovenous p. a venous pulse in the neck having an accentuated a wave during atrial systole, owing to increased force of contraction of the right atrium; a characteristic of tricuspid stenosis.
biferious p. pulsus bisferiens.
bigeminal p. a pulse in which beats occur as two in rapid succession separated from the following pair by a longer interval; it is usually related to regularly occurring ventricular premature beats.
bisferious p. pulsus bisferiens.
bounding p. strong p.
brachial p. one felt over the brachial artery at the inner aspect of the elbow.
cannonball p. Corrigan p.
capillary p. Quincke p.
carotid p. the pulse in the carotid artery; tracings of it can be used in timing the phases of the cardiac cycle.

FIGURE 8-3 Example of a noun, *pulse,* showing some adjective entries associated with the noun. (From *Dorland's illustrated medical dictionary,* ed 31, Philadelphia, Saunders, 2009.)

8-1 SELF-STUDY

DIRECTIONS: Try the following exercises to get some experience with cross-references. Say the word aloud to become familiar with the sound just as though the word were dictated. Write down the word you are researching and check the word sounder file in Appendix B if you need help writing it. Next, write the noun that accompanies the word you need to research. Look for that key word in the dictionary, and under it look for the word you are researching; correct your spelling if necesssry; then write the correct spelling. Remember to write these freshly researched words in your own word book.

Explanation of pronunciation: long vowels (e.g., ā as in *date*), short vowels (e.g., â as in *apple*), short stress mark ("), and long stress (in capital letters).

EXAMPLE

First word dictated	*Second word dictated*	*Look under*	*Spelling*
KROOR-al	ligament	ligament	crural
1. bĭ-PĔN-āt	muscle		
2. pī″-lo-MŌtor	nerve		
3. mĭ-en-TĔR-ik	reflex		
4. ŏs	pĕr″-o-NĒum		
5. SHĬL-erz	test		
6. lăb-i-RĬN-thĭn	symptom		
7. HŌR-nerz	syndrome		
8. de-KŬbi-tus	paralysis		
9. tĭk	dū-lū-RŪ		
10. ĕss-mark	bandage		
11. pe-NAHRZ	maneuver		
12. săl″-i-SĬL-ik	acid		
13. dī-KRŎT-ik	pulse		
14. BAHR-to-linz	duct		
15. văs	spi-RAH-lē		
16. dĭff″-the-RĬT-ik	membrane		
17. ĭd″-e-o-PĂTH-ik	disease		
18. SKĬR-us	carcinoma		
19. TŬni-kah	ăd″-vĕn-TĬSH-ē-ah		
20. PŌums	syndrome		

Please turn to p. 445 in Appendix A for the answers to these problems.

MEDICAL WORD BOOKS AND MEDICAL SPELLERS

Medical word books that are used as spellers are available in two formats: a single, comprehensive book divided according to all medical specialties with additional lists, and a dictionary-style word or phrase book. Many of the books are available as computer software. The books are inexpensive and compact, and they provide a simple method of locating a term quickly because the words are alphabetically arranged. Remember that when you use a medical word speller, you will have to find the word again in the dictionary if you have any doubt that you have selected the correct word. Insertion of a perfectly spelled *wrong* word is a major error. With the correct spelling in hand, however, your dictionary search is easy.

Word books list common and uncommon medical terms without definitions to ease the burden of searching through many books. A good example is *Sloane's Medical Word Book* by Ellen Drake, CMT. This book is divided into three major parts. The first covers anatomy, general medical and surgical terms, radionuclides, chemotherapeutic agents, experimental drugs for immune diseases, and laboratory terms. The second part is divided into 15 specialties or organ systems; words are listed so that the familiar term leads to the unfamiliar term, which is given as a subentry. The third part gives abbreviations and symbols, combining forms, and rules for forming plurals. It is quicker and easier to use a book arranged by specialty because the number of available words is limited. For example, if the troublesome unknown word concerns the eye, you could locate it quickly and easily by searching through the ophthalmology section in this type of book.

A regular medical speller has the same general format as a dictionary but has no definitions, and, again, the dictionary must be used after you find the word if you need any verification. These books are valuable if you are transcribing in a specialty or transcribing many specialized reports. Because the terms are well organized in these books, the time needed to find a specific word is greatly reduced. Almost every medical specialty has its own speller reference. Specialty reference books can be found for cardiology, dentistry, dermatology, gastroenterology, immunology/acquired immunodeficiency syndrome (AIDS), internal medicine, laboratory medicine, neonatology, neurology and neurosurgery, obstetrics and gynecology, oncology/hematology, ophthalmology, oral and maxillofacial surgery, orthopedics, otorhinolaryngology, pathology, pediatrics, pharmaceuticals, plastic surgery, podiatry, psychiatry, radiology and nuclear medicine, rehabilitation/physical therapy, speech/language/hearing, surgery, and urology. There is even a reference book for exotic, weird, and obscure words (*Vera Pyle's Current Medical Terminology*).

Some of the publishers of the most popular and useful word books are as follows:

Elsevier Publishing, Inc.
3251 Riverport Lane
Maryland Heights, MO 63043
1-800-325-4177
Fax 1-800-535-9935
www.elsevier.com

F.A. Davis Co.
1915 Arch Street
Philadelphia, PA 19103
1-800-323-3555, extension 1000
Fax 215-440-3016
www.fadavis.com

Health Professions Institute
PO Box 801
Modesto, CA 95353
209-551-2112
Fax 209-551-0404
www.hpisum.com

Lippincott Williams & Wilkins
351 West Camden Street
Baltimore, MD 21201
1-800-882-0483
Fax 800-447-8438
www.lww.com

Medical word books or general medical speller books by no means completely list all medical terms, and you could still encounter a problem when a new term or slang expression is dictated. When you initially consult a general medical word book, read the preface first so that you will learn how to find the terms; each book has a unique format. Format and style guides are also available to show you how to set up reports, how to properly transcribe numbers, and so on. Do not forget that your medical terminology textbook and most of this book are meant to be used as reference books as well.

USING REFERENCE BOOKS

Using reference books is easy if you follow these steps:

1. Make an attempt to spell the target word; write it out (use the Sound and Word Finder table if necessary).
2. Write down the words or phrases that accompany the word.
3. Try to get a sense of the word, abbreviation, or phrase for which you are looking. Determine the type of the word. Is it used as a verb or as a noun? Do you need the plural form? Do you know the specialty or body part involved? For instance, if you are transcribing an operative report, does the word have to do with operative procedures, techniques, anesthesia, positioning of the patient, sutures and equipment, or a body part or function? Then you will know whether to select a reference for a surgical term or a body system term. If it is for body system, then you ask yourself which system.
4. Select a reference. Read the introduction and front matter along with the instructions about how to use the reference. Check the table of contents and other features to see how the book is set up if this is your first opportunity to use this reference or if you have forgotten exactly how it is set up.
   Learn about the main entries and subentries. Remember that there are many tables in books listing muscles, bones, arteries, abbreviations, units of measurement, and so on.
5. Go to the section you have chosen and begin your search.
6. If appropriate, verify your selection with a dictionary.
7. Record the word accurately in your own reference book.
8. Return the book carefully to its proper storage place.

8-2 PRACTICE TEST

DIRECTIONS: This exercise will help you further develop research skills for finding the correct spelling of a technical word. A set of reference books is listed. Each question gives a target word, sometimes within a phrase; the word is underlined and spelled correctly. That phrase is your first clue as to which reference book you should select. Remember this fact, not just for this practice but in real research. An MT often zeroes in on a word by trying to spell it one way or another and forgets all about the other *known* words that can help.

▶ Record which reference book you would select if you needed to find the word or phrase to verify spelling, capitalization, punctuation, or meaning.
▶ Write your choice of focus first.
▶ Select and record the letter that identifies the book from the list of references given.
▶ Write down the section of that book to which you will turn. There may be several methods to your research, and so you could make more than one selection and write down any comments you feel are necessary.

Reference Book List

A Comprehensive drug book
B Drug speller
C Abbreviation book
D Medical speller with words listed by body systems
E Full-size medical dictionary
F Standard English dictionary
G English word speller
H Comprehensive medical speller
I Book of eponyms
J Medical phrase book
K Surgical word book
L Style guide
M Your textbook: *Medical Transcription: Techniques and Procedures*
N Your own reference notebook
O Other (please name)

If you have any of these types of books available, write the name of that book next to the corresponding type of reference listed. This step will reinforce your understanding of how and when to use these books. For instance, after the general term *D Medical speller with words listed by body systems* you could have written *Sloane's Medical Word Book* and after *O Other* you could have written *Vera Pyle's Current Medical Terminology*.

EXAMPLE

After the diagnosis of benign prostatic hypertrophy was made, a **TURP** was scheduled.

What is your first focus? <u>Abbreviation</u>

First Choice: Book <u>C</u> Section <u>T, the first letter of the abbreviation</u>

What is your second focus? <u>any male problem</u>

Second Choice: Book <u>D</u> Section <u>male</u>

Comment: <u>I actually have that abbreviation in my own reference notebook   (N).</u>

NOTE: If you could not see the word and it was unfamiliar to you, all you would hear would be *turp*. The best reference now would be reference D; the worst, reference E. You are looking for words that begin with *t*. The dictionary is seldom the first choice.

1. The patient sustained a <u>Colles'</u> fracture.

   What is your first focus? _____

   First Choice: Book _____   Section _____

   What is your second focus? _____

   Second Choice: Book _____   Section _____

   Third Choice: Book _____   Section _____

   Comment: _____

2. She recently relocated here from <u>Albuquerque</u>, New Mexico.

   What is your first focus? _____

   First Choice: Book _____   Section _____

   What is your second focus? _____

   Second Choice: Book _____   Section _____

   Comment: _____

3. with the employment of the <u>Castroviejo</u> scissors

   What is your first focus? _____

   First Choice: Book _____   Section _____

   What is your second focus? _____

   Second Choice: Book _____   Section _____

   Third Choice: Book _____   Section _____

   Comment: _____

4. I do not think that <u>extirpation</u> surgery will be needed.

   What is your first focus? _____

   First Choice: Book _____   Section _____

   What is your second focus? _____

   Second Choice: Book _____   Section _____

   Third Choice: Book _____   Section _____

   Comment: _____

5. You cannot understand whether the speaker said <u>15 mg or 50 mg</u> of a drug.

   What is your first focus? _____

   First Choice: Book _____   Section _____

   What is your second focus? _____

   Second Choice: Book _____   Section _____

   Comment: _____

6. There was a great deal of <u>mucous</u> discharge.

What is your first focus? _____

First Choice: Book ____   Section ____

What is your second focus? _____

Second Choice: Book ____   Section ____

Comment: _____

7. There was considerable narrowing at the <u>pylorus</u>, with some reflux into the stomach.

What is your first focus? _____

First Choice: Book ____   Section ____

What is your second focus? _____

Second Choice: Book ____   Section ____

Comment: _____

8. A <u>D&C</u> was performed after the spontaneous abortion.

What is your first focus? _____

First Choice: Book ____   Section ____

What is your second focus? _____

Second Choice: Book ____   Section ____

Comment: _____

9. The patient experienced receptive <u>aphasia</u> after her last stroke.

What is your first focus? _____

First Choice: Book ____   Section ____

What is your second focus? _____

Second Choice: Book ____   Section ____

Comment: _____

10. There was a small patch of <u>eczema</u> inside her right elbow.

What is your first focus? _____

First Choice: Book ____   Section ____

What is your second focus? _____

Second Choice: Book ____   Section ____

Comment: _____

11. Blood pressure was <u>120 over 80.</u>

What is your first focus? _____

First Choice: Book ____   Section ____

What is your second focus? _____

Second Choice: Book ____   Section ____

Comment: _____

8

CHAPTER

12. The pH was "<u>seven oh</u>."

What is your first focus? _____

First Choice: Book _____   Section _____

What is your second focus? _____

Second Choice: Book _____   Section _____

Comment: _____

13. Diagnosis: <u>Mycobacterium</u> tuberculosis.

What is your first focus? _____

First Choice: Book _____   Section _____

What is your second focus? _____

Second Choice: Book _____   Section _____

Comment: _____

14. Examination of the ears: <u>TMs</u> intact

What is your first focus? _____

First Choice: Book _____   Section _____

What is your second focus? _____

Second Choice: Book _____   Section _____

Comment: _____

15. Eyes: <u>PERRLA</u>

What is your first focus? _____

First Choice: Book _____   Section _____

What is your second focus? _____

Second Choice: Book _____   Section _____

Comment: _____

Please turn to p. 445 in Appendix A for the answers to these problems.

Right now you are really focusing on reference books, and perhaps you are thinking you might like to add some to your own reference library. Now is not a good time to rush out and buy books, but it is an excellent time to research books and think about those that you would like to add to your collection. Keep your eyes open for used books; when a new edition of a good book becomes available, the old one could still be fine for a beginner, and you can buy a used one or even a new copy of the old edition from the publisher at a great discount. A drug book published in 2008 will be just fine for you in 2011 if it is a good book to begin with.

SOFTWARE SPELLCHECKER

As mentioned, spellcheckers have their limitations. A spellchecker can only tell you whether the word you select is spelled correctly. For example, the sentences *Its knot all ways rite any whey* and *Its only a machine* would appear to be without error when checked for accuracy. Therefore, it is up to you to decide what is correct and what makes sense with regard to selection of noun, adjective, homonym, and meaning. After you see your selection of word choices, research each one by using the method you have just practiced. It is up to you to decide if it is quicker for you to use a specialty book or a dictionary first. Your words will be clustered in either reference.

What do you do if none of your selections are correct or you find no suggestions made at all? First, after carefully listening again to the word, make a different guess at the spelling. Do not forget to consult the Sound and Word Finder table. The first few letters of your guessed words may be totally off. Consider *fizz-e-cull exam* as your mystery word. *Fizz* is very different from *phys*. Second, if you cannot find the word, use the second word, in this case, *exam,* to help you research. Third, if you are still unsuccessful, leave a complete flag. (See Chapter 7, pp. 187 and 188.) Finally, never make a "good guess." As time goes by and with more and more experience, you will become quicker and more confident. Never accept the spelling of a word given by a dictator or anyone else until you have verified the spelling with one of your reference books.

The next area that the spellchecker cannot help you with is homonyms. Chapter 10 helps you discover how to solve some of the problems with those confusing word pairs.

JOURNALS AND NEWSLETTERS

Journals and newsletters provide up-to-date information on new words or words coined as the words and terms are born, before the words or terms appear in standard reference books. As a working MT, you are wise to have access to such publications to obtain information on new terminology and pharmaceuticals as well as articles of interest to a practicing MT. Examples of such publications include the following:

Health Data Matrix, the business and technology journal of AHDI and CDIA, published bimonthly by
Association for Healthcare Documentation Integrity
4230 Kiernan Avenue, Suite 130
Modesto, CA 95356
Telephone: 800-982-2182 and 209-527-9620
Email: AHDI@AHDI.org
Website: www.ahdionline.org

Plexus, published bimonthly by
Association for Healthcare Documentation Integrity
4230 Kiernan Avenue, Suite 130
Modesto, CA 95356
Telephone: 800-982-2182 and 209-527-9620
Email: AHDI@AHDI.org
Website: www.ahdionline.org

For The Record, committed to enhancing the health information profession, published biweekly by
For the Record
3801 Schuylkill Road
Spring City, PA 19475

e-Perspectives, a quarterly free online journal published by
Health Professions Institute
PO Box 801
Modesto, CA 95353
Website: www.hpisum.com.

Advance for Health Information Professionals, a free monthly on-line journal
Telephone: 800-355-1088
Website: www.advanceweb.com/him

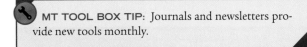

MT TOOL BOX TIP: Journals and newsletters provide new tools monthly.

MEDICAL SPELLING

Many medical terms of Greek derivation are difficult to spell. Those that start with a silent letter cause particular problems because you cannot locate them in the dictionary unless you know which phonetic sounds are likely to begin with a silent consonant.

Here is a list of some typical Greek and other unusual word beginnings, along with their phonetic sounds and an example of a word in which each is used.

SPELLING AT BEGINNING OF WORD	PHONETIC SOUND	EXAMPLE
pn	n	pneumonia (nu-MŌnya)
ps	s	psychiatric (sī-kē-ĂT-rik)
pn	n	pneumal (NŪmall)
pt	t	ptosis (TŌsis)
pt	t	ptarmus (TAHR-mis)
ct	t	ctetology (te-TŎL-o-jē)
cn	n	cnemis (NĒmis)
gn	n	gnathalgia (năth-ĂL-je-ah)
mn	n	mnemonic (ne-MŎN-ik)
ps	p	psoriatic (sōr-ē-ĂT-ik)
kn	n	knuckle (NŬK-ul)
eu	you	euphoria (yū-FŌR-ē-ah)

Medical terms of Greek derivation can also have silent letters in the middle of the word. Notice the silent *g* in *phlegm* (flĕm) and the silent second *h* in *hemorrhoid* (HĔM-o-royd). Furthermore, the *ch* combination makes the *k* sound, as in *key,* and the *ph* combination makes the *f* sound, as in *find.*

Two other Greek combinations are *ae* and *oe*. In modern American English use, they often become simply *e*. For example, *anaesthesia* is now written as *anesthesia* and *orthopaedic* as *orthopedic*. (However, when corresponding with the American Academy of Orthopaedic Surgeons [AAOS], use the *ae* spelling.) The suffix *coele* is now written as *-cele,* as in the word *rectocele*.

Some prefixes sound similar in dictation. Watch out for *ante/anti, para/peri, inter/intra, hyper/hypo,* and *super/supra.* Refer to Appendix B for help with these troublemakers.

Last, six Greek suffixes cause spelling problems for the beginning MT. They are *-rrhagia* (RĀ-jē-ah), -rrha-phy (RĀ-fē), -rrhexis (RĚK-sis), -rrhea (RĒ-ah), *-rrhage* (rij), and *-rrhoid* (royd). You will notice the double *r*, but you will hear only one. Memorize these.

REMINDER: Refer to Appendix B, Sound and Word Finder Table, for some phonetic clues when you encounter the possibility of a silent letter.

8-3 PRACTICE TEST

DIRECTIONS: Before beginning this practice test, read and review the Sound and Word Finder Table in Appendix B. The left column indicates how certain words would sound when dictated. See if you can spell them correctly by using your medical dictionary as a reference. Refer to the Sound and Word Finder table for help in looking up the words.

Explanation of pronunciation: long vowels (e.g., ā as in *date*), short vowels (e.g., ă as in *apple*), short stress mark ("), and long stress (in capital letters).

EXAMPLE

Phonetic sound	Remember the silent letter(s)	Spelling
sū″dō-lŭk-SĀ-shŭn	p_____	pseudoluxation
1. năth″-ō-DĬN-ē-ah		
2. tĕ-RĬJ-ē-ŭm		
3. nŭ-MĂT-ĭk		
4. NĒmē-ăl		
5. NŎK-nē		
6. zănk		
7. HĔM-or-ĭj		
8. kăk″-o-JŪsē-ah		
9. mĕt″-ro-RĔK-sis		
10. mĕn″-o-mĕt-ro-RĀ-jē-ah		

The answers are in Appendix A, p. 447.

COMPOUND WORDS

Compounds consist of two or more separate words and/or phrases that are used as a single word, often with the help of a hyphen to join them. A common dilemma is whether certain compound words are written as one or two words and are hyphenated. This problem occurs with English words as well as with medical words. Often, there are no specific rules to follow for these compound words other than those applicable to hyphenation and word division. For example, no rule explains why *shin bone* is two words and *cheekbone* is one word. There is really no logic to determine whether a word is open, hyphenated, or written as one word. Consider the following:

second-degree burn (adjective)
second degree (noun)
decision-making (adjective)
decision making (noun)
A-V block (adjective)
sickle cell anemia (noun)
half-life
clean-cut

toll-free

long-standing

paper-thin

likelihood

Windows-based (adjective)

likewise

nevertheless

panic-stricken

on-screen

spellchecker

healthcare

website

Combining Forms

Another confusing issue is compound medical terms that combine nouns and combine adjectives. For example, the physician dictates what sounds like two adjectives: *tracheal bronchial tree*. The MT types it incorrectly as *tracheal-bronchial tree* and then correctly as *tracheobronchial tree*. An example of a compound noun is *oral pharynx*, which typed correctly is *oropharynx*. Always consult the dictionary for help when you are unsure about compound words. The following phrases are written as one word. They could be heard or perceived as a combination of modifier plus noun, but they are combined modifiers. The spellchecker often rejects some newer compounds, and so after you have researched the word carefully, "teach" your program the new combination.

You hear	Properly transcribed
electric shock therapy	electroshock therapy
cardial esophageal junction	cardioesophageal junction
gastral intestinal hemorrhage	gastrointestinal hemorrhage
cardial respiratory system	cardiorespiratory system
tracheal bronchial tree	tracheobronchial tree
anterior lateral position	anterolateral position
posterior lateral position	posterolateral position

The following words could be heard or perceived as compound modifiers, but they are not; they should be typed as separate words. Never combine the modifier with the noun.

medial rectus muscle	(*not* mediorectus)
articular cartilage	(*not* articulocartilage)
palpebral fissure	(*not* palpebrofissure)
jugular venous	(*not* jugulovenous)

The following are combined because they have a prefix-plus-root combination and should not be separated:

You hear	Properly transcribed
para hilar mass	parahilar mass
extra ocular movement	extraocular movement
post operative recovery	postoperative recovery
peri anal skin	perianal skin

The following word combinations (and many more) are written and understood as one word.

You hear	Properly transcribed
patent *air way*	patent *airway*
still born infant	*stillborn* infant
normal *eye sight*	normal *eyesight*
oral pharynx	*oropharynx*
normal tensive	*normotensive*
electric cautery	*electrocautery*
nasal labial	*nasolabial*

Some words that begin with the prefix *re-* have a different meaning when they are hyphenated. Be careful to use the correct hyphenated or unhyphenated version. Often there is a slight spoken shift in emphasis to the *re-* when the hyphenated version is correct, but not always.

The word *presents* (pre-ZENTS) is used as a clinical expression to describe the patient's arrival in a medical setting, for example, office, emergency department, urgent care center. When the patient returns, the term *re-presents* could be used.

EXAMPLES

The patient *re-presented* to the clinic at this time after an unexplained fall early this morning. (*Spelling the word unhyphenated would be incorrect.*)

Dr. Cho *re-treated* the inflamed area. (*Treated it again*)

She *retreated* to Hawaii for a vacation.

I will *re-collect* the medical records from the outpatient department. (*Collect again*)

He had to *recollect* the operative procedure. (*Notice the slight change in pronunciation of* recollect *from* re-collect.)

Meg *re-marked* the x-ray cassette. (*Marked it again*)

Mrs. Avery *remarked* to me about the lengthy cell-phone call.

Please *re-sort* the ledger cards. (*Sort again*)

She had to *resort* to asking the parents to leave the treatment area.

Also

re-cover (cover again) *recover*

re-create (create again) *recreate*

re-present (present again) *represent*

re-sign (sign again) *resign*

re-formed (formed again) *reformed*

8-4 SELF-STUDY

DIRECTIONS: Underline the correct single word, two words, or hyphenated word combination.

1. The *femoral-popliteal/femoropopliteal* pulse was full and bounding.

2. The patient continued to have some pain in the *ante-cardium/antecardium/ante cardium*.

3. Mr. Johnson had a CVA *(cerebral vascular accident/cerebrovascular accident)*.

4. The patient was diagnosed with *muscular dystrophy/musculodystrophy*.

5. Please check the *metatarsal-phalangeal/metatarsophalangeal* joint again.

6. She returned for her *bi manual/by manual/bimanual* examination.

7. The *musculo-cutaneous/muscular cutaneous/musculocutaneous* nerve innervates the *forearm/fore arm*.

8. She has been scheduled for a cesarean section because of a positive *fetal-pelvic/fetopelvic/fetal pelvic* index.

9. The patient entered the hospital for repair of a *vesicocolonic/vesical colonic/vesical-colonic* fistula.

10. There is a shadow in the right *costal-chondral/costochondral/costo-chondral* area.

11. We encountered the infiltrate throughout the *tracheal bronchial/tracheal-bronchial/tracheobronchial* tree.

12. When I was able to see the patient, he was *in extremis/inextremis/in-extremis*.

13. The patient was placed on the table in *dorsosacral/dorsal sacral/dorsal-sacral* position.

14. The admitting diagnosis is *corpulmonale/cor pulmonale/cor-pulmonale*.

15. I am scheduled to perform an *ileoconduit/ileal-conduit/ileal conduit* the first thing in the morning.

The answers are given in Appendix A, p. 447.

 8-5 SELF-STUDY

DIRECTIONS: The following self-test includes some frequently encountered compound words. Indicate your answer by writing the corresponding letter in the blank provided. First, use your medical dictionary; then, if you are unable to find the word, check your English dictionary.

EXAMPLE

	(a) gallbladder	(b) gall-bladder	(c) gall bladder	<u> a </u>
1.	(a) nosedrops	(b) nose drops	(c) nose-drops	_____
2.	(a) chickenpox	(b) chicken pox	(c) chicken-pox	_____
3.	(a) reexamine	(b) re-examine	(c) re examine	_____
4.	(a) herpes virus	(b) herpesvirus	(c) herpes-virus	_____
5.	(a) nailplate	(b) nail-plate	(c) nail plate	_____
6.	(a) finger nail	(b) finger-nail	(c) fingernail	_____
7.	(a) lidlag	(b) lid lag	(c) lid-lag	_____
8.	(a) pacemaker	(b) pace maker	(c) pace-maker	_____
9.	(a) ear drum	(b) ear-drum	(c) eardrum	_____
10.	(a) ear wax	(b) ear-wax	(c) earwax	_____

Check your answers in Appendix A, p. 447.

FRENCH MEDICAL WORDS

French words are difficult to pronounce for English-speaking people because different sounds are given to the letters. Furthermore, some physicians do not attempt to use the French pronunciation but instead pronounce the word as though it were English. The following are some commonly used French medical terms with their pronunciation in French, with an occasional English version. Practice these words by repeating them aloud. Refer to *Medical Transcription Guide Do's & Don'ts,* 3rd edition, by Marcy Diehl, for a comprehensive guide to French words used in medical reports.

ballottement	(bah-LŎT-maw) or (bah-LŎT-ment)
bougie	(bū-ZHĒ) or (BŪzhē, BŪjē)
bougienage	(bū-zhē-NAHZH)
bruit	(brwē) or (brūt)
café-au-lait	(kah-FÃ-ō-LÃ)
chancre	(SHĂNG-ker)
contrecoup, contracoup	(kŏn-tra-KŪ)
cul-de-sac	(KŬL-de-sahk)
curette, curet	(kū-RĚT)
débridement	(da-BRĒD-maw) or (de-BRĬD-ment)
douche	(dūsh)
fourchette	(fōr-SHĔT)
gastrogavage	(găs″-trō-gah-VAHZH)
gastrolavage	(găs″-trō-lah-VAHZH)
grand mal	(grahn MAHL)
lavage	(lah-VAHZH) or (LĂV-ij)
milieu	(mē-LŪ) or (mēl′ YU)
peau d'orange	(pō-do-RAHNJ)
perléche	(per-LĔSH)
petit mal	(pe-TĒ MAHL)
poudrage	(pū-DRAHZH)
rale	(rahl)
Roux-en-Y	(RŪen-wī)
tic douloureux	(tĭk dū-lŭ-RŪ)
triage	(trē-AHZH)

SPELLING THE NAMES OF DRUGS

Drug names are going to be a major part of your transcripts because they are mentioned early in a physician's first encounter with a patient either in the hospital, clinic, office, or emergency department and become part of the patient's medical history as expressed in the first chart note, consultation, or history and physical. You not only must identify and spell a drug correctly but also must learn which drug names are capitalized, hyphenated, and/or compounded. You must also know how to confirm drug dosages when they are dictated. Here are some general terms for drugs:

▶ Prescription drugs: Prescription drugs require a physician's authorization in writing or by telephone to the pharmacy in order to be dispensed to the patient.

▶ OTC drugs: Over-the-counter (OTC) drugs may be purchased without a prescription. Some OTC drugs were formerly prescription drugs.

▶ Controlled substance drugs: Controlled substances are a special classification of drugs (often abused, such as narcotics and hypnotics), regulated by the Drug Enforcement Administration (DEA). Licensed physicians must have a special narcotics license issued by the DEA to prescribe these drugs; prescriptions for them are written on special numbered pads and are not filled or refilled in the same manner as other drugs.

A drug has three different names: the *chemical name* is the long and often complicated formula for the drug; the *generic* (or nonproprietary) *name* is usually a short, single name; and the *brand name* is the proprietary name of the drug copyrighted by the manufacturer. Popular drugs have several brand names because each manufacturer gives the drug a different identity. You can often spot a brand name by the superscript ® before or after it. Most brand names begin with a capital letter. When you research the spelling of a drug name, it is difficult to know when drug names are generic or brand unless the reference book used shows both. If a physician dictates a report about a drug used in a clinical trial, this situation also may present a problem. Sometimes the spelling of a drug name used in trials has changed by the time the pharmaceutical company announces that the drug is available by prescription. Naming of drugs is very complex, and a great deal of work is done to keep the names from looking or sounding alike. Many drug errors are caused by confusion about drug names. Drug names should never be abbreviated.

Look at the following list of everyday items to help you differentiate between the brand name for an item (capitalized) and the generic name for the same item (not capitalized).

BRAND NAME	GENERIC NAME
Scotch tape	cellophane tape
Kleenex	facial tissue
Xerox	photocopy
Schwinn	bicycle

Now look at the brand names, generic name, and chemical name for the bronchodilator *albuterol sulfate*.

▶ Brand names
  AccuNeb
  Combivent
  DuoNeb
  Proventil HFA
  Ventolin HFA
▶ Chemical name
  α^1-[(*tert*-Butylamino) methyl]-4-hydroxy-*m*-xylene-α, α'-diol sulfate
▶ Generic name
  albuterol sulfate

On the other hand, a *generic drug* is one that is marketed only under its generic name. It may or may not have a corresponding brand-name counterpart. Generic drugs are often less expensive than the corresponding brand-name drug.

Drug names also include words that describe trade-marked forms of how drugs are packaged, dosage form, and delivery systems (e.g., *Captabs, Spansule, Wyseal*). An excellent reference list for the packaging and dosage forms appears in Appendix B. Make a copy of this list to place in your personal reference notebook. The list does not appear elsewhere in this handy single-page format.

> 🔧 **MT TOOL BOX TIP:** Your personal notebook is one of your most valuable reference tools.

Notice that *only* the first letter of most brand-name drugs is capitalized, except for a few unusual exceptions, such as *NegGram* and *pHisoHex*. Most hyphenated brand names also have a capital letter after the hyphen, as in *Ser-Ap-Es* or *Slo-Phyllin* (alternately pronounced as either "sa-LAW-fa-lin" or "slow-fill-in"). A generic term is not capitalized. Some drug names can appear either capitalized or in lowercase, such as the word *penicillin*. However, if the physician dictates a certain type of penicillin, such as *Penicillin-VK*, the term should always be capitalized. When dictated, the brand name *Kay Ciel* is often mistakenly transcribed as *KCl*, the abbreviation for potassium chloride. Later you can look up *Kay Ciel* to see why it is prescribed. Some similar brand names end in different letters, such as *Urispas, Anaspaz,* and *Cystospaz.* Another common spelling mistake occurs when the generic drug *phenytoin* is typed because the *y* is not usually pronounced. Physicians commonly pronounce *lozenger* for the word *lozenge*—there is no final *r*. Sometimes you can use other information about a drug to help you discern which drug name you are hearing: If the name sounds like *Cylex, Celexa,* and *Salex,* and you know that the name you need is "acne cream" prescribed for the patient, you research each drug, and you select *Salex*. If the drug sounds like *Fosamax* or *Flomax* and 0.4 mg is the dosage, you research these two drugs and you know it is *Flomax*. Further confirmation is the patient's diagnosis of benign prostatic hyperplasia.

To refresh your memory of what you learned in Chapters 3 and 4, here are some general guidelines on typing information about medications.

It is not always necessary to follow the idiosyncratic capitalizations, abbreviations, numbers, hyphens, or slash marks of some drug names unless your employer prefers it. It is important for you to know your employer's expectations in this instance.

EXAMPLES

Neotabs (Neo-Tabs), Esgic Plus (Esgic-Plus), Hydrodiuril (HydroDIURIL), Rhogam (RhoGAM), Antivert 50 (Antivert/50), DHE 45 (D.H.E. 45), Phisohex (pHisoHex), Neggram (NegGram), ATS (A/T/S), Chlortrimeton (Chlor-Trimeton), Klorcon 25 (Klor-Con/25).

When a transcribed document contains a list of drugs, commas should separate them.

EXAMPLE

The patient has been taking Cardizem CD, Mevacor, and Persantine.

When metric units of measure are used with numerals, the metric term is abbreviated, and it is not followed by a period except at the end of a sentence.

EXAMPLE

The patient has been taking Lanoxin 0.25 *mg*, Calan SR 180 *mg*, and Ery-Tab 350 *mg*.

As you learned in Chapter 3, when several drugs are listed with dosages given, the units are separated by commas and with semicolons or periods if there are internal commas. Instructions on when and how the medication is to be taken are preferably typed in lowercase with periods separating the initials.

EXAMPLE

Medications include Tenex 1 mg p.o. bedtime, Lasix 20 mg p.o. q.d., Clinoril 200 mg p.o. b.i.d., and NitroTab 0.3 mg sublingually p.r.n. chest pain.

> **MT TOOL BOX TIP:** Strength of drug must be 100% accurate.

If a drug name can be either generic or brand and most of the other medications listed in the dictation are brand names, then capitalize the drug name in question. If a list of drugs is all generic, then assume that the medication that could be either brand or generic is generic. The fact that brand names for drugs are always capitalized and that generic names are not presents a difficult problem to the beginning MT. Fortunately, help in the form of word books that specialize in listing only drug terms is available. Some books show whether a drug is generic or brand and what type of drug it is (e.g., narcotic, laxative, diet aid, hormone). The use of such books speeds location of the term because complicated and detailed drug information is not included.

> 🔧 **MT TOOL BOX TIP:** Drug books ensure good tool use when transcribing drug names.

Reliable Drug Reference Books

Do not trust the dictator or a friend who spells the drug term for you; just use that source as the first place to *begin* your research to the correct spelling. Always confirm drug names you find on the Internet with a reliable drug reference as well. Randy Drake, a well-known author of drug reference books and journal articles says this about Web research:

> *If you use the Web as a reference source, you can usually find multiple ways to spell just about anything. The problem is that you can't tell which is right and which is wrong. Misspellings of drug names abound. You can find* levothyroid *all over the Web, for example, but* levothyroid *does not exist anywhere in the world, neither now or in the past. The correct spelling is* Levothroid *(without a y). Google doesn't spell anything; Google is a search engine that indexes words found on Web pages. The main problem is that Google finds and indexes everything that appears everywhere on the Wild, Wild Web (what do you think "www" stands for?)*

PHYSICIANS' DESK REFERENCE (PDR)

Most physicians who belong to the American Medical Association receive the *Physicians' Desk Reference (PDR)* because of their membership; others may purchase it for drug referencing. This reference book lists only those drugs that the pharmaceutical companies pay to have listed, and therefore not all drugs are included. Most physicians refer to the PDR and have a copy in their offices. However, the PDR is a bit complicated to use and is not always the most effective tool for spelling assistance. Because it could be the only one available for your use or a more comprehensive research tool is needed, it is discussed first here.

The PDR is divided into five color-coded sections to facilitate use. However, these sections can vary in color in different editions, and the titles can also vary slightly in wording. The PDR consists of the following color-coded sections (only sections preceded by an asterisk are used by the MT):

Section 1 (white): Manufacturers' Index (alphabetical list that includes names, addresses, telephone numbers, and emergency contacts).

*Section 2 (pink): Brand and Generic Name Index (alphabetical list of integrated brand and generic names).

*Section 3 (blue): Product Category Index (list of all fully described drugs by prescribing category).

Section 4 (gray): Product Identification Section (full-color, actual-size photos of tablets and capsules). This section also has pictures of a variety of other dosage forms and packages. It is arranged alphabetically by manufacturer's name.

*Section 5 (white): Product Information (provides prescribing information on drugs). This section is the main section of the book and includes more than 3000 pharmaceutical listings. It is arranged in alphabetical order by manufacturer's name.

In addition to indicating the spellings of drugs, the PDR lists injectable materials used in radiographic procedures and the brand names of products used for laboratory and skin tests. When a physician dictates an unfamiliar drug name, refer first to the Brand and Generic Name Index to see whether you can find the proper spelling and decide whether the word should be capitalized or in lowercase. This section is a listing of all the brand and generic names of drugs. The horizontal diamond symbol (◆) preceding a drug name indicates that a photograph appears in the Product Identification Section (gray).

If you are using an older edition of the PDR and you cannot find the dictated drug name in the Brand and Generic Name Index, check next to see whether it is in the Generic and Chemical Name Index as a heading. (This is a term used in older editions of the PDR.) If you find it in this section as a heading, you will know that it is a generic name and is not capitalized.

Although some generic names have been adopted by drug manufacturers as brand names, use the generic form when transcribing unless the dictator wishes otherwise. At times physicians prescribe a generic drug instead of a brand-name drug because generic drugs are usually less expensive. Furthermore, in some medical writing, generic names are used rather than the brand names. Some drug references are formatted in such a way that brand and generic names appear capitalized. If you are in doubt about a generic name, check a good medical dictionary, which will list most generic drug names. There is also a *PDR for Herbal Medicines*.

After looking up and locating a drug name that is difficult to spell because it does not follow common phonetic rules, write the name in your notebook in two places: the phonetic location and the correct alphabetical location.

EXAMPLE

Eucerin

"Ucerin," see *Eucerin*

Clinical Pharmacology

Clinical Pharmacology is the primary drug information and medication management resource for most of the largest retail pharmacy chains and consultant pharmacy corporations in the United States, many United States pharmaceutical and medical schools, more than 700 hospitals, well-known health information websites, and hundreds of thousands of healthcare professionals and consumers worldwide.

The general format for a *brand name* entry is:

Entry ⓒᴬᴺ form(s) ℞/oTc *designated use* [generics] dosages ᒺsound-alike(s)

|_#1_||_#2_||_#3_||_#4_||_____#5_____||_#6_||_#7_||_____#8_____|

1. The drug name (in bold), which almost always starts with a capital letter.
2. If a brand is not marketed in the U.S., an icon designates the country where it is available. Canadian brands are designated by ⓒᴬᴺ.
3. The form of administration; e.g., tablets, capsules, syrup. (Sometimes these words are slurred by the dictator, causing confusion regarding the name.)
4. The ℞ or oTc status. A few drugs may be either ℞ or oTc depending on strength or various state laws.
5. The designated use in italics as for generics. These are more complete or less complete as supplied by the individual drug companies.
6. The brackets that follow contain the generic names of the active ingredients to which the reader may refer for further information.
7. Dosage information follows the generics. For multi-ingredient drugs, a bullet separates the dosages of each ingredient, listed in the same order as the generics. For example,

    Darvon Compound 65 Pulvules (capsules) ℞ *narcotic analgesic; antipyretic* [propoxyphene HCl; aspirin; caffeine] 65•389•32.4 mg

shows a three-ingredient product containing 65 mg propoxyphene HCl, 389 mg aspirin, and 32.4 mg caffeine.

Some drugs may have more than one strength, indicated by a comma in the dosage field:

    Norpace caplules ℞ *antiarrhythmic* [disopyramide phosphate] 100, 150 mg

A semicolon in the dosage field separates either different products listed together, such as:

    Pred Mild; Pred Forte eye drop suspension ℞ *coticosteroidal anti-inflammatory* [prednisolone acetate] 0.12%; 1%

or different delivery forms:

    Phenergan tablets, suppositories, injection ℞ *antihistamine; sedative; antiemetic; motion sickness relief* [promethazine HCl] 12.5, 25, 50 mg; 12.5, 25 mg; 25, 50 mg/mL or 15 mL

(Note that all three delivery forms of Phenergan come in multiple strengths.)

Liquid delivery forms show the strength per usual dose where appropriae. Thus injectables and drops are usually shown per milliliter (mL), with oral liquids and syrups shown per 5 mL or 15 mL.

The ≟ symbol indicates that dosage information has not been supplied by the manufacturer for one or more ingredients.

The ≛ symbol is used when a value *cannot* be given because the generic entry refers to multiple ingredients.

8. Sound-alike drugs follow the "ear" icon.

FIGURE 8-4 "Notes on Using the Text" from *Saunders Pharmaceutical Word Book.* This is the general format for a brand name entry. (From Drake E: *Saunders pharmaceutical word book 2010,* St Louis, Saunders, 2010.)

Written by pharmacists who have been formally trained in drug information, *Clinical Pharmacology* provides up-to-date, peer-reviewed, clinically relevant information on all United States prescription drugs, as well as off-label uses and dosage, herbal supplements, nutritional and over-the-counter products, and new and investigational drugs.

American Drug Index and Quick Look Drug Book

Another drug reference book is the *American Drug Index* (published annually by Facts and Comparisons). In this book, official generic drug names are preceded by a dot. Every trade name has a manufacturer's name in parentheses after the name of the drug. If a manufacturer's name does not appear there, the drug is generic and should be typed in lowercase, regardless of whether there is a dot. This is not an easy reference to use. A word book that makes it easier and quicker to find the spelling of generic or brand drug terms is *Quick Look Drug Book* (published by Lippincott Williams & Wilkins).

The Saunders Pharmaceutical Word Book

The best solution for MTs is *The Saunders Pharmaceutical Word Book* by Ellen Drake, CMT and Randy Drake, written specifically for MTs by a certified MT who recognized the need for a quick, easy, and reliable source for spelling and capitalization of both generic and brand names of drugs. The book lists each drug's use and how the drug is commonly prescribed. The final section of the book features a list of sound-alike drug names and a list of the most commonly prescribed drugs. The book is updated annually. This reference includes the names of herbal remedies and lists drugs that have been discontinued. This final section of the book is very valuable when the physician sees a patient who has used a drug in the past and the drug is mentioned in the report. See Figures 8-4 and 8-5 for an excellent guide to the use of *Saunders Pharmaceutical Word Book*. This also is a lesson in drugs, which is very interesting

H 9600 SR sustained-release caplets ℞ *decongestant; expectorant* [pseudoephedrine HCl; guaifenesin] 90•600 mg

H₁ blockers *a class of antihistamines* [also called: histamine H₁ antagonists]

H₂ blockers *a class of gastrointestinal antisecretory agents* [also called: histamine H₂ antagonists]

²H (deuterium) [see: deuterium oxide]

H₂¹⁵O [see: water O 15]

³H (tritium) [see: tritiated water]

HAART (highly active antiretroviral therapy) *multi-drug therapy given to HIV-positive patients to prevent progression to AIDS; a generic term applied to several different anti-HIV protocols*

hachimycin INN, BAN

HAD (hexamethylmelamine, Adriamycin, DDP) *chemotherapy protocol*

hafnium *element (Hf)*

Hair Booster Vitamin tablets OTC *vitamin/mineral/iron supplement* [multiple B vitamins & minerals; iron; folic acid] ⚥•18•0.4 mg

FIGURE 8-5 A typical page from the *Saunders Pharmaceutical Word Book* showing the beginning of the H section of listings for both brand and generic names of drugs. (From Drake E: *Saunders pharmaceutical word book 2010*, St Louis, Saunders, 2010.)

and serves as a reminder that one should always read the instructions for the use of a reference book before trying to use it.

Finally, keep up-to-date on drug names so you will recognize a name even if you cannot spell it.

Peptic Ulcer and Gastric Reflux Agents (cont.)
sucralfate
Tagamet
tridihexethyl chloride
Tritec
Zantac
Zantac EFFERdose
Zantac GELdose

Peripheral Vasodilators
Cerespan
cilostazol
Cyclan
cyclandelate
Cyclo-Prostin
Cyclospasmol
epoprostenol
Ethaquin
Ethatab
ethaverine HCl
Ethavex-100
Flolan
flunarizine HCl
Genabid
Isovex
isoxsuprine HCl
Lipo-Nicin/100
Lipo-Nicin/300
niacin (vitamin B$_3$)
Niacor
Niaspan
Nicolar
nicotinic acid (vitamin B$_3$)
papaverine HCl
Pavabid
Pavagen TD
Pavarine
Pavased
Pavatine
Paverolan
pentoxifylline
Pletal
Priscoline HCl
Sibelium
tolazoline HCl
Trental
Vasodilan
Voxsuprine

Plasma Expanders [see: Blood Expanders and Substitutes]

Platelet Aggregation Inhibitors
[see also: Cardiac Agents]
abciximab
Aggrastat
Aggrenox
Apo-Ticlopidine (CAN)
aspirin
cilostazol
clopidogrel bisulfate
dipyridamole
Easprin
eptifibatide
Gen-Ticlodipine (CAN)
Integrilin
Persantine
Plavix
Pletal
ReoPro
Ticlid
ticlopidine HCl
tirofiban HCl
vitamin E
ZORprin
Progestins [see: Sex Hormones, Progestins]

Prostatic Hyperplasia Agents
Apo-Terazosin (CAN)
Cardura
doxazosin mesylate
finasteride
Flomax
HP-4
Hytrin
Novo-Terazosin (CAN)
PPRT-321
Proscar
tamsulosin HCl
terazosin HCl
Psoriasis [see: Dermatological Preparations, Psoriasis Agents]

Indications

FIGURE 8-6 A typical page from the Indications section of the *Saunders Pharmaceutical Xref Book* by Drake and Drake. (From Drake R, Drake E: *Saunders pharmaceutical xref book*, Philadelphia, Saunders, 2003.)

8-6 PRACTICE TEST

DIRECTIONS: To become better acquainted with the drug references, complete the following exercises:

1. Give the name of the section in the *PDR* that can help you to spell a brand-name drug.

   _____

2. The following are generic drug names. Write in the first brand name listed for each one.

   a. diazepam in tablet form _____

   b. carisoprodol with codeine tablets _____

   c. simvastatin _____

   d. lovastatin _____

   e. atenolol _____

   f. warfarin sodium _____

3. The dictator has indicated either 15 mg or 50 mg of the drug amoxapine. You check your drug reference and select_____ mg. How do you know this is correct? _____

4. You are not sure if the dictator has prescribed *Flu*madine or *flu*tamide for the treatment of the patient's in*flu*enza. You check with your drug reference and select _____. The alternative drug is a treatment for _____.

5. What would you do if you were unsure of these or other selections? _____

6. Write in the generic name for each brand name given.

Brand Name	*Generic Name*
a. Prilosec	_____
b. Dilantin Kapseals	_____
c. Plavix tablets	_____
d. Tofranil	_____
e. Pyridium	_____
f. Fosamax	_____

7. What other drug names could be confused with *Pyridium?* _____

Answers are in Appendix A, p. 447.

 8-7 REVIEW TEST

DIRECTIONS: The physician has dictated these 10 brand or generic drug names in a research paper. See whether you can determine the correct spelling for each by referring to your drug reference books. Be sure to begin all brand names with a capital letter and all generic names with a lowercase letter. Type the first drug name listed if there is more than one. Type your answers on a separate sheet of paper.

Drug Name Phonetics

1. eye-bu-PRO-fen
2. die-AS-a-pam
3. NEM-bu-tal so-D-um
4. ZY-lo-kane

5. AL-PRA-so-lam
6. MED-rawl
7. BEN-zoe-kane

8. KLO-na-dene
9. MACK-ROW-bid
10. a-TEN-oh-lal

WEBSITES

As you have no doubt already discovered, hundreds of websites are available to assist in your research. In general, you must be careful when using websites for research because it is difficult to verify accuracy unless you are familiar with the originator of the site. Always double-check your reference. The following sites should be reliable at this time. You should add to this list as other students or MTs recommend reliable sites. Be very selective and careful in your choice of a site. An unreliable site not only misleads you but also can cause you to select an incorrect word. How do you recognize a reliable site? You check its source. Use only professional sources, such as these provided. Be sure to "bookmark" your favorite sites on your home computer, and make a list in your notebook of those you want to use in the classroom.

Professional Organizations

Association for Healthcare Documentation Integrity
www.ahdionline.org

Health Professions Institute
www.hpisum.com

American Health Information Management Association
www.ahima.org

American Medical Association
http://webapps.ama-assn.org/doctorfinder/home.html

Hospital List

www.hospital-data.com

Drug References

www.pdrhealth.com
www.rxlist.com (This site permits fuzzy searches, and you can search by indications.)

Sutures

www.ussdgsutures.com

Encyclopedias, Dictionaries, Thesauruses, Quotations

www.onelook.com (Allows wildcard searches: you give a few letters at the beginning, middle, or end of a word.)
http://mtbot.com/links/index.php
http://www.mtstars.com
http://dictionary.refrence.com/brouse
www.nlm.nih.gov/medlineplus/mplusdictionary.html
www.whonamedit.com (Eponyms.)
www.bartleby.com/107/ *(Gray's Anatomy.)*
www.stedmans.com/section.cfm/45
www.dorlands.com

Medical Questions

www.medhelp.org
www.omnimedicalsearch.com
www.ask.com

8-8 REVIEW TEST

DIRECTIONS: Using the websites listed, or those with which you are familiar and trust, complete the following exercise.

▸ Check each of the target mystery words by using two or three sites.
▸ Write down the correct word on a separate sheet of paper.
▸ Record which of the sites produced your target word most easily and fastest.

The words are listed as "sounds like."

1. The patient was in a "fyug" state.
2. She was scheduled for "tor-a-fur" chemotherapy.*
3. The patient just moved here from "oh-high."
4. I encountered a "paw-city" of understandable speech.
5. There is not much left in my "arm-a-men-t…" (end sound missing) to try and help this patient.
6. We need to order a chest "rent-gen-a-gram" before he is admitted to the hospital.
7. She was administered a "poo-dental" block before delivery.

*HINT: If you have trouble finding this, check with the Sound and Word Finder table in Appendix B and then look in Vera Pyle's *Current Medical Terminology.*

MT TOOL BOX TIP: Taking frequent breaks when you are studying and working is a tool for good health.

LABORATORY TERMINOLOGY AND NORMAL VALUES

Even an accomplished MT can have difficulty when the physician dictates laboratory results. The sequence of numbers, metric terms, abbreviations, and development of short-form expressions all sound like a foreign language. Some of the short forms are acceptable and are typed as dictated. A list of short forms is shown in Appendix B.

EXAMPLES

bands	basos	blasts	eos	monos
polys	pro time	segs	stabs	

However, other laboratory slang expressions or short forms that are dictated must always be spelled out.

EXAMPLES

bili for *bilirubin*

B strep for *beta-hemolytic streptococcus*

coags for *coagulation studies*

crit for *hematocrit*

diff for *differential* (blood cells seen in smear examined to obtain a white blood cell count)

lytes for *electrolytes*

H&H for *hemoglobin and hematocrit*

The word *milliequivalent* is often mispronounced as *mill-equivalent,* and its abbreviation is unusual and is typed *mEq.*

Dictation of a report for a urine specimen could list the appearance, color, and odor along with the specific gravity, dictated as *ten ten* or *one oh one oh* and typed with a decimal as *1.010.* Urine is examined under the microscope with a *high-power field* (hpf), not a *high-powered field;* findings include bacteria, crystals and urates, blood, white blood cells, ketones, glucose, bile, protein, and uric acid.

Normal laboratory values for many tests vary from one laboratory to another, depending on the type of equipment used. Appendix B gives additional information on laboratory terminology and *approximate* normal values so that you will know whether the information dictated is abnormal or within the normal reference range. The following Review Test will help you become more familiar with the terminology and numbers and thus overcome difficulty in transcribing such information.

 MT TOOL BOX TIP: Proper lab values are critical to document integrity.

 ## 8-9 REVIEW TEST

DIRECTIONS: The physician has dictated the following laboratory values. You have been asked to verify the numbers and report whether they are high (H), low (L), or within normal reference range or within normal limits (WNL). Please refer to Appendix B, Laboratory Terminology and Normal Values, beginning on p. 501, to help you obtain the answers. Write your answers in the blanks provided. The abbreviations include some of the ones you will hear and see in reports, and so you may also have to refer to the list of brief forms on pp. 466-512 to see what these tests are.

1. The first test report is a CBC (complete blood count) for a 55-year-old male patient. This report will include a listing of hemoglobin value, a red blood cell count, a white blood cell count (with a differential count), a hematocrit, and a platelet count.

Test Performed	Values Given	Normal Values	Results are H, L, or WNL
EXAMPLE			
hemoglobin	16	14.0–18.0 g/dL	WNL
hematocrit	39%	_____	_____
red blood cell count	5.1 million	_____	_____
white blood cell count	15,100	_____	_____
polys	71.4%	_____	_____
lymphs	23%	_____	_____
eos	1.5%	_____	_____

monos	4%	_____	_____
basos	0.1%	_____	_____
platelets	175,000	_____	_____

2. The second patient had a urinalysis:

Test Performed	Values Given	Normal Values	Results are H, L, or WNL
pH	5.6	_____	_____
specific gravity	1.020	_____	_____
protein	negative	_____	_____
glucose	negative	_____	_____
hemoglobin	negative	_____	_____
casts	none	_____	_____
RBCs (hpf)	none	_____	_____
crystals	few	_____	_____
WBCs (hpf)	2	_____	_____

3. The third patient, a young woman, had some blood tests. Her hemoglobin and hematocrit (H&H), a 2-hour fasting blood glucose (GTT), and triglyceride level were determined. She also had a total serum cholesterol test.

Test Performed	Values Given	Normal Values	Results are H, L, or WNL
hemoglobin	8.1	_____	_____
hematocrit	28%	_____	_____
triglycerides, serum	160 mg	_____	_____
GTT	130	_____	_____
cholesterol, total serum	245	_____	_____

✔ 8-10 REVIEW TEST

CLASSROOM GROUP RESEARCH SKILLS TEST

DIRECTIONS: Using your reference skills and any books available to you for research, fill in the blank with the italicized mystery word. The word is written in phonetics as you might hear it. If there is not enough information about the mystery word, write a comment concerning it. Pairs or teams of students can work on this together with the instructor's permission. In actual practice, you often need the "ears" of another MT to help with a difficult word. If you have the Internet available in the classroom and the instructor permits, follow up your book search with an Internet search and compare results. You could establish a contest with another student using book referencing versus the Internet.

EXAMPLE

Heart: Clear to *pee-en-ay.*

Answer: <u>P&A</u>

Research done using: <u>looked in an abbreviation book/looked in a book featuring the cardiovascular system</u>

Meaning of what you found: <u>percussion and auscultation</u>

1. There was *SO-as* muscle involvement.

   Answer: _____

   Research done using: _____

   What does this muscle flex? _____

2. A *bun-nell* hand drill was then utilized.

   Answer: _____

   Research done using: _____

3. He has been employed by the *corn-wallis corporation* for the last nine years.

   Answer: _____

   Research done using: _____

4. He has just moved to this area after living in *shree lanka* for the last three years.

   Answer: _____

   Research done using: _____

5. Gastrointestinal: Stool tested *GWAY-ak* positive.

   Answer: _____

   Research done using: _____

   What did this test mean? _____

6. There was a normally placed *HI-oyd* bone.

   Answer: _____

   Research done using: _____

   Where is this bone located? _____

7. The *VAS-tus me-de-AL-is* in the right leg was damaged.

   Answer: _____

   Research done using: _____

   Where in the right leg is it specifically located? _____

8. An *ace* inhibitor was prescribed for her hypertension.

   Answer: _____

   Research done using: _____

   What is the meaning of the word? _____

9. The patient is *es-pee* hysterectomy.

   Answer: _____

   Research done using: _____

   What is the meaning of the word? _____

10. There was a *ka-LA-zee-on* on the medial aspect of the right eyelid.

    Answer: _____

    Research done using: _____

    What is a common term (synonym) for the word? _____

11. Skin test revealed sensitivity to *Coccidioides* _____?

    "can't understand second part."

    Answer: _____

    Research done using: _____

12. Review of Systems: CR: Two-pillow *or-THOP-nee-a.* (*Be careful with this word, because it is often mispronounced or-THOB-nee-a. Speakers seldom say that hard* p.)

    Answer: _____

    Research done using: _____

    What does this word mean? _____

13. Chief complaint: *par-o-NIK-e-ah,* left great toe.

    Answer: _____

    Research done using: _____

    Where in the left great toe is the problem specifically? _____

14. The *dor-SA-lis PEED-es* pulses were intact.

    Answer: _____

    Research done using: _____

    Where are these pulses? _____

15. Diagnosis: *os-eh-LOP-see-ah.* (*The patient is seeing a neurologist for an eye problem.*)

    Answer: _____

    Research done using: _____

CHAPTER 9

Word Endings: Plurals, Nouns, and Adjectives

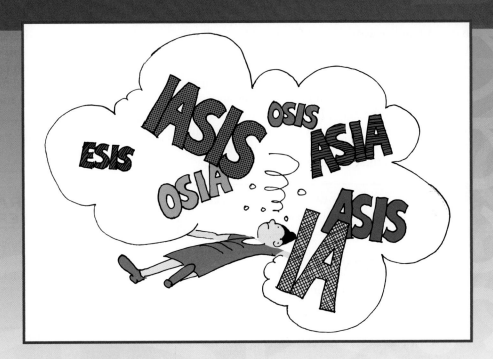

OBJECTIVES

After reading this chapter and completing the exercises, you should be able to

1. Explain the rules for making medical and English words plural.
2. Identify adjective and noun endings.
3. Construct plural and adjective endings of medical terms.
4. Recognize when you need to substitute the proper part of speech for a dictated word.

INTRODUCTION

Word endings are emphasized in this textbook because they can cause problems for both beginning and experienced medical transcriptionists (MTs) when transcribing medical documents. Some dictators tend to "swallow up" the endings of words as they dictate or dictate a singular ending when the context of the sentence indicates a plural form should be used. The spelling of plural forms of Latin and Greek words does not follow English rules. Therefore, it is important to become familiar with these differences. You will also learn that some of the Latin and Greek words have been Anglicized and have English plural endings.

In addition to Latin and Greek endings, you will learn the difference between noun endings and adjective endings. In the examples and exercises presented, some of the most common words dictated in medical reports are introduced so that you can have experience in working with these words.

 MT TOOL BOX TIP: Word endings are tools to understand the part of speech of a word.

VOCABULARY

Adjective: Word used to limit or qualify a noun.

EXAMPLE

This is a *well-developed* and *well-nourished young Hispanic* boy.

Noun: Name of a person, place, or thing.

EXAMPLE

This is a well-developed and well-nourished young Hispanic *boy*.

Plural: Noun that refers to more than one.

EXAMPLE

No *x-rays* are available for review.

Singular: Noun that refers to only one.

EXAMPLE

No *x-ray* is available for review.

Suffix: Letter or group of letters added to the end of a word to give it grammatical function or to form a new word.

EXAMPLE

Diagno*sis:* Cellu*litis,* left arm.

PLURAL ENDINGS

Medical terms, as you know from previous study, stem mainly from Greek and Latin. The rules to make these words plural differ from the rules for forming English plurals. You must know these rules and the few variations. If the physician dictates a plural form that is unfamiliar to you, check it in a medical dictionary to be sure of the ending. In current usage, many terms have English plural endings, and it is good policy to use an English plural whenever one is available. There is a wide variation in dictation styles, however, and you will notice that some physicians dictate Latin or Greek endings even though English ones are acceptable. Be sure to use the preferred plural form when it is needed, even if it sounded as though a singular form was dictated.

 MT TOOL BOX TIP: English and medical plural forms are must-have tools.

FORMING PLURALS OF MEDICAL TERMS

This summary showing how to form plurals is also in Appendix B. You can tear it out and insert it in your personal notebook for quick reference.

Plural Form Synopsis

SINGULAR ENDING	EXAMPLE	PLURAL ENDING	EXAMPLE
-a	bursa	-ae (pronounce *ae* as ī	bursae
-us	alveolus	-i	alveoli
-um	labium	-a	labia
-ma	carcinoma	-mata	carcinomata
-on	criterion	-a	criteria
-is	anastomosis	-es	anastomoses
-ix	appendix	-ices	appendices
-ex	apex	-ices	apices
-ax	thorax	-aces	thoraces
-en	foramen	-ina	foramina
-nx	phalanx	-nges	phalanges
-yx	calyx	-yces	calyces

The following are some rules for making medical terms plural.

RULE 9.1 When a Greek- or Latin-based word ends in *-um*, form the plural by changing the *um* to *a* (pronounced "ah").

EXAMPLE

labium becomes *labia*

The following words are often seen with incorrect plural forms:

diverticulum becomes *diverticula*, **not** *diverticulae* or *diverticuli*

septum becomes *septa*, **not** *septae* or *septi*

haustrum becomes *haustra*, **not** *haustrae*

(Be sure to add these to your notebook.)

 9-1 SELF-STUDY

DIRECTIONS: Read each of the following sentences and choose the correct singular or plural form. To reinforce learning the correct spelling, write the word you choose on the blank line. Use your medical dictionary as a reference, if necessary.

1. A culture (medium/media) was prepared.　　　　　　　　　　　　　　　　　　_____

2. The Table of Culture (Medium/Media) had a typographical error in the spelling of "Mycoplasma."　　　　　　　　　　　　　　　　　　_____

3. The right and left (acetabulum/acetabula) showed mild degeneration.　　　　_____

4. Mark Evans had four (diverticulum/diverticula/diverticuli) noted during the colonoscopy.　　　　　　　　　　　　　　　　　　_____

5. The (ischium/ischia) on the left showed a fracture line on the x-ray.　　　　_____

Check your answers with those given on p. 448 in Appendix A.

RULE 9.2 When a Greek- or Latin-based word ends in -*a*, form the plural by adding an *e* (variably pronounced ī, ē, or ā).*

EXAMPLE

vertebra becomes *vertebrae*

 9-2 SELF-STUDY

DIRECTIONS: Read each of the following sentences and choose the correct singular or plural form. To reinforce learning the correct spelling, write the word you choose on the blank line. Use your medical dictionary as a reference, if necessary.

1. The patient's right shoulder (bursa/bursae) was injected with cortisone.　　_____

2. The (pleura/pleurae) of both lungs were filled with fluid.　　　　　　　　_____

3. The posterior pleura overlying the (aorta/aortae) was incised.　　　　　　_____

4. The remaining attachments of the muscle at the base of the (lamina/laminae) were removed.　　　　　　　　　　　　　　　　　　_____

5. The infant had congenital defects of the right and left (maxilla/maxillae).　_____

Check your answers with those given on p. 448 in Appendix A.

---

*Dictionaries do not agree on pronunciation.

RULE 9.3 When a Greek- or Latin-based word ends in *-us*, form the plural by changing the *us* to *i* (pronounced *eye*).

EXAMPLE

coccus becomes *cocci*

EXCEPTIONS: Some take the English plural *es:*

plexus becomes *plexuses*

fetus becomes *fetuses*

sinus becomes *sinuses*

Others take the following forms:

corpus becomes *corpora*

viscus becomes *viscera*

genus becomes *genera*

opus becomes *opera*

ulcus becomes *ulcera*

meatus stays *meatus* or becomes *meatuses*

syllabus becomes *syllabuses* or *syllabi*

The following do not change in the plural form:

arcus decubitus ductus hiatus introitus processus

The following English words also do not change:

apparatus consensus status

9-3 SELF-STUDY

DIRECTIONS: Read each of the following sentences and choose the correct singular or plural form. On the blank line, write the word you choose, to reinforce spelling. Use your medical dictionary as a reference, if necessary.

1. This patient was diagnosed as having pneumonia, as she has an acute inflammation and infection of the (alveolus/alveoli). _____

2. The tumor apparently originated at the left main (bronchus/bronchi) and extends peripherally. _____

3. Specimen consists of an irregular black (calculus/calculi) that measures 5 mm in maximum dimension. _____

4. A scraping from the skin lesion on the dorsal aspect of the left foot was sent for a test for (fungus/fungi). _____

5. Leg length was measured from the medial (malleolus, malleoli) to the crest of the (ileum/ilium/ilia). _____ and _____

Check your answers with those given on p. 448 in Appendix A.

RULE 9.4 When a Greek- or Latin-based word ends in *-is*, form the plural by changing the *is* to *es* (pronounced ēz or ēs).

EXAMPLE

urinalysis becomes *urinalyses*

EXCEPTIONS:

iris becomes *irides*

-itis becomes *-itides*

epididymis becomes *epididymides*

femoris becomes *femora*

9-4 SELF-STUDY

DIRECTIONS: Read each of the following sentences and choose the correct singular or plural form. To reinforce learning the correct spelling, write the word you choose on the blank line. Use your medical dictionary as a reference, if necessary.

1. The rectal stump was considered to be quite adequate for (anastomosis/anastomoses). _____

2. (Diagnosis/Diagnoses): 1. Amyotrophic lateral sclerosis. 2. Ventilatory insufficiency. _____

3. An (ecchymosis/ecchymoses) was noted on examination of the right arm. _____

4. The x-ray film revealed an (exostosis/exostoses) on the distal end of the femur. _____

5. The patient's (prognosis/prognoses) is poor. _____

Check your answers with those given on p. 448 in Appendix A.

 ## 9-5 PRACTICE TEST

DIRECTIONS: Underline the correct word in parentheses in each sentence.

1. The (bacteria/bacterium) in question were *Escherichia coli.*

2. He applied for help before a true (crises/crisis) occurred.

3. Eyes: (Conjunctiva/Conjunctivae) clear; (sclerae/sclera) clear.

4. I did not receive a course (syllabus/syllabuses/syllabi) for either of the classes I was taking.

5. The body scan showed one bone and two liver (metastasis/metastases).

6. After removal of the dumbbell cyst, the (glomerulus/glomeruli) of the left kidney did not function.

7. The (bases/basis) of both lungs were involved.

8. Most of the abdominal (viscus/viscera) (was, were) involved.

9. He is hoping that most of the (larvae/larva) have been destroyed.

10. Progesterone is produced by the (corpus/corpora) luteum.

11. First the uterus and then the right (adnexa/adnexum) (were/was) viewed through the laparoscope.

Check your answers with those given on p. 448 in Appendix A.

RULE 9.5 When a Greek- or Latin-based word ends in *-ax*, *-ix*, or *-yx*, form the plural by changing the *x* to *c* and add *es*.

EXAMPLES

appendix becomes *appendices*

thorax becomes *thoraces*

calyx or *calix* becomes *calyces* or *calices*

RULE 9.6 When a Greek- or Latin-based word ends in *-ex*, form the plural by changing the *ex* to *ices*.

EXAMPLES

apex becomes *apices*

index becomes *indices*

RULE 9.7 When a Greek- or Latin-based word ends in *-en*, form the plural by changing the *en* to *ina*.

EXAMPLE

foramen becomes *foramina*

RULE 9.8 When a Greek- or Latin-based word ends in *-ma*, form the plural by changing the *ma* to *mata*.

EXAMPLE

carcinoma becomes *carcinomata*

NOTE: With this ending, it is also permissible to add an *s* to the singular.

EXAMPLE

carcinomas

RULE 9.9 When a Greek- or Latin-based word ends in *-nx*, form the plural by changing the *x* to *g* and add *es*.

EXAMPLE

phalanx becomes *phalanges*

RULE 9.10 When a Greek- or Latin-based word ends in *-on*, form the plural by changing the *on* to *a*.

EXAMPLES

criterion becomes *criteria*

phenomenon becomes *phenomena*

zygion becomes *zygia*

 MT TOOL BOX TIP: Taking frequent breaks when you are studying and working is a tool for health.

9-6 SELF-STUDY

DIRECTIONS: Read each of the following sentences and choose the correct singular or plural form. To reinforce learning the correct spelling, write the word you choose on the blank line. Use your medical dictionary as a reference, if necessary.

1. A Pap smear report stated minimal dysplasia of the (cervix/cervices). _____

2. The patient's blood pressure of 200/100 was a symptom of her tumor of the (cortex/cortices) of the adrenal gland. _____

3. The (lumen/lumens/lumina) of the catheters had defects, so they were returned to the manufacturer. _____ or _____

4. The male anatomy has two (epididymis/epididymides). _____

5. Obstruction of the (larynx/larynges) was caused by a benign growth. _____

6. There were many (fibroma/fibromata/fibromas) that formed in the soft tissue of the upper thigh. _____ or _____

Check your answers with those given on p. 449 in Appendix A.

Exceptions to Rules for Plural Ending

The words in the following list form plurals in irregular ways:

caput becomes *capita*
cornu becomes *cornua*
femur becomes *femora*
os, which has two meanings, becomes *ora* for mouths or *ossa* for bones
paries becomes *parietes*
pons becomes *pontes*
vas becomes *vasa*
glans becomes *glandes*
dens becomes *dentes*
comedo becomes *comedones*
lentigo becomes *lentigines*

NOTE: Add these to your personal notebook.

BASIC RULES FOR PLURAL ENGLISH WORDS

The plurals of many English medical terms are formed by applying the basic rules for forming plurals of English nouns.

RULE 9.11 The plural is generally formed by adding *s* to the singular.

EXAMPLES

myelogram	myelogram*s*
bronchoscope	bronchoscope*s*
disease	disease*s*

RULE 9.12 When a noun ends in *-s, -x, -ch, -sh,* or *-z,* add *es* to the singular.

EXAMPLES

stress	stress*es*
crutch	crutch*es*
fax	fax*es*
patch	patch*es*
mash	mash*es*

EXCEPTION:

os ora   os ossa

When the *ch* makes a *k* sound, just add an *s.*

stomach	stomach*s*

RULE 9.13 When a noun ends in *-y* preceded by a consonant, change the *y* to *i* and add *es.*

EXAMPLES

mammoplasty	mammoplast*ies*
ovary	ovar*ies*
artery	arter*ies*
therapy	therap*ies*
policy	polic*ies*

RULE 9.14 When a noun ends in *-y* preceded by a vowel, add an *s* to the singular word.

EXAMPLES

attorney	attorney*s*
boy	boy*s*
delay	delay*s*

NOTE: There are only a few of these nouns.

RULE 9.15 Nouns ending in *-o* preceded by a vowel form their plurals by adding *s* to the singular.

EXAMPLES

tattoo	tattoo*s*
ratio	ratio*s*

When a noun ends in *-o* preceded by a consonant, in most cases, add *es* to the singular.

EXAMPLES

tomato	tomato*es*
mulatto	mulatto*es*

However, some nouns ending in *-o* preceded by a consonant add an *s* to the singular.

EXAMPLES

embryo	embryo*s*
placebo	placebo*s*

Finally, some nouns ending in *-o* preceded by a consonant have two plural forms.

EXAMPLES

zero	zero*s*	zero*es*
innuendo	innuendo*s*	innuendo*es*
vertigo	vertigo*s*	vertigo*es*

EXCEPTIONS:

comedo	comedo*nes*
lentigo	lentig*ines*

NOTE: It is important to have an up-to-date spellchecking system to catch these variations for you.

RULE 9.16 Most nouns that end in *-f* or *-fe* are made plural by changing the *f* or *fe* to *ves*.

EXAMPLES

scarf	scar*ves*	calf	cal*ves*
life	li*ves*	knife	kni*ves*

RULE 9.17 The plurals of hyphenated or compound words are formed on the main element of the compound.

EXAMPLES

hanger-on	hanger*s*-on
mother-in-law	mother*s*-in-law
surgeon general	surgeon*s* general

editor in chief	editor*s* in chief
rule of thumb	rule*s* of thumb
go-between	go-between*s*
fingerbreadth	fingerbreadth*s*
followup	followup*s*
two-by-two	two-by-two*s*
flashback	flashback*s*
tablespoonful	tablespoonful*s*
cupful	cupful*s*

Some compound nouns have two recognized plural forms.

EXAMPLE: *attorney general*

attorneys general or **attorney generals**

RULE 9.18 Some nouns form irregular plurals by changing letters within the word.

EXAMPLE

woman	wom*en*
child	child*ren*
foot	f*ee*t
ox	ox*en*
mouse	m*ice*

EXCEPTION: Use the term *mouse devices* when discussing computers.

RULE 9.19 Form the plural of most abbreviations and numbers by adding an *s* to the singular.

EXAMPLES

TM	TM*s*	MD	MD*s*
DTR	DTR*s*	HMO	HMO*s*
Dr	Dr*s*	CMT	CMT*s*

She moved here in the 1990s.

His mother is in her 80s and needs home-health care.

He was able to do his 6's and 7's.

However, abbreviations for weights and measures are not made plural; singular verbs are used with them.

EXAMPLES

3 cc   5 mL   2.5 mg

Mrs Seitz weighs 56 *kg*.

There *was* 2 *mL* drawn up in the syringe.

The incision is 5 *cm* long.

9-7 SELF-STUDY

DIRECTIONS: Practice these endings by changing the nouns to both foreign and English plurals. Fill in the blanks.

1. The head of the femur fits into the *acetabulum.* A human has two _____ or

    _____.

2. An *antrum* is a cavity or chamber. The patient has fluid in three sinus _____ or

    _____.

3. The *aorta* is one of the main arteries of the body. We do not have two _____or

    _____.

4. Some books have an *appendix.* Many large reference books have several _____ or

    _____.

5. *Axilla* means armpit. He had cysts of both _____ or _____.

6. The first *biopsy* was of the skin from Mrs Aver's arm, but the second and third _____ were of
   the skin from her knee and thigh.

7. She has basal cell *carcinoma,* but previously she had two other types of _____ or

    _____ of the thyroid and kidney.

8. *Comedo* is another word for "blackhead." The teenager came in with many _____ or

    _____.

9. The *conjunctiva* protects our eyes from dust and dirt. We have two _____ or

    _____ in our anatomy.

10. The thigh bone is called the *femur.* We have two _____ or _____ in
    our anatomy.

11. *Foramen* means opening or passage. We have numerous _____ or

    _____ throughout our skeletal anatomy.

Check your answers with those given on p. 449 in Appendix A.

RULE 9.20 Form the plural of proper nouns that end in *-s, -sh, -ch, -x,* or *-z* by adding *es.* For all others, form the plural by adding *s.*

EXAMPLES

Wood: the Wood*s*	Wing: the Wing*s*
Woods: the Woods*es*	Fox: the Fox*es*
Davis: the Davis*es*	Bush: the Bush*es*
Gomez: the Gomez*es*	March: the March*es*
Graves: the Graves*es*	Brown: the Brown*s*

Omit the *es* if it makes the word difficult to pronounce.

EXAMPLE

Brandoffs: the Brandoffs (not the Brandoff*es*)

Never change the spelling of a surname to make it plural.

EXAMPLES

Wolf:	the Wolf*s* (not the Wolves)
Rothchild:	the Rothchild*s* (not the Rothchildren)

RULE 9.21 To form the plural of French words that end in *-eau* and *-eu,* add an *x.*

EXAMPLES

milieu (singular): *milieux* (plural)

rouleau (singular): *rouleaux* (plural)

RULE 9.22 To form the plural of Italian words that end in *-o,* change the *o* to an *i.*

EXAMPLE

virtuoso (singular) *virtuosi* (plural)

RULE 9.23 Some English and medical nouns can be used as singular or plural.

EXAMPLES

biceps	facies	triceps	caries	series	none
scissors	data (this has become accepted use)				

The following are used chiefly in the plural:

adnexa	feces	forceps	genitalia	assets
cramps	tongs	measles	menses	dues
scabies	fauces	hiccups	tweezers	odds
bends	chills	clothes	agenda	errata

The following are always singular:

ascites	herpes	lues	news	lens	pons	facies

NOUN ENDINGS

There are many more noun endings to medical terms than adjective endings. For example, consider the words *microscope, microscopic,* and *microscopy.*

1. The *-scope* on the end of *microscope* tells us two things about the word:
   - It is a noun.
   - It is an instrument.
2. The *-scopic* on the end of *microscopic* tells us two things:
   - It is an adjective.
   - It means pertaining to an examination.
3. The *-scopy* on the end of *microscopy* tells us two things:
   - It is a noun.
   - It means the process of examining.

Notice how these endings have changed the meaning of the word. If the speaker slurs the ends of words, you can see how difficult it is to determine which way to spell the word unless you know the meaning of how the word is used in context. Dictated phrases with the term *bilateral* in front of a noun (a procedure) may confuse the transcriptionist about deciding whether to make the noun plural. The noun should be plural; for example, *bilateral mastectomy* should be typed *bilateral mastectomies.* A list of some of the most frequently used noun endings, their meanings, and an example of how each is used is found below.

Noun Endings

ENDING	MEANING	EXAMPLE
-algia	pain	neuralgia
-ase	an enzyme	phosphatase
-asia, -asis	condition or state of	phlegmasia
-esis		hypophonesis
-osia, -osis		synarthrosis
-ia,* -iasis		calcemia, cholelithiasis
-ation, -tion, ion	act of	disarticulation
-ectomy	excision, the process of cutting out	hysterectomy
-emia	condition of the blood	leukemia
-er	agent	ultrasonographer
-gram	record tracing (record)	cardiogram
-graph	instrument to record	cardiograph
-graphy	process or action of recording	cardiography
-ician, -ist	person who specializes in, agent, person who practices	physician, allergist
-ism	condition or theory	mutism
-itis	inflammation	cystitis
-ity	expression of quality	clarity, obesity
-meter	instrument that measures	thermometer
-metry	process of measuring	optometry
-ologist	person who studies, specialist in disease of	endocrinologist
-ology	study of, science of	endocrinology
-oma	tumor, a morbid condition	carcinoma
-or	denoting an agent, doer, a person; a quality or condition	objector, error, horror
-pen, -penia	need, deficiency, poverty	leukopenia
-scope	an instrument for visual examination	cytoscope
-scopy	process, action, examination	cytoscopy

*Many Greek nouns that end in *-ia* appear in English with *-y* instead of *-ia.*

Continued

Noun Endings—cont'd

ENDING	MEANING	EXAMPLE
-stomy, -stoma, -ostomy	an artificial opening	colostomy, stomata
-tom, -tome	an instrument for cutting	microtome
-tomy, -otomy	a cutting into, incision	meatotomy
-um, -us	pertaining to	diverticulum, digitus
-y	process or action	acromegaly

ADJECTIVE ENDINGS

As you recall from the vocabulary in the introduction to this chapter, a word that qualifies or restricts the meaning of a noun is called an adjective. Example: "A *small* cyst was present at the olecranon process." Medical terms can have either English or Latin adjective endings, and in certain instances, the choice in spelling can confuse the MT. For example, *mucus* is a noun, whereas *mucous* is an adjective. *Mucous* describes a kind of membrane and is therefore an adjective; *mucus* is the membrane's secretion and is therefore a noun. These words are pronounced exactly alike, so the transcriptionist must see how the word is used in the sentence to determine its spelling.

In many instances, the medical dictionary does not list the adjective form. It is therefore vital to know the noun and be able to convert it to an adjective on the basis of what you hear being dictated. For example, if the speaker says "HI-lar," you look in the dictionary and find the noun *hilum*. You then recognize that -*ar* has to fit on the root *hil*- and come up with *hilar*.

See the list below for the most common adjective endings with their literal translations and examples of how they appear in medical terms. You will notice that a few of these adjective endings are interchangeable with the noun forms (designated by daggers).

Adjective Endings

ENDING	MEANING	EXAMPLE
-able, -ible	capable of, able to be, fit or likely	friable, digestible
-ac	characteristic of, relating to, affected by or having	cardiac
-al, -alis*	of or pertaining to, belonging to	oral, brachialis
-ar, -ary	pertaining to, belonging to, showing	ocular, elementary
-ate	possessing or characterized by, caused by	quadrate
-ery, -ary†	one who, that which, place where, relating to, engaging in or performing	surgery, capillary
-ic, -icus*	dealing with, pertaining to, connected with, resembling	organic, cephalicus
-id	signifying, state of, condition, marked by, giving to showing	viscid
-ive	having power to, have the quality of	palliative
-oid	like or resembling	sphenoid
-ory†	having the nature of	circulatory
-ous, -ose	to be full of, marked by, given to, having the quality of	squamous, adipose

*These are Latin endings and can usually be found in a medical dictionary under the headings of veins, arteries, nerves, ligaments, and so on.
†Many Greek nouns that end in -*ia* appear in English with -*y* instead of -*ia*.

9-8 SELF-STUDY

DIRECTIONS: Now see whether you can identify the following endings by indicating whether the word is an adjective or a noun. State whether the *nouns* have singular or plural endings. Adjectives are not found in singular or plural forms.

	Adjective or Noun	*Singular or Plural*
EXAMPLES		
derm*oid*	adjective	
lymph*omas*	noun	plural
1. sphygmomano*meter*		
2. arthr*algias*		
3. lumbosacr*al*		
4. progn*oses*		
5. cyto*penia*		
6. entop*ic*		
7. rhin*itis*		
8. annul*ar*		
9. glyc*emia*		
10. laparo*tomy*		

Check your answers with those given in Appendix A on p. 449.

9-9 REVIEW TEST

DIRECTIONS: Make these nouns into plurals and then into adjectives. Use your English dictionary to help.

Noun	*Greek or Latin Plural*	*English Plural*	*Adjective*
EXAMPLE			
axilla	axillae	axillas	axillary
1. cranium			
2. focus			
3. caput			
4. pelvimeter			
5. prognosis			
6. lingua			
7. pelvis			
8. phalanx			

DIRECTIONS: Convert these adjectives into nouns. First, locate the noun in a reference. Then spell out the medical term that the physician dictated as an adjective.

The Physician Has Dictated an Adjective That Sounds Like	The Spelling of the Adjective Is	The Noun Is
EXAMPLE		
AN-yu-lar	annular	annulus or anulus or anus
9. VIS-er-al		
10. kar'-de-o-GRAF-ik		
11. kil'-o-MET-rik		
12. sis'-to-SKOP-ik		
13. in-FEK-shus		
14. an'-es-THET-ik		
15. du'-o-DE-nal		
16. kon'-di-LO-mah-toid		
17. BRONG-ke-al		
18. FEE-kal		
19. AB-sest		
20. her-PET-ik		

★ 9-10 FINAL REVIEW

In this multiple-choice test, you will review some of the things you have learned in this chapter.

DIRECTIONS: Select the best answer and write the letter describing that answer on the line provided.

1. Which of the following nouns always takes a plural verb? _____
   a. viscus
   b. bruit
   c. cul-de-sac
   d. adnexa

2. Which is the plural form of *epididymis*? _____
   a. epididymides
   b. epididymae
   c. epididymites
   d. epididymi

3. To form the plural of a noun that ends in -*y* preceded by a consonant _____
   a. add an *s*
   b. add *es*
   c. change the *y* to *i* and add *es*
   d. nouns that end in -*y* do not take the plural form

4. The foreign plural of the word *foramen* is _____
   a. foramens
   b. foramina
   c. foramans
   d. forameni

5. Which of the following words is an unusual plural form? _____
   a. corpora
   b. data
   c. femora
   d. carcinomata

DIRECTIONS: From the following groups, select the set that is incorrectly expressed. Write the correct singular or plural that belongs with the set.

6. a. spermatozoon—spermatozoa
   b. thorax—thoraces
   c. acetabulum—acetabula
   d. placebo—placeboes
   Incorrect set: _____   Word needed is: _____

7. a. focus—foci
   b. lumen—lumata
   c. nevus—nevi
   d. hernia—hernias
   Incorrect set: _____   Word needed is: _____

8. a. cornu—cornua
   b. rugus—rugae
   c. alveolus—alveoli
   d. comedo—comedones
   Incorrect set: _____   Word needed is: _____

9. a. prognosis—prognoses
   b. fornix—fornixes
   c. base—bases
   d. hilum—hila
   Incorrect set: _____   Word needed is: _____

10. a. meniscus—menisci
   b. bacterium—bacteria
   c. sequela—sequels
   d. arthritis—arthritides
   Incorrect set: _____   Word needed is: _____

Grammar Review

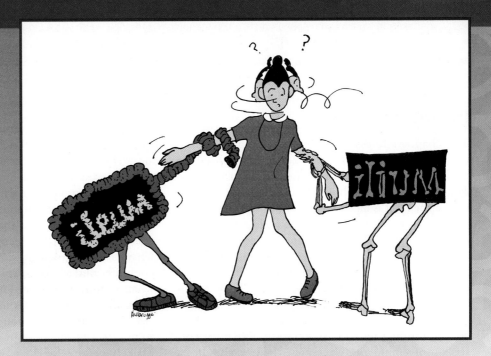

OBJECTIVES

After reading this chapter and completing the exercises, you should be able to

1. Identify and understand similar sounding words that are grammatically different in meaning and use.
2. Match nouns and pronouns with proper singular or plural verbs.
3. Recognize collective nouns.
4. Recast sentences with dangling or misplaced modifiers.
5. Select and use parallel parts of speech in a sentence or list construction.
6. Demonstrate the ability to select proper pronouns.
7. Recognize word hazards.

Note from the Author

You asked for this chapter. No, maybe not you personally, but those who have gone before you and needed just a little help getting their grammar skills back because it had been a while since grade school and all those drills. When I first started teaching, I thought it was a waste of time to discuss grammar, because, after all, we were just transcribing what someone else was saying, and surely they were speaking in perfect sentences. Well, not quite. Maybe what someone else thought he or she was saying or imagined should be said or may have thought about saying... you know what I mean. Then there was the reaction "Did I hear what I thought I heard?" or "Does that mean what I think it means?" or simply "What was that?" Add all of that to the things the medical transcriptionist (MT) does not know are out there that can snag his or her fingers as they gently pluck the keyboard. Now you have another challenge for your skills in working with speech recognition technology, requiring you to be even more alert to inadvertent "misspeak." Take it slowly. Enjoy.

INTRODUCTION

This chapter addresses a difficult problem in medical transcription: grammar. Grammar consists of the use of the proper words, put together in the proper way, to perfectly express a thought. Although MTs should transcribe what is dictated, it is important to keep the rules of proper grammar in mind and to conform to them at all times. Perhaps the dictator does not make a word exactly clear, or the verb in the sentence is said so long after the subject is dictated that the verb does not match the subject in number. There could be a misunderstanding in what the transcriptionist thought was said, or there just could be a slip in concentration after a lot of dictation. When the correction of grammar is necessary, the text should be edited only to the extent that it does not change the intended meaning. When a statement is ambiguous, the astute dictation editor recognizes the discrepancy and queries the dictator. When the intended meaning is clear but the text is grammatically faulty, it is vital that corrections be made to enhance clarity and readability.

HOMONYMS AND OTHER CONFUSING WORD PAIRS

Homonyms are the most difficult of the "word demons" in both English and medical words, and a good deal of experience is necessary for the MT to choose the correct term. Homonyms, as you recall, are words that are similar in pronunciation but different in meaning and spelling. A few English examples are *hair/hare,* *weak/week,* and *too/two/to.* When you hear these words dictated, you know which one to choose because you know its meaning. But what happens when you do not even know that a homonym exists and you choose a correctly spelled word that is the homonym of the correct word? This problem is one of the main challenges in speech recognition technology because the computer and program submit a word that matches what "it thinks" was heard. You must learn to spot this error and correct it. This next set of words and exercises is meant to make you aware of these words and to put you on the alert for the many more that exist. Mastery of some of the more challenging homonyms can save you time and possibly embarrassment. You will be confronted by homonyms throughout your career as a medical transcriptionist. (A list of common medical homonyms and confusing word pairs, showing their pronunciation and meaning and the words that sound similar to them, is found in Appendix B. Also in Appendix B is a list of regular English homonym pairs.) As an introduction, complete a brief diagnostic test covering some of the most common English homonyms and confusing word pairs.

 MT TOOL BOX TIP: Own all the common medical and English homonyms for a perfect grammar tool.

10-1 DIAGNOSTIC TEST

DIRECTIONS: In the following sentences, you will find an underlined word. That word is or is not the correct selection for the sentence. If you think the word is correct, write C in the space at the end of the sentence. If you think the underlined word has been substituted for a homonym or for a word that is often confused with the target word, then write the correct word in the blank at the end of the sentence.

EXAMPLE

The <u>advise</u> that Dr Blake gave was excellent. <u>advice</u>

1. The patient <u>past</u> the kidney stone with ease. _____

2. The patient becomes out of <u>breathe</u> when walking up a flight of stairs. _____

3. You may <u>cite</u> that article as your reference. _____

4. The patient began to <u>loose</u> weight. _____

5. The patient's <u>principle</u> complaint was pain. _____

6. The patient's condition is now stable and <u>stationary</u>. _____

7. Proofread your work carefully; <u>than</u> you can vouch for <u>its</u> accuracy.

   _____ and _____

8. We did not know <u>who's</u> instrument bag was found in the corridor. _____

9. <u>You're</u> office is <u>to</u> far from the hospital. _____ and _____

10. The old medical building was <u>razed</u> to make room for a new hospital. _____

11. The patient has completed one <u>coarse</u> of radiation treatment after her mastectomy. _____

12. The tubes were traced out to the fimbriae to doubly identify <u>they're</u> anatomy. _____

13. We have permission to <u>except</u> the subpoena when it is served. _____

14. The <u>principle</u> reason for the trip was to search for a new hospital <u>sight</u>.

    _____ and _____

15. After nine hours in surgery, Dr Cho performed another procedure without a <u>brake</u>. _____

16. He quickly sorted out the <u>correspondents</u> he wanted to take with him. _____

17. He is the <u>soul</u> support of a very large family. _____

18. <u>There</u> bringing the accident case to the emergency room. _____

19. Never take your spell-checker for <u>granite</u>. _____

20. Our supply of letterhead <u>stationery</u> is nearly depleted. _____

    You had some help here. What if you were not alerted to the place where there was a possible error? Worse yet is a paragraph that you are quickly scanning. Many of the words in the previous questions simply do not register because the "sound" of them makes sense in what we are reading. Practice now by training your eyes to stop seeing what might be said and really look at each word.

    Try this set now by selecting the incorrect word and writing the correct word at the end of the sentence. Write C in the blank if the sentence is correct as written.

21. You need to very the highs and lows in that speech model. _____

22. Clinical trails will begin with a group of disparate patients. _____

23. There is no oversite provided from the remote location. _____

24. It was deemed unnecessary to report the incidence to risk management. _____

25. We need to pay attention to the contents of the sentence as dictated. _____

26. The patient assisted in calling 9-1-1. _____

27. If it does not make since, concentrate on an alternative word. _____

28. She complains of vomiting and lose stools. _____

29. The infant was delivered from a frank breach position. _____

30. A single bridal suture was incorporated in the closure. _____

The answers are on p. 449 in Appendix A.

WORD-CHOICE PAIRS

The following sets of words are not in strict alphabetical order but are featured in loose alphabetical order so that you know where to look when you have to check back to find a reference. This chapter might as well begin with one of the most difficult of all word-choice pairs. After you have conquered the effects of *affect* and *effect,* the rest of the chapter will hold no more terrors for you!

Affect-Effect

The first step in having power over *affect* and *effect* is to determine how the word in question is being used in the sentence: as a noun or as a verb.

 MT TOOL BOX TIP: *Effect* and *affect*—a difficult tool to learn to use properly.

effect: result (noun)

EXAMPLE

Estrogen *effect* appears adequate for her age.

affect: to influence (verb)

EXAMPLE

The surgeon doubted that this finding would *affect* the final diagnosis.

These examples are how these words are used most of the time. But the big problem arises when you encounter the exceptions for each of these words.

EXCEPTION: *effect* used as a verb. The word *effect* is used as a verb in the context of power, creation, and administration.

EXAMPLE

He single-handedly *effected* the changes in our department.

EXCEPTION: *affect* used as a noun. The word *affect* is seldom used as a noun in everyday speech. In psychiatry, the noun *affect* (ĂF-fĕct) refers to the emotional reactions associated with an experience and is generally qualified by an adjective.

EXAMPLE

The patient had a *blunted affect.*

Now you can begin to exercise power over this set. The first step when you encounter one of them is to firmly determine whether it is a noun or a verb. In doing so, you make the correct word choice, and the sentence is accurate. Because the exception for *affect* is so narrow, after you memorize the exception, this usage is no longer a problem. Now just the final hurdle is left: when you use *effect* as a verb. In fact, this last issue is usually the one to cause the problem. You can answer it by doing the following:

1. You decide you need a verb choice.
2. Now you examine just how this verb is going to be used. Remember that in general, you will select *affect;* now you have to see whether the exception is correct.
3. Does the use of *affect* denote power and so on? If not, that is the end of the thinking process. If it does, then your choice changes to *effect.*

Consider how long that took to explain, and you could still be unsure. That situation is one of the reasons for the problem. You come up with a word, and yet you are unsure, and the longer you sit and think and ponder and worry, the harder the word choice becomes. The final decision is to choose something, anything, and get going! What you want to do is get past all of the thinking and pondering and be able to choose the correct word right away. Never just "choose something." Practice!

10-2 SELF-STUDY

DIRECTIONS: In the following sentences, first decide whether the target word is being used as a noun (n) or a verb (v) and write that choice in the first blank. Second, make your word choice and write that in the second blank. If you are making your choice because of an exception to the rule, write in E (for exception) with your word choice.

1. She had mixed feelings during her pregnancy as to what (effect/affect) the child would have on her.
   n-v _____ choice _____

2. He had some continuing (effects/affects) of atrophy.
   n-v _____ choice _____

3. The patient was in restraints, unresponsive, with a flat (effect/affect).
   n-v _____ choice _____

4. Men and women are equally (effected/affected). n-v _____ choice _____

5. The catheters were removed, and hemostasis was (effected/affected) with pressure.
   n-v _____ choice _____

6. Versed is a preoperative tranquilizer that has an amnesiac (effect/affect) postoperatively.
   n-v _____ choice _____

7. In this case, the weather did not seem to (effect/affect) his symptoms.
   n-v _____ choice _____

8. This silent epidemic will (effect/affect) millions.
   n-v _____ choice _____

9. I doubt that repeated thoracentesis will (effect/affect) her effusion much.
   n-v _____ choice _____

10. Benadryl has the (effect/affect) of making one drowsy.
   n-v _____ choice _____

The answers are on p. 449 in Appendix A.

A–An

a: article used with a word that begins with a consonant or that sounds like a consonant and with some initialisms

EXAMPLES

a transcript   *a* mistake   *a* one-day turnover   *a* CBC

an: article used with a word that begins with a vowel sound and with some initialisms

EXAMPLES

an hour   *an* eight-hour work day   *an* outcome
an abbreviation   *an* MD degree   *an* EKG

Abduction–Adduction–Addiction

abduction (abduct): draw away from the median of the body or one of its parts

EXAMPLES

Abduction was limited to 15° from the midline.

He was unable to *abduct* his right thumb.

An "a-b-duction"* surgery was performed.

adduction (adduct): movement toward the midline

---

*The dictator may use this form to be sure that the MT understood *abduction* and will transcribe *abduction*.

EXAMPLES

He wanted to improve his ability to *adduct* his right thumb.

An "a-d-duction" procedure will help this patient immensely.

(Transcribed *adduction* procedure)

addiction: physical and/or psychological dependence on a substance

EXAMPLE

Her *addiction* to alchohol was now said to be under control.

Abrasion–Aberration

abrasion: a scraping away of the surface

EXAMPLE

She came in with multiple *abrasions* and contusions.

aberration: a deviation from the normal course

EXAMPLE

We have to consider that this new symptom is an *aberration* in the usual course of this disease.

Absorption–Adsorption–Abruption

absorption: a soaking up, assimilation

EXAMPLE

There was rapid *absorption* of the drug into the system.

adsorption: attachment of one substance to the surface of another substance

EXAMPLE

Adsorption of the poison by the charcoal helped rid the patient's body of the toxin.

abruption: a tearing away or detachment

EXAMPLE

She experienced a placental *abruption* during her seventh month.

Accept–Except

accept: to receive or to take

EXAMPLE

His family could not *accept* his diagnosis.

except: to leave out

EXAMPLE

His family understood everything *except* the diagnosis.

Adapt–Adopt

adapt: to modify

EXAMPLE

He was able to *adapt* the instrument for this procedure.

adopt: to take as one's own

EXAMPLE

I plan to *adopt* the positive attitude held by the quality assurance manager.

Adherence–Adherents

adherence: holding fast to and following closely; sticking fast; a faithful attachment

EXAMPLE

The *adherence* of the bandage caused a rash to break out.

adherents: followers or believers of an advocate

EXAMPLE

Many people at the hospital are *adherents* to his line of thinking.

Advise–Advice

advise: to counsel, to notify (verb)

EXAMPLE

Dr Blake will *advise* her to have surgery.

advice: a recommendation (noun)

EXAMPLE

The quality assurance manager gave her good *advice*.

Aid–Aide

aid: a form of help (noun); to help or assist (verb)

EXAMPLE

We need to readjust her hearing *aid*.

aide: a person who helps or assists (noun)

EXAMPLE

They are going to find a home health *aide* for her to help with the housework.

Allusion–Illusion

allusion: an indirect reference

EXAMPLE

I got the point when she made an *allusion* to the fact that we were late again this morning.

illusion: a deception or misleading impression

EXAMPLE

Combing his hair over the bald spot fails to give the *illusion* that he has a full head of hair!

Already–All Ready

already: previously

EXAMPLE

The transcription had *already* been done by the night shift.

all ready: completely prepared or ready

EXAMPLE

They were *all ready* for the surgery to begin.

Alternately–Alternatively

alternately: by turns (alternating)

EXAMPLE

He was *alternately* discouraged and hopeful.

alternatively: offering a possible choice (an alternative)

EXAMPLE

Alternatively, there is the question of doing nothing at all.

Altogether–All Together

altogether: wholly, entirely, completely (adverb)

EXAMPLE

The two medical cases are *altogether* different.

all together: collectively, in a group

EXAMPLE

We must leave for the clinic tour *all together.*

Apposition–Opposition

apposition: placement of things in proximity

EXAMPLE

Wound edges were placed in *apposition* before suturing.

opposition: a contrary action or condition

EXAMPLE

The consultant's *opposition* delayed the patient's discharge from the hospital.

Appraise–Apprise

appraise: to evaluate or size up

EXAMPLE

The consultant was asked to *appraise* more than his current problem.

apprise: to inform

EXAMPLE

He asked Dr Wilson to *apprise* the residents of the new surgical team rotation.

Assure–Ensure–Insure

assure: provide positive information; implies removal of doubt

EXAMPLE

We will do all that we can to *assure* your family of the favorable prognosis.

ensure: make certain

EXAMPLE

He cannot *ensure* the results of this procedure.

insure: take precautions beforehand

EXAMPLE

She plans to *insure* her travel arrangements this time.

Awhile–A While

awhile: briefly (adverb)

EXAMPLE

We must wait *awhile* before we will be able to see the patient.

a while: a space of time (noun)

EXAMPLE

It took *a while* for him to telephone the diagnosis to the charge nurse.

Bad–Badly

bad: unfavorable (an adjective; acceptable when discussing illness)

EXAMPLE

The patient has felt *bad* for several days. (Substitute *sick* for *bad* to catch this usage.)

badly: unacceptably (an adverb; describes how something is done)

EXAMPLE

She performed *badly* and was eventually fired.

Beside–Besides

beside: by the side of

EXAMPLE

He sat *beside* the patient.

besides: in addition to, moreover

EXAMPLE

Besides, he was not on call.

Bolus–Bullous

bolus: a concentrated mass of pharmaceutical preparation administered all at once

EXAMPLE

We prepared a chemotherapy *bolus* of several drugs to be injected intravenously.

bullous: in reference to bullae, which are large vesicles containing fluid

EXAMPLE

Many *bullous* sacs were scattered throughout the pleura.

Breech–Breach

breech: buttocks; a part of a gun

EXAMPLE

The infant was delivered from a frank *breech* position.

breach: a gap or break

EXAMPLE

We continued the discussion in order to avoid a *breach* in communication.

Bridle–Bridal

bridle: referring to part of the tack for a horse; a loop,(noun); to hold back or control (verb)

EXAMPLE

A single *bridle* suture was placed.

bridal: of or relating to a bride or a wedding

EXAMPLE

We finished our work early so that we could attend the *bridal* shower together.

Checkup–Check Up

checkup: a careful inspection (noun)

EXAMPLE

The physician reminded the patient that it was time for a thorough *checkup.*

check up: to perform an examination (verb)

EXAMPLE

We *check up* on patients at least four times a day.

Chord–Cord

chord: series of musical notes

EXAMPLE

He refused to leave until the final *chord* was played.

HINT: A chord with an *h* is the one you *hear.*

cord: strands twisted together (e.g., spinal cord, umbilical cord, vocal cord); a cable; a unit of measurement of wood

EXAMPLE

The vocal *cords* were viewed with indirect mirror laryngoscopy.

Cite–Sight–Site

See *Sight.*

Compare To–Compare With

compare to: to liken dissimilar things

EXAMPLE

The pace in the emergency department was frantic, *compared to* the placid movements of the triage clerk.

compare with: to liken similar things

EXAMPLE

Compared with the rotation in the abdominal surgery unit, the rotation in orthopedic surgery was a breeze.

Complement–Compliment

complement: that which completes; a substance or group of substances found in normal blood serum

EXAMPLES

Massage therapy was a *complement* to the physical therapy.

A *complement* fixation was ordered as part of the laboratory work.

compliment: admiration or praise

EXAMPLE

He gave a *compliment* to each member of the committee for their prompt response.

Continual–Continuous

continual: repetitive, recurring

EXAMPLE

She made *continual* visits to the emergency department.

continuous: unbroken, without interruption

EXAMPLE

Her stay with the child was *continuous,* lasting throughout the visiting hours.

Devise–Device

devise: to form (verb)

EXAMPLE

Dr Johnson wanted to *devise* a plan for the family to follow when they took the child home.

device: a contrivance (noun)

EXAMPLE

He was able to make a *device* that permitted the child to learn to stand and walk with a normal stance.

Dilate–Dilation–Dilatation

dilate: to expand or open (verb)

EXAMPLE

The pupils were able to fully *dilate.*

dilation: the act of dilating

EXAMPLE

She was scheduled for *dilation* of her esophagus.

dilatation: the condition of being stretched or dilated

EXAMPLE

He discovered that the *dilatation* was not as uncomfortable as he imagined.

Disc–Disk

disc/disk: a flat, round, plate-like structure

disc: used when making reference to the eye; it is the term preferred by some orthopaedic surgeons

disk: all other uses of this term

EXAMPLES

The patient's diagnosis was papilledema, which is a swollen optic *disc.*

Ms Evans' surgery today is to repair a herniated intervertebral *disk.*

You need to be careful when inserting the *disk* into your computer

Discrete–Discreet

discrete: separate

EXAMPLE

The patient had total involvement of the right fallopian tube and a *discrete* mass on the right ovary.

discreet: wise, showing good judgment

EXAMPLE

He was being very *discreet* in keeping the medical files locked.

HINT: A mnemonic device for remembering the difference between these two is that the *t* separates the *e*'s in *discrete* (meaning separate).

Disinterested–Uninterested

disinterested: impartial

EXAMPLE

We are going to need a *disinterested* party here to make the final decision.

uninterested: unconcerned, indifferent

EXAMPLE

We could not understand why the parents seemed so *uninterested* in followup care.

Dysphagia–Dysphasia–Dysplasia

dysphagia: difficulty swallowing

EXAMPLE

She had *dysphagia* after her esophageal dilation.

dysphasia: impairment of speech faculty

EXAMPLE

After he had a stroke, Mr James had *dysphasia* for six months.

dysplasia: poorly formed

EXAMPLE

The child continues to have problems because of his spinal *dysplasia.*

Elicit–Illicit

elicit: to draw forth (verb)

EXAMPLE

He attempted to *elicit* the appropriate response.

illicit: unlawful (adjective)

EXAMPLE

It is *illicit* to give out information concerning a child without written permission from the parents or guardian.

e.g.–i.e

e.g.: for example (followed by a comma)

EXAMPLE

We asked for clarification of the work hours (*e.g.,* who can plan on overtime, who will work on holidays, who is available for per diem). (Note use of the comma.)

i.e.: that is

EXAMPLE

I noticed only one difference (*i.e.,* the increased strength in her right biceps).

(Note the use of the comma.) The same function can often be accomplished with a colon.

EXAMPLE

I noticed only one difference: the increased strength in her right biceps.

Emigrate–Immigrate (Emigrant–Immigrant)

emigrate: to leave one's country to reside elsewhere (emigrant: a person who emigrates)

EXAMPLE

He has yet to decide whether he wishes to *emigrate* from Scotland.

immigrate: to enter a country where the person is not a native, for permanent residence (immigrant: a person who immigrates)

EXAMPLE

The entire family recently *immigrated* to the United States from Russia.

HINT: To help you remember: emigrant as in *exit;* immigrant as in *in.*

Eminent–Imminent–Immanent

eminent: famous, superior

EXAMPLE

The speaker was the *eminent* surgeon Dr Sidney Battencourt.

imminent: impending, about to happen

EXAMPLE

He continues to be very fearful of his *imminent* demise.

immanent: present, dwelling within

EXAMPLE

She was very serene, relating to me that perfect peace was always *immanent.*

Enervated–Innervated

enervated: to be weakened, debilitated

EXAMPLE

He was *enervated* by just a few steps to the bathroom.

innervated: to be supplied with nerves

EXAMPLE

That part of the arm is *innervated* by the ulnar nerve.

Etiology–Ideology

etiology: all the possible causes of a disease or problem

EXAMPLE

The *etiology* of the syndrome is still undetermined.

ideology: a systematic group of concepts; theories of a program

EXAMPLE

We were unable to get a clear picture of the primary *ideology* of his group.

Every Day–Everyday

every day: each day

EXAMPLE

I will see the patient *every day.*

everyday: ordinary

EXAMPLE

She is unable to do her *everyday* chores.

Every One–Everyone

every one: each one (singular)

EXAMPLE

Every one of the diagnoses was ruled out.

everyone: all persons (plural)

EXAMPLE

Everyone was present at the board meeting.

Please look at the last two sets of words. In the next review, you could encounter those words along with other word sets that follow the same pattern. Note how one part of the set is used as a whole word and one part is used as two words. These words are as follows: *any one–anyone, any way–anyway, any time–anytime, some day–someday, some time–sometime, any more–anymore, any thing–anything.*

10-3 SELF-STUDY

DIRECTIONS: Please underline the word or word pair that is correct in each sentence.

1. The four hospital visits cost $450 (altogether/all together).
2. We should learn how to operate within the network system (altogether/all together).
3. At this hospital, (anyone/any one) is entitled to incentive pay when doing medical transcription.
4. The laboratory information is outdated, but type it into the chart note (anyway/any way).
5. Is there (anyway/any way) you can have the history and physical faxed by the end of the shift?
6. (Although/All though) it is Friday, we still have to put in some overtime.
7. Is it (alright/all right) to turn in the discharge summary a day late?
8. The cholecystectomy is scheduled for (someday/some day) next week.
9. She knows that (someday/some day) she will be in charge of quality assurance.
10. The medical records and medical transcription supervisors are finally (already/all ready) to announce the new incentive policy.
11. The radiology report was (already/all ready) filed in the medical record when the physician asked for it.
12. Dr Gordon should be able to see you (anytime/any time) in February.
13. The emergency department services are open for your use (anytime/any time).
14. He has certain clothes for (everyday/every day) wear and surgical scrubs for work.
15. For (sometime/some time) now, he has been dictating his medical reports on a digital recorder.
16. The consultation reports were sent (sometime/some time) last week.
17. The senior staff do not get (anymore/any more) incentive raises.
18. Is there (anything/any thing) Dr Avery can get you for your headache?

The answers are on p. 450 in Appendix A.

Farther–Further

farther: to or at a more distant or remote point in space (distance) or time

EXAMPLE

The patient cannot walk farther than halfway down the hall.

further: additional

EXAMPLE

I do not believe that *further* tests need to be carried out at this time.

Fewer–Less

fewer: smaller quantity referring to number of persons or things

EXAMPLE

There were *fewer* members of the surgical team than we had anticipated.

less: smaller quantity referring to volume or mass

EXAMPLE

I was able to draw *less* fluid on thoracentesis than planned.

Followup–Follow Up–Follow-up

followup: the care given to a patient after a procedure (e.g., surgical or diagnostic procedure), office call, or treatment for an accident or illness (noun); pertaining to care given to a patient after a specific medical service was performed (adjective)

EXAMPLE

She was scheduled for daily *followup* in the hospital.

follow up: to provide patient care, such as reexamination or brief history after the patient's illness, accident, or procedure (verb)

EXAMPLE

I will want to *follow up* this problem daily for the next week at least.

follow-up: occurring after an office call or treatment for an accident or illness (adjective)

EXAMPLE

Her *follow-up* examination was scheduled as early as possible (also *followup*).

Formerly–Formally

formerly: earlier (states when)

EXAMPLE

He was *formerly* a patient in the Green Valley Sanitarium.

formally: officially (states how)

EXAMPLE

He was *formally* greeted by the president of the association.

Imply–Infer

imply: hint at, insinuate; what the speaker suggests

EXAMPLE

We were afraid that he would *imply* that the tumor was cancerous.

infer: presume from what another said or wrote, to draw a conclusion

EXAMPLE

From your response, I *infer* that you are angry.

NOTE: Infer is what the listener takes in or perceives the speaker to be saying.

In Toto–Total

in toto: totally; referring to a specimen sample in which an entire piece of tissue is submitted (adverb)

EXAMPLE

The specimen was removed and sent to pathology *in toto*.

total: entire, the whole (noun or adjective)

EXAMPLE

The patient had *total* involvement of the right fallopian tube within the mass.

Incidence–Incidents

incidence: frequency

EXAMPLE

The *incidence* of accidents on the ward has greatly decreased.

incidents: subordinate to something else, consequences or events

EXAMPLE

That is likely to be one of the unfortunate *incidents* to expect when alcohol is mixed with driving an automobile.

Last–Latest

last: final

EXAMPLE

It was his *last* request.

latest: most recent

EXAMPLE

The *latest* diagnosis is pelvic inflammatory disease.

Lie–Lay

lie: a falsehood (noun); to utter a falsehood (verb) (not a problem, grammar-wise, that is)

lie: to recline (verb) (the most incorrectly used verb in English)

EXAMPLE

I asked the patient to *lie* on the examining table. *(recline, present tense, now)*

PROBLEM: The past tense of *lie* is *lay*, which we will consider next. The verb *lie* is an intransitive verb: it never takes an object.

lay: to place (This is a transitive verb: it always takes an object; we have to have something to place.)

EXAMPLE

I asked her to *lay* the dictionary on the table. *(place)*

PROBLEM: The present tense of *lay* is the same as the past tense of *lie*.

Now take a look at all the principal parts of *lie*: lie, lay, lain, lying.

EXAMPLE

The patient was asked to *lie* on the table; he *lay* there a long time; he has *lain* there too long in the past and knows he will be *lying* here again in the future.

Look at the principal parts of *lay*: lay, laid, laid, laying (place).

EXAMPLE

I asked her to *lay* the dictionary on the table. I do not like it to be *laid* on the printer, where it has been *laid* often in the past. The students are fond of *laying* it there because it is closer to the monitor and the keyboard.

Here is a hint to help you choose the correct version of the word: substitute the word *place* for your word. If it works, then *lay* or one of its principal parts fits. If it does not fit, then *lie* or one of its principal parts fits. (In brief, *lay* = place and *lie* = recline.)

EXAMPLES

I need to (lie/lay) this heavy box down. (*place* the box? Yes. Therefore, it is *lay* the box.)

The nurse said he (lay/laid) awake most of the night. (*placed* awake? No. Therefore, it is *lay* awake.)

Yesterday I (lay/laid) the medical records on the top of the filing cabinet. (*placed* the records? Yes. Therefore, it is *laid*.)

He had been (lying/laying) tile for the past several years. (*placing* tile? Yes. Therefore, it is *laying*.)

She has never been accused of (lying/laying) down on the job. (*placing* down? No. Therefore, it is *lying*.)

Like–As If

like: similar to

EXAMPLE

Her face is *like* a mask.

as if: as though

EXAMPLE

She felt *as if* she would not be able to continue working until the end of the shift.

Lose–Loose

lose: sacrifice; to suffer a loss (verb)

EXAMPLE

He was afraid he would *lose* his concentration with the music playing.

loose: relaxed (adjective), not pressed close together

EXAMPLE

She complained of nausea and *loose* stools.

Maybe–May Be

maybe: possibly (adverb)

EXAMPLE

Maybe you could ask him about it before we get our hopes up.

may be: perhaps is (verb)

EXAMPLE

He *may be* ready to authorize a raise for everyone.

Most–Majority

most: nearly all

EXAMPLE

Most of us wanted to begin work earlier; John was a holdout.

majority: the number greater than half a total (used with things that can be counted)

EXAMPLE

The *majority* of the voters said no to the proposal. *Most* of the eligible voters sent in ballots.

Nauseated–Nauseous

nauseated: feeling queasy

EXAMPLE

He has been *nauseated* since he woke up this morning.

nauseous: causing nausea

EXAMPLE

The fumes were nauseous.

Navel–Naval

navel: the umbilicus

EXAMPLE

There was an exquisitely tender spot just to the right of the *navel*.

naval: having to do with a navy, ships, or sailing

EXAMPLE

A huge *naval* deployment was planned for the end of the year.

CHAPTER 10

 10-4 SELF-STUDY

DIRECTIONS: Underline the word or word pair enclosed in parentheses that fits the meaning of the sentence.

1. The vocal (chords/cords) were viewed by using indirect mirror laryngoscopy.

2. It seemed (like/as if) he would begin the procedure unassisted.

3. There is no one (besides/beside) the family to give consent.

4. Please remember that you were asked to (accept/except) my (advise/advice).

5. I was concerned because the mole did not have any (discrete/discreet) margins.

6. We could not (elicit/illicit) any information from the patient because we could not speak his language.

7. (Further/Farther) workup on this patient will be required. I did not mean to (infer/imply) that the diagnosis was being questioned.

8. Please (lay/lie) a pillow on the examining table before you ask the patient to (lie/lay) down.

9. The catheters were removed, and hemostasis was (affected/effected) with pressure.

10. The long-term (affects/effects) of the drug are unknown.

11. A single (bridal/bridle) suture was placed.

12. The (etiology/ideology) of his condition is unknown at this time.

13. After careful consideration of the patient's remarks, I must (imply/infer) that he has no intention of following our plans.

14. She had noticed the pain radiating from the area just to the right of the (naval/navel).

The answers are on p. 450 in Appendix A.

Only One of–The Only One of–One of

NOTE: This distinction is not easy, so take some time with it.

the only one of: used with a singular verb

EXAMPLE
He is *the only one of* the surgeons who *was* available.

only one of, one of: used with a plural verb

EXAMPLES
He is *only one of* the surgeons who *were* available.
She is *one of* those who *were* always eager to respond.

Opposition
See *Apposition.*

Palette–Palate–Pallet
palette: an artist's paint board

EXAMPLE
Her work is said to be the results of her wide and wonderful *palette.*

palate: the roof of the mouth; taste

EXAMPLE
He was able to close the hare lip and cleft *palate* with ease.

pallet: a bed; a platform for moving materials

EXAMPLE
The *pallet* slipped and fell, and a splinter flew into her hand.

HINT: *Because the word you most likely will be transcribing will be* palate, *just remember it is the word with one* l *and one* t.

Past–Passed
past: recent or preceding (adjective)

EXAMPLE
Nothing in his *past* history indicated that he was at risk.

passed: approved or to go beyond (verb)

EXAMPLE
The ambulance *passed* us as we hurried to the hospital.

Persons–People
persons: emphasizes the individual

EXAMPLE
She is one of those *persons* who never say anything bad about anyone else.

people: an undifferentiated group

EXAMPLE
He recommended that two *people* should be appointed to the committee.

Plane–Plain
plane: a level or grade (noun); to level (verb)

EXAMPLE
His professional life has always been on a high *plane.*

plain: simple; not pretty; clear (adjective)

EXAMPLE
Plain x-rays of the abdomen were ordered.

Principle–Principal
principle: rule, regulation

EXAMPLE

We have a new class in the *principles* of medical ethics.

principal: main, head

EXAMPLE

We need to turn our attention to the *principal* diagnosis.

Proceed–Precede

proceed: advance, continue

EXAMPLE

She must *proceed* with her initial assessment.

precede: to be earlier than, to go before

EXAMPLE

History taking *precedes* the physical examination except in an emergency.

Recur–Reoccur

reoccur: no such word exists

recur: repeat, return

EXAMPLE

He was frightened that his symptoms would *recur* during his holiday.

Regardless–Irregardless

irregardless: an incorrect form; do not use

regardless: despite

EXAMPLE

Regardless of our advice, he checked himself out of the hospital.

Regime–Regimen–Regiment

regime: a period of rule or form of government

EXAMPLE

Nothing much can be planned during this *regime*.

regimen: a systematic schedule set up to improve or maintain the health of a patient

EXAMPLE

The patient has a strict *regimen* to follow as soon as he is discharged.

regiment: a military unit

Repeat–Repeated

repeat: to say or perform again

EXAMPLE

We need to *repeat* the sonographic study as soon as possible.

repeated: occurring again and again

EXAMPLE

She had *repeated* bouts of doubling-up pain.

Root–Route

root: underlying support; origin or source

EXAMPLE

The cannula was placed near the *root* of the aortic valve.

route: a line of travel

EXAMPLE

The *route* between the surgery suite and the recovery room is nearly blocked with ladders and paint cans.

Sit–Sat–Set

sit: to assume a particular position; does not take an object (sit, sat, sat)

EXAMPLE

We had no idea how long she would *sit* there.

sat: the past tense of sit

EXAMPLE

He *sat* in the emergency department for three hours before being seen.

set: to place; takes an object (the past tense is set)

EXAMPLE

Please *set* the Mayo stand closer to the work area.

EXCEPTIONS: The sun *sets,* and milk and pudding *set.*

Sight–Site–Cite

sight: vision

EXAMPLE

Her *sight* was greatly improved after the cataract surgery.

site: location

EXAMPLE

The *site* of the injury was extensive.

cite: quote

EXAMPLE

He can *cite* that regulation in the hospital bylaws.

Sometime–Some Time–Sometimes

sometime: at some unspecified time

EXAMPLE

We need to consider doing a complete physical examination *sometime*.

some time: a period of time

EXAMPLE

I do think we have *some time* to indulge in "watchful waiting."

sometimes: now and then

EXAMPLE

He takes a walk *sometimes* after his evening meal.

Super–Supra

super: as a prefix, means over, above; used mainly with everyday word roots

EXAMPLE

I have a *super*abundance of medical records waiting to be signed off.

NOTE: The term *supernumerary cysts* is not really an exception, more a lay term.

supra: as a prefix, means over, above; used mainly with medical word roots

EXAMPLE

There is tenderness in the *supra*pubic area.

Then–Than

then: at that time (adverb)

EXAMPLE

We *then* closed the incision with #3-0 Dacron.

than: a word used in comparing or contrasting (conjunction)

EXAMPLE

Don has always proofread on screen faster *than* I have.

Tortuous–Torturous

tortuous: winding, full of turns, tricky

EXAMPLE

His right ankle was fractured on a *tortuous* ski trail.

torturous: painful, very unpleasant

EXAMPLE

He spent a *torturous* time waiting to be rescued.

Worse–Worst

worse: bad or ill to a greater degree

EXAMPLE

By morning, the patient was feeling much *worse*.

worst: bad or ill to the greatest degree

EXAMPLE

I am sorry, but it is the *worst* possible diagnosis.

10-5 SELF-STUDY

DIRECTIONS: Underline the proper word or words enclosed in parentheses that are correct for the given sentence.

1. He was first seen in the emergency department with (supersternal/suprasternal) pain.

2. The hay fever symptoms (reoccur/recur) each spring.

3. (Irregardless/Regardless) of the consequences, he reported what he had witnessed.

4. The patient was left (sitting/setting) there entirely too long; he should have been (lying/laying) down.

5. Her (site/cite/sight) was (affected/effected) by the injury to her eye.

6. She presented in the office with one of the (worse/worst) cases of poison oak that I have ever encountered.

7. We will discuss his medication and exercise (regimen/regiment) again when he returns for (followup/follow up).

8. He has (past/passed) the 5-year mark in his recovery.

9. It was finally determined that there was nerve (root/route) inflammation.

10. (Then/Than) we decided that we must wait (some time/sometime) for further healing to take place.

11. She was really (innervated/enervated) when she saw that the huge backlog of records was still not cleared.

12. It always makes me (nauseated/nauseous) when I stay in the animal laboratory too long.

13. (Further/Farther) workup on this patient will be required.

14. I did not mean to (infer/imply) that the diagnosis was being questioned.

15. It was a long, complicated, and (tortuous/torturous) procedure.

16. We asked her to (proceed/precede) with her discussions with possible organ donors.

17. The catheters were removed, and hemostasis was (affected/effected) with pressure.

18. The long-term (affects/effects) of the drug are unknown.

19. The patient was basically unresponsive, with a flat (affect/effect).

20. That Dorland's has (lain/laid/lay) there all day without anyone picking it up.

The answers are on p. 450 in Appendix A.

Which–That
Do not use in reference to persons.

that: a relative pronoun that introduces a restrictive clause; not enclosed in commas

EXAMPLE
The instruments *that* you sterilized were not returned to the drawer.

which: a relative pronoun that introduces a nonrestrictive clause; enclosed in commas

EXAMPLE
The instruments, *which* you sterilized, were not returned to the drawer.

Use *which* and *that* for things and *who, whose,* and *whom* for persons.

EXAMPLES
She is the patient *who* needed to be seen immediately.
This is the pacemaker *that* I am using on Mrs Silvanis.
This pacemaker, *which* we found was not defective, was used on Mrs Silvanis.

Who–Whom
Who and *whoever* are used as subjects. *Whom* and *whomever* are used as objects.
To determine the correct form, first separate the clause containing the target word and disregard the rest of the sentence. If *he, she,* or *they* would be correct, use *who* or *whoever.* If *him, her,* or *them* would be correct, use *whom* or *whomever.*

EXAMPLES
(Who/Whom) did you say was on call?

1. Separate the clause: *who/whom* was on call.
2. Substitute the helper pronouns: *he/she* was on call.
3. Select *who.*

The internist, the only one (whom/who) we had a pager number for, arrived immediately.
1. Separate the clause: we had a pager number for *whom/who.*
2. Substitute the helper pronouns: we had a pager number for *him/her.*
3. Select *whom.*

Who–Whom and Verb Forms with Only One of–The Only One of–One of
the only one of: used with a singular verb

EXAMPLE
He is *the only one of* the surgeons *who was* available.
The only one of the staff *whom we invited* was Dr Berry.

only one of, one of: used with a plural verb

EXAMPLES
He is *only one of* the surgeons *who were* available.
She is *one of* those *who were* always eager to respond.

Workup–Work Up
workup: the diagnostic study (noun)

EXAMPLE
He has to perform the *workup* on about six more patients before he begins rounds.

work up: to perform the history and/or physical examination (verb)

EXAMPLE
She will *work up* each of the patients for the attending physician.

10-6 SELF-STUDY

DIRECTIONS: Please underline the word or words enclosed in parentheses that are correct.

1. Please consult (whoever/whomever) is on call.

2. She is the one (who/whom) they called to (work up/workup) the patients before surgery.

3. The patient (who/whom) you have just discharged called the office.

4. The patient (who/whom) just fainted was standing by the door.

5. There is a suspicious nodule on the (superclavicular/supraclavicular) node.

6. Please call (whoever/whomever) you think would arrive quickly.

7. (Whom/Who) did he say was on call?

8. It was a far more extensive surgery (then/than) I had anticipated.

9. She is the one (who/whom) I understand they consulted.

10. She could not have arrived in the emergency department at a (worst/worse) time.

11. No one can remember (who/whom) is the anesthesiologist on call.

12. Give this to (whomever/whoever) will complete the (workup/work up.)

13. The third floor, (which/that) is the pediatric ward, was affected by a power failure.

14. All of the patients (which/who/whom) had been waiting had to be told they could not be seen.

15. We need someone (who/whom) would be available for per diem transcription.

The answers are on p. 451 in Appendix A.

 # 10-7 PRACTICE TEST

Another test? This time, no review. Here are some words that have not been discussed. However, Appendix B includes a list of medical homonyms if you need help. Try first to see whether you can figure the answers out on your own.

DIRECTIONS: Select the word from the left column that will correctly complete each sentence in the right column.

aura
aural

1. The ear is concerned with the acoustic or _____ sense.
2. Betsy Blake complained of having an _____ before her epileptic attacks.

ora
oral

3. Valium is an _____ medication.
4. The _____ serrata is the serrated margin of the retina in the anterior part of the eyeball.

hypertension
antihypertension
hypotension

5. Mr Yoshida's blood pressure was 165/90, indicating _____.
6. Mrs Lockhard had a blood pressure reading of 100/60, which is a condition of _____.
7. ProAmatine is a drug that produces an increase in blood pressure because the patient is experiencing _____.

amenorrhea
menorrhea
dysmenorrhea
menorrhagia
metrorrhagia

8. Her chief complaint was _____, meaning absence of menses.
9. One of Miss Mason's signs was abnormal uterine bleeding between periods, a condition called _____.

antiseptic
asepsis
aseptic
sepsis
septic

10. The surgical instruments must be _____ at all times.
11. The laboratory report indicated pus-forming microorganisms in the blood, a condition of _____.

palpitation
palpation

12. She has had no further episodes of _____ of the heart.
13. The physician examined the area by _____ and felt a small cyst.

tract
track

14. He was seen in consultation by Dr Friedman, who performed an upper gastrointestinal _____ endoscopy and found nothing unusual.

instillation
installation

15. Before the _____ of a general anesthetic, a KUB examination was performed.

ileum
ilium

16. There is a small mass in the lumen of the terminal _____.

The answers are on p. 451 in Appendix A.

ADJECTIVE MODIFIERS

If necessary, review the noun and adjective word endings in Chapter 9. Be sure that you use an adjective to modify a noun.

EXAMPLES

An *aortic* aneurysm (*Not* aorta *aneurysm*)

The *mucous* membrane (*Not* mucus *membrane*)

The *urethral* meatus (*Not* urethra *meatus*)

A *hemorrhagic* episode (*Not* hemorrhage *episode*)

ANTECEDENTS

Each pronoun must have a clear antecedent; if it does not, substitute a noun for it.

EXAMPLES

Dr Johnson observed the operation on Mr Spokes, after which *he* was taken to the recovery room.

You would assume that Mr Spokes was taken to the recovery room, but the sentence is unclear.

Recast: Dr Johnson observed the operation on Mr Spokes, after which the patient was taken to the recovery room.

Pull the patient's record; notify the doctor of the emergency; then give *him* the record.

You would guess that the physician is to receive the record, but this action is unclear.

Recast: Pull the patient's record; notify the doctor of the emergency; give *the doctor* the record.

 MT TOOL BOX TIP: Hold on to your antecedents to make sentences make sense.

COLLECTIVE NOUNS

Collective nouns include words such as *team, class, committee, group, couple, family, jury, number, set, variety,* and *staff* and units of measure and sums of money. These nouns take a singular verb when thought of together as a group or set.

Look at *number* as a collective noun that can be either singular or plural. When *number* is preceded by *the*, it takes a singular verb. When *number* is preceded by *a*, it takes a plural verb.

EXAMPLES

The number of white blood cells in the sample *is* alarming.

A large number of white blood cells *are* needed for the sampling.

EXAMPLES

Then *450 mg* of clindamycin *was* prescribed by the clinic physician.

This *group* of diagnoses *is* proposed.

The *review of systems was* negative.

He thought that *$500 was* a lot of money.

Only *20%* of the fluid *was* removed.

When the individuals making up the group are considered, then a plural verb is used.

EXAMPLES

The family *were crowded* into the small room.

The jury *were overcome* by the fumes in the hallway.

The couple, as well as the child, *were reassured.*

DANGLING CONSTRUCTIONS AND MISPLACED MODIFIERS

Words, phrases, or clauses may all be modifiers. Misplaced modifiers occur when the writer does not make clear what is being modified. In some instances, the word being modified may be missing altogether, and so the modifier "dangles." Misplaced modifying words or phrases often produce humorous results. Therefore, you must reconstruct or recast the sentence so that all the parts are in agreement. Ambiguous or illogical placement of a modifier can usually be avoided by placing the modifier close to the word it modifies.

EXAMPLES

Walking down the road, the ambulance passed me.

Recast: The ambulance passed me as I was walking down the road.

Before the patients are placed on gurneys, they are thoroughly scrubbed.

Recast: The gurneys are thoroughly scrubbed before patients are placed on them.

After recovering from a coma, the physician reassured him.

Recast: After the patient recovered from the coma, the physician reassured him.

He was referred to a urologist with advanced pyelonephritis.

Recast: He had advanced pyelonephritis and was referred to a urologist.

INDEFINITE PRONOUNS AND VERBS

Indefinite pronouns such as *anybody, anyone, each, everyone, nobody, no one, somebody,* and *someone* are usually singular.

EXAMPLES

Nobody is on the roster to work the p.m. shift.

Everyone is invited to attend the utilization review meeting.

No one is going to take responsibility for leaving the file unlocked.

I hope that *everybody is* happy.

The indefinite pronouns *both, others, several, many,* and *few* are plural.

EXAMPLE

Several possibilities are apparent for the resolution of the problem.

These are easy because the pronoun itself indicates more than one. However, the indefinite pronouns *more, most, none, all, any,* and *some* may be singular or plural depending on how they are used. Often, they too are employed with a singular or plural noun.

EXAMPLES

Most of our class *is* taking the RMT exam on the same weekend.

Most of the medical transcriptionists where I work *are* certified.

None can be singular and plural. When *none* refers to a group, use a singular or a plural verb, depending on what is to be emphasized. When *none* means *not a single one,* use a singular verb.

EXAMPLE

None of our staff *was* available to serve on the safety committee. *(Not one)*

When *none* means *not any* or *no part of,* use a plural verb.

EXAMPLE

None of our staff *were* available to serve on the safety committee. *(Not any)*

PARALLEL STRUCTURE

Parallel ideas must be expressed in parallel form in a sentence. This rule applies to lists as well. Each part of speech (adjective, noun, verb, and so on) must be matched in parallel structure.

 MT TOOL BOX TIP: Parallel lists—a tool for good structure.

EXAMPLE

Learning to write is a challenge and interesting.

Here *writing* is described with an adjective *(interesting)* and with a noun *(challenge).* It would be better to use two adjectives and change the sentence.

Recast: Learning to write is challenging and interesting.

Because lists are often used in the reports, remember to match nouns with nouns, verbs with verbs, and so on.

EXAMPLE: *a poorly constructed list*

Considerations for your workstation include the following:

▶ Get a comfortable, adjustable chair.

▶ You should have a glare-protected screen.

- Ergonomic keyboards help prevent injury.
- It is important to have adequate room lighting.
- Be sure that your reference placement is convenient.
- If you need it, an adjustable footrest is helpful.
- Adequate storage for your personal things.
- Keep the environment quiet or use white noise.
- Moderate temperature.

Recast: Considerations for your workstation include the following:

- a comfortable, adjustable chair
- a glare-protected screen
- an ergonomic keyboard
- adequate room lighting
- convenient reference placement
- an adjustable footrest
- adequate storage
- a quiet environment (or white noise)
- moderate temperature

EXAMPLES

To be accurate and meeting your production level are important here.

Recast: To be accurate and to meet your production level are important here.

Or: It is important to be accurate and to meet your production level here.

Pull the patient's record, notifying the doctor of the emergency, then give the record to him and be sure to relate any information you have received.

Recast: Pull the patient's record; notify the doctor of the emergency; give the record to *the doctor;* and relate any information you have received.

Notice also, that the antecedent for the pronoun *him* was unclear, and so a noun was substituted.

The pairs *either-or, neither-nor, not only–but also,* and *both-and* are called *correlative conjunctions,* and elements on both sides must match.

EXAMPLES

Either I get this correct *or* I resign myself to going over the entire chapter again.

Neither the consultant *nor* the family physician was prepared for the outcome.

Not only the emergency department *but also* the urgent care center was overwhelmed by the crisis.

Both the full-time staff *and* the per diem staff were pleased with the raise.

She does not agree to have radiation nor chemotherapy. *(Poor)*

Recast: She will agree to *neither* radiation *nor* chemotherapy.

PERSONAL PRONOUNS

The appropriate pronoun is selected on the basis of its position in the sentence.

Pronouns Used as the Subject of the Sentence: *I, You, He, She, We, They*

EXAMPLES

Dr Johnson and *I* prepared the rotation schedule together.

NOTE: Mention yourself second if you are included.

The residents and *we* could not agree on it, however.

Pronouns Used as the Objects of Verbs and Prepositions: *Me, You, Him, Her, Us, Them*

EXAMPLES

She asked *him* to deliver the report to *her* and *me.* (The pronoun *him* is the object of the verb. The pronouns *her* and *me* are the objects of the preposition.)

She gave the reports to *them* and *us.*

Just between *you* and *me,* these often cause *me* to pause.

NOTE: Sentences that contain a linking verb in the form of *to be (am, is, are, were, was, will be, been, become)* do not take a direct object. The object of such a verb is called a *predicate complement.* These linking verbs may join a plural subject with a singular complement or a singular subject with a plural complement. You must be sure that the verb agrees with the subject.

EXAMPLES

It *is* I.

That could not have *been* she who called.

Dr Jones said it *was* he whom we saw.

I know that Robert said it *was* we who made all the noise, but I know it *was* they.

HELP: How do you check this usage? Ask who made the noise. *We* did or *they* did. Some writers avoid the problem and rewrite the sentence.

I know that Robert said we made the noise, but I know they did.

Dr Jones said that the person we saw was Michael.

Pronouns and Contractions

Be sure to make the correct choice. Spell out your contraction, and you will be sure.

their	they're	*(they are)*
its	it's	*(it is)*
whose	who's	*(who is* or *who has)*

Reflexive Pronouns: *Myself, Herself, Ourselves, Yourself, Himself, Itself, Yourselves, Themselves*

Reflexive pronouns are used to emphasize or to refer to the subject of the sentence.

EXAMPLES

She *herself* did not realize what was going on until too late.

You call *yourself* an artist?

The physician *herself* called that in.

They all considered *themselves* lucky to be alive.

I made that spelling error all by *myself!*

Give that to him and *myself*. *(Incorrect)*

Give that to him and *me*. *(Correct)*

Adrianna and *myself* made that decision. *(Incorrect)*

Myself and Adrianna made that decision. *(Incorrect)*

Adrianna and *I* made that decision. *(Correct)*

PLURALS AND SINGULARS

You learned how to form the plurals of nouns in previous chapters. Now you have to be sure that you are matching the nouns properly with plural verbs.

Compound subjects take a plural verb.

EXAMPLE

The patient and his parents *were* accommodated quickly by the night supervisor.

Plural subjects take a plural verb. (Find the subject of the sentence, not just the word close to the verb.)

EXAMPLES

The *conjunctivae were* bilaterally inflamed.

Fifteen *members* of the board *were* present.

Sections of the cervical tissue *show* mild dysplasia.

The *urinalysis was* negative, as *were* the *chest x-ray* and *drug screen*.

Singular subjects take a singular verb. (Find the subject of the sentence, not just the word close to the verb.)

EXAMPLES

The *cost* of the diagnostic procedures *is* increasing.

The scalene node *biopsy is* scheduled for tomorrow morning.

The Language of Medicine, along with three other texts, *is* recommended for study.

Bronchoscopy of the right upper lobe bronchus, right lower lobe bronchus, and left lower lobe bronchus *is* scheduled to precede the thoracotomy.

The *child*, as well as his parents, *was reassured*.

The *admission workup* (CBC, urinalysis, and chest x-ray) *was* carried out the previous day.

Collective nouns (team, group, committee, units of measurement) take a singular verb.

EXAMPLES

Then *450 mg* of clindamycin was *prescribed* by the clinic physician.

This *group* of diagnoses *is proposed*.

The *review of systems was* negative.

Only *20%* of the fluid *was examined*.

Parts of a compound subject joined by *or* or *nor* take a singular verb when the subjects are singular.

EXAMPLES

Neither the primary care physician *nor* the consultant *was* available to confirm a "do not resuscitate" order.

Either the nursing home *or* the skilled nursing facility *is* her destination.

Parts of a compound subject joined by *or* or *nor* take a plural verb when the subjects are plural or *the subject closest to the verb is plural*.

EXAMPLES

Neither the *Dorland's* nor the specialty reference books *were* available.

Neither the specialty reference books nor the *Dorland's was* available.

Either the residents or the doctor on call *was* responsible for the change in the rotation.

Either the pathology reports or the operative report *is* left to be transcribed.

Neither the consultants nor the referring physician *was* sure when the seizure occurred.

Neither the referring physician nor the consultants *were* sure when the seizure occurred.

Parts of a compound subject joined by *not only–but also* take a singular verb when the subject closest to the verb is singular. Use a plural verb when the subject closest to the verb is plural.

EXAMPLES

We found that not only the oviducts but also the uterus *was* involved.

We found that not only the uterus but also the oviducts *were* involved.

PLURAL PRONOUNS WITH SINGULAR ANTECEDENTS

To avoid sexist language, use of plural pronouns with singular antecedents is becoming acceptable, thereby avoiding the tedious repetition of *his or her* and so on.

Do attempt to recast the sentence, if you can, to avoid this construction.

EXAMPLES

Poor: *Each* medical transcriptionist must have *their* own books and research materials.

Better: *All* medical transcriptionists must have *their* own books and research materials.

Poor: *Every one* of the participants enjoyed learning a new method to proofread *their* own on-screen documents.

Better: The *participants* enjoyed learning a new method to proofread *their* own on-screen documents.

SENTENCE STRUCTURE

Use complete sentences when transcribing most reports. Clipped sentences are correct, however, when dictated in chart notes (progress reports) or in the history and physical examination. In general, the missing words are suggested, and you can insert them easily.

EXAMPLES

Clipped: Chest clear to percussion and auscultation.

Expanded clipped (for physical examination note): Chest: Clear to percussion and auscultation.

Complete (for a formal document): The chest is clear to percussion and auscultation.

Clipped: Closed with 3-0 silk sutures.

Complete: The incision was closed with 3-0 silk sutures.

Be sure the sentence says what you know the speaker intended.

EXAMPLES

He went to the emergency department in Douglas, where they told him that he had chest discomfort.

Intended: He went to the emergency department in Douglas because he had chest discomfort.

She has well-documented diabetic retinopathy with hemorrhages throughout both *lung* fields.

Intended: She has well-documented diabetic retinopathy with hemorrhages throughout both *eye* fields.

He *has some* transient ischemic event, resulting in the loss of his *eye* for a short time.

Intended: He *had a* transient ischemic event, resulting in the loss of his *vision* for a short time.

Mrs Johnson was diagnosed with diabetes mellitus.

Intended: Mrs Johnson's diagnosis was diabetes mellitus.

Or: Mrs Johnson's problem was diagnosed as diabetes. (*A disease, not a patient, is diagnosed.*)

There is sublingular or submandibular swelling.

Intended: There is *no* sublingular or submandibular swelling. (*Left out the word* no.)

He was late because he had to see the bullet wound in the emergency department.

Intended: He was late because he had to see the patient with the bullet wound in the emergency department. (*Patients are not referred to as their problem.*)

TENSE OF VERBS

The tense of a verb indicates if something is happening now (present tense), has happened in the past (past tense), or is planned for the future (future tense).

Past tense is used in the history part of a report, operative reports, in discharge summaries, and in discussing patients who have died.

EXAMPLES

The patient *has had* sciatica on the left side for the past 2 years.

The patient *complained* of pain in the epigastrium that radiated into the right lower quadrant. There *was* no rebound tenderness when I examined her.

NOTE: This second sentence became part of her history.

Incorrect: The patient *was* seen yesterday and *is* doing well.

Correct: The patient *was* seen yesterday and *was* doing well.

In medical dictation, both the present tense and historic present tense (where the dictator uses the present to explain something that actually occurred in the past) are used, and both past and present tense verbs may occur in the same sentence.

Present tense is used in physical examination reports. Generally one finds a combination of past, present, and future tenses occurring in the complete examination of the patient which includes the history, the examination, and plans for future care.

EXAMPLES

The patient *is* sure she wants to continue under my care. (Historic present tense)

The patient *has had* left sciatica for the past two years; this condition *is* now exacerbated. (combination of past and present tenses)

PLAN: The patient *is to be seen* again in one week. (future tense)

Heart: There *is* normal sinus rhythm.

Abdomen: It *is* flat. There *is* no rebound tenderness.

Because the physical examination report is generally dictated in clipped sentences, this example generally appears as follows:

Heart: Normal sinus rhythm.
Abdomen: Flat. No rebound tenderness.

Do not use clipped sentences in formal documents (e.g., letters, medicolegal documents).

PROPER TERMS FOR PERSONS

In descriptions of persons, patients should be described as infants, boys, girls, men, or women. Terms to avoid are *male* and *female* used as nouns.

neonate	birth to 1 month
newborn	birth to 1 month
infant	1 month to 1 year
child	1 to 12 years
boy/girl	1 to 12 years
adolescent	13 to 17 years
teenager	13 to 17 years
adult	man or woman aged 18 years or older

10-8 PRACTICE TEST

DIRECTIONS: Retype the following sentences, making any corrections if necessary. If the sentence is correct as written (be careful), just write C after the number of the question. Please double-space your answer sheet for ease of grading. Your answers do not need to appear exactly as these are written, but all of the elements of the problem should be corrected, with no new incorrect elements added.

EXAMPLE

He also had a vasectomy and a tonsillectomy as a child.

Corrected: He had a tonsillectomy as a child; he also has had a vasectomy.

1. In the past, she was admitted once and apparently underwent a stress test that was negative in Ohio.

2. He denied any history of angiograms done.

3. It was felt that the afterload reduction would not be significant enough to affect her hemodynamically.

4. She either knocked her head on the fence or she fell to the ground.

5. There was a 35-minute lapse between when the mother called and the arrival of the ambulance.

6. Neither the patient nor his parents or friends seemed to be aware of the risks involved.

7. Review of systems otherwise is complete but negative.

8. The teenage patient (that/who/whom) we saw in the office yesterday expired in the emergency department last night.

9. Dr Jamieson, Dr Gonzales, and (myself/me/I) were selected as new members of the anesthesiology team.

10. There were 30 patients involved in our double-blind study, and three are being examined each day.

11. She (is/was) to be seen in followup but (is/was) unable to keep her appointment.

12. The patient was involved in an automobile accident while 5 months pregnant with a taxi.

13. The patient was transferred to the surgery suite with her films in good condition.

14. The hospital utilization committee reviewed (their/its/it's) discharge policy at yesterday's meeting.

15. On the pathology report, sections 1 through 4 (are/were) labeled "tissue from uterine fundus."

16. We all wondered about whom the new interns were.

17. Whomever the physician calls in consultation will have trouble with her.

18. The patient will (follow up/followup/follow-up) with (me/myself) next week.

19. A degree of gasping and snoring as well as mouth breathing are further noted.

20. The circumflex artery as well as its branches are thought to be free of any irregularities or lesions.

Check your answers in Appendix A, p. 451.

10-9 REVIEW TEST

DIRECTIONS: Rewrite the following sentences, correcting any grammatical errors you may find. Type the reconstructed sentence on a separate sheet of paper. You may submit more than one version if necessary. If you think that the question is correct as written, write **C** after the number of the question.

1. Moldering away in the hospital basement for several years, Nancy found the missing microfilm.

2. We noticed recent callous on the x-ray.

3. 1200 mL of serosanguineous fluid were aspirated from the abdomen's cavity.

4. The panel was polled individually.

5. Each of the members of the committee were notified of the change.

6. Every one of these instruments have been carefully tested.

7. The voice recognition system is accurate, easy, and performs slowly.

8. He would neither call an ambulance nor would he go to the acute care center.

9. Aurora was sure it was them that arrived at the meeting late.

10. She had only 6 pregnancies.

11. A venous hum and bruit was heard on auscultation.

12. They accused the doctor and I of a breach of confidentiality.

13. No one knows about this but he and I.

14. A lengthy surgery, panhysterectomy and vesicourethropexy, are scheduled early tomorrow.

15. The patient complained of burning on urination, but there is no urgency or frequency.

16. No rales, rubs, thrills, murmurs, or venous hum is heard on auscultation.

 10-10 FINAL REVIEW

1. Select the incorrect sentence: _____
   a. He is the young man whom you recall was involved in the accident.
   b. Ask the patient to lie down on the table.
   c. The sharp's container was not sitting on the shelf properly.
   d. The drug was an excellent complement to the other modalities utilized.

2. Select the incorrect sentence: _____
   a. It's not the correct instrument.
   b. He is the one who was to be admitted immediately.
   c. *Dorland's* dictionary, along with three other references, is sitting on my desk.
   d. He has past the 5-year mark in his recovery.

3. Which of the following is *incorrectly* expressed? _____
   a. The long-term affects of the disease are unknown.
   b. The patient's affect was blunted.
   c. Wound closure was effected swiftly.
   d. The patient's renal function was adversely affected.

CHAPTER 10

4. Indicate the incorrect sentence: _____
   a. Each of the members of the committee was notified of the change.
   b. The diagnosis of three of our staff members is listed on the report.
   c. Every one of these instruments has been carefully tested.
   d. Mary's gift, tablecloth, napkins, and napkin rings, were lovely.

5. Which of the following sentences shows *correct* subject-verb agreement? _____
   a. The age and sex of the patient causes variation in the normal range of laboratory values.
   b. Inspection of the upper extremities show scattered small abrasions.
   c. Examination of sections of both right and left lung shows severe vascular congestion.
   d. We have no way of telling what the exact relationship of this mass to the subclavian vein and subclavian artery are.

6. Which sentence is incorrect? _____
   a. There was total involvement of the right fallopian tube with a discrete mass on the right ovary.
   b. I asked her to be discreet about this conversation.
   c. Initially, the single, discreet nodule was isolated from the mass.
   d. Please keep a discrete distance.

CHAPTER **11**

Outpatient Medical Chart Notes and Daily Progress Notes

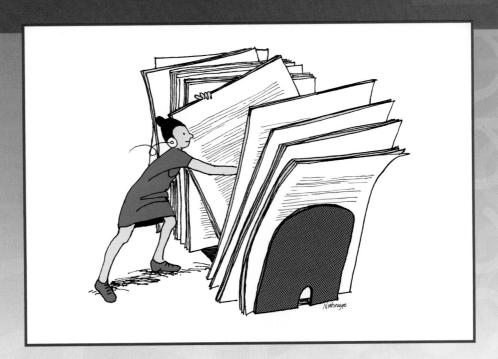

OBJECTIVES

After reading this chapter and working the exercises, you should be able to

1. Explain the necessity of transcribing accurate patient progress notes.
2. Demonstrate the proper procedure and format for transcribing medical chart notes and progress notes.
3. Use the different methods employed in transcribing entries into medical records.
4. Recognize and correct any erroneous entries made in the medical record.
5. List the basic information found in patient notes in emergency department, medical office, and clinic records.
6. Identify the key components of the electronic medical record and the traditional paper document.
7. Discuss the importance of medical record notes to the billing cycle.

Note from the Author

With this chapter, you begin to work with some very interesting documents. These medical record notes are like miniature biographies that give details of a patient's health, good or bad, which become the short health story of his or her life during the present and immediate past. These narrative notes provide the details of our health, which significantly shapes who we are, and the shape of the patient's life is acutely visible to you. Some of these stories are very sad, others are full of promise, and most are simply the day-in and day-out continuation of lives as they are being lived. I hope you learn to feel, as I did, very privileged to share in the care of the patient even in this small way by carefully transcribing this special narrative as a documentation specialist.

INTRODUCTION

Medical record notes (also called *chart notes, outpatient notes,* or *progress notes*) are the formal or informal notes taken by the physician when he or she meets with or examines a patient in the office, clinic, acute care center, or emergency department. These notes are a part of the patient's permanent medical record; as you recall from Chapter 1, medical records are vital in patient care. Although medical records are used mainly to assist the physician with care of the patient, they can be reviewed by attorneys, other physicians, insurance companies, or the court. It is essential that they be neat, accurate, and complete.

"Accurate" means that they are transcribed as dictated, and "complete" requires that they be dated and signed or initialed by the dictator. It is hard to insist that the physician sign or initial the records, but you might overcome the physician's reluctance by making it easier to do so: for example, by typing a line at the end of each chart entry for the signature or initials. Then, at the end of the shift or the day, all of the reports can be stacked in a convenient area for signing. It is important that entries be reviewed and signed in a timely manner.

> **MT TOOL BOX TIP:** Complete, accurate, and timely documentation—a tool to own.

For a chart to be admissible as evidence in court, the party dictating or writing entries must be able to attest that they were true and correct at the time they were written. The best indication of that is the physician's signature or initials at the end of each typed note. The hospital insists that the physician sign all dictated material and all entries he or she makes on the patient's hospital record; failure to do so could result in a loss of hospital staff privileges.

Furthermore, before copies of records leave the facility, the originals must be checked for accuracy; if the originals were not signed before, they must be signed immediately. Any liability of the medical transcriptionist (MT) personally is of small significance unless there are unusual

circumstances, such as negligence, willfulness, or malice. A physician cannot easily shift the blame to another person because the faulty records are his or her responsibility as long as the proper procedure for release of information has been established. If an MT is at fault in recording improperly, the supervisor or office manager has the right to discharge the MT for not meeting job expectations. This possibility is a peril for the careless worker.

At one time, physicians handwrote daily progress entries into the patient's hospital medical record. In office or clinic situations, some physicians never dictate chart notes, preferring to enter them into the patient's record in longhand. Although it is not essential that medical records be typed, it is best to do so. Obviously, typed notes are easier to read. When more than one physician is involved in patient care, such as in a large office or clinic, it is essential that all notes be easy to read with no risk of misinterpretation. Some physicians are utilizing the electronic medical record and using a pull-down menu to select from a variety of prompts by pointing and clicking from a collection of items that pertain to the exam or visit. This method does not provide the narration that makes up the full story about the patient nor does it provide the reasoning behind medical decisions.

This chapter is not concerned with electronic records or longhand notes but rather with learning the process of taking chart notes from the equipment and transcribing the notes properly into the patient's record. In the hospital, clinic, or office setting, in which notes become part of the electronic medical record, they must be typed. If written out, the notes may be copied and typed. The electronic medical record is a database that tracks vital data and *ideally* replaces paper with computer screens that are clear, easy-to-read, accurate, and accessible. It supports the entry of all patient care variables with appropriate default choices and maintains clinical care pathways. Users may enter text notes by selecting standard phrases and sentences. The notes are then fully edited to create documents that accurately record the observations of the physicians or nursing staff. Document-based electronic medical records maximize office efficiencies by managing data to replace the outdated paper chart. The system is fast, accurate, and easy to use. Even complex patient encounters are quickly and precisely documented. Regardless of format, text entries or templates should follow fundamental principles for the quality of the entry. Many hospitals are scanning progress notes and other forms into the EHR, which enhances patient care and provides clearer communication. Special attention needs to be given to format and styles used in preparation of any document that will be scanned into the EHR; some formats will not scan. The MT must ensure that guidelines for these records are followed carefully to improve the flow of data into the record and ensure that it is usable.

Even though the electronic age brings new variables to the recording of the most basic encounter with the patient, it does not change the foundation, which is that records must be maintained in a manner that follows applicable regulations, accreditation standards, and legal standards.

Persons dictating and those transcribing or editing records must follow established guidelines:

▶ Identify the patient by name and health record number when applicable on every page in the record or computerized record screen, every form, and every computerized printout.

▶ Make entries as soon as possible after an event or observation is made. (Entries are never made in advance.)

▶ Include a complete date and time on every entry.

▶ Use black ink for written entries. You must ensure that these are legible.

▶ Use specific language; avoid vague or generalized language.

▶ Record objective facts, not what is presumed.

▶ Document what can be seen, heard, touched, and/or smelled.

▶ Describe signs or symptoms.

▶ Use quotation marks when quoting the patient.

▶ Document the patient's response to care.

▶ Use only abbreviations approved by the organization.

The physician should try to dictate as soon as the patient visit is complete and the details are still fresh. Some physicians have also found it helpful to dictate notes at the patient's bedside or with the patient present in the office or in the emergency department. This practice gives the examiner the opportunity to ask for any details that may have been overlooked in the initial history taking; it also provides an opportunity to reinstruct the patient about medications or to explain the purpose of tests and the expected results. An advantage to the patient is the ability to hear the same information repeated into the dictation equipment, reinforcing what was previously discussed. The patient also gets another opportunity to ask questions or even provide additional pieces of information. Importantly, patients

get a better understanding of the amount of time spent under the physician's care.

Emergency department chart notes are dictated as the patient is being seen. They are usually transcribed on a STAT (immediate) basis. The items dictated into a chart note vary and can include all or only some of the following: an account of the health history of the patient and the patient's family, the findings on physical examination, the signs or symptoms occurring while the patient is under observation, and the medication and treatments the patient receives or those recommended. This information can be set off by individual topics, such as the *chief complaint (CC)*, the reason the patient is visiting the doctor or emergency department; the *history (HX)* of the complaint; the *physical examination (PX)*; the *treatment (RX)* recommended by the physician; and the physician's *impression (IMP)* or *diagnosis (DX)* of the problem. Abbreviations are used very freely in chart notes. Refer again to the list of abbreviations in Appendix B. In addition, a brief general list is provided for you to refer to as you begin your assignments.

The office-based MT works with dictated progress notes made when the patient is seen in the office, at home, or in the specialty clinic, with reference made to admissions and discharges from the hospital or a nursing facility. Notes are also made when the physician is called in to see an established patient in the emergency department. Telephone conversations with the patient or with other physicians treating the patient may also be recorded.

GENERAL PRINCIPLES FOR COMPLETE DOCUMENTATION IN MEDICAL RECORDS

An office-based MT needs to be aware of the general principles for complete documentation of medical records to ensure that these notes are written or transcribed into the record, documenting services for which the provider of care expects to be paid. To provide documentation of services rendered, you must know what billing codes are used by the facility for the service documented. The nature and amount of physician work and documentation vary by the type of service performed, the place of the service, and the status of the patient (new or established). These general principles are applicable to all types of medical and surgical services in all settings. The billing and diagnosis codes reported on the health insurance claim form must be supported by the documentation in the record.

The MT can be very helpful to the billing and coding department because Recovery Audit Contractors (RACs) from the Centers for Medicare and Medicaid Services could scrutinize billings at any time. The MT can review the transcript to define justification for each charge and can identify documents that do not have sufficiently detailed information, flagging them for review by the coding supervisor. Most coding is based on the transcribed report so documentation is critical. Coding is not the responsibility of the MT; it is the responsibility of the coder. Education and coordination between the two professions is necessary.

The following is a general outline of the principles through which payments are made. It is important to observe that these components are documented and to alert your employer when they are **not** mentioned. In addition, the following describes the information that is generally found in these records and helps you set it up in a logical manner.

1. The records must be complete and legible.
2. Each patient encounter should include the following documentation:
   ▸ date
   ▸ reason for the encounter
   ▸ history, physical examination, prior diagnostic test results
   ▸ diagnosis (assessment, impression)
   ▸ plan for care
   ▸ name of the observer
3. Rationale for ordering diagnostic or other services should be documented or inferred.
4. Health risk factors should be identified.
5. Progress, response to treatment, changes in treatment, and revision of diagnosis should be documented.

Seven components are used when describing the level of services for evaluation and management of the patient. The level of care given determines how many of these components are used. Therefore, it is important that they are documented when done. The components may be listed as separate elements of the history, or they may be included in the history of the present illness.

 MT TOOL BOX TIP: Accuracy is a tool for which there is no substitute—keep it sharp.

History

The history includes the
▸ CC: Chief Complaint. The CC describes the symptom, problem, or condition that is the reason for the encounter and must be clearly described and documented in the record.
▸ HPI: History of Present Illness. The HPI is the chronological description of the development of the patient's present illness from the first sign and/or symptom or from the previous encounter to the present.
▸ PFSH: Past, Family, and/or Social History. The PFSH is a review of the patient's past illnesses, operations, injuries, and treatments; a review of medical events

in the patient's family, including diseases that could be hereditary; and a review of past and current activities in which the patient was or is engaged.
▸ ROS: Review of Systems. A problem-pertinent ROS is an inquiry about the system directly related to the problems identified in the HPI. The patient's positive responses and pertinent negatives (i.e., all the things the patient does not have wrong) related to the problem are documented. Signs or symptoms the patient might be experiencing or has experienced are identified, including constitutional symptoms (fever, weight loss, fatigue); integumentary (skin and/or breast); eyes, ears, nose, and throat; mouth; cardiovascular; respiratory; gastrointestinal; genitourinary; musculoskeletal; neurologic; psychiatric; endocrine; hematologic/lymphatic; and allergic/immunologic.

The ROS and PFSH may be recorded by an ancillary staff member or on a form completed by the patient. When directly related to the problem identified in the HPI, the time spent with the patient in history taking, care, examination, counseling, and coordination of services should also be documented. Attention should be directed to recording the time spent talking to the family, nursing facility, caregivers, and so on.

Examination

The extent of the examination performed and documented depends on clinical judgment and the nature of the presenting problems. Examinations range from limited to complete. Depending on the level of services performed, there are four types of examinations:

1. **Problem focused**: a limited examination of the affected body area or system.
2. **Expanded**: a limited examination of the affected body area or system and other symptomatic or related systems.
3. **Detailed**: an extended examination of the affected body area and other symptomatic or related systems.
4. **Comprehensive**: a general multisystem examination or a complete examination of a single system.

Charges for care rendered are based on the precise level of services performed combined with the type of medical decision-making as discussed in the following.

Medical Decision Making

There are four types of medical decision making. They are measured by the number of possible diagnoses or management options that must be considered; the complexity of medical records, tests, and other information that must be obtained, reviewed, and analyzed; the risk of significant complications associated with the problem or problems; the diagnostic procedures; and/or possible management options. They are as follows:

1. **Straightforward**
   ▸ self-limited or minor problem

2. **Low complexity**
   - two or more self-limited or minor problems
   - stable chronic illness
   - acute uncomplicated illness or injury
3. **Moderate complexity**
   - one or more chronic illnesses with mild exacerbation, progression, or side effects of treatment
   - two or more stable chronic illnesses
   - undiagnosed new problem
   - acute illness
   - acute complicated injury
4. **High complexity**
   - one or more chronic illnesses with severe exacerbation, progression, or side effects of treatment
   - acute or chronic illness or injuries that pose a threat to life or bodily function

Counseling and Coordination of Care

When counseling and/or coordination of care involves more than 50% of the physician/patient/family encounter time in the office, outpatient setting, hospital, or nursing facility, the total length of time of the encounter (face-to-face) must be documented, and the record should describe the counseling and/or activities to coordinate care.

NEW PATIENT, OFFICE

When a patient comes into the office or specialty clinic for the initial visit, a chart is prepared. These charts vary, just as physicians and their medical specialties vary. Therefore, this section examines the broad methods of record preparation; you can easily apply these instructions to the method used by your employer. There really is no "best" way to keep medical records

INFORMATION REQUIRED FOR CASE HISTORY FILE

Date..........

Patient.......... Date of Birth.......... Age..........
(Mr., Mrs., Miss, Master) First Name Initial Last Name

Name of Husband, Wife or Parent.......... Home Phone..........

Home Address.......... If Military, Serial No. Soc. Sec. No..........

Patient Employed By:..........
City or Town Zip Code

Business Address..........

Occupation.......... Business Phone..........

Husband or Wife Employed by:..........

Business Address..........
City or Town Zip Code

Occupation.......... Business Phone..........

Name of nearest relative not named above (indicate relationship)..........

Address..........

Insured by:.......... Group No.......... Member No..........

Recommended by:.......... Former Physician..........

If patient is a minor
Give name of person legally responsible:..........

I hereby authorize and request the .... Insurance Company to pay the amount due me in my pending claim for medical expense Benefits directly to ....MD

Date.......... Signature..........

A

FIGURE 11-1 A, Example of a social data sheet.

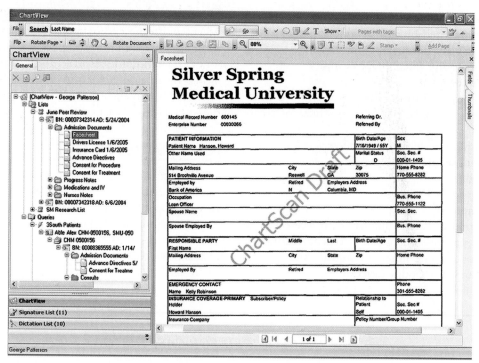

FIGURE 11-1, cont'd B, Screen shot of patient demographic data. **(B,** Courtesy of 3M Health Information Systems, Inc.)

other than neat, accurate, complete, and timely (made as soon as possible after the patient is seen).

The patient completes a social data sheet during the initial visit (Figure 11-1). These data sheets also vary according to the wishes of the individual physician's medical practice, the facility, or the staff. This information is then used to prepare the accounting file for the patient, as well as to supply the initial information for the patient's medical record. Some offices transfer all of this information to the initial page of the medical record; others take the barest minimum (complete name and birth date or age). Medical consultants often want to have the name and telephone number of the referring physician listed. It is important for you to learn exactly what information your employer wants transferred from the social data sheet to this initial chart page.

Figures 11-2 to 11-6 illustrate a variety of chart paper styles. Some physicians have special paper printed for notes, others purchase chart paper from medical printing supply houses, but most prefer plain 8½ × 11 inch paper. Special paper with small illustrations of body parts printed in the margins (see Figure 11-6) is often used in emergency departments, private medical offices, dental offices, and specialty offices (e.g., gynecologists, ophthalmologists, orthopedic surgeons, urologists, and medicolegal specialists). These forms are then fed into a laser printer.

After the initial information is transferred from the patient's social data sheet, the medical records administrator dates the chart paper by using a date stamp or making the entry in longhand. The date may be written out, abbreviated, or written in numerals. The paper is then placed into a labeled file folder or a clipboard and presented to the physician at the time the patient is seen.

At the conclusion of the visit, the physician writes the notes in the chart, dictates them to be transcribed into the chart, or dictates a separate document that takes the place of the chart entry. This document can be a formal history and physical examination report (which you will learn to prepare in Chapter 12), it may be a formal report to an attorney or workers' compensation company, or it may be a consultation report to the physician who referred the patient to the office (see Figure 11-2, entry of 2-8-XX). If the dictator prefers not to make a chart entry and dictates a document, as just discussed, to take the place of the entry, you will transcribe the document and make a note of it in the patient's record where the normal chart entry belongs. In Figure 11-2, the MT (mlo) made the entry "2-8-XX See letter to Dr Wong mlo"; thus, the physician needs only to review that letter for a summary of the February 8 office visit. This practice precludes dictating the same material twice. Another method of communication is to dictate a complete chart note and indicate that a copy of the note should be sent to the referring physician.

You can type this entry or write it in longhand. Always follow *your* personal chart entry with *your* initials written in longhand.

February 7, 20XX See note to Dr. Normington mlo

(also correct)

Feb. 7, 20XX See note to Dr. Normington mlo

Mary Neidgrinhaus   DOB: 06/11/XX

REF: Yuen Wong, MD
555-527-8765

12/18/20XX
HX: This 4-1/2-year-old girl has been having URIs beginning in October 200X. She
             has had several of these infections since that time and has been seen by another
             otolaryngologist who recommended that she have surgery including an
             adenotonsillectomy and bilateral myringotomies with tubes. The mother desired
             another opinion, and the family doctor referred her to me.

ALLERGIES: AMPICILLIN and SEPTRA

PX: Well-developed and well-nourished girl in no acute distress.
VS: Pulse: 84/min. Resp: 20/min. Temp: 98.8° axillary.
HEENT: Eyes: PERRLA. EOMs normal. Ears: The right TM was retracted and slightly
             injected. The left TM was retracted but not injected. Both canals were negative.
             Nose: The nasal septum was roughly in the midline. Mucous membrane lining
             somewhat pale and slightly swollen. Throat: Tonsils were +3 and very cryptic,
NECK: There were tonsillar nodes palpable in both anterior cervical triangles.

CHEST: Lungs: Clear to P& A. Heart: Regular rate and rhythm; no murmurs.

IMP: 1. Hypertrophy of tonsils and adenoids.
             2. Bilateral recurrent serous otitis media.

RX: Dimetapp elixir 20 mL 1 teaspoon q.i.d.

mlo   Gene M. Kasten, MD

12/28/20XX   Right ear improved; no change in the left. Mother still does not want surgery.
RX   Alacol syrup 30 mL 1/2 teaspoon q.i.d.

mlo   Gene M. Kasten, MD

1-3-XX   Mother telephoned: Alacol "not working." Called in
             Tri-Tuss syrup 30 mL 1/2t q.id. per Dr. Kasten. grt

01/14/200X   No improvement in left ear. Right ear significantly the same as when last seen.
             Mother now approves surgery for removal of the tonsils and adenoids and
             bilateral myringotomies with tube insertions.

mlo   Gene M. Kasten, MD

01/15/200X   *See copy of History and Physical dictated for View of the Lakes Memorial*
             Outpatient Center.

2-6-XX   Pt. admitted to VOL outpatient 0600 grt
2-8-xx   See letter to Dr. Wong mlo

FIGURE 11-2 Example of a typical chart note with a variety of visits listed. Notice how the "allergy" is handled in the note of December 18.

KARL ROBRECHT, MD
INTERNAL MEDICINE
555 LAKE VIEW DRIVE
BAY VILLAGE, OHIO 44140

Name				Date
Legal Address				Tel. No.
Local Address				Tel. No.
Birthplace		Age	Sex	Marital Status
Occupation	Employer	Address		Tel. No.
Nearest Relative, or Guardian (Relationship)		Address		Tel. No.
Occupation	Employer	Address		Tel. No.
Referred by		Address		Tel. No.
Insurance Company		Address		Policy No./Type

PHYSICAL EXAMINATION

Height _____ Weight _____ T _____ P _____ General Appearance _____

Eyes _____ Vision Recorded on Sight Screener _____

Ears _____ Hearing: rt _____ lt _____

Teeth _____ Nose _____

Throat _____ Thyroid _____

Skin _____ Scars _____

Heart _____ BP _____

Lungs _____

Breasts _____

Abdomen _____

Rectum _____ Hernia _____

Extremities _____

Nervous System _____

Reflexes _____

Personality _____

Hygiene _____

Remarks _____

FIGURE 11-3 Example of medical office chart paper, initial visit.

EMERGENCY DEPARTMENT RECORD

Holly P. Woodsen

CHART REQUESTED

LOCATION	DATE	TIME REGISTERED	TRIAGE TIME	AM ☐ PM ☐	OUTPT ☐	INPT ☐
202	11/29/0X	11:32				

ARRIVED ▶ [X] WALKED ☐ WC ☐ AMB ☐ PARA AMB ☐ OTHER

ACCOMPANIED BY ▶ ☐ ALONE ☐ SPOUSE ☐ PARENT ☐ FRIEND ☐ RELATIVE

PATIENT'S ADDRESS

1335 11th Street
Mt. Channel, YY 54321

HOME PHONE 619 278-6489
WORK PHONE 619 278-6489

RELATIVE TO CONTACT / PHONE

PRIMARY CARE CLINIC 221

PERSONAL PHYSICIAN W.A. Berry

AGE 027	SEX F	TEMP 99.7	BLOOD PRESSURE 111/76	PULSE 87	RESP 20	WEIGHT (Peds)	CURRENT MEDICATIONS ∅

DRUG SENSITIVITY ☐ NO [X] YES   IF YES, SPECIFY DRUG PCN   LMP   LAST TETANUS

	✓	
CBC WBC		
CBC H&H		
Lytes		
Bun/Creat		
Glucose/Acet		
Amylase		
U/A		
C&S____		
Preg Test		
CPK		
CXR		
Abd Ser/KUB		
ABG		
Peak Flow		
Pulse Ox		
EKG		

Visual Acuity OD (R)____ OS (L)____

CHIEF COMPLAINT   (IF INJURY - WHERE AND HOW DID IT OCCUR?)   ASSAULTED by boyfriend

TIME OF INITIAL EXAM

HISTORY AND EXAM

S: 27 y/o female who presents to the ER after an alter-cation. Pt reports that she was driving her car, her boyfriend was in the front passenger seat. The pt reported to me that she reached across and struck him on the chest, and that he responded by punching her on the right side of her face three times. Pt was driving the car and apparently did not lose consciousness and did not lose control of the car. She denies being struck in the chest or abdomen.

Incident has been reported to the police by nursing staff.

O: She is awake, alert and appropriate. Head and face appear atraumatic, no STS or ecchymosis is noted. The neck is supple. Pupils midposition and reactive, EOMs are intact. Full ROM to the mandible, no malocclusion. No chest wall or bony pelvic tenderness.

A: Facial contusions.

P: Reassurance. Ice. ASA. Tylenol. Soft diet as needed. Re-exam for persistent pain or malocclusion.

DISABILITY ☐ NO ☐ YES   IF YES, GIVE RETURN TO WORK DATE

SPECIFY   ED PHYSICIAN

CONDITION AT DISCHARGE (CHECK ALL THAT APPLY)
☐ UNCHANGED ☐ ALERT/ORIENTED ☐ ON CRUTCHES ☐ DOA ▶
☐ ASYMPTOMATIC ☐ AMBULATORY ☐ EXPIRED ☐ OTHER ▶

INSTRUCTIONS TO PATIENT
☐ WRITTEN ▶
☐ VERBAL   SPECIFY,

DISPOSITION (CHECK ALL THAT APPLY)   SERVICE & FLOOR   DOCTOR, DATE, LOCATION, TIME   TIME
☐ RETURN PRN ☐ WORK ☐ ADMITTED ▶   ☐ REFERRED TO ▶
☐ HOME ☐ HOLDING ☐ TRANSFERRED ▶   ☐ RETURN TO ▶

FIGURE 11-4 Example of an emergency department chart note illustrating minimum heads and SOAP format.

Name _Donald Grenco_   Age _68_

Date _09-28-XX_

HT _5'6"_   WT _243_   BP ® _46/78_

T _96.5_   P _85_   R

ALLERGIES

NKA

C C SOB X months "worse

Dyspnea: Rest _Yes_
          Exercise

since stroke
last year"

Had CVA last Nov

Wt ↑ 9 lb.

CURRENT MEDICATIONS:

Orthopnea: ⊖

Cough: ⊖

Sputum: ⊖

Wheezing: _Yes_

Fever: ⊖

Chest Pain: ⊖

Edema: _Yes_

Wt. Change: ↑ 9 lb since 7-14-XX

Smoking: ⊖

Last CXR:

Last Oximetry: _today_

Last Spiro: _7-14-XX_

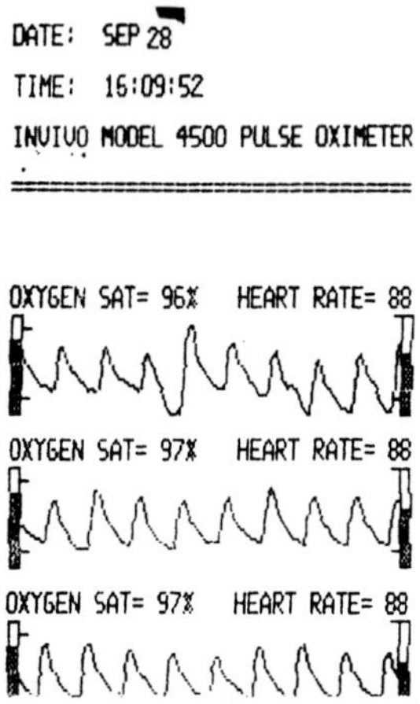

DATE: SEP 28
TIME: 16:09:52
INVIVO MODEL 4500 PULSE OXIMETER
================================

OXYGEN SAT= 96%   HEART RATE= 88

OXYGEN SAT= 97%   HEART RATE= 88

OXYGEN SAT= 97%   HEART RATE= 88

This 68-year-old patient had a CVA last November and reports that he is "weak all over." Very SOB with minimal exertion. Sleeps poorly. Very sleepy during the day.
HEENT: Negative.
Neck: Supple.
Heart: Regular rhythm.
Extremities: 2+ ankle edema.
Impression: Diabetes. Restrictive lung disease.
? Sleep disorder.
Plan: Sleep evaluation.
Get hospital records from November of last year.

WAB/lar

FIGURE 11-5 Example of a chart note from a pulmonary specialist's office illustrating personalized chart paper and a combination of written and transcribed notes. Notice the copy of the oxygen saturation rate combined with the chart note.

Allergic to PCN

EAR NOSE & THROAT

Kingersley, Margaret O.
Patient's name

Address: 145 West Cuyamaca, Roseland Hills, XX
Tel No. 555-9743   Referred by: Dept. of Rehabilitation

Insurance Rehab   Date: 1-9-XX
Age: 60   Sex: F

CC: This is a 60-year-old pt who was seen in the office on May 15, 200X, on referral from the Department of Rehabilitation.

HX: I obtained a history from the patient that she has been aware of hearing loss in both ears, worse in the left ear, since about 1998. She was first tested in Dr. Victor Goodhill's office at the University Clinic in 1999, and at that time showed a bilateral sensorineural deafness worse in the left ear. Because there was some asymmetry of her hearing, mastoid and middle ear tomograms were performed and these were normal. She also had a ENG, which was also normal.

Beginning in 1999, she was fitted with first, a hearing aid in her left ear, and later one in her right ear, and these are in-the-ear types. She states that she does not find them very satisfactory, in most situations, unless it is very quiet.

The pt does report some tinnitus in both ears, which has been present for a number of years. She is unable to describe this noise.

The pt has no problems with vertigo.

JHJ/ro

FIGURE 11-6 Example of a chart note from an ear, nose, and throat specialist illustrating the use of personalized chart paper with diagramed body parts.

ESTABLISHED PATIENT, OFFICE

Although the initial visit notes are usually lengthy, subsequent or followup notes can be as brief as a few lines. They vary according to the patient's complaint and type of visit to the office. For example, an entry for an established patient being seen in the office for a followup visit after the patient had a myringotomy could well read as shown in the 5-5-OX and 5-12-OX entries on the following chart note:

EXAMPLE

Tammy O. Beckley   BD: 02-15-0X

5-1-0X   Sunday, 0315 hours. Patient seen in ER complaining of pain, a.d. x 3 d. PX revealed fluid and pus. Temp. 101°.

ADVICE: Myringotomy.

DIAGNOSIS: Otitis media, right.

tat   Julian Cooke-Dieter, MD

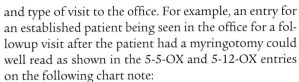

5/2/0X Admit 0600 Mercy SurgiCenter tat
5/2/0X Right myringotomy with aspiration. Discharged 1015 hours. tat

5-5-0X   No pain right ear. Pt. Progressing. Return 1 week. Temp. 99°.

tat   Julian Cooke-Dieter, MD

5-12-0X   Temp normal; no fluid, no pus, no pain. Return p.r.n.

tat   Julian Cooke-Dieter, MD

The use of special paper in your printer makes these notes very easy to handle. Several companies manufacture pressure-sensitive paper for transcribing medical notes. This paper comes in a variety of forms, such as a continuous sheet of paper folded or on a roll. It is placed behind the pin-feed printer where the regular paper is placed or is fed into the laser printer when needed. The MT simply types the patient's name, date, and dictation, leaving a space at the end for the dictator's signature or initials. Each note is typed without removal of paper from the printer. Then, when the transcript is finished, the entire sheet is cut off and given to the dictator for signature. This method makes it easier for the physician as well, because individual charts do not have to be opened and signed. This method of transcribing notes is particularly helpful when dictation is sent out of the office and the medical records do not accompany it. After approval, the notes are cut apart with a paper cutter or scissors or they are separated at the perforations (Figure 11-7, A). The backing is peeled off of each one, and the note is then placed on the next blank space on the progress sheet so as not to obliterate the information previously entered (see Figure 11-7, B). See Figure 11-8, p. 285, which illustrates several patient notes on a sheet of pressure-sensitive paper. After signature placement, these will be cut apart and placed in the individual records at the next available spot on the chart paper.

Again, the physician may dictate a followup letter to the referring physician at this point, rather than making a regular entry note. As new pages are added, the patient's name must be typed on the top of the page. There is no reason why you cannot continue the notes to the back of the chart paper, and some offices do so to prevent the medical record from becoming bulky. Other physicians prefer to use only one side of the chart paper. The second and all subsequent pages of the progress notes are headed up with the patient's name. If you must continue a chart entry to the following page in the middle of an entry, be sure to type *continued* at the bottom of the beginning page and head up the following page with the date of the chart entry and the word *continued*, as well as the patient's name.

Figures 11-5, 11-6, and 11-8 through 11-11 show examples of medical office progress notes. Please turn to Appendix C on Evolve to examine a variety of office, clinic, emergency department, and urgent care center records as well.

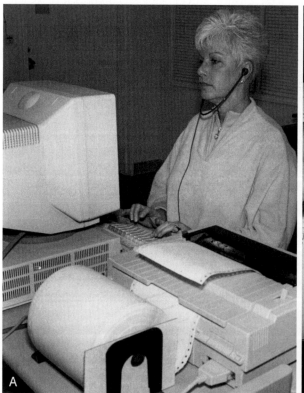
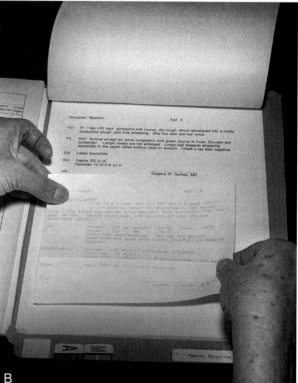

FIGURE 11-7 A, MT using Pat Systems pressure-sensitive paper on a roll. **B,** Demonstration of ease of placing the pressure-sensitive paper onto the existing chart note in the medical record. (**A,** Paper courtesy of Pat Systems [www.transpaper.com/howitworks.htm]. **B,** Photograph courtesy of John Dixon, Grossmont College, San Diego, Calif.)

Barbara Anne Noonan
07/07/XX

The patient returns today feeling rather poorly. She was admitted to the GrandView Hospital for fluid accumulation, which came on rather suddenly last week. Fluid has been removed but the patient is still short of breath. No chest pain and no hemoptysis.

On examination, the patient looks progressively sicker than when first seen. Ankles are quite swollen. Moderately short of breath at rest. P&A of the lungs reveal probable fluid accumulation along the right base. The liver is still prominent and hard.

It would seem advisable that radiation therapy stop at this point. I am not sure what, if any, palliation we have afforded the lady, but I do not think her general situation would permit further radiation to curative doses. This was discussed with her and her husband. It was with some relief as she accepted my recommendation.
LR/do

_____

John W. Issabel
07/07/XX

Patient's weight is up slightly at 124 pounds. Requires 4-6 Dilaudid a day, about the same as he has been taking earlier. Pain is a little better, still localized to soft tissues about 3 cm to the right of the midline at about the level of C7. His wife notices some return of night sweats, though no symptoms of this were noted by the patient and he has not measured his temperature. He is otherwise feeling well.

To exam, he looks better than he has looked on previous visits here. There are no palpable nodes. He has tan skin reaction over both ports, more so on the posterior than anterior. Chest is clear to percussion and auscultation. No distinct bone tenderness. No palpable axillary masses or liver masses. No peripheral cyanosis or edema.

PLAN: Chest x-ray with films on the right side, upper chest. Liver function test, CBC. Return here 1 month and to see Dr. Tu on 7/11/XX. I have asked that he keep track of his temperature twice a day in the interim.
LR/do

_____

Edward Fredrickson
07/07/XX

Bilateral femur and hip films show only osteoporosis. Will consider for palliative treatment should reproducible pain persist.
LR/do

_____

Herbert Frenay
07/07/XX

Mr. Frenay returns to be sure that his groin has healed up following significant reaction from radiation treatments.

On exam, he has no adenopathy in the area. There is some edema. The skin has healed well. There is also distal edema of the lower extremity, which is quite significant and I'm sure related to the combination of radiation and surgery. He has seen Dr. Hoffman, and Dr. Hoffman has given him a Jobst stocking for this. He will follow up with Dr. Hoffman and here only on a p.r.n. basis.
LR/do

_____

FIGURE 11-8 Chart notes on four patients transcribed onto pressure-sensitive paper. After the notes are signed by the dictator, they will be cut apart just above each patient's name and placed in the individual charts.

Flanaghan, Michael R.   AGE: 82

March 17, 20XX

SUBJECTIVE: Patient presented complaining of insomnia, weakness, and
                 shortness of breath. Described Hx of progressive dyspnea on
                 exertion over a 2- to 3-year period.

OBJECTIVE: BP110. Pulse 120 and regular. Visible neck vein distention at 45
                 degrees elevation; rales at both lung bases. Cardiac examination
                 revealed an enlarged heart with PMI felt at the midclavicular line.
                 Sounds were distant, but a systolic murmur was described.

ECG: Sinus tachycardia, left axis deviation, and right bundle branch block.

ECHO: Enlarged left ventricle and calcified and stenotic aortic valve. Left
                 ventricular hypertrophy also demonstrated.

ASSESSMENT: 1. Calcified aortic stenosis.
                 2. Congestive heart failure.

PLAN: 1. Admit to hospital.
                 2. Treat with sodium restriction, digitalis, diuretic.

_____

mlo   Joseph D. Becquer, MD

FIGURE 11-9 Sample chart note showing the SOAP method.

These examples of chart entries that you have just examined are not intended to show *exactly* how to type entries but rather to indicate a variety of methods used by different MTs. At this point, you will not be able to determine exactly how a chart is to be typed, because your employer could have definite guidelines for you to follow. For now, and to practice, try to achieve a readable note. Do not combine all the information, but pull out the main topics. In one style, you do not bring the line of typing back to the left margin until the third line, so that the date and topics will stand out clearly; the third and subsequent lines may be brought back to the left margin or blocked under the first two lines.

(See Figures 11-9 and 11-11 for this method.) Establish a clean, easy-to-read format for progress notes.

The following actual chart note *appears* to have a format, but the format does not contribute to ease of reading or scanning. The patient's name is not appropriately placed. Nothing is gained by having a tab setting after the date in this manner, which leaves a great deal of space that serves no purpose. The use of boldface works better when subtopics are found within text. Avoid the overuse of double-spacing, full caps, boldface, and underlining. The style selected needs a purpose: a new topic, an alert, an emphasis, an outline, and white space.

EXAMPLE: *Poor format*

5-4-XX   ERMA WONG returns today wearing her shoulder immobilizer. She is having difficulty sleeping at night and finds the Vicodin is quite helpful for that. Examination reveals ecchymosis of the arm, elbow, and forearm as her hematoma is resolving. She has normal neurovascular examination and normal appearance of her right hand.

X- RAYS: AP and lateral x-rays of the right shoulder were obtained. Interpretation: The x-rays show severe osteoporosis. There is impaction of the humeral head fracture. There has been slight change with further impaction since her previous x-rays. There is no displacement of the tuberosity fragment.

IMPRESSION: Satisfactory course with an unstable proximal humerus. Fracture of the right dominant upper extremity and severe osteoporosis.

RECOMMENDATIONS: The patient will remain in her shoulder immobilizer and will have her use of the right upper extremity severely limited until such time that more stability is obtained by progressive healing. Will return for followup examination and x-rays in 10 days. Hopefully, we will be able to start some early pendulum exercises at that time.

RFV:bmg

EXAMPLE: *Improved format*

Erma Wong

5-4-XX   Patient returns today wearing her shoulder immobilizer. She is having difficulty sleeping at night and finds the Vicodin is quite helpful for that.

PX: Ecchymosis of the arm, elbow, and forearm as her hematoma is resolving. She has normal neurovascular examination and normal appearance of her right hand.

X- RAYS: AP and lateral x-rays of the right shoulder were obtained. Interpretation: The x-rays show **severe osteoporosis**. There is impaction of the humeral head fracture. There has been slight change with further impaction since her previous x-rays. There is no displacement of the tuberosity fragment.

DX: 1. Satisfactory course with an unstable proximal humerus.
           2. Fracture of the right dominant upper extremity.
           3. Severe osteoporosis.

RX: The patient will remain in her shoulder immobilizer and will have her use of the right upper extremity severely limited until such time that more stability is obtained by progressive healing. Will return for followup examination and x-rays in 10 days. Hopefully, we will be able to start some early pendulum exercises at that time.

RFV:bmg

Flanaghan, Michael R.   AGE: 82

March 17, 20XX

HX: Patient presented complaining of insomnia, weakness, and shortness of breath. Described HX of progressive dyspnea on exertion over a 2- to 3-year period.

PX: BP: 110. Pulse120 and regular. Visible neck vein distention at 45 degrees elevation; rales at both lung bases. Cardiac examination revealed an enlarged heart with PMI felt at the midclavicular line. Sounds were distant, but a systolic murmur was described.

ECG: Sinus tachycardia, left axis deviation, and right bundle branch block.

ECHO: Enlarged left ventricle and calcified and stenotic aortic valve. Left ventricular hypertrophy also demonstrated.

DX: 1. Calcified aortic stenosis.
             2. Congestive heart failure.

RX: 1. Admit to hospital.
             2. Treat with sodium restriction, digitalis, diuretic.

_____
Joseph D. Becquer, MD/gmc

FIGURE 11-10 Sample chart note showing the HX (history), PX (physical examination), DX (diagnosis), RX (treatment) method.

11

CHAPTER

CHART NOTE, EMERGENCY DEPARTMENT VISIT

In the emergency department, the triage nurse determines the sequence in which patients will see a physician. Laboratory tests, radiographs, and simple tests may be ordered at this time by the triage nurse. At this point, the level of care is determined and may be described as the following:

▶ *Nonurgent care* involves routine care that could have taken place in a physician's office during office hours. This care is often provided for patients who have no physician. Problems include mild flu symptoms, earache, and prescription refills. Admission to the hospital is unlikely. If the emergency department is busy, these patients may be referred to a nearby urgent care center.

▶ *Urgent care* involves care necessitating basic emergency services. Problems include lacerations, acute flu symptoms, mild shortness of breath, broken bones, threatened abortion, and rectal bleeding. Admission to the hospital is possible.

▶ *Emergency care* involves care requiring immediate attention of the physician. Problems include chest pain, stroke, acute trauma, acute shortness of breath, respiratory arrest, and conditions necessitating cardiopulmonary resuscitation. Admission to the hospital is likely.

The patient, family member, or person bringing the patient to the department completes the social data information sheet (see Figure 11-1). If the patient is brought in by emergency vehicle, the vehicle personnel generally provide some of the necessary information. Care is not withheld during the gathering of this information; often, care is begun while other personnel interview family or friends for the social history. Initial caregivers handwrite notes as the history is taken from the patient or from persons with the patient. A nurse or technician initially assesses the patient and handwrites notes or inputs data by computer. When the physician sees the patient, he or she usually handwrites a brief initial impression and orders to be carried out (i.e., medications, laboratory tests, radiographs, and treatment). At this point, dictation may begin.

Norman O. Brockman   Age: 4

JUL 2 6 200X   The patient is a white male, age 4, who came in to see me today
                    with a history of yellow discharge in the right ear, a fever and a
sore throat of 2 days' duration. His oral temperature was 100. The pharynx was injected, the
tonsils inflamed, and there was crusted purulent material seen in the right ear canal. The
tympanic membrane was normal.

DIAGNOSIS: Tonsillitis and otitis externa.

Medication: Erythrocin 400 mg q.4 h.

tr   Michael R. Stearn, MD

JUL 2 7 200X   After 24 hours of therapy, the patient was afebrile and comfortable.
                    Temperature is 99°. The throat was slightly reddened, the ear
canals were dry, and both TMs normal.

tr   Michael R. Stearn, MD

AUG 2 200X   Followup exam showed him to be completely asymptomatic and
                    free of unusual physical findings. The drug was discontinued at this
                    time.

tr   Michael R. Stearn, MD

OCT 1 9 200X   Stepped on a piece of glass. Cleansed wound. Mother said Norman
                    had tetanus booster just 6 weeks ago in Boyd Hospital ER after a
dog bite. Patient not to return unless problem develops.

tr   Michael R. Stearn, MD

OCT 3 0 200X   Patient caught right index finger in car door 2 mos days ago; finger
                    became inflamed, red, swollen yesterday. Today there is
seropurulent discharge present; no lymphangitis visible. Distal phalanx is involved.

Advice: Hot compress to right hand t.i.d. To return in 24 hours if no change.

DIAGNOSIS: Cellulitis, right index finger, distal phalanx.

tr   Michael R. Stearn, MD

FIGURE 11-11 Example of a chart note with two properly made corrections.

Reilly, Randa   ER D&T: 10/08/XX   DOB: 03/26/XX

CC: Head pain, post fall.

S: This 25-year-old patient presents with a HX of falling from a horse into a heavy wooden fence, breaking the fence. Patient complains primarily of head pain, neck pain, right knee pain, and some mild coccyx pain. There was a brief loss of consciousness observed by her brother and regaining of consciousness with repetitive questioning. Thereafter, she again lost consciousness for a short period of time. Patient has been slow to answer questions and has been noted to have repetitive questions since the accident.

O: Patient in no acute distress. Appears to be stable with C-collar and rigid back board.
      HEENT: Minimal tears in the occipital area. Pupils equal and reactive. EOMs full.
      Ears: TMs without blood.
      NECK: C-collar in place, with a tenderness over the mid C-spine bony area without obvious swelling or deformity. (C-collar left in place.)
      CHEST: Nontender to compression. Equal breath sounds. Heart regular rhythm.
      ABDOMEN: Soft. Nontender.
      EXTREMITIES: Moves all four well. There is mild tenderness on palpitation over the right patella but no instability, no limitation of ROM. Cranial nerves II-VII intact. No meds.

A: Mild concussion.

P: CT of the head after C-spine is clear. Home with head injury instructions. Recheck with private doctor in 1-2 days or return here p.r.n. with any change in mental status.

Kip I. Praycroft, MD/ref

FIGURE 11-12 Example of an emergency department chart note done in the SOAP format.

The dictator indicates if the dictation is STAT (to be transcribed immediately). This dictation can be done with a handheld recorder or with a telephone hardwired to the dictation system. (See Chapter 2 for handheld recording devices, which are placed on computers to be downloaded, as well as other electronic devices to carry out this function.) Dictation for patients requiring admission or transfer must be delivered directly to the MT in some manner. See Figures 11-4 and 11-12 to 11-14 for examples of notes dictated from the emergency department. Additional emergency department notes are in Appendix C on Evolve.

After the release of the patient, the physician writes (or dictates) a formal diagnosis and updates, appends, or completes the dictation. These notes are generally brief, and format can vary with the dictator. Some dictators ask for boldface headings for each section, whereas others prefer the condensed story format.

The urgent care center does not triage patients but provides care in the order in which patients arrive.

The center refers the patient to the emergency department if necessary. The following hints will give you ideas for office, emergency department, and urgent care center chart notes.

TRANSCRIPTION HINTS

1. Enter the patient's complete name. Double-check the spelling of the name, and verify ID numbers accompanying the patient's name.
2. Date every entry with the month, day, and year. These can be spelled out, abbreviated, or made with a date stamp. The time of day that the patient was examined is often required as well.
3. Single-space and keep the margins narrow (not less than 1/2 inch, however). Double-space between topics or major headings.
4. Condense the note to conserve space. Use phrases rather than complete sentences, and use abbreviations when dictated and appropriate.

EMERGENCY DEPARTMENT RECORD	CHART REQUEST		

LOCATION	DATE	TIME REGISTERED	TRIAGE TIME	OUTPT.	INPT.	NAME
202	10-08-XX	2:45 ☐AM ☒PM	☐AM ☐PM	☐	☐	REILLY, RANDA O

ARRIVED	☐ WALKED	☐ WC	☐ AMB	☐ PARA AMB	☐ OTHER
ACCOMPANIED BY	☐ ALONE	☐ SPOUSE	☐ PARENT	☐ FRIEND	☐ RELATIVE

PATIENT'S ADDRESS	MED. REC. NO.	BIRTHDATE
3228 East Main, Century City, XX 12345		11-10-XX

HOME TELEPHONE	WORK TELEPHONE	PRIMARY CARE CLINIC	PERSONAL PHYSICIAN
(800) 654-9863	( )		John Lambert, MD

AGE	SEX	TEMP.	B.P.	PULSE	RESP.	WEIGHT (Peds)	CHIEF COMPLAINT
25	F	98.7	120.70				Head pain, post fall

ALLERGIES	MEDICATIONS
	none

S: This 25-year-old patient presents with a HX of falling from a horse into a heavy wooden fence, breaking the fence. Patient complains primarily of head pain, neck pain, right knee pain, and some mild coccyx pain. There was a brief loss of consciousness observed by her brother and regaining of consciousness with repetitive questioning. Thereafter, she again lost consciousness for a short period of time. Patient has been slow to answer questions and has been noted to have repetitive questions since the accident.

O: Patient in no acute distress. Appears to be stable with C-collar and rigid back board.
HEENT: Minimal tears in the occipital area. Pupils equal and reactive. EOMs full. Ears: TMs without blood.
NECK: C-collar in place, with a tenderness over the mid C-spine bony area without obvious swelling or deformity. (C-collar left in place.)
CHEST: Nontender to compression. Equal breath sounds. Heart regular rhythm.
ABDOMEN: Soft. Nontender.
EXTREMITIES: Moves all four well. There is mild tenderness on palpitation over the right patella but no instability, no limitation of ROM. Cranial nerves II-VII intact. No meds.

A: Mild concussion.

P: CT of the head after C-spine is clear. Home with head injury instructions. Recheck with private doctor in 1-2 days or return here p.r.n. with any change in mental status.

D: 10-08-XX
T: 10-08-XX
amd

ED PHYSICIAN	DATE
(signature)	10-08-XX

NS-7672 (9-95)

FIGURE 11-13 Example of an emergency department note done in the SOAP format on special chart paper used in the emergency department. See Figure 11-12 for the same note transcribed on plain paper.

Patient Name: Windemere, Malago
Med Rec No: 8742-A
Date of Service: 11/06/XX

EMERGENCY DEPARTMENT REPORT
County Trauma and Emergency Center, 8735 Zion Avenue, Benson, XX 99000

TIME OF EXAMINATION: 3:15 a.m.

CHIEF COMPLAINT: Left eye redness and discharge.

HISTORY OF PRESENT ILLNESS: This is a 57-year-old male who was in his usual state of health until yesterday. He began to have some sore throat. He also noted that while mowing the lawn he felt some discomfort in the left eye as if there was something in his eye. The patient was wearing wrap-around sunglasses while he was mowing his lawn and does not specifically remember anything going into his eye. He denies any changes in vision. He denies any fever, chest pain, or cough. He denies any nausea or vomiting. He does not wear contacts or glasses.

PAST MEDICAL HISTORY: None.

ALLERGIES: PENICILLIN.

MEDICATIONS: He takes no medicines.

PHYSICAL EXAMINATION
VITAL SIGNS: Temperature 97.0, blood pressure 113/73, pulse 90, and respiratory rate 18. **HEENT**: His acuity on the right is 20/20 and on the left is 20/25. The left eye is markedly injected, and there is a moderate amount of yellow purulent discharge noted. On slit-lamp examination, the discharge is again noted. No foreign bodies are noted when the eyelids are flipped. The anterior chamber is clear. On fluorescein staining, there is no ulceration or abrasion noted. The right eye is clear except for some mild conjunctival erythema. The oropharynx is clear, without exudate. **NECK**: Supple, without cervical lymphadenopathy. No stridor is noted.

DISPOSITION
1.   Nonsteroidal anti-inflammatory drugs for pain and Vicodin for more severe pain.
2.   Sulamyd drops in both eyes 4 times a day for the next 5 days.
3.   Conjunctivitis instructions.
4.   The patient should follow up with the emergency department if he does not have improvement in his symptoms in the next 36-48 hours or if he has any visual changes, vomiting, is unable to tolerate p.o., or has any other problems. He will nevertheless follow up with his primary care physician as needed.

DIAGNOSIS: Likely viral illness with viral conjunctivitis and pharyngitis; however, bacterial conjunctivitis cannot be ruled out.

EMERGENCY DEPARTMENT REPORT
Page 1 of 2

This is not an official document unless signed by physician.

8735 Zion Avenue • Benson, XX 99000 • Telephone (555) 876-9876

FIGURE 11-14 Example of an emergency department chart note done in expanded format.

EXAMPLE

Dictated: Today's date is November 11, 20XX, and this is a chart note on Nancy Marques, a 32-year-old female who came in today in follow up to an upper respiratory tract infection either viral or secondary to mycoplasma. She is much better except that she has had a chronic cough now for about ten days. The ears, nose, and throat are normal, and the sinuses are nontender. The lymph nodes are normal and the lungs are clear. The diagnosis is postviral cough. I have given her a prescription for Hycodan five to ten milliliters for up to ten days and then observation. If the cough is still present in two weeks, I will consider steroid trial.

Transcribed

Nancy Marques   Age: 32

November 11, 20XX

HPI: Followup upper respiratory tract infection, either viral or secondary to mycoplasma.
        She is much better except for chronic cough for 10 days.

PX: ENT: Normal. Sinuses: Nontender. Lymph nodes: Normal. Lungs: Clear.

DX: Postviral cough.

RX: Hycodan 5 to10 mL for 10 days and then observation. If cough present in 2 weeks, I will consider steroid trial.

ntw   _____
                       Mary Laudenslayer, MD

This example is sharp looking and easy to read, and specific data can be immediately located. However, it is not that quick and simple for the transcriptionist, because you cannot type exactly what is heard; instead, you must stop and analyze at the same time, being sure that all data are recorded. Practice and experience, however, make this format fast and interesting.

Another format example for the same dictation:

Nancy Marques   Age: 32

November 11, 20XX

HPI

Followup upper respiratory tract infection, either viral or secondary to mycoplasma.

She is much better except for chronic cough for 10 days.

PX

ENT: Normal. Sinuses: Nontender. Lymph nodes: Normal. Lungs: Clear.

DX

Postviral cough.

RX

Hycodan 5-10 mL for 10 days and then observation. If cough present in 2 weeks, I will consider steroid trial.

ntw   _____
                       Mary Laudenslayer, MD

5. Make outline headings on all but very brief entries. These headings will vary according to the physician's style. Some physicians use the *SOAP* method or variations, described as follows (see Figures 11-9 and 11-12):

   ▶ S: This signifies *subjective. Subjective* means from the patient's point of view. This is the reason the patient is seeking care. It is the main problem necessitating care (also called *chief complaint*).

   ▶ O: This refers to *objective,* or the physician's point of view, and what is found on physical examination, x-ray film, or laboratory work: the clinical evidence.

   ▶ A: This refers to *assessment,* or what the examiner thinks could be or is wrong with the patient according to the information gathered: the diagnosis.

   ▶ P: This refers to *plan,* or what the physician plans to do or advises the patient to do: laboratory tests, surgery, medications, referral to another practitioner, treatment, management, and so forth.

There are variations on this style. Some dictators begin with the chief complaint (CC), and others leave out one or more of the headings. Headings are either abbreviated or spelled out. Be consistent in your choice. It is very important that the note be explicit and complete. Because the encounter with the patient is the basis for reimbursement from insurance companies, some physicians want to include additional entries to reflect the *nature* (N) of the presenting problem; the *counseling* or *coordination of care* (C) that is involved, particularly when these two areas make up more than half of the time of the visit; and the *medical decision making* (M). These items are often difficult for the coder or reviewer to find in the note, and this kind of information is vital in determining the level of service performed during a patient encounter as described earlier.

Another format choice could include the following:

   ▶ CC: This refers to the *chief complaint* (the same as *subjective* in the SOAP format).

   ▶ PX (also PE): This refers to the *physical examination* (the same as *objective* in the SOAP format).

   ▶ DX: This refers to the *diagnosis, impression* (IMP), or *assessment* (the same as *assessment* in the SOAP format).

   ▶ RX: This abbreviation for *prescription* is used for the advice or plans for the patient (the same as *Plan* in the SOAP format). See Figure 11-10.

Other titles, such as LAB or X-RAY, can be used as headings. Multiple-physician practices, clinics, and hospitals often use the problem-oriented medical record (POMR) format, which is a problem list with corresponding numbered progress notes. In brief, this format includes the following areas:

- ▶ Database: The chief complaint, the history of this complaint, a review of the body systems, physical examination, and laboratory work.
- ▶ Problem list: A numbered list of every problem that the patient has that necessitates further investigation.
- ▶ Treatment plan: Numbered list to correspond with each item on the problem list.
- ▶ Notes: Numbered progress notes to correspond with each item on the problem list.

6. Use abbreviations and symbols freely as the dictator wishes, but be sure that the abbreviations are standard and acceptable. (Remember that the records could be viewed by persons outside the office or hospital.) Abbreviations save space, and notes should be as concise as possible.
7. Insert indentations to make topics stand out. Type the main topics in full caps. Use boldface when it is helpful or requested by the dictator.
8. Underline and type drug allergies in full caps or in boldface.
9. Initial the entry just as you initial any other document that you type or transcribe. Initials can be placed at the left margin or after the dictator's name or initials.
10. Type a signature line or leave sufficient space for the dictator's signature or initials.
11. In the medical office, check daily about the previous day's house calls, emergency department calls, and hospital admissions or discharges, so that the charts can be pulled and these entries made.
12. Finally, forget the format for a moment and remember that detailed and accurate documentation is essential to justify any treatment rendered. The level of care must be obvious and the MT can be alert for insufficient documentation that could cause a RAC denial. Be alert for any errors, such as a mix up of *left/right*, lab values out of range, incorrect dosages, misstatements, and so forth. Know what should be documented and check to be sure it is.

Examine all the figures again for typing format. Look closely at the variety of examples in Appendix C on Evolve.

These are some common abbreviations found frequently in office chart notes. You can use these as well as those found in Appendix B as you complete the following assignments.

anPX	annual examination
BP	blood pressure
Bx	biopsy
CBC	complete blood cell count
CC	chief complaint
consult	consultation

CPX	complete physical examination
DKA	did not keep appointment
DNS	did not show (keep appointment)
DOB	date of birth
Dx (DX)	diagnosis
FUO	fever of unknown origin
Fx (FX)	fracture
H&P	history and physical examination
Hx (HX)	history
IMP	impression
inj	injection
NKA	no known allergies
PE	physical examination
?	"?" suggests a problem (for example, "?pg" is "question of being pregnant"; "?flu" is "possible flu"; "?hernia" is "possible hernia"; and so on)
PH	past history
PO	postoperative
PRE	preoperative or prepartum
pre-op	preoperative examination
pt	patient
Px (PX)	physical examination
R/O	rule out
sig.	directions
STAT	immediately
TPR	temperature, pulse, respirations
Tx (TX)	treatment
VS	vital signs

MAKING CORRECTIONS

Errors in handwritten chart notes are corrected as follows: Draw a line through the error, making sure the inaccurate information is legible and being careful not to obliterate it. Make the correct notation either above or below the error, wherever there is room, and date and initial the entry. Do not write over your error, do not erase the error, do not try to "fix" the error, and do not attempt to blot it out with heavy applications of ink or self-adhesive typing strips.

Errors that are made while the entry is being transcribed are corrected just as you would correct any other material. Errors found subsequently are corrected in longhand by following the previously described procedures. However, it is not necessary to date errors when they are made or discovered on the same day as they are entered; just correct and initial the error.

See Figure 11-11, p. 289, for an example of chart notes with entry errors properly corrected. Notice that these corrections are not dated, which indicates that they were made on the day of the entry. Correcting errors on an electronically signed report requires an addendum explaining the change(s) made on the previous transcript. The new report is then signed within the EHR.

11-1 SELF-STUDY

DIRECTIONS: Retype the following material into chart note format, as illustrated in Figure 11-10.

The date is October 10, 20XX. The patient is Anthony Frishman. Tony is now 12-1/2 years old. He underwent bilateral triple arthrodesis in August 20XX. He is out of his splints and doing well. His foot rests are a bit long, and his feet are not touching them. He has no major complaints as far as his feet are concerned. Exam: He has a long c-curve to the right, which may be slightly increased clinically since last x-rayed in June 20XX when it was twenty-five degrees. His feet are in neutral position as far as equinus. There is a slight varus inclination. X-rays: multiple views of his feet demonstrate fusion bilaterally of the triple staples. Diagnosis is limb girdle dystrophy. The plan is to return to clinic in one to two months for sitting SP spine x-ray. Also we will obtain pulmonary function test at that time. Karl T. Robrecht, MD.

After you have completed this assignment, turn to Appendix A, p. 453, for one version of this transcript.

11-2 PRACTICE TEST

DIRECTIONS: Retype the following information as an emergency department report for Eugene W. Gomez, MD. Use the current date, minimum chart note heading, and plain (unlined) 8½ 11 inch paper. See Chapter 5 for help with numbers and abbreviations.

The patient's name is Maryellen Mawson.

Note: this is a six year old who has had a three week history of polydipsia polyuria polyphagia and weight loss. the child has become progressively more lethargic over the past twenty four hours and twelve hours ago the parents noticed she was breathing rapidly. physical examination reveals height one hundred twenty seven centimeters weight thirty three kilograms temperature ninety nine degrees fahrenheit pulse one hundred twelve and blood pressure ninety five over seventy. the child was semicomatose. she has dry mucous membranes but good skin turgor and full peripheral pulses. a stat lab report shows sodium one hundred thirty eight milliequivalents

per liter, potassium three point three milliequivalents per liter chloride ninety seven milliequivalents per liter and a total carbon dioxide of five milliequivalents per liter. blood glucose is seven
hundred milligrams percent. plan is to admit stat to childrens hospital.

After you complete this, see Appendix A, p. 453, for one version of this transcript.

 11-3 REVIEW TEST

DIRECTIONS: Carefully examine the examples of chart notes that have been illustrated and retype the following information as office chart notes for your employer, Laurel R. Denison, MD. You can use the minimum chart note heading, plain (unlined) 8½ × 11 inch paper, format of your choice, and standard abbreviations where applicable. Use today's date. Please notice that these are notes about several patients; therefore, each patient should have a separate sheet of paper.

1. *Gustavo deVargas.* Birthdate 3-3-34. Patient had onset of persistent vomiting five days ago. He does not appear seriously ill. The abdomen remains flat and there is no tenderness or rigidity; no masses are palpable; bowel sounds are scarce. X-ray of the abdomen yesterday revealed a four centimeter, ill-defined, round mass in the right upper quadrant and loops of small bowel containing air. Subsequent x-rays, including some taken today, revealed that this rounded mass persists, is quite well outlined on some of the x-rays, and is now in the left lower quadrant. There is small bowel distention in relation to the mass, which suggests that the mass is a loop of small bowel with gaseous distention proximal to it. It is questionable whether there is any gas in the colon. Rectal examination is negative. Impression: intestinal obstruction due to ingested foreign body. Advice: laparotomy.
2. *Mrs Esther Conway.* Age thirty-three. Patient complains of constant dribbling, wetting at night, uses fifteen pads a day. Urinalysis: specific gravity one point zero, few bacteria, few urates. Diagnosis: urinary incontinence. Patient is to return in four days for diagnostic testing.
3. *Robin Vincenti.* Age twenty-seven. Patient complains of having had the flu and headache and of being tired. Unable to go to work today. Exam shows weakness of left hand. Hyperreflexia on the left. X-ray shows cardiomegaly and slight pulmonary congestion. Impression: post flu syndrome, transient ischemic attack; possible CVA. Patient to return in four days and may return to work in approximately one week.
4. *Marissa Weeks.* Age seventeen. CC: thrown from a horse. Px: numerous contusions, tenderness in thoracic region, x-ray ordered. Dx: compression fracture of "tee twelve." Rx: patient referred to Edward Harrison, orthopedic specialist.
5. *William Santee.* Age thirteen. (Make your entry showing a letter was dictated rather than a chart entry made [see Figure 6-1, pp. 150–153, for the actual letter that was dictated and transcribed]. You do not type this letter; you prepare a chart note in reference to this letter. Use February 7 as your date rather than today's date.)

 11-4 REVIEW TEST

DIRECTIONS: Using the instructions given for the 11-3 Review Test, type the following information into the patients' charts that you previously prepared. Use a date four days from the date you used for Review Test 11-3.

Remember that in actual practice you no longer have these records, and so you would make your transcripts one right after another, and they would be cut and pasted to the original. You can use cellophane tape to tape your entry to the appropriate document to reenact this procedure.

1. *Gustavo deVargas.* Patient telephoned office today and agreed to laparotomy. He is to be admitted to Valley Presbyterian Hospital tomorrow afternoon at 3 for surgery the following day.
2. Secretary: Please make your own entry into the chart showing that Mr deVargas was admitted to the hospital on the appropriate day.

3. *Robin Vincenti.* Chest clear to P&A. X-ray is clear and shows normal heart silhouette. Full use of left hand; no residual pain or weakness. Plans to return to work tomorrow.
4. *Mrs Esther Conway.* Intravenous pyelogram and cystoscopy revealed multiple fistulae of bladder with two openings into urinary bladder and copious leakage into vagina. Continued to work. Diagnosis: multiple vesicovaginal fistulae. To be admitted to the hospital for repair.
5. Secretary: Please make your own entry into the chart for day of admission, four days from her last visit, into University Hospital for Mrs Conway.

 11-5 SELF-STUDY

DIRECTIONS: In the following chart note, the entry of "left thoracotomy" should read "right thoracotomy." You discover the error on February 1, 20XX. Please correct it.

Brad Philman   **Age: 47**

1-13-20XX Pt admitted to Good Sam for bronchoscopy and possible left thoracotomy and

pleural poudrage.

Please look in Appendix A, p. 453, for the proper correction technique.

 11-6 REVIEW TEST

DIRECTIONS: Imagine that you are typing the following notes on pressure-sensitive paper. Do not forget to leave a little space between the notes so they can be cut apart, but do not cut your notes apart. Use today's date. Use the SOAP format for chart note 5. Your employer is Catherine R. Schultz, MD.

1. *Lupe Morales.* Lump, right breast. Patient found this lump four weeks ago. It has increased in size rapidly, she says. She also has a lump under her right arm. Ordered mammograms. Diagnosis: Possible carcinoma of the breast.
2. *Adeline Pierson.* CC: pain and swelling over the right wrist. Hx: The patient states that while she was working as a waitress she was lifting and carrying a tray of dishes and it slipped, resulting in pain and swelling over the radial side of the distal radius of her right wrist. This was found to be a ganglion and was aspirated by another physician. However, it has recurred and is larger than before. She wishes this surgically removed. Her past general health has been good. She has had no serious illnesses and no surgeries. She takes no medications. Allergies: None known.
3. *Peter Barton.* PO followup. Incision looks good, some slight swelling and tenderness.
4. *Kellis McNeil.* CC: Right inguinal hernia. Hx: Patient first noticed that he had a right inguinal hernia because of pain there approximately one week ago. He presents with a very tender right inguinal ring. The hernia was reduced but readily protruded. PH: The patient had an umbilical hernia repair eight years ago. He had a hemorrhoidectomy four years ago. Drugs: Valium five milligrams t.i.d. Advice: Right herniorrhaphy.
5. *Arnott B. Weeks.* stiff finger joints. patient says more severe after sleeping or nonuse. general fatigue stopped, occurred again in last two weeks. stopped drinking, some weight loss. on exam there is swelling and pain around joints of fingers. symmetrical involvement. bp is one hundred forty four over eighty five pulse is sixty seven weight is one hundred seventy eight.
   x-ray: narrowed joint space, osteoporosis at joint. uric acid: four point two. rheumatoid arthritis. aspirin ten grains q.i.d., phenylbutazone one hundred milligrams qid, number twenty eight. return one month.

11-7 REVIEW TEST

DIRECTIONS: Transcribe the following notes for the emergency department. Use the SOAP format or any variation that is appropriate and easy to read. The dictator is Marc Nielsen, MD. The date is May 1, 20XX.

Colleen Lynkins is a thirty-three-year-old female whose chief complaint is upper mid back pain. The patient woke up tonight with upper mid back pain. Patient states that she has a new mattress. There is no history of trauma or other insults. She had spontaneous pneumothorax twice in the past year. Had tubal ligation ten years ago. She states that she cannot be pregnant. Physical examination: NKA. Temperature is ninety-eight. Blood pressure is one hundred ten over eighty. The chest is clear. The heart is in regular rhythm. The abdomen is soft. Extremities were nonneurological. Central nervous system is intact. Head and neck are benign. Plan. Chest x-ray and proceed.

11-8 REVIEW TEST

DIRECTIONS: See Review Test 11-3, Project 1, chart note for Gustavo deVargas. Use the SOAP method and prepare the chart note for Dr Denison.

11-9 SELF-STUDY

DIRECTIONS: Use your computer and briefly list the various components of a chart note. (Hint: Try for seven different entries.) The answers are on p. 454 in Appendix A.

CHAPTER 12

Preparation of a History and Physical Examination Report

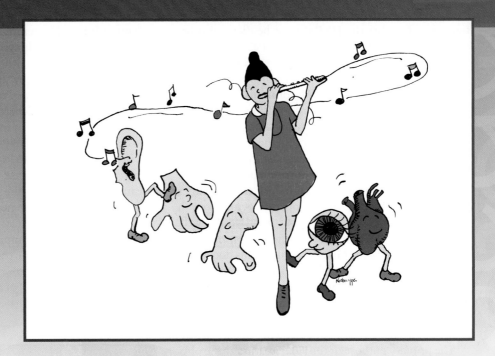

OBJECTIVES

After reading this chapter and completing the exercises, you should be able to

1. Identify the various mechanical formats used to prepare a history and physical examination report.
2. Explain why certain information is obtained from the patient and recorded.
3. Describe the different ways of gathering and dictating vital medical data.
4. Prepare formal history and physical examination reports by using a variety of styles.
5. Explain why the H&P is considered a high-priority document.

INTRODUCTION

The history and physical examination report (H&P) is the first in a set of documents referred to as the *Basic Four* or the *Big Four*. These are the four main documents transcribed in a hospital setting: the H&P, operative report, discharge summary, and consultation report. The H&P takes priority in transcription because it must be on the patient's chart/record before certain other procedures can be carried out. In fact, surgery can be held up until the H&P is in the record. It is also important to realize that the H&P cannot be dictated more than 30 days before a procedure. If this happens, it must be updated by the physician. In the previous chapter, you learned how an H&P is set up in its condensed form: the chart note. The SOAP format is a miniature H&P with the S (subjective) portion taking the place of the history; the O (objective) portion taking the place of the physical examination (PX or PE); the A (assessment) portion taking the place of the diagnostic portion of the examination; and the P (plan) portion taking the place of the outlined future treatment. In fact, the guidelines titled "General Principles for Complete Documentation in Medical Records" on p. 275 apply to the H&P as well. Some physicians dictate an H&P in lieu of an initial chart note. Because the hospital requires this document to be in the patient's hospital record before surgery, surgeons document history and physical examination findings on the preoperative visit with a patient, and some trauma surgeons, likewise, prefer a more complete H&P to the SOAP chart note in the emergency department.

The primary purpose of the H&P is to assist the physician in making a diagnosis on which the patient's care and treatment will be based. There are no precise rules for exactly how a history is documented or a physical examination is carried out, nor is there an exact format for recording the data gathered. Rules and formats vary, just as the personalities of the dictators vary. However, most physicians, regardless of medical specialty, approach the evaluation of a patient in a similar manner.

All patients, when initially seen, need to give the physician a complete history of their problems and be examined. How many questions they are asked, the types of questions, and the body area emphasized are determined both by the problem and by the medical specialty involved. For example, a patient with chest pain who is seeing a cardiologist will have far more attention paid to the chest than to the bladder and bowels. A patient with a hearing problem does not expect an extensive examination of the abdomen or extremities. However, when a patient is scheduled for a major operative procedure or has symptoms that suggest a complex systemic illness, all body systems are examined to some extent.

You will need to know how to transcribe an H&P if you perform acute-care transcription or outpatient clinic and emergency department transcription. If you transcribe for a surgical or medical specialist, you could also be required to type H&Ps. As with chart notes, some physicians write their H&Ps in longhand. There is certainly no requirement that H&Ps be typed. However, because they are part of the patient's medical record, it is important that they be neat, readable, complete, and accurate.

The H&P serves an important function as a diary of what has happened to the patient in the past, a plan for care in the present, the physical condition at the time of the examination, and an outline of how the patient can be helped in the future.

 MT TOOL BOX TIP: Complete, accurate, and timely documentation—a tool to own.

FORMATS AND STYLES

Begin with a screen shot of a transcription platform featuring an H&P.

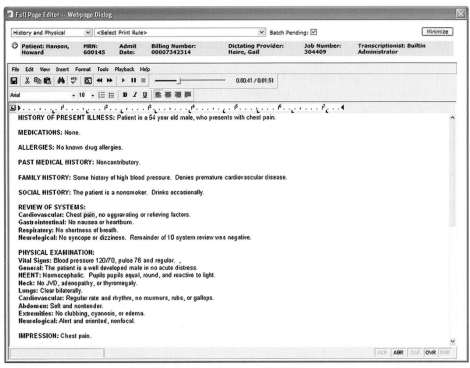

Screen shot showing transcription platform for H & P. (Courtesy of 3M Health Information Systems, Inc. © 3M. All rights reserved.)

Several formats are used for typing an H&P. There is no "best" style or method, but each hospital, clinic, or medical office should adopt a standard outline. A standard format is mandatory when the documents you transcribe become part of any electronic health record (EHR), and the format must be compatible with that platform. You will learn that the "run-on" format meets some of the criteria at this time. However, if the medical office or clinic prefers other styles or formats, you need to know how to prepare them as well. Responsibility for designing the format for the hospital belongs to the hospital forms committee. The hospital generally accepts the H&P prepared by the MT as long as the format falls within the general guidelines of the hospital's style. At present, studies are being done to help determine a workable standard format for H&Ps, as well as for the documents you will study in Chapter 13. It is expected that any standard format will resemble the run-on format illustrated in this chapter. This format is the fastest and easiest to complete and is the recommended style in many institutions.

Most MTs who transcribe H&Ps on a regular basis make a template, macro, or boilerplate of a typical H&P. By using these "normals," the MT is ready to transcribe the H&P, the outline is in place, narrow 1/2- to 3/4-inch margins are set, tab stops, if necessary, are set up, and any required fields are established; all that is necessary is to "fill in the blanks." Parts of the outline not needed are simply deleted during transcription. If a new topic is given, it is added at this time. A copy of this macro, template, or boilerplate also acts as a prompt for dictators so that they will remember to obtain and dictate vital data.

EXAMPLE

Patient name
HISTORY
    CHIEF COMPLAINT
    PRESENT ILLNESS
    PAST HISTORY
    OPERATIONS
    MEDICATIONS
    HABITS
    ALLERGIES
SOCIAL
FAMILY HISTORY
REVIEW OF SYSTEMS
    SKIN
    HEENT
    NECK
    CR
    GI
    GU
    GYN
    NM

dictator's name

MT's initials
D:
T:

12
CHAPTER

This example is not meant to be a format but to illustrate the topics and subtopics to expect in a format. When you fill in the outline during transcription, you may leave in the prompt for patient's name and type the name after it, but usually you simply overwrite the prompt and insert the patient's name. These are called "stops" or "tokens." You may add any other social demographics needed, such as hospital number and name of referring physician. You place your reference initials at the prompt indicated with "initials." What you do not see on the template are the commands for narrow margins, tab stops, and pause commands (which is where the cursor would position itself to permit you to enter the necessary data). If you have not yet learned to make a macro, start with something less complicated for practice. In many settings, the dictation system is interfaced with the hospital demographic database, and the patient's demographic information and/or statistics are filled in automatically at the top of the report, and you begin to type with the first dictated material. It is

vital that you double-check the demographics at this point to make sure that they do indeed refer to this dictation.

Just as you examined the formats for letter setup, you will now examine the formats for setting up an H&P. Actual wording of the outline itself varies, too, but that and the data that go into the report are discussed later. Keeping the facts in the proper sequence, spacing them properly, and entering them accurately make the work of transcribing interesting and challenging.

Usually the data for the history are obtained first. The following examples and guides for typing histories are also observed when you are typing the physical examination report. Always check with your client for the preferred style. You might never use some of these outlines again, but if you do need to use them for some client at some time, you will be familiar with them. You will also learn to appreciate the more straightforward styles. There are many suggestions and advice for streamlining the format, but document authors and MTs might prefer their own style regardless of recommendations.

Basic Block Format Report Style

(Figure 12-1)

Statistical Data: As determined by the medical facility.
In some transcription services, the entire statistical heading is printed for the MT to include the patient's name, identification number, physician, date, and so on. Examples are illustrated for you in Appendix C on Evolve.

Title: *History* or *Personal History* centered on the page.
Typed in all capital letters.

Main Topic Titles: Typed in all capital letters.
Each main topic on a line by itself.
Begun flush at left margin.

Main Topic Data: Begun on line under main topic title.
Single-spaced.
Double-space between the last line of one main topic data and the first line of the next main topic data.

Subtopic Titles: Typed in all capital letters, followed by a colon if data follows on the same line.

Subtopic Data: Begun on the *same* line as subtopic title or directly below it.
Single-space between subtopics. All lines begin flush at the left margin.
Double-space after last subtopic before a new main topic.

Margins: Narrow (1/2 inch to 3/4 inch is appropriate).

Close: Three blank spaces for signature.
Dictator's typed name.
Double space.
MT's initials or code number.
Date of dictation (D).
Date of transcription (T).

de Mars, Verna Marie   Hospital # 76-83-06

HISTORY

CHIEF COMPLAINT
Prolapse and bleeding after each bowel movement for the past 3-4 months.

PRESENT ILLNESS
This 78-year-old white female says she usually has 3 bowel movements a day in small amounts, and there has been a recent change in the frequency, size, and type of bowel movement she has been having. She is also having some pain and irritation in this area. She has had no previous anorectal surgery or rectal infection. She denies any blood in the stool itself.

PAST HISTORY
ILLNESSES
The patient had polio at age 8 from which she has made a remarkable recovery. Apparently, she was paralyzed in both lower extremities and now has adequate use of these. She has no other serious illnesses.
ALLERGIES
ALLERGIC TO PENICILLIN. She denies any other drug or food allergies.
MEDICATIONS
None.
OPERATIONS
Herniorrhaphy, 25 years ago.
SOCIAL
She does not smoke or drink. She lives with her husband, who is an invalid and for whom she cares. She is a retired former municipal court judge.

FAMILY HISTORY
One brother died of cancer of the throat; another has cancer of the kidney.

REVIEW OF SYSTEMS
SKIN: No rashes or jaundice.
HEENT: Unremarkable.
CR: No history of chest pain, shortness of breath, or pedal edema. She has had some mild hypertension in the past but is not under any medical supervision, nor is she taking any medication for this.
GI: Weight is stable. See Present Illness.
OB-GYN: Gravida 2 para 2. Climacteric at age 46; no sequelae.
EXTREMITIES: No edema.
NEUROLOGIC: Unremarkable.

Cortland M. Struthers, MD

jrt
D: 5/17/20XX
T: 5/20/20XX

FIGURE 12-1 Example of a history transcribed in basic block format.

12

CHAPTER

Modified Block Format Report Style

(Figure 12-2)

			Question:	How does this differ from Basic Block?
Statistical Data:	As determined by the medical facility.		**Answer:**	Subtopics are not in full caps.

Statistical Data: As determined by the medical facility.

Title: *History* or *Personal History* centered on the page.
Typed in all capital letters.

Main Topic Titles: Typed in all capital letters.
Begun flush at left margin.
Double-space between main topics.

Subtopic Titles: First word capitalized; title followed by a colon if text continues on the same line.

Data: Begun on the *same* line as the subtopic title.
Single-spaced.
Single-space between subtopics and double-space after last subtopic before the new main topic title.
Double-space between the last line of one main-topic data and the first line of the next main topic.

Margins: Narrow (1/2 inch to 3/4 inch).

Close: Three blank spaces for signature.
Dictator's typed name.
Double space.
MT's initials or code number.
Date of dictation (D).
Date of transcription (T).

Question: How does this differ from Basic Block?
Answer: Subtopics are not in full caps.
Data for subtopics are on the same line as the topic itself.
ROS is identical.
Takes up less space on page.

de Mars, Verna Marie   Hospital # 76-83-06

HISTORY

CHIEF COMPLAINT
Prolapse and bleeding after each bowel movement for the past 3-4 months.

PRESENT ILLNESS
This 78-year-old white female says she usually has 3 bowel movements a day in small amounts, and there has been a recent change in the frequency, size, and type of bowel movement she has been having. She is also having some pain and irritation in this area. She has had no previous anorectal surgery or rectal infection. She denies any blood in the stool itself.

PAST HISTORY
Illnesses: The patient had polio at age 8 from which she has made a remarkable recovery. Apparently, she was paralyzed in both lower extremities and now has adequate use of these. She has no other serious illnesses.
Allergies: ALLERGIC TO PENICILLIN. She denies any other drug or food allergies.
Medications: None.
Operations: Herniorrhaphy, 25 years ago.
Social: She does not smoke or drink. She lives with her husband, who is an invalid and for whom she cares. She is a retired former municipal court judge.
Family History: One brother died of cancer of the throat; another has cancer of the kidney.

REVIEW OF SYSTEMS
SKIN: No rashes or jaundice.
HEENT: Unremarkable.
CR: No history of chest pain, shortness of breath, or pedal edema. She has had some mild hypertension in the past but is not under any medical supervision, nor is she taking any medication for this.
GI: Weight is stable. See Present Illness.
OB-GYN: Gravida 2 para 2. Climacteric at age 46; no sequelae.
EXTREMITIES: No edema.
NEUROLOGIC: Unremarkable.

Cortland M. Struthers, MD

jrt
D: 5/17/20XX
T: 5/20/20XX

FIGURE 12-2 Example of a history transcribed in modified block format.

Run-on Modified Block Report Style
(Figure 12-3)

Statistical Data: As determined by the medical facility.

Title: *History* or *Personal History* centered on the page or flush with the left margin.
Typed in all capital letters.

Main Topic Titles: Typed in all capital letters, followed by a colon.
Begun flush with the left margin.
Double-space between main topics.

Subtopic Titles: Capitalized and followed by a colon if text continues on the same line.

Data: Begun on the *same* line as topic or subtopic title.
Single-spaced.

Margins: Narrow (1/2 inch to 3/4 inch).

Close: Three blank spaces for signature.
Dictator's typed name.
Double space.
MT's initials or code number.
Date of dictation (D).
Date of transcription (T).

Question:	How does this differ from Basic Block or Modified Block?
Answer:	Data for main topic shares line with topic title.
	Subtopic titles are not in full caps.
	Data for subtopics are run in with the topic itself.
	ROS data is run in.
	Takes up less space on page than previous two.

COMMENT: This style is not as easy to read as others illustrated and one has to wade through some data to find exactly what is wanted.

de Mars, Verna Marie
76-83-06

HISTORY

CHIEF COMPLAINT: Prolapse and bleeding after each bowel movement for the past 3-4 months.

PRESENT ILLNESS: This 78-year-old white female says she usually has 3 bowel movements a day in small amounts, and there has been a recent change in the frequency, size, and type of bowel movement she has been having. She is also having some pain and irritation in this area. She has had no previous anorectal surgery or rectal infection. She denies any blood in the stool itself.

PAST HISTORY: Illnesses: The patient had polio at age 8 from which she has made a remarkable recovery. Apparently, she was paralyzed in both lower extremities and now has adequate use of these. She has no other serious illnesses. Allergies: ALLERGIC TO PENICILLIN. She denies any other drug or food allergies. Medications: None. Operations: Herniorrhaphy, 25 years ago. Social: She does not smoke or drink. She lives with her husband, who is an invalid and for whom she cares. She is a retired former municpal court judge.

FAMILY HISTORY: One brother died of cancer of the throat; another has cancer of the kidney.

REVIEW OF SYSTEMS: Skin: No rashes or jaundice. HEENT: Unremarkable. CR: No history of chest pain, shortness of breath, or pedal edema. She has had some mild hypertension in the past but is not under any medical supervision, nor is she taking any medication for this. GI: Weight is stable. See Present Illness. OB-GYN: Gravida 2 para 2. Climacteric at age 46; no sequelae. Extremities: No edema. Neurologic: Unremarkable.

Cortland M. Struthers, MD

jrt
D: 5/17/20XX
T: 5/20/20XX

FIGURE 12-3 Example of a history transcribed in modified run-on block format.

Tabulated Block Report Style

(Figure 12-4)

Statistical Data: As determined by the medical facility.

Title: *History* or *Personal History* centered on the page.
Typed in all capital letters.

Main Topic Titles: Typed in all capital letters, followed by a colon unless it is on the line alone (such as *Past History* and *Review of Systems* in Figure 12-4). Begun flush at left margin. Double-space between main topics.

Subtopic Titles: Typed in full capitals, followed by a colon if text continues on the same line.

Data: Begun on the *same* line as the topic or subtopic title.
Data input begun two tab stops after the heading. (Tabbing and blocking are determined by the length of the longest title in the history: Review of Systems. All other data are tabbed and blocked to this same point under the previous line. The initial tab at this place is adequate for all data to be evenly blocked. The "block indent" feature of software programs is very helpful in this format.) Begin typing on the same line as the topic or subtopic title after the appropriate tab is reached.
Single-spaced.
Single-space between subtopics and double-space after last subtopic before the new main topic title.
Double-space between the last line of one main-topic data and the first line of the next main topic.

Margins: Narrow (1/2 inch to 3/4 inch).

Close: Three blank spaces for signature.
Dictator's typed name.
Double space.
MT's initials or code number.
Date of dictation (D).
Date of transcription (T).

COMMENT: Some MTs use a variation of this style by bringing the third and subsequent lines of the blocked data back to the left margin. This saves space when the data is lengthy (Figure 12-5, *Present Illness* and *Family History*). Neither of these styles would be acceptable to use with facilities that prefer run-on format styles. However, these styles are often used in private medical facilities that do not use electronic record platforms. It is easy to read but not as easy to type.

---

de Mars, Verna Marie   Hospital # 76-83-06

HISTORY

CHIEF COMPLAINT: Prolapse and bleeding after each bowel movement for the past 3-4 months.

PRESENT ILLNESS: This 78-year-old white female says she usually has 3 bowel movements a day in
                      small amounts, and there has been a recent change in the frequency, size, and type
                      of bowel movement she has been having. She is also having some pain and
                      irritation in this area. She has had no previous anorectal surgery or rectal infection.
                      She denies any blood in the stool itself.

PAST HISTORY
ILLNESSES: The patient had polio at age 8 from which she has made a remarkable recovery.
                      Apparently, she was paralyzed in both lower extremities and now has adequate use
                      of these. She has no other serious illnesses.
ALLERGIES: ALLERGIC TO PENICILLIN. She denies any other drug or food allergies.
MEDICATIONS: None.
OPERATIONS: Herniorrhaphy, 25 years ago.
SOCIAL: She does not smoke or drink. She lives with her husband, who is an invalid and for
                      whom she cares. She is a retired former municpal court judge.

FAMILY HISTORY: One brother died of cancer of the throat; another has cancer of the kidney.

REVIEW OF SYSTEMS
SKIN: No rashes or jaundice.
HEENT: Unremarkable.
CR: No history of chest pain, shortness of breath, or pedal edema. She has had some
                      mild hypertension in the past but is not under any medical supervision, nor is she
                      taking any medication for this.
GI: Weight is stable. See Present Illness.
OB-GYN: Gravida 2 para 2. Climacteric at age 46; no sequelae.
EXTREMITIES: No edema.
NEUROLOGIC: Unremarkable.

Cortland M. Struthers, MD

jrt
D: 5/17/20XX
T: 5/20/20XX

FIGURE 12-4 Example of a history transcribed in tabulated block format.

de Mars, Verna Marie   Hospital # 76-83-06

HISTORY

CHIEF COMPLAINT: Prolapse and bleeding after each bowel movement for the past
3-4 months.

PRESENT ILLNESS: This 78-year-old white female says she usually has 3 bowel movements a
day in small amounts, and there has been a recent change in the
frequency, size, and type of bowel movement she has been having. She is also having some
pain and irritation in this area. She has had no previous anorectal surgery or rectal infection. She
denies any blood in the stool itself.

PAST HISTORY
ILLNESSES: The patient had polio at age 8 from which she has made a remarkable
recovery. Apparently, she was paralyzed in both lower extremities and
now has adequate use of these. She has no other serious illnesses.

ALLERGIES: <u>ALLERGIC TO PENICILLIN</u>. She denies any other drug or food allergies.

MEDICATIONS: Fosamax 70 mg once a week, Synthroid 50 mg daily.

OPERATIONS: T & A in childhood; herniorrhaphy 25 years ago.

SOCIAL: She does not smoke or drink. She lives with her husband, who is an invalid
and for whom she cares. She is a retired former municpal court judge.

FAMILY HISTORY: She has four children, living and well. One child died in childhood in an
automobile accident. Her mother died at age 91 of a CVA; her father died
at age 89 of natural causes. She has two siblings, living and well; one brother died of carcinoma of
the liver when he was 64. She had a maternal aunt who died of carcinoma of the breast.

REVIEW OF SYSTEMS
SKIN: No rashes or jaundice.
HEENT: Unremarkable.
CR: No history of chest pain, shortness of breath, or pedal edema. She has had
some mild hypertension in the past but is not under any medical
Supervision, nor is she taking any medication for this.
GI: Weight is stable. See Present Illness.
OB-GYN: Gravida 5 para 5. Climacteric at age 46; no sequelae.
EXTREMITIES: No edema.
NEUROLOGIC: Unremarkable.

Cortland M. Struthers, MD

jrt
D: 5/17/20XX
T: 5/20/20XX

FIGURE 12-5 Example of a history transcribed in indented block format.

THE HISTORY

The physician obtains information for the history by questioning the patient or the family or persons accompanying the patient when the patient is unable to provide the history. A carefully documented history directs the focus of the physical examination and assists with making the final diagnosis.

Now briefly examine each part of the outline. You can look at the examples and see how it develops.

Statistical Data

Statistical data always include the name of the patient and any other means of identification that the hospital, office, or clinic uses. This part can include the patient's *medical record number (MRN),* age, room number, date of admission, account number, and referring physician; the dictator's name; and the names of anyone who is to receive a copy of the dictation. This material could be preprinted on forms at the time of admission. The material can be preentered for the MT on the H&P macro when the dictation is downloaded. If these data are preinserted on your document, always double check all data for accuracy.

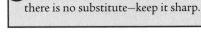

MT TOOL BOX TIP: Accuracy is a tool for which there is no substitute—keep it sharp.

Chief Complaint

Most facilities prefer spelled-out main headings and abbreviated subtopic headings. The SOAP format is an exception, but its use is confined to chart notes. The chief complaint (abbreviated CC) is a description of what symptom or sign caused the patient to go to the physician, emergency department, or hospital. It is usually brief, can be specific or vague, and can be dictated in the patient's own words. The nature of the patient's complaints gives focus and direction to the H&P. If there is a list of complaints, the complaints are usually dictated in the order of importance.

Present Illness

Present illness (abbreviated PI) is also called *History of Chief Complaint* or *History of Present Illness* (abbreviated HPI). The patient's problem is discussed in detail, with emphasis on duration and severity. The patient relates the details he or she feels are significant, and the physician inquires whether they are related to other symptoms or events. If the patient has been treated by another physician for the same or a similar problem, this treatment is discussed, along with the possible diagnosis and additional treatment prescribed.

Past History

Past history (abbreviated PH) begins with the patient's childhood and includes all previous medical history with reference to chronic diseases and conditions not directly related to the present condition; past injuries, including fractures, wounds, burns, trauma, and injuries from falls or accidents (including industrial accidents and injuries); illnesses; and surgical procedures. This main topic is generally broken down into subtopics as follows.

HABITS

This subtopic includes information about the patient's usual lifestyle, including exercise, recreation, and the use of alcohol, tobacco, and drugs (both prescription and recreational). The dictator could use a separate topic for drugs the patient has taken recently or is currently taking and call this subtopic *Medications.*

EXAMPLE

HABITS: The patient is a social drinker. He has a 30-year history of smoking a half-pack of cigarettes a day.

DISEASES

This subtopic includes both childhood and adult diseases and any resulting complications.

EXAMPLE

DISEASES: Usual childhood diseases without sequelae.

OPERATIONS

All surgical procedures, dates, and sequelae are recorded in this subtopic. This subtopic may also be called *Surgeries.*

EXAMPLE

SURGERIES: She broke her right thumb in 2009 and had it repaired.

ALLERGIES

This subtopic includes any reactions the patient has to drugs, food, or the environment. Many physicians and/or facilities direct the MT to boldface, underline, or type in all capital letters a positive reply to a query regarding a drug allergy.

EXAMPLES

ALLERGIES: The patient denies any drug or environmental allergies.

ALLERGIES: ALLERGIC TO PENICILLIN AND TETRACYCLINE.

12

CHAPTER

SOCIAL HISTORY

The socioeconomic status of the patient is noted in this subtopic. It includes his or her occupation, profession, or trade; recreational interests; home environment; and marital status.

GYNECOLOGIC (WHEN THE PATIENT IS A WOMAN)

In this subtopic, the number of pregnancies, deliveries, complications, living children, and abortions and sexual activity are noted, along with times of menarche and menopause and any problems with the menses.

Prolonged investigation of any one or more of these topics is made, depending on the patient's chief complaint. Some dictators use some or all of the topics listed; others group all of these data into a brief paragraph titled *Past History*. You will also notice that physicians list many negative replies to some of these items; for example, "The patient *denies* any allergies or drug sensitivities"; "There is *no* history of familial disease"; or "The patient *does not* use drugs or alcohol." These expressions are recorded after the listed topic. This last sentence would read as follows on your transcript:

EXAMPLE

MEDICATIONS: No use of drugs or alcohol.

Dictated: The patient denies allergies to drugs.

Transcribed: ALLERGIES: Denies allergies to drugs.

Family History

The state of health of the patient's parents, siblings, and grandparents is discussed under this topic. If any of these family members are deceased, the age and cause of death are often recorded. Inquiry is made concerning certain diseases that tend to be familial, such as tuberculosis, diabetes, epilepsy, carcinoma, and heart disease. The place and circumstances of the patient's birth might also be noteworthy.

EXAMPLE

FAMILY HISTORY: Father and mother are living and well. He has two sisters alive and well, and he had one brother who died at age 20 as the result of an automobile accident.

Review of Systems

This topic is also called *Systemic Review, Functional Inquiry,* and *Inventory by Systems.* The review of systems is an oral review conducted in question-and-answer style with the patient, as stated, of all the body systems to ensure that nothing has been overlooked. The absence or presence of problems is noted. Again, a variety of methods are used for typing this information. In general, the physician reviews by starting at the top of the body and going through the body systems, ending with the nervous or musculoskeletal system. The physician dictates the data as a single paragraph with no headings or breaks the data down into subtopics. The subtopics used are as follows, along with the abbreviations commonly used and accepted.

SKIN

This subtopic includes eruptions, rashes, itches, discolorations, dryness, and scaling. Sometimes the dictator dictates "quote" and "unquote" or "end quote" around a response from the patient. This practice indicates that the patient has made a decision about the problem that may or may not be correct, particularly when the dictator has asked whether another physician had treated the patient for this condition or whether patient had treated himself or herself.

EXAMPLE

Dictated: No rashes or scaling, but the patient says that he has had *quote* psoriasis in the past *unquote.*

Transcribed: SKIN: No rashes or scaling, but the patient says that he has had "psoriasis" in the past.

NOTE: Sometimes you could be left on your own to decide where the quotes start and stop with the dictator saying, *He has had quote psoriasis in the past.* Either way, you will place the quotation marks where they logically belong.

HAIR

This subtopic includes changes in its texture or distribution, loss of hair, and excessive hair.

HEENT

This subtopic pertains to head, eyes, ears, nose, and throat. Additional subtopics could be added, or a single, all-inclusive paragraph could be used.

Eyes. This section includes vision problems such as glaucoma, scotoma, conjunctivitis, trachoma, pain, discharge, redness, fields, use of glasses, blurring, double vision, seeing spots or rings around lights, watering, itching, and abnormal sensitivity to light.

Ears. This section includes hearing loss, discharge, dizziness, syncope, tinnitus, pain, and condition of the tympanic membranes.

Nose. This section includes discharges, sense of smell, colds, allergies, and epistaxis.

Mouth and Throat. This section includes condition of teeth, dental hygiene, dentures, gums, difficulty in swallowing, hoarseness, sore throat, postnasal drip, and choking.

Neck. This section includes the thyroid and movement of the neck.

NOTE: Some dictators say "head and neck" and place HEENT and neck problems in one paragraph.

CARDIORESPIRATORY (CR)

CR refers to both the cardiovascular and the respiratory systems. The cardiovascular problems can include chest pain and its severity, tachycardia, bradycardia, heart murmurs, heart attacks, palpitations, high blood pressure, and varicose veins. Closely related respiratory problems include the sequelae of heart problems, dyspnea, orthopnea, shortness of breath, edema, hemoptysis, and pneumonia.

GASTROINTESTINAL (GI)

The GI subtopic includes abdominal pain of any type or severity, appetite, indigestion, dysphagia, anorexia, vomiting, hematemesis, change in weight or diet, change in bowel habits, melena, flatus, diarrhea, constipation, and jaundice.

GENITOURINARY (GU)

The GU subtopic includes dysuria, nocturia, hematuria, urgency, frequency, pyuria, oliguria, incontinence, hesitancy, urinary dribbling, discharge, lumbar pain, stones, and sexually transmitted diseases.

GYNECOLOGIC (GYN)

The GYN subtopic includes menarche, flow, dysmenorrhea, menorrhagia, metrorrhagia, dyspareunia, leukorrhea, use of contraceptives, obstetric history, pregnancies, deliveries, and abortions. *Gravida* followed by a number refers to the number of pregnancies, including ectopic pregnancies, hydatidiform moles, abortions, and normal pregnancies. *Para* followed by a number refers to the number of deliveries after the 20th week of gestation (live birth or stillbirth, single or multiple, vaginal or cesarean) and does not correspond to the number of infants born.

EXAMPLE

GYN: Gravida 3 para 2 abortus 0.

NEUROPSYCHIATRIC (NP)

The NP subtopic includes syncope, headache, vertigo, pain, scotomata, paralysis, ataxia, convulsion, and emotional state.

MUSCULOSKELETAL (MS)

The MS subtopic includes pain, stiffness, limitation of movement, and fractures.

Sometimes there is nothing noteworthy to add to the history in the systemic review (it was covered adequately in the history as related), and so the dictator says, "Systemic review is essentially negative." This expression is typed after the outline topic.

EXAMPLE

REVIEW OF SYSTEMS: Essentially negative.

The actual structuring of the paragraphs is the responsibility of the MT, and therefore this basic understanding of a history will aid you. The physician may not dictate the outline, so you must be able to recognize each body part that he or she is discussing so that you can choose the appropriate topic or subtopic.

If the history continues to a second page, type the word "continued" in parentheses after the last typed line on the first page. On the second page, beginning at the left margin, repeat the statistical data from the first page and add the heading *History, page 2*. This step is often difficult to carry out correctly, and you should use the print preview on your computer to ensure that these headings appear in the correct place. If your work is printed off site, or is designated for an EHR, you could be asked not to type "continued" on the bottom of your page.

Before you begin your first assignment, briefly review the illustrated histories.

12-1 SELF-STUDY

DIRECTIONS: Retype the following data into history outline by using the basic block format. See p. 303 and Figure 12-1.

▶ Begin each exercise by setting the right and left margins at 0.5, which means a change from the default setting of 1.0. Be sure that the right margin is not justified.

▶ Reexamine the outline directions once again (p. 302).

▶ The patient's name and other statistical data can be set up as you desire. Be alert to topic changes and proper mechanics. Remember to use proper grammar, punctuation, abbreviations, capitalization, and figures as required.

The patient is Geoffrey Paul Hawkins. The dictating physician is Paul R. Elsner, MD. The material was dictated yesterday. The patient's hospital ID number is 54-98-10. His chief complaint is abdominal pains and vomiting since three a.m. Present Illness: This eleven and a half year old white male, who was perfectly well yesterday and last evening, awoke from his sleep with vomiting at three a.m. today. This was followed by nausea, which has been severe, together with a little bile coming up, but no great amount of continued vomiting. There is severe, recurrent, doubling-up type cramping to time of admission at ten this morning. There has been no recent upper respiratory tract infection, no prior similar episode, no history of recurrent constipation or diarrhea. Patient's last bowel movement was yesterday and of normal quality. His mother reports that he eats sunflower seeds to excess and may have done so yesterday. Past History: Patient was born at home with midwife delivery, uncomplicated. He has had the usual immunizations for childhood. There has been no prior hospitalization, no tonsillectomy, no surgery, no fracture. He has had stitches a couple of times in the office. Family History: Mother is thirty-five and at the present time is under treatment for cancer of the breast. She reports that she had surgery and is on chemotherapy at the present time. She has not been given radiation. Father is age forty, living and well. There are two sisters, both older than the patient, both living and well. They both had appendectomies, one of which had ruptured. There are a maternal great niece, uncle and paternal grandmother who have had diabetes. There is no diabetes in the immediate family and no other history of familial disorders, such as bleeding, anemia, tuberculosis, heart disease. Personal History: The patient has no known drug allergies, has not been on any medication at the present time. Grade six, but does poorly. Seems to be the class clown according to his mother. He has no hobbies. Systemic Review: HEENT: There has been a muscle in one eye which has been off for years; Dr McMannis is following this. His vision is good, hearing is normal. CR: No known murmurs. No chronic cough, no recent cough, no dyspnea. GI: No prior GI difficulty. No food allergies. No chronic or recurrent constipation. GU: No nocturia, no enuresis, no GU infection. NM: No history of head injury, no history of polio, paralysis, meningitis, or numbness.

Check your work in Appendix A, p. 455, Pay close attention to format.

12-2 PRACTICE TEST

DIRECTIONS: Retype the following data into a history outline by using tabulated block format. Be alert to topic changes. Remember that the dictator might not follow the exact wording or format given in the sample outlines (see Figure 12-4).

▶ Change left and right margin settings to 0.5.
▶ Clear all tabs and set new tab stop at 2.0.

The patient is Joseph R. Balentine. The report was dictated on 11/06/XX and transcribed the same day. The dictating physician is Benjamin B. Abboud. He requests that a copy be sent to Stuart L. Paulson, MD. The patient's ID number is 423-12-22. His chief complaint: the patient is a 25 year old male complaining of recurring epistaxis. Present Illness: the patient reports that yesterday he had onset of epistaxis in the left side of his nose. This was intermittent throughout the day and at four thirty this morning, he came to the ER. Past History: Allergies: None. Illnesses: The patient had a collapsed lung about five years ago and subsequently had surgery, but does not know the exact etiology of the problem or the exact name of the surgery. There is no bleeding history except for PI. Medications: None. Family History: Essentially unremarkable. Father, mother, siblings are all well and healthy. Review of Systems: Skin: No rashes or jaundice. HEENT: See PI. CR: See past history. No history of pneumonia, tuberculosis, chronic cough, or hemoptysis. No history of pedal edema. GI: Weight is stable. He denies any nausea, vomiting, diarrhea, or food intolerance. GU: No history of GU tract infections, dysuria, hematuria, pyuria. Endocrine: no polyuria or polydipsia. Neurologic: no history of psychiatric disorder.

A transcript for this appears in Appendix A, p. 456.

THE PHYSICAL EXAMINATION

A thorough physical examination comprises an examination and complete assessment of all body systems. It is usually done after the history is documented and includes an inspection of the body, beginning with the head and concluding with the feet (cephalocaudal). An analysis of the subjective findings that were taken down during the history documentation and review of systems indicates the extent of the physical examination of different body parts that is required. For example, extensive complaints regarding the cardiovascular system will result in intensive examination of the lungs and heart.

Four basic procedures are included in the complete physical examination report:
1. Inspection: looking at the body.
2. Palpation: feeling various parts and organs.
3. Percussion: listening to the sounds produced when a particular region is tapped (percussed).
4. Auscultation: listening to body sounds.

The style and format for the physical examination report are identical to those for the history. Be consistent and follow the same style you use for the history when you type the physical examination report. The physical examination report is typed on a separate sheet of paper with full headings, but, again, in run-on format, you simply continue on the same sheet. The first example is run-on format, showing you both a history and a physical examination report.

Follow the same guidelines as illustrated in the history section for typing the physical examination report.

These two documents, the history and the physical examination, are actually prepared as a single document. They are separated into two documents in this chapter to teach them one at a time as separate functions for you to master.

Physical Examination, Basic Block Format

Follow the format illustrated for typing the history. The statistical data are repeated on the new page, and the title *Physical Examination* could be centered on the page, typed in full capital letters. Figure 12-6 is an example of a physical examination report typed in basic block format. Figure 12-7 is an example of a H&P typed in basic block format. Normally, the H&P is typed as a single document like this.

History and Physical, Run-On Format

Examples of a combined H&P in run-on format are shown in Figure 12-8. Note the preferred line-up when there is more than one diagnosis. Notice as well, that only a single page is needed for the H&P in run-on format in contrast to the basic block shown in Figure 12-7. In fact, if you need to save both time and space, the diagnoses would be typed in a block form similar to the previous sections of data. This is not a preferred solution, but it is one that is used.

Physical Examination, Tabulated Block Format

Follow the format illustrated for typing the history. The statistical information is repeated on the new page, and the title *Physical Examination* is centered on the page, typed in full capital letters. When the history and the physical examination are prepared as usual, in one continuous document, type "History" beginning at the left margin and type the word "Physical" to introduce that section, again at the left margin. Use all capital letters. Figure 12-9 is an

---

de Mars, Verna Marie
76-83-06

PHYSICAL EXAMINATION

GENERAL
This is a 78-year-old, well-developed, well-nourished, slightly obese white woman in no acute distress. She is alert and oriented to time, place, and person.

VITAL SIGNS
PULSE: 76/min. BP: 130/80. RESP: 12. TEMPERATURE: 99°.

HEENT: EYES: Pupils equal and react to light and accommodation. EOMs intact. Sclerae white. Fundi not visualized.
EARS: Hearing and drums are normal. MOUTH: The teeth are in poor repair. Several bridges are present. The tongue protrudes in the midline with some questionable deviation to the right. Uvula projects upward on elicitation of the gag reflex. No lesions of the mucous membranes.
NECK: Supple, with some limitation of motion to the right. No masses present. The carotid pulsations are equal, with no bruit. There is no neck vein distention and no thyromegaly. The trachea is deviated slightly to the right.
CHEST: No increase in AP diameter. LUNGS: Clear to P&A. HEART: Quiet precordium. Normal sinus rhythm, without murmurs, rubs, or gallops. Heart sounds appear normal and to split physiologically. No S4 heard.
ABDOMEN: Flat, without scars. No organomegaly. Liver, kidneys, and spleen not palpable. Tympanic to percussion. The bowel sounds are normoactive.
PELVIC: Deferred.
RECTAL: On anoscopy, there is an exophytic, soft, easily movable mass encompassing one half the circumference of the rectum directly at the dentate line. Full sigmoidoscopic examination to 25 cm was unremarkable.
EXTREMITIES: Range of motion is within normal limits. No pedal edema. All pulses appear equal and full bilaterally. No evidence of chronic arterial or venous disease.
NEUROLOGICAL: Cranial nerves II-XII appear grossly intact. There are no pathological reflexes demonstrated. Reflexes within normal limits.

IMPRESSION: Rectal tumor.

Cortland M. Struthers, MD

jrt
D: 5/17/20XX
T: 5/20/20XX

FIGURE 12-6 Example of a physical examination report transcribed in basic block format.

example of a physical examination typed in modified block format.

Physical Examination, Indented Format

Follow the format illustrated for typing the history. The statistical data are repeated on the new page, and the title *Physical Examination* is centered on the page, typed in all capital letters. Again, this is usually prepared as one continuous document.

THE OUTLINE

The physical examination is the examiner's objective (*O* in the SOAP method) observations of abnormalities or signs of the illness or injury. Part of this observation was taking place while the history was being taken from the patient but is recorded now.

As you did with the history, briefly examine each part of the outline used in the physical examination report. You type the statistical data just as you did for the history and the heading *Physical Examination*. Now, begin with the topics.

General

The "General" topic includes the general appearance and nutritional state of the patient, body build, alertness, personal hygiene, general state of health, age, height, weight, and race. It may include the emotional condition (euphoric, lethargic, distracted, well-oriented, agitated).

Vital Signs

Vital signs include the temperature, pulse, respiration, and blood pressure. Most often, however, this information is included with the previous topic.

Morris G Heslop

527-98-6540

Date: March 7, 20XX

Room 631-A

HISTORY

CHIEF COMPLAINT: Acute onset, severe abdominal pain and indigestion.

PRESENT ILLNESS: This 41-year-old male patient presented to Fletcher Hills Memorial Emergency Room at approximately 12 o'clock on Friday, March 6, 20XX, complaining of a gaseous feeling in his upper abdomen, radiating to the right side and down to the right lower quadrant of the abdomen. The patient is a pilot for Atlantic-Pacific Airlines. Last night, approximately 6 p.m., he had a spaghetti dinner in Denver, Colorado, and was restless approximately 5-6 hours later; and while he did not have diarrhea, he felt bloating and indigestion, which was relieved to a very small extent by Maalox. He continued to have increasing discomfort in his upper abdomen with radiation to the back, between the shoulder blades, but there was no vomiting, diarrhea, or fever. He became quite sweaty and pale while flying and had the copilot take over.

PAST HISTORY
OPERATIONS: The patient had a herniorrhaphy 2 years ago at Fletcher Memorial and an appendectomy as a teenager.
ALLERGIES: None.
HABITS: He does not smoke. The only alcohol intake is occasional wine with meals. No current drugs or medications.

FAMILY HISTORY: There is no family history of importance.

REVIEW OF SYSTEMS
EENT: No double vision. No ringing of the ears. No headache.
GI: No weight change. No change in bowel habits or any blood in the bowel movements.
GU: No difficulty urinating; no blood in the urine.
CR: Denies any chest pain or radiation of any type of pain into his left hand or arm over to the shoulders.

PHYSICAL EXAMINATION
GENERAL: The patient is an alert, cooperative male clutching at the right lower portion of his abdomen at times during the interview. He says that this is still uncomfortable. Pulse: 78 and regular. BP: 116/80. Temperature: 98.6. Afebrile.

(continued)

FIGURE 12-7 Example of a history and physical examination report transcribed in basic block format.

Morris G Heslop
527-98-6540
Room 631-A
Date: March 7, 20XX
HISTORY and Physical Examination, Page 2

HEENT: React to L&A. No AV nicking. Ears are normal. Pharynx is normal.
NECK: No thyroid enlargement or bruit noted.
CHEST: Heart tones are normal.
ABDOMEN: On pressure in the epigastrium, he complains of a little discomfort more to the
right side of the abdomen, and on pressure in the right lower quadrant, he does wince.
Bowel sounds are hypoactive, and there is no palpable liver, kidneys, spleen. There is no
rebound on percussion. There is no inguinal hernia.
GENITALIA: Testicles are normal
RECTAL: No heat, and there is no blood in the bowel movements on gross examination.
There is no diarrhea present.
NEUROMUSCULAR: Biceps, triceps, Achilles, patellar reflexes are normal. Range of motion of
all extremities is normal. There is no pedal edema, and pedal pulses are normal.

DIAGNOSES
1. Possible acute cholecystitis.
2. Possible food poisoning.
3. Possible early, penetrating ulcer.
4. Rule out pancreatitis.

PLAN OF DIRECTION: X-rays, ulcer-type diet, ECG, 2-hour urine amylase.

Frank O. Bodner, MD

ref
D: 3-7-XX
T: 3-7-XX

FIGURE 12-7, cont'd Notice the preferred stacked style for the diagnoses.

HEENT (or Head and Neck)

Information on the head, eyes, ears, nose, and throat is included in this topic. After the main heading abbreviation, the individual subtopics are pulled out and typed in either outline or paragraph form, depending on the emphasis placed on all or each. The personal wishes of either the dictator or the MT also determine which method is used; both methods were illustrated for you in the previous examples. These subtopics include the following.

HEAD

This subtopic includes shape, color, and texture of the skin and hair.

EYES

This subtopic includes the sclerae, corneas, conjunctivae, fundi, reaction of the pupils to light and accommodation (PERLA or PERRLA), extraocular movements (EOMs), and visual acuity and fields.

EARS

Canals, ossicles, tympanic membranes (TMs), hearing, and discharge are included in this subtopic.

NOSE

This subtopic includes airway, septum, and sinuses.

MOUTH AND THROAT

This subtopic includes teeth, gums, lips, tongue, salivary glands, tonsils, dentures, palate, uvula, and mucosa.

NECK

This subtopic includes contour, mobility, lymph nodes, thyroid size and shape, position of trachea, carotid pulses, and neck vein distention. "Neck" is often used as a main topic. If the dictator dictates "HEENT" and then "Neck," use "Neck" as a main topic. If "Head and Neck" are dictated, then "Neck" is a subtopic.

Morris G. Heslop
527-98-6540
Room 631-A

March 7, 20XX

HISTORY

CHIEF COMPLAINT: Acute onset, severe abdominal pain and indigestion.
PRESENT ILLNESS: This 41-year-old male patient presented to Fletcher Hills Memorial Emergency Room at approximately 12 o'clock on Friday, March 6, 200X, complaining of a gaseous feeling in his upper abdomen, radiating to the right side and down to the right lower quadrant of the abdomen. The patient is a pilot for Atlantic-Pacific Airlines. Last night, approximately 6 p.m., he had a spaghetti dinner in Denver, Colorado, and was restless approximately 5-6 hours later; and while he did not have diarrhea, he felt bloating and indigestion, which was relieved to a very small extent by Maalox. He continued to have increasing discomfort in his upper abdomen with radiation to the back, between the shoulder blades; but there was no vomiting, diarrhea, or fever. He became quite sweaty and pale while flying and had the copilot take over.
PAST HISTORY: Operations: The patient had a herniorrhaphy 2 years ago at Fletcher Memorial and an appendectomy as a teenager. Allergies: None. Habits: He does not smoke. The only alcohol intake is occasional wine with meals. No current drugs or medications.
FAMILY HISTORY: There is no family history of importance.
REVIEW OF SYSTEMS: EENT: No double vision. No ringing of the ears. No headache. GI: No weight change. No change in bowel habits or any blood in the bowel movements. GU: No difficulty urinating; no blood in the urine. CR: Denies any chest pain or radiation of any type of pain into his left hand or arm over to the shoulders.

PHYSICAL EXAMINATION

GENERAL: The patient is an alert, cooperative male clutching at the right lower portion of his abdomen at times during the interview. He says that this is still uncomfortable. Pulse: 78 and regular. BP: 116/80. Temperature: 98.6. Afebrile.
HEENT: React to L&A. No AV nicking. Ears are normal. Pharynx is normal.
NECK: No thyroid enlargement or bruit noted.
CHEST: Heart tones are normal.
ABDOMEN: On pressure in the epigastrium, he complains of a little discomfort more to the right side of the abdomen, and on pressure in the right lower quadrant, he does wince. Bowel sounds are hypoactive, and there is no palpable liver, kidneys, spleen. There is no rebound on percussion. There is no inguinal hernia.
GENITALIA: Testicles are normal.
RECTAL: No heat, and there is no blood in the bowel movements on gross examination. There is no diarrhea present.
NEUROMUSCULAR: Biceps, triceps, Achilles, patellar reflexes are normal. Range of motion of all extremities is normal. There is no pedal edema, and pedal pulses are normal.

DIAGNOSES
1. Possible acute cholecystitis.
2. Possible food poisoning.
3. Possible early, penetrating ulcer.
4. Rule out pancreatitis.

PLAN OF DIRECTION: X-rays, ulcer-type diet, ECG, 2-hour urine amylase.

Frank O. Bodner, MD
ref
D: 3-7-XX
T: 3-7-XX

FIGURE 12-8 Example of a physical examination report transcribed in run-on format.

Chest

The next main topic is the chest, which is often divided into the subtopics of heart and lungs. This section includes the shape, symmetry, expansion, and breasts.

LUNGS

This subtopic includes breath sounds, expansion, fields, resonance, and adventitious sounds (rales, rhonchi, wheezes, rubs, stridor).

HEART

This subtopic includes rhythm (sinus rhythm), borders, silhouette, rate, murmurs, rubs, gallops, heaves, lifts, thrills, and palpitations.

Abdomen

This topic includes the symmetry, shape, contour, bowel sounds, tenderness, rigidity, guarding, herniation, and palpation of the liver, spleen, and kidneys.

de Mars, Verna Marie   Hospital # 76-83-06

PHYSICAL EXAMINATION

GENERAL: This is a 78-year-old, well-developed, well-nourished, slightly obese white woman in no acute distress. She is alert and oriented to time, place, and person.

VITAL SIGNS: PULSE: 76/min. BP: 130/80. RESP: 12. TEMPERATURE: 99°.

HEENT
EYES: Pupils equal and react to light and accommodation. EOMs intact. Sclerae white. Fundi not visualized.
EARS: Hearing and drums are normal.
MOUTH: The teeth are in poor repair. Several bridges are present. The tongue protrudes in the midline with some questionable deviation to the right. Uvula projects upward on elicitation of the gag reflex. No lesions of the mucous membranes.

NECK: Supple, with some limitation of motion to the right. No masses present. The carotid pulsations are equal, with no bruit. There is no neck vein distention and no thyromegaly. The trachea is deviated slightly to the right.

CHEST: No increase in AP diameter.
LUNGS: Clear to P&A.
HEART: Quiet precordium. Normal sinus rhythm, without murmurs, rubs, or gallops. Heart sounds appear normal and to split physiologically. No S4 heard.

ABDOMEN: Flat, without scars. No organomegaly. Liver, kidneys, and spleen not palpable. Tympanic to percussion. The bowel sounds are normoactive.

PELVIC: Deferred.

RECTAL: On anoscopy, there is an exophytic, soft, easily movable mass encompassing one half the circumference of the rectum directly at the dentate line. Full sigmoidoscopic examination to 25 cm was unremarkable.

EXTREMITIES: Range of motion is within normal limits. No pedal edema. All pulses appear equal and full bilaterally. No evidence of chronic arterial or venous disease.

NEUROLOGICAL: Cranial nerves II-XII appear grossly intact. There are no pathological reflexes demonstrated. Reflexes within normal limits.

IMPRESSION: Rectal tumor.

Cortland M. Struthers, MD

jrt
D: 5/17/20XX
T: 5/20/20XX

FIGURE 12-9 Example of a physical examination report transcribed in modified block format.

Genitalia (or Pelvic or Genitourinary)

In female patients, this topic includes external genitalia (vulva), Skene and Bartholin glands, introitus, vagina, cervix, uterus, adnexa, discharge, escutcheon, urethral meatus, perineum, and anus. In male patients, it includes the prostate (which also can be listed under "Rectal"), testes, epididymides, penis, lesions, and discharge.

Rectal

This topic includes anus, sphincter tone, perineum, and hemorrhoids.

Extremities

This topic includes bones, joints, movement, color, temperature, edema, and varicosities. Sometimes the reflexes and pulses are included in this section.

Neurologic

Reflexes, cranial nerves, orientation in all three spheres (time, place, person), signs (Babinski, Brudzinski, Hoffmann, Kernig, Romberg, Strunsky), station, and gait are included in this topic.

Diagnosis (Impression, Assessment, or Conclusion)

The diagnosis includes a provisional or final diagnosis, which is the conclusion the examiner has reached on the basis of the history he or she has documented and the examination just concluded. It can be an explanation for the patient's problem, the identification or explanation of a disease process, or the actual name of a disease. Diagnostic studies can be ordered (such as radiographs, electrocardiography, blood workup) before a final diagnosis is made. These are generally typed in lined-up format when there is more than one diagnosis (see Figure 12-8).

> **NOTE:** Do not use abbreviations in the diagnosis part of the medical record.

Treatment (or Recommendation)

This topic includes the plan of treatment and can include a course of medications or indicate surgery or some of the diagnostic studies mentioned earlier.

THE DATA

The physician either dictates the data in narrative form without topics or subtopics or dictates the topics and subtopics for you. You will use the proper topic as soon as reference is made to it, no matter how it is dictated.

EXAMPLE

Dictated: The abdomen is scaphoid. There are no masses or rigidity.

Transcribed: ABDOMEN: Scaphoid, no masses or rigidity.

On the other hand, some medical records protocols require everything in sentence form. In this case, you would type

> ABDOMEN: The abdomen is scaphoid; there are no masses or rigidity.

Always ask your client for the preferred format and style.

When transcribing physical examination reports, you should be prepared to write a tactful note to the physician or your supervisor if the dictator leaves out a vital part of the examination; for example, a hysterectomy is the contemplated procedure and the pelvic examination was not dictated. Be alert to laboratory values so that you recognize where a decimal point belongs when it is not dictated. (Laboratory values are given in Appendix B.) Critical thinking requires that you be alert and aware of the information you are transcribing to be sure that there are no omissions or inadvertent data. Some MTs have expressed a hesitancy to call a perceived error to the attention of the client or supervisor, in the misplaced notion that they cannot be so forward as to point this out. The opposite is true. It is hoped that you will not let something enter the record if there is any doubt of its accuracy.

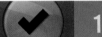 **12-3** REVIEW TEST

DIRECTIONS: Retype the following data into physical examination outline by using the run-on modified block format with no spacing between topics. Be alert to proper grammar and punctuation.

▸ This information is the physical examination for the patient, Geoffrey Paul Hawkins, in Self-Study 12-1.

The patient is a well developed, well nourished white male who appears his age of eleven and a half. He is of moderately small stature but is well tanned from being in the sun. He appears to be in no acute distress but is quite apprehensive. The skin is warm and dry, well tanned; no jaundice, no lesions. The pupils are round, regular and equal; react to light and accommodation. No icterus seen. Conjunctivae normal. Ears: drums pearly, hearing is good to spoken voice. Nose: septum straight. No lesions. The mouth and throat are benign. The tonsils are small and the teeth are in good repair. The neck is supple. The thyroid is not enlarged. There is no remarkable lymphadenopathy. Trachea is in the midline with no tug. The lungs are clear to percussion and auscultation. Heart: regular sinus rhythm, no murmurs heard. A2 is louder than P2. The abdomen is scaphoid with no scars. Patient indicates midepigastric tenderness. Peristalsis is audible and possibly slightly hyperactive but very close to average in intensity. There is some tenderness, mainly in the right upper quadrant. Both left and right lower quadrants appear to be soft with no rebound present. Equivocal Murphy punch tenderness is present. No CVA tenderness. Genitalia: Testes down, no penile lesions. Rectal: There is stool in the ampulla. Sphincter tone is good. Patient complains of some tenderness in both vaults, but no masses found. Skeletal: No gross bone or joint anomalies. Neurologic: No motor or sensory loss found. Deep tendon reflexes active and equal. Toe signs down. Pedal pulses palpable. Impression: Abdominal pain, etiology unproved, but probable gastroenteritis. Rule out early appendicitis.

12-4 REVIEW TEST

DIRECTIONS: Retype the following data into physical examination outline by using the basic block format. Be alert to proper grammar and punctuation. This patient, Joseph R. Balentine, is the one you had for Practice Test 12-2.

The patient is a well-developed, muscular, slightly pale young man in somewhat acute distress secondary to the apprehension and bleeding. Blood pressure is one hundred ten over seventy. Pulse is seventy four. Respirations are sixteen. HEENT: Head is normocephalic. Eyes are round, regular and equal and bilaterally react to light and accommodation. There is bilateral cerumen in the ears, TMs are normal. The right nasal cavity was somewhat congested to the nasopharynx. There is active bleeding from the left nasal cavity. There are no palpable nodes in the neck, and the thyroid is in the midline. The chest is symmetric; normal male breasts. The lungs are clear bilaterally, no rales or wheezes. There is a pneumonectomy scar, left anterolateral chest. The heart is normal in size. There is normal sinus rhythm, no murmurs, thrills, or rubs. The abdomen is soft, no tenderness. The rectal exam is deferred. The extremities are symmetrical, no cyanosis, edema, or deformities. There is normal range of motion. Reflexes are physiological. Pulses are two plus and equal bilaterally. There is no cranial or neurological deficit. The impression is left posterior epistaxis, recurrent.

12-5 PRACTICE TEST

DIRECTIONS: Retype the following data into correct H&P form. The patient is Lily Mae Jenkins, and the dictator is Philip D. Quince. He wants copies sent to Dr Willow Moran and Dr Gordon Bender. The patient's clinic number is 5980-A. Please use run-on basic block format and today's date. Be alert to proper grammar and punctuation.

The chief complaint is rectal bleeding, one day. Present illness: This ninety-year-old lady has been looking after her own personal affairs and living with her daughter for the last three years. Last night, she had a bowel movement that had some bright red blood mixed in with it. This morning, she had another bowel movement, and it consisted mostly of bright-red blood. She has a history of gallbladder disease, dating back over 50 years. She refused to have her gallbladder taken out but has been on a low fat diet ever since that time. Her daughter describes numerous gallbladder attacks, lasting for several days, consisting of severe, right upper quadrant pain. She has had occasional, intermittent right lower quadrant pain that does not seem similar to the gallbladder attacks. Past history: Operations: In 1997 she had enucleation of the left eye. She had surgery in 2005 for glaucoma in the right eye. Medical: 1986, Colles fracture, right wrist. 1990s severe arthritis of her spine. Medications: patient is presently taking Evista 60 mg per day, Plavix 75 mg every morning, Indocin, one tablet, t.i.d. She takes Bufferin p.r.n. for pain. She takes nitroglycerin two to three tablets a week for chest pain and has done so for five years. Both of her parents lived until their nineties. She had six children: one died at age three as the result of injuries sustained in an automobile accident; one died at age 56 of carcinoma of the breast. Otherwise, the family history is unremarkable. There are four children who are alive and well. Functional inquiry: HEENT: Hearing in her right ear is absent. Hearing in her left ear is decreased. There is an artificial eye in the left and there is only slight vision in her right eye if one comes exactly in the middle of her visual field. Patient has been edentulous for several years. Chest: Nonsmoker. CV: Patient has had angina for over five years and abnormal cardiograms for the last three. She is cold all of the time and is constantly bundling herself up in an effort to keep warm. GI: Her bowel movements have been normal. See history of present illness. GU: She has no history of any bladder or kidney infections, despite the fact that she had a history of kidney failure last year. NM: Patient has shooting, severe pains up her spine that are relatively incapaci-tating, but she manages to keep going by just taking Bufferin. Physical examination: This is a ninety year old black woman in no obvious distress, who is hard of hearing but can answer ques-tions. HEENT: The ears: There is wax in both ears. The drums, beyond the wax, appear within normal limits. There is no hearing in the right ear and only slight hearing in the left. The left eye is artificial. The right eye is pinpoint. There is no scarring in the right eye, consistent with an iridectomy. She has a cataract in the right eye, as well. Nose is unremarkable. Mouth is eden-tulous. Neck: There are no carotid bruits. No jugular venous distention. Thyroid is palpable and unremarkable. Range of motion of the neck is generally slightly restricted. Chest is clear to percussion and auscultation. Heart: The apical beat is not palpable. There is some tenderness over the costochondral cartilages on the left side. The heart size is not enlarged to percussion. There is muffled heart sound. There is no third or fourth heart sound. There are no murmurs heard in the supine position. Breasts are palpable and there are no masses noted. Abdomen is soft. There are marked senile keratoses over the abdominal wall. There is some diffuse tender-ness on deep palpation over the cecum in the right lower quadrant. There is no other tenderness noted or abnormal bowel sounds noted in the abdomen. Bowel sounds are within normal limits. Pelvic: Not done. Rectal: Full sigmoidoscopic examination to twenty five centimeters revealed fresh blood in the sigmoid area with no obvious bleeding source noted. Extremities: There is essentially no motion in the back. Range of motion of the hips is within normal limits and pain-less. There is only a plus one dorsalis pedis on the right; otherwise, there are no peripheral pulses present. There is marked coldness of both feet. Central nervous system: The patient's strength is within normal limits. The reflexes are within normal limits. Coordination is not tested. There is an involuntary shaking, consistent with the diagnosis of old Parkinson disease. Impression: Acute gastrointestinal hemorrhage, etiology not yet diagnosed. Chronic cholecystitis. Severe osteoarthritis of spine. Arteriosclerotic heart disease with angina pectoris.

See Appendix A, p. 457, for the proper response to this assignment.

12-6 SELF-STUDY

DIRECTIONS: Please answer the following questions by referring to the figures in this chapter. Answer here or on a separate sheet of paper as your instructor directs.

Using Figure 12-1

1. Under the subtopic "Allergies": why is "allergic to penicillin" typed in capital letters?

_____

2. Under the subtopic "Neurologic": what does "unremarkable" mean?

_____

3. Under "GI": why is "Present Illness" capitalized? _____

4. Under "OB-GYN": what does "climacteric" mean?

Using Figure 12-8

5. Under "Present Illness": why is "between the shoulder blades" set apart by a comma and a semicolon?

_____

6. Under "General": what does "afebrile" mean? _____

7. Under "Family History": what does it mean when it is said that "there is no family history of importance"?

_____

8. Under "HEENT": what does "L&A" mean? _____

9. Under "Neuromuscular": why did the MT not abbreviate that as "NM"?

_____

Using Figure 12-9

10. Under "Eyes": why is "sclerae" not written as "sclera," "fundi" not written as "fundus," and EOMs not written as "EOM" or "eom"?_____

_____

11. Under "Neurological": why are the Roman numerals used to describe the cranial nerves two through twelve?

_____

Using Figure 12-10

12. Under "Recommendation": why not use the standard abbreviation "T&A" instead of "tonsillectomy and adenoidectomy"? _____

Using Figures 12-1, 12-2, 12-3, and 12-4 (All Have Identical Material)

13. Which one is the most attractive? _____

14. Which one is easiest to read? _____

15. Which one was the easiest to type? (You have typed all three formats, and so you should have an opinion about this one, too.) _____

See Appendix A, p. 459, for the answers to these questions.

12-7 REVIEW TEST

DIRECTIONS: Retype the following data into correct H&P form. The patient is J. J. "Kip" Siegler. The physician is Felix Rios, MD. Use today's date and the format of your choice. Please indicate which format you have selected for your assignment by writing the name of the format on the top of your page.

The chief complaint is right-sided, abdominal pain, eight hours duration. The present illness is as follows: this is the first Brookside Hospital admission for this twenty-four year old unemployed carpenter who was in his usual state of excellent health until approximately eight hours prior to admission when he developed some high, transverse midepigastric abdominal pain following completion of a Chinese meal. The pain became progressively more intense and gradually, over the following four hours, localized in the right lower quadrant. One hour prior to admission, while preparing to come to the hospital, the patient had one episode of emesis. The patient denies any subsequent nausea and diarrhea but has been "constipated" for the past two days. The past medical history: Serious injuries: None. Surgery: None. Illnesses: None. Allergies: Assorted pollens, undetermined. Medications: None. Smoke: None. Alcohol: Very infrequently. Immunizations: None in the past four years. The father is deceased, age twenty-one, apparent suicide. The mother is living and well, age forty-one. One sister, age twenty-two, living and well. The patient is married and has one child and has been unemployed for the past six months. He spends most of his time refurbishing an old sailboat. Systemic review is unremarkable. On physical examination there is an alert, oriented Caucasian male in very mild abdominal distress, lying supine with his right hip flexed. His temperature is one hundred one point two degrees, pulse is eighty eight, respirations twenty, blood pressure is one hundred thirty over seventy eight. The skin is warm and moist without pallor, icterus, or cyanosis. There are no acute lesions or petechiae. Tympanic membranes are clear. Pupils are equal and reactive to light. Conjunctivae are mildly injected. Nares, likewise mildly injected. Pharynx and mouth, likewise, very minimally injected, without evidence of purulent debris. The neck is supple, without cervical adenopathy. The lungs are clear to auscultation and percussion. The heart rhythm is regular without murmurs or enlargement. The abdomen is somewhat protuberant with absent bowel sounds, with moderate tenderness and guarding in the right lower quadrant without rebound.

There is also very mild tenderness in the right "See vee a" area. There are no apparent herniae determined in the supine position. Rectal: Prostate is normal. There is moderate to exquisite tenderness in the right quadrant. Stool is brown, and HemeSelect is negative. Genitalia: Patient is circumcised. Testicles are bilaterally descended, appear normal in size and shape. Extremities: No deformities or edema. Neurologic: Deep tendon reflexes are two plus bilaterally. Diagnosis: Acute appendicitis.

Roland, Jamie T.
543098
June 8, 20XX

Copy: Robert R. Shoemaker, MD

SHORT-STAY RECORD

HISTORY:	Patient is a 6-year-old male complaining of frequent episodes of tonsillitis. He has missed several weeks of school this spring because of infections. He is a constant mouth breather.He snores loudly at night. He has constant nasal obstruction. There is no history of earaches.
PAST HISTORY:	There are no allergies. Bleeding history: None. Operations: None. Illnesses: None.Medications: Vitamins, iron. Has been on penicillin for resolution of symptoms. Family history: Noncontributory.

PHYSICAL EXAMINATION

SKIN:	No rashes.
EENT:	Ears: TMs and canals appeared normal. Nose: Congested posteriorly but not anteriorly. Throat: Very large cryptic tonsils meeting in the midline.
NECK:	Numerous palpable nodes.
CHEST:	Lungs: Clear to percussion and auscultation. Heart: Not enlarged; normal sinus rhythm; no murmurs.
ABDOMEN:	Soft, nontender.
EXTREMITIES:	Full range of motion.
NEUROLOGICAL:	Completely normal.
IMPRESSION:	Chronic hypertrophic tonsils and adenoids with recurrent infections.
RECOMMENDATION:	Tonsillectomy and adenoidectomy.

sd/321

_____
Dolores R. Nelson, MD

D: 06/08/20XX
T: 06/08/20XX

FIGURE 12-10 Example of a short-stay record transcribed in tabulated block format.

SHORT-STAY RECORD

When a patient is being sent to an outpatient surgical or diagnostic center, a shortened form of the H&P record is acceptable in most facilities. This form is appropriate for many diagnostic procedures and minor operative procedures. The statistical data would be the same as those required on the longer forms, but the description of the patient's condition and the physical examination report could be considerably condensed. Again, this document must be on the record before any procedures can begin.

Figure 12-11 is an example of a short-stay record set up in modified basic block format.

Roland, Jamie T.
54-30-98
June 8, 20XX

Copy: Robert R. Shoemaker, MD

SHORT-STAY RECORD

HISTORY
Patient is a 6-year-old male complaining of frequent episodes of tonsillitis. He has missed several weeks of school this spring because of infections. He is a constant mouth breather. He snores loudly at night. He has constant nasal obstruction. There is no history of earaches.

PAST HISTORY
There are no allergies. Bleeding history: None. Operations: None. Illnesses: None. Medications: Vitamins, iron. Has been on penicillin for resolution of symptoms. Family history: Noncontributory.

PHYSICAL EXAMINATION
SKIN: No rashes.
EENT: Ears: TMs and canals appeared normal. Nose: Congested posteriorly but not anteriorly. Throat: Very large cryptic tonsils meeting in the midline. Neck: Numerous palpable nodes.
CHEST: Lungs: Clear to percussion and auscultation. Heart: Not enlarged; normal sinus rhythm; no murmurs.
ABDOMEN: Soft, nontender.
EXTREMITIES: Full range of motion.
NEUROLOGICAL: Completely normal.

IMPRESSION: Chronic hypertrophic tonsils and adenoids with recurrent infections.

RECOMMENDATION: Tonsillectomy and adenoidectomy.

Dolores R. Nelson, MD

sd/321
D: 06/08/20XX
T: 06/08/20XX

FIGURE 12-11 Example of a short-stay record transcribed in modified basic block format.

INTERVAL HISTORY

If a patient returns to the hospital within a month of being discharged and has the same complaint, a complete H&P does not have to be written for the patient. However, an interval history (or interval note) is completed to describe what has happened to the patient since discharge. The complete statistical data are used, but the medical information is considerably briefer, with emphasis on the present complaint and interval history. The physical examination report would include any new findings since the previous examination and can include a brief check on vital body systems. A more extensive examination would be done in the area in which symptoms prompted the readmission to the hospital.

Figure 12-12 is an example of an interval history note.

Please go to Appendix C on Evolve and examine the variety of documents prepared as history and physical examinations.

Benita L. Martinez   March 17, 20XX
09-74-12
INTERVAL HISTORY

PRESENT COMPLAINT
This is a 45-year-old female who the 1st of March had a Roux-en-Y gastrojejunostomy done for a reflux bile gastritis. Postoperatively, she did moderately well; however, she began to evidence signs of anastomotic obstruction that got persistently worse. Upper GI series was done 4 days ago, which showed an almost complete obstruction of the anastomosis. Patient is now being admitted for decompression of her stomach and revision of the gastrojejunostomy.

PAST HISTORY
Regional family; see old chart.

PHYSICAL EXAMINATION
Well-developed, well-nourished, but nervous white female in no acute distress.

HEENT
Eyes: React to L&A. Ears: Canals and membranes normal. Nose: Negative.

NECK
Supple, with no masses, no enlargement of glands. Thyroid: Not palpable.

LUNGS
Clear to percussion and auscultation.

HEART
Rhythm and rate normal. No murmurs. No enlargements.

ABDOMEN
Recent bilateral, subcostal incision, well-healed. No other abdominal masses.

PELVIC
Not done.

EXTREMITIES
Negative.

IMPRESSION
Gastrojejunal anastomotic obstruction.

ADVICE
1. Decompression by Levin tube.
2. Re-resection and anastomose March 18, 20XX.

William B. Dixon, MD

mlo
D: 3/17/XX
T: 3/17/XX

FIGURE 12-12 Example of an interval history transcribed in basic block format.

12-8 REVIEW TEST

DIRECTIONS: You have the following material in a report titled *History and Physical*. Please write the name of the position in the report where that material would be transcribed. This position could be called the "title" of the paragraph involved.

EXAMPLE

The patient is a 32-year-old woman who is 5 feet 9 inches tall and weighs 297 pounds. The patient has been morbidly obese for several years and has tried to lose weight conservatively, and her efforts have failed.

Title: *Chief Complaint* or *History of Present Illness,* depending on what comes first.

1. clear to P&A, with no rales or wheezes

   Title: _____

2. 1+ protein and rare bacteria

   Title: _____

3. Soft, nontender, with no palpable mass and normal bowel sounds

   Title: _____

4. Scaphoid

   Title: _____

5. No rales, rhonchi, or extra sounds

   Title: _____

6. Trachea is midline; thyroid not palpable

   Title: _____

7. Symmetric deep tendon reflexes; cranial nerves and cerebellar examination intact

   Title: _____

8. Denies any history of diabetes mellitus or hypertension

   Title: _____

9. Does not smoke, drink, or use illicit drugs

   Title: _____

10. Her maternal grandmother has Reiter syndrome

    Title: _____

11. No JVD, carotid bruit, lymphadenopathy, or thyromegaly

    Title: _____

12. Alert, oriented times three

    Title: _____

13. Fracture, open, right mid femur

    Title: _____

14. Regular sinus rhythm

    Title: _____

15. Edentulous

Title: _____

16. Her first psychiatric treatment was in 1998 for depression

Title: _____

17. The patient reports that she was dizzy when she took Haldol

Title: _____

18. Noncontributory

Title: _____

19. Temperature 98.7, pulse 100, respiratory rate 18, blood pressure 128/98

Title: _____

20. Deferred

Title: _____

21. TMs intact

Title: _____

22. No rashes

Title: _____

23. Vitamins, iron. Has been on penicillin for resolution of symptoms

Title: _____

24. Full range of motion

Title: _____

25. No nocturia, dysuria, splitting or deviation of the stream

Title: _____

★ 12-9 FINAL REVIEW

DIRECTIONS: You hear this dictation at the end of your H&P. Please transcribe it properly. Be careful to check the spelling and capitalization of the drug names as well as the dosages dictated; there are three errors to correct.

Current medications topamax two hundred milligrams twice a day depakote five hundred milligrams twice a day dalmane thirty milligrams at bedtime risperdal twenty two milligrams three at bedtime tegretol two hundred milligrams three times a day verapamil one hundred twenty milligrams halftablet twice a day zebeta five milligrams half tablet twice a day singular ten milligrams once a day protonix forty milligrams once a day provera two point five milligrams once a day premarin one point two five milligrams once a day allegra ten milligrams once a day nasonex spray "pee-are-en" atrovent two puffs three times a day

12

CHAPTER

CHAPTER 13

Preparation of Miscellaneous Medical Reports

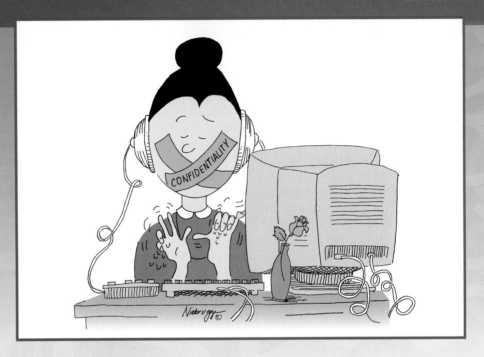

OBJECTIVES

After reading this chapter and completing the exercises, you should be able to

1. Identify the kind of information that appears in various medical reports.
2. Prepare a discharge summary, operative report, pathology report, radiology report, consultation report, autopsy protocol, and medicolegal report.
3. Know how to find acceptable formats for a variety of reports and medical documents.
4. Recognize the usefulness of a standard macro within a document.
5. Recognize the names of operative procedures, instruments, types of anesthesia, and suture materials, and be familiar with how these terms should be transcribed.
6. Identify any missing documentation that is required in a complete report.

INTRODUCTION

This chapter continues instruction for the preparation of "the basic four": the history and physical examination (H&P) report (see Chapter 12), operative report, consultation report, and discharge summary. These as well as a variety of other patient reports are transcribed by medical transcriptionists (MTs) or editors for the hospital or the facility or service contracted by the hospital. Occasionally, a physician wants the MT who works for the office or clinic to transcribe some of these reports; in some medical facilities, the department MT transcribes the documents for that department only. For example, the pathology department could have laboratory reports and autopsy reports transcribed in the department. Consultation reports could be transcribed in the hospital or physician's office, and medicolegal reports are usually done by the private medical office MT or transcription service employed. Some services hire MTs with a legal background, as well as a medical background, and they specialize in transcription of medicolegal reports. Private transcription agencies are prepared to transcribe a variety of medical documents. Because you do not know where you will seek employment, it is important for you to be prepared to transcribe the many different types of medical reports with various requirements.

With proper consents and authorizations, reports are sent to consultants who participated in the management of the patient, to insurance companies who want background information on patients, to third-party carriers for claims reimbursement, to referring physicians, and to the Social Security Administration to assess a patient for total disability.

Accuracy and readability are the most important factors emphasized in reference to format. All headings and subheadings must follow the same format; therefore, it is important to determine how you will set up the report before you begin. Topics of equal importance are given equal emphasis through the use of capital letters, lowercase letters, spacing, centering, and so on. The figures in this chapter give you a glimpse of possible headings; each physician/dictator/client chooses different words to emphasize. The sequence of the topic words may also be reversed in some dictations. The general guideline is to transcribe exactly the sequence that is dictated and to determine the words requiring the most emphasis for major headings and those requiring less emphasis for subheadings. In some institutions, forms with preprinted headings necessitate that you reformat the dictation so that it is typed in the sequence given on the forms. In Appendix C on Evolve, there is an operational policy for individuals to consult when they select a format (see Figure C-44). As mentioned in previous chapters, various professional groups have joined in an effort to standardize report formats.

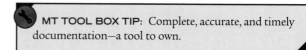

MT TOOL BOX TIP: Complete, accurate, and timely documentation—a tool to own.

DISCHARGE SUMMARIES

A discharge summary (clinical resumé or final progress note) is required for each patient discharged from a hospital and must be completed within 30 days of patient discharge. It contains some of the same information found in the patient's H&P report with the addition of the reason for admission, clearly stated admitting and discharge diagnoses, operations performed, significant findings including laboratory and x-ray studies, consultations, hospital course, and condition of the patient on discharge, including medications with dose and frequency, instructions for continuing care and therapy, possible complications that may occur, and possibly a date for a followup office visit. The condition of the patient on discharge should be stated in terms that enable a specific measurable comparison with the condition on admission; the use of vague terminology such as "improved" should be avoided. If a resident or intern (house staff physician) dictates the discharge summary, it is usually approved by the attending physician (attending staff physician). They need not be too long but should be complete enough to fully justify diagnoses. The discharge summary may affect many areas of the hospital including the revenue cycle management, compliance, and continuity of care. If the patient or a legally qualified representative has provided written authorization, a copy of the discharge summary should be sent to any known medical practitioner or medical facility responsible for followup care of the patient. Often, discharge summaries for patients being transferred are transcribed on a STAT basis. If STAT material is processed at an offsite location, a facsimile is placed with the medical record and is replaced with the original report when the original is delivered to the facility. One of the advantages of the use of the electronic medical record is that the document is available for immediate use. Upon their request, patients can be provided with a copy of their discharge instructions and procedures at the time of discharge. Just being aware of the requirements of the discharge summary will alert the MT to oversee the completed version and alert the QA supervisor if it does not contain vital components.

In the case of a patient's death, a summary statement should be added to the record either as a final progress note or as a separate resumé. This final note should give the reason for admission, findings and

Evans, Cornelia Elizabeth
97-32-11
July 16, 20XX

DISCHARGE SUMMARY

ADMISSION DATE: June 14, 20XX   DISCHARGE DATE: July 15, 20XX

HISTORY OF PRESENT ILLNESS
This 19-year-old black female nulligravida was admitted to the hospital on June 14, 200X, with fever of 102°, left lower quadrant pain, vaginal discharge, constipation, and a tender left adnexal mass. Her past history and family history were unremarkable. Present pain had started 2 to 3 weeks prior to admission. Her periods were irregular, with the latest period starting on May 30, 20XX, and lasting for 6 days. She had taken contraceptive pills in the past but had stopped because she was not sexually active.

PHYSICAL EXAMINATION
She appeared well developed and well nourished and in mild distress. The only positive physical findings were limited to the abdomen and pelvis. Her abdomen was mildly distended, and it was tender, especially in the left lower quadrant. At pelvic examination, the cervix was tender on motion, and the uterus was of normal size, retroverted, and somewhat fixed. There was a tender cystic mass, about 4 to 5 cm, in the left adnexa. Rectal examination was negative.

ADMITTING DIAGNOSES
Probable pelvic inflammatory disease (PID).
Rule out ectopic pregnancy.

LABORATORY DATA ON ADMISSION
Hemoglobin 8.8, hematocrit 26.5, WBC 8100 with 80 segs and 18 lymphs. Sedimentation rate 100 mm in 1 hour. Sickle cell prep+ (turned out to be a trait). Urinalysis normal. Electrolytes normal. SMA-12 normal. Chest x-ray negative. A 2-hour UCG negative.

HOSPITAL COURSE AND TREATMENT
Initially, she was given cephalothin 2 g IV q.6 h. and kanamycin 0.5 g 1M b.i.d. Over the next 2 days, the patient's condition improved. Her pain decreased, and her temperature came down to normal in the morning and spiked to 101° in the evening. Repeat CBC showed hemoglobin 7.8, hematocrit 23.5. The pregnancy test was negative. On the 2nd night following admission, she spiked to 104°. The patient was started on antituberculosis treatment consisting of isoniazid 300 mg per day, ethambutol 600 mg b.i.d., and rifampin 600 mg daily. She became afebrile on the 6th postoperative day and was discharged on July 15, 20XX, in good condition. She will be seen in the office in 1 week.

SURGICAL PROCEDURES
Biopsy of omentum for frozen section; culture specimens.

DISCHARGE DIAGNOSIS
Genital tuberculosis.

Harold B. Cooper, MD

amd
D:7/15/20XX
T:7/16/20XX

FIGURE 13-1 Discharge summary, basic block format. (Under *ADMITTING DIAGNOSES*, "PID" was dictated, and the MT spelled out the diagnosis and put the abbreviation in parentheses.)

hospital course, events leading to the patient's death, details of the patient's condition prior to death, and time of death.

Figures 13-1 and 13-2 are examples of complete discharge summaries, showing appearance, formats, and content. The formats discussed follow those illustrated in detail in Chapter 12. See p. 351 for a brief synopsis of the three basic report styles. You can always return to Chapter 12 if you want a more detailed outline. However, with the experience you gained in that chapter, you probably will only need to examine the

figures in this chapter and Appendix C on Evolve to prepare your assignments.

OPERATIVE REPORTS

Whenever a surgical procedure is performed in the hospital, an outpatient surgical center, or a clinic, an operative report should be dictated to the medical record immediately after surgery. The following is the transcription platform screen shot of an operative report:

Transcription platform for operative report. (Courtesy of 3M Health Information Systems, Inc. © 3M. All rights reserved.)

The parts of the report are dictated in sequential order:

1. Preoperative diagnosis(es)
2. Postoperative diagnosis(es)
3. Name of procedure(s)
4. Name of surgeon(s)
5. Name of assistant(s), if any.

The report should contain a description of findings, technical procedures used, and specimens removed. If the postoperative diagnosis is the same as the preoperative diagnosis, repeat the preoperative diagnosis exactly. (Frequently the dictator will say "same" for the postoperative diagnosis. The word "same" is not transcribed; the preoperative diagnosis is transcribed again after the words *Postoperative diagnosis*).

The body of the report is a narrative of the procedure details and findings and contains the type of anesthetic, incision, instruments used, drains, packs, closure, sponge count, tissue removed or altered, materials removed or inserted, blood loss and replacement, wound status, complications or unusual events, and condition of the patient on leaving the surgical area. The completed operative report must be authenticated by the surgeon either with a manual or electronic signature and filed in the medical record as soon as possible after surgery. When a delay in transcription or filing occurs, a comprehensive operative progress note should be entered in the medical record immediately after surgery to provide pertinent information for other physicians who attend the patient. If a patient requires additional surgery after the initial surgery has been completed, the report can be transcribed on a STAT basis.

See Figure 13-3, *A,* and figure above for examples of operative reports. Notice in Figure 13-3 that the first paragraph is one long paragraph. Although this format seems awkward, this is how many surgeons dictate their operative records. However, some hospitals require that surgeons separate the report into subheadings, such as *Anesthesia, Incision, Findings, Procedure, Closure,* and so on. In designating suture material size, see Chapter 5, Rule 5.18. Figure 13-3, *B,* illustrates another format for an operative report with a slight variation in style. See Appendix C on Evolve for examples of additional variations in format. Operative reports are more difficult to transcribe than other documents because of the thousands of procedures that are performed, the many instruments named during the procedure, the types and names of suture materials, the placement (position) of the patient on the operating table, the type and substance used for anesthesia, and the types of incisions and closures made. The format itself for this document is simple and straightforward (Figure 13-4).

PATHOLOGY REPORTS

As an MT, you can specialize by typing pathology or radiology reports. Pathology MTs work in laboratories, hospital medical laboratories, and coroners' offices. A variety of job duties other than transcription

---

COLLEGE MEDICAL CENTER

1000 North Main Street · College Town, XY 12345-0001· PHONE: (013} 123-4567 FAX: (013) 130-4599

DISCHARGE SUMMARY

DATE OF ADMISSION: July 9, 20XX   DATE OF DISCHARGE: July 15, 20XX

ADMITTING DIAGNOSES
1. Pneumonia.
2. Hypertension.
3. History of congestive heart failure.
4. Menopause.

BRIEF HISTORY
This is a 67-year-old woman with a complaint of chest tightness who was seen at Smith-Davis Urgent Care and was found to have bilateral pneumonia and hypoxemia. The patient was subsequently transferred to College Medical for admission.

HOSPITAL COURSE
The patient was admitted and placed on antibiotics and oxygen supplement. The patient improved, showing gradual resolution of hypoxemia. The patient was discharged in stable condition.

DISCHARGE DIAGNOSES
1. Pneumonia.
2. Hypertension.
3. History of congestive heart failure.
4. Menopause.

PROGNOSIS
Good. Discharged on medications. Ceftin 125 mg b.i.d. for 7 days. The patient is to follow up with Dr Darnell in one week.

Raul Garcia, MD

RG:mlt
D: 7/15/20XX
T: 7/15/20XX

DISCHARGE SUMMARY

PT. NAME:	MONTEZ, MARIA LOUISE
IDNO:	IT-890480 598
ROOM NO:	598
ATTENDING:	RAUL GARCIA, MD

FIGURE 13-2 Discharge summary, basic block format. The bottom of the report illustrates the method used at some hospitals to insert the patient's identifying data.

exist: giving reports via the telephone; filing; retrieving diagnoses from *Systematized Nomenclature of Human and Veterinary Medicine (SNOMED) International, Current Procedural Terminology (CPT),* and *International Classification of Diseases, Tenth Revision, Clinical Modification (ICD-10-CM)* coding; keeping tumor and autopsy logs; typing statistical reports; delivering reports; sorting and delivering mail; labeling and filing specimens; maintaining cross files; preparing procedure manuals throughout the laboratory; and performing other miscellaneous laboratory tasks, depending on the size of the workplace and the number of pathologists on the staff. Some of the departments in the laboratory include histology, chemistry, hematology, microbiology/bacteriology, immunology, and blood bank. Pathology consists of two divisions: anatomical (surgical and autopsy) and clinical (blood bank, microbiology, hematology, and chemistry).

When a surgical procedure is performed to remove tissue or fluid from the body, the pathologist could examine these specimens to determine the nature and extent of the disease. In some instances, a pathologist renders his or her opinion before the sutures are placed, as in the event of a malignant tumor, in which case more extensive surgery may be required. This tissue examination, or biopsy report, is called a *pathology*

Patient: Elaine J. Silverman Hospital Number 84-32-11
Room Number: 1308
Date: June 20, 20XX

OPERATIVE REPORT

PREOPERATIVE DIAGNOSES

1. Menorrhagia.
2. Chronic pelvic inflammatory disease.
3. Perineal relaxation.

POSTOPERATIVE DIAGNOSES

1. Menorrhagia.
2. Chronic pelvic inflammatory disease.
3. Perineal relaxation.

OPERATION

1. Total abdominal hysterectomy.
2. Lysis of pelvic adhesions.
3. Bilateral salpingo-oophorectomy.
4. Appendectomy.
5. Posterior colpoplasty.

PROCEDURE

Under general anesthesia, the patient was prepared and draped for abdominal operation. The abdomen was opened through a Pfannenstiel incision, and examination of the upper abdomen was entirely normal. Examination of the pelvis revealed an enlarged uterus. The uterus was 3 degrees retroverted and adhered to the cul-de-sac. Both tubes and ovaries were involved in an inflammatory mass, with extensive adhesions to the lateral pelvic wall on both sides. The tubes revealed evidence of chronic pelvic inflammatory disease. The omentum was also attached to the fundus and to the left adnexa. The omentum was dissected by means of blunt and sharp dissection; the dissection was carried to each adnexa, freeing both tubes and ovaries by means of blunt and sharp dissection. The uterus was found to be approximately 2 times enlarged after freeing all the adhesions. The uterovesical fold of peritoneum was then incised in an elliptical manner, bladder was dissected off the lower uterine segment. The round ligament and the infundibulopelvic ligament on each side were identified, clamped, cut, and ligated. The uterine artery on each side was clamped, cut, and doubly ligated. Paracervical fascia was developed. Heaney clamps were placed on the cardinal ligaments, and the cardinal ligaments were cut, and the pedicles ligated. The vagina was circumscribed; the uterus, both tubes, and ovaries were removed from the operative field. The cardinal ligaments were then sutured into the lateral angles of the vagina by means of interrupted sutures; the vagina was then closed with continuous over-and-over sutures. The paracervical fascia was sutured into place with interrupted figure-of-eight suture; the lateral suture incorporated the stumps of the uterine arteries; the pelvis was then reperitonealized with a continuous length of GI 2-0 atraumatic suture. Appendix was identified, and appendectomy was done in the usual manner. The appendiceal stump was cauterized with phenol and neutralized with alcohol. Re-examination of the pelvis at this time revealed all bleeding well controlled. The abdominal wall was then closed in layers, and the skin was approximated with camelback clips. During the procedure, the patient received 1 unit of blood. Patient was then prepared for vaginal surgery.

Patient was placed in lithotomy position, prepared, and draped. Posterior colpoplasty was begun for repair of rectocele and perineal relaxation. The posterior vaginal mucosa was dissected from the perirectal fascia; the excess posterior vaginal mucosa was excised, and the perirectal fascia was brought together with continuous interlocking suture of 0 chromic. The posterior vaginal mucosa was closed with continuous interlocking suture of 0 chromic. Perineal body was closed with subcutaneous subcuticular stitch. There was a correct sponge count. The patient withstood the operation well. Patient left the operating room in good condition.

Harold B. Cooper, MD

ftr
D: 6-20 20XX
T: 6-22-20XX

FIGURE 13-3 A, Operative report, basic block format.

Patient: Elaine J. Silverman
Hospital Number 84-32-11

Date: June 20, 200X
Room Number: 1308

OPERATIVE REPORT

PREOPERATIVE DIAGNOSES:
1. Menorrhagia
2. Chronic pelvic inflammatory disease
3. Perineal relaxation

POSTOPERATIVE DIAGNOSES:
1. Menorrhagia
2. Chronic pelvic inflammatory disease
3. Perineal relaxation

OPERATION:
1. Total abdominal hysterectomy
2. Lysis of pelvic adhesions
3. Bilateral salpingo-oophorectomy
4. Appendectomy
5. Posterior colpoplasty

PROCEDURE: Under general anesthesia, the patient was prepared and draped for abdominal operation. The abdomen was opened through a Pfannenstiel incision, and examination of the upper abdomen was entirely normal. Examination of the pelvis revealed an enlarged uterus. The uterus was 3 degrees retroverted and adhered to the cul-de-sac. Both tubes and ovaries were involved in an inflammatory mass, with extensive adhesions to the lateral pelvic wall on both sides. The tubes revealed evidence of chronic pelvic inflammatory disease. The omentum was also attached to the fundus and to the left adnexa. The omentum was dissected by means of blunt and sharp dissection; the dissection was carried to each adnexa, freeing both tubes and ovaries by means of blunt and sharp dissection. The uterus was found to be approximately 2 times enlarged after freeing all the adhesions. The uterovesical fold of peritoneum was then incised in an elliptical manner, bladder was dissected off the lower uterine segment. The round ligament and the infundibulopelvic ligament on each side were identified, clamped, cut, and ligated. The uterine artery on each side was clamped, cut, and doubly ligated. Paracervical fascia was developed. Heaney clamps were placed on the cardinal ligaments, and the cardinal ligaments were cut, and the pedicles ligated. The vagina was circumscribed; the uterus, both tubes, and ovaries were removed from the operative field. The cardinal ligaments were then sutured into the lateral angles of the vagina by means of interrupted sutures; the vagina was then closed with continuous over-and-over sutures. The paracervical fascia was sutured into place with interrupted figure-of-eight suture; the lateral suture incorporated the stumps of the uterine arteries; the pelvis was then reperitonealized with a continuous length of GI 2-0 atraumatic suture. Appendix was identified, and appendectomy was done in the usual manner. The appendiceal stump was cauterized with phenol and neutralized with alcohol. Re-examination of the pelvis at this time revealed all bleeding well controlled. The abdominal wall was then closed in layers, and the skin was approximated with camelback clips. During the procedure, the patient received 1 unit of blood. Patient was then prepared for vaginal surgery.

Patient was placed in lithotomy position, prepared, and draped. Posterior colpoplasty was begun for repair of rectocele and perineal relaxation. The posterior vaginal mucosa was dissected from the perirectal fascia; the excess posterior vaginal mucosa was excised, and the perirectal fascia was brought together with continuous interlocking suture of 0 chromic. The posterior vaginal mucosa was closed with continuous interlocking suture of 0 chromic. Perineal body was closed with subcutaneous subcuticular stitch. There was a correct sponge count. The patient withstood the operation well. Patient left the operating room in good condition.

Harold B. Cooper, MD

ftr
D: 6-20-20XX
T: 6-22-20XX

College Park Hospital
321 College Park Circle
Woods Creek, XX 98765

FIGURE 13-3, cont'd B, Operative report, variation on basic block.

report or *tissue report* (Figure 13-5). It consists of a *gross description* of the specimen submitted, which means the way the specimen looks to the naked eye before the specimen is prepared for microscopic study. The *microscopic description* is the description of the tissue after it has been prepared and carefully examined under the microscope. The *diagnosis* is then given. Often, the gross descriptions *(grosses)* of all of the surgical specimens are dictated, transcribed, and given to the pathologist, who then dictates the microscopic descriptions *(micros)*. These are transcribed, and the completed pathology reports are given to the pathologist for

TUFTS MEDICAL CENTER OUTPATIENT CARE

PATIENT: Ouddy, Busaba
DATE: 11/15/XX
SURGEON: Henry D. Sousa, DPM
ANESTHESIOLOGIST: Jeffrey B. Morgan, MD
ANESTHESIA: 10 mL of equally mixed 2% Xylocaine plain and 0.5% Marcaine plain.
PROCEDURE TIME: The operation began at 0730 and ended at 0815.

OPERATIVE REPORT

PREOPERATIVE DIAGNOSIS: Hallux limitus, right foot.
POSTOPERATIVE DIAGNOSIS: Hallux limitus, right foot.
OPERATION PERFORMED: Cheilectomy, first metatarsophalangeal joint, right foot.

OPERATIVE TECHNIQUE IN DETAIL: The patient was brought to the operating room and placed in the supine position. Anesthesia was achieved with the use of the aforementioned anesthesia distributed in a Mayo block to the right foot. Following sterile preparation, application of Betadine solution, and sterile draping, with hemostasis obtained by the placement of a tourniquet to the level of the ankle and inflated to 250 mmHg, the following surgical procedures were performed: A linear incision was placed on the dorsal aspect of the right foot medial to the extensor hallucis longus tendon. This incision began proximally at the mid shaft of the first metatarsal and extended distally to the midshaft of the first proximal phalanx. The wound edges were underscored, and all vital structures were retracted. Superficial bleeders were coagulated with the use of a Bovie unit. The incision was deepened via anatomical dissection to the level of the capsule and periosteal structures about the first metatarsophalangeal joint. Using an incision that paralleled the initial skin incision, the capsule and periosteal structures were dissected free, delivering the dorsal exostosis that was located on the first metatarsal and proximal phalanx into the surgical site. At this time, the first metatarsophalangeal joint was inspected, and there were free-floating ossicles that were excised from the wound sites. The cartilage was noted to have central erosions located on both the head of the first metatarsal and base of the proximal phalanx. The bony exostosis that was present on the medial dorsolateral aspect of the first metatarsal head and base of the proximal phalanx were resected entirely. The surgical site was then flushed with copious amounts of sterile saline, inspected, and found to be free of debris. The hypertropic synovium was then excised. The surgical site was then freed further with the use of a scoop. The surgical site was then flushed again with copious amounts of sterile saline, inspected, and found to be free of debris. The surgical site was then remodeled to make a more normal-appearing metatarsal head and base of the proximal phalanx. The surgical site was then again flushed with copious amounts of sterile saline, inspected, and found to be free of debris. The patient was then placed through a range of motion and was noted to have 70 degrees of motion at the time of the surgical procedure. This was in comparison to 40 degrees preoperatively, with the last 15 degrees of that 40 degrees being painful. The surgical site was then reapposed with the periosteum and capsular structures closed via 3-0 PDS. The subcutaneous tissues were closed in layers using simple interrupted sutures of 4-0 Vicryl. The skin edges were reapposed using subcutaneous stitching of 4-0 Prolene. The surgical site was then further maintained using tincture of benzoin and Steri-Strips. The surgical site was then covered with a dry, sterile dressing consisting of Adaptic, 3 x 3 Huffs, and a 3-inch roll of Kling. Tourniquet was released. Capillary filling time was noted to return to digits 1 through 5 on the right foot within normal limits. Prior to application of the dressing, 1 mL of Soluspan was injected into the surgical site. Dressing was further maintained using 3-inch Coban.

Patient tolerated surgical procedure well and left the operating room with vital signs stable.

HENRY D. SOUSA, DPM
reo
D: 11|15/XX
T: 11|15/XX

FIGURE 13-4 Operative report, modified block run-on format. Note that the dictator is a podiatrist.

signature. A copy of the report is given to each physician involved in the case, and a copy is retained in the laboratory. The original is placed in the patient's medical record.

In addition to tissue and tumor reports, a pathology MT may type second-opinion reports, fine-needle aspiration reports, muscle biopsy reports, renal biopsy reports, bone marrow examination reports, autopsy reports, forensic reports, and coroner reports. Pathology reports must be completed within 24 hours.

Pathologists usually dictate in the present tense because they interpret the pathologic findings as they look at the specimen. The history is in past tense, and the findings are in present tense. Each dictation includes certain headings, but the headings are not always used and are not always in the same sequence.

In pathology dictation, it is often the nonmedical term that puzzles the novice MT because it can be difficult to understand the mechanics behind the dictated words. A common phrase encountered and

```
                    College Hospital
             2345 College Hospital Boulevard
                  Wood Creek, XX 98765

                   PATHOLOGY REPORT

Date:  June 20, 20XX
Patient: Elaine J. Silverman
Room No. 130S

Physician: Harold B. Cooper, MD

Pathology No. 430211

SPECIMEN SUBMITTED
Tumor, right axilla.

GROSS DESCRIPTION
Specimen A consists of an oval mass of yellow fibroadipose tissue measuring 4 x 3 x 2 cm. On cut section, there
are some small, soft, pliable areas of gray apparent lymph node alternating with adipose tissue. A frozen section
consultation at time of surgery was delivered as NO EVIDENCE OF MALIGNANCY on frozen section, to await
permanent section for final diagnosis. Majority of the specimen will be submitted for microscopic examination.

Specimen B consists of an oval mass of yellow soft tissue measuring 2.5 x 2.5 x 1.5 cm. On cut section, there is a
thin rim of pink to tan-brown lymphatic tissue and the mid portion appears to be adipose tissue. A pathological
consultation at time of surgery was delivered as no suspicious areas noted and to await permanent sections for
final diagnosis. The entire specimen will be submitted for microscopic examination.

RTW:wfr

MICROSCOPIC DESCRIPTION

Specimen A sections show fibroadipose tissue and nine fragments of lymph nodes. The lymph nodes show areas
with prominent germinal centers and moderate sinus histiocytosis. There appears to be some increased
vascularity and reactive endothelial cells seen. There is no evidence of malignancy.

Specimen B sections show adipose tissue and 5 lymph node fragments. These 5 portions of lymph nodes show
reactive changes including sinus histiocytosis. There is no evidence of malignancy.

DIAGNOSIS

A & B: TUMOR, RIGHT AXILLA: SHOWING 14 LYMPH NODE FRAGMENTS WITH REACTIVE
CHANGES AND NO EVIDENCE OF MALIGNANCY.




Shirlely T. Nason, MD

STN:wrf
D:  6-18-20XX
T:  6-18-20XX
```

FIGURE 13-5 Pathology report, basic block format.

typed incorrectly is "The specimen is submitted in toto." This statement means that the entire specimen is submitted by the pathologist for further processing. Because many pathologic terms cannot be found in standard references, always obtain a good word reference book or pathology/laboratory medicine dictionary if a great deal of your transcription deals with pathology. Macros of standard dictated material are very useful in this specialty. See Appendix C on Evolve for some examples.

RADIOLOGY AND IMAGING REPORTS

As mentioned previously, another way of specializing is to become a radiology MT for a group of radiologists or for the radiology department in a hospital.

An x-ray report (Figure 13-6) is a description of the findings and interpretations of the radiologist who reviews the x-ray films taken of a patient. These can be bone and joint films, soft tissue films, or special studies

College Hospital
4567 Broad Avenue
Woodland Hills, XY 12345

Radiology Report

Examination Date:	June 14, 20XX	Patient Name:	Elaine J. Silverman
Date Reported:	June 14, 20XX	X-ray No.:	43200
Physician:	Harold B. Cooper, MD	Age:	19
Examination:	PA Chest, Abdomen	Hospital No.:	80-32-11

FINDINGS

PA CHEST: Upright PA view of chest shows the lung fields are clear, without evidence of an active process. Heart size is normal.

There is no evidence of pneumoperitoneum.

IMPRESSION: NEGATIVE CHEST.

ABDOMEN: Flat and upright views of the abdomen show a normal gas pattern without evidence of obstruction or ileus. There are no calcifications or abnormal masses noted.

IMPRESSION: NEGATIVE STUDY.

Radiologist _____
                          Marian B. Skinner, MD

wpd
D: 06-14-XX
T: 06-14-XX

FIGURE 13-6 Radiology report, tabulated block format.

of the internal organs that require the patient to take contrast medium (dye) orally or by injection. The contrast medium is radiolucent (permitting the passage of some roentgen rays) or radiopaque (not permitting the passage of roentgen rays). For assistance in spelling the types of contrast media, refer to the back of the current *Physicians' Desk Reference (PDR),* which has a comprehensive reference list. An examination of an organ with radioactive isotopes is called a *scan.* Radiologists' reports may change from present to past tense within the body of a document. As a rule, the procedure was performed (past tense), and the findings are given in the present tense. At some facilities, each physician has a set of normal phrases or paragraphs saved electronically in the form of macros or normals. The physician may choose to dictate the radiologic examination and say, "Add note N1," or "Use my normal chest" to access one of these phrases; if necessary, the phrase can be edited, depending on the case dictated.

Technology has produced methods to view structures in dimension (stereoscopy) or in layers (tomography). Through the use of x-rays with computers, a specific slice of the abdomen, chest, or head can be seen; this imaging technique is called *computed tomography* (CT) or *CT scanning.* A process for measuring temperature by photographically recording infrared radiations emanating from the surface of the body is called *thermography.* Use of high-frequency sound waves without the use of x-rays can give a composite picture of an area; the image is called a *sonogram* or an *echogram.* A system that produces sectional images of the body without the use of x-rays is *magnetic resonance imaging* (MRI), also called *nuclear magnetic resonance* (NMR) *imaging* (Figure 13-7). In this method, a band of radio frequencies and a range of magnetic field strengths are used, so that information is obtained simultaneously from a large number of points in a volume. The information is processed by a computer with the use of mathematical techniques similar to those used to form CT images.

Some facilities provide radiotherapy for treatment or palliation of malignant tumors, so radiotherapy summaries become part of the patient's medical record. Nuclear medicine diagnostic and therapeutic procedures require reports (Figure 13-8) stating the interpretations, consultation, and therapy (e.g., specific preparation of the patient, identity, date, and amount of radiopharmaceutical used).

The radiology report provides preliminary information and the type of x-ray films taken or the x-ray examination performed for example; "Chest x-ray, PA and lateral," at the top of the report. To avoid confusion, the date in the heading should reflect the date of service rather than the date of dictation. Dictation and transcription dates are best placed at the end of the

GrandView Magnetic Imaging Center
4500 River Road
Center City, XY 12345
(813) 647-0980

INTERPRETATION

PATIENT: Jeffrey P. Clauson   AGE: 27
NUMBER: 430-34-1276   DATE: August 30, 20XX

MAGNETIC RESONANCE IMAGING, CERVICAL SPINE

HISTORY
Cervical radiculopathy

TECHNIQUE
Sag. GE 600/30/23. MR, 43 Nex, 5 mm, CC.
Sag. SE 500/24. MR, 4 Nex, 5 mm, CC.
Ax. SE 1000/30. HR, 2 Nex, 5 mm, CC.

FINDINGS
The sagittal sequences cover from the lower posterior fossa to approximately T4-5. The axial sequence covered from the upper odontoid process through mid T1.

There is mild reversal of normal lordotic curve of the cervical spine.

The C2-3 and C3-4 interspaces are normal.

There is posterior osteophyte formation projecting broadly across the anterior aspect of the spinal canal at C4-5 level. On the sagittal sequences, this appears to contact the cord. There is no deformity identified with the cord to indicate compression. The foramina are patent.

The C5-6 level is unremarkable aside from some narrowing of the anterior subarachnoid space, probably a result of mild spurring and the effect of the reversal of the normal lordotic curve.

At C6-7 there are degenerative disk changes with disk space narrowing and osteophyte formation. There is no cord compression, although there is moderate left foraminal stenosis.

The C7-T1 level demonstrates moderate left foraminal stenosis.

There is either spur or disk bulge at the T1-2 level This was only seen on the sagittal sequences. The abnormality appears to contact the cord but does not appear to cause any compression. There are no additional extradural abnormalities. There are no intradural extramedullary lesions. The cord is normal without abnormal intensity to indicate the presence of infarction or mass, and there is no evidence of a syrinx. This is mentioned in that the cerebellar tonsils project somewhat below the foramen magnum indicating the possibility of a Chiari II malformation.

IMPRESSION

CEREBRAL SPONDYLOSIS AS DESCRIBED ABOVE. PROBABLE CHIARI II MALFORMATION. NO CORD SYRINX.

Jason B. Iverson, MD
rmt

FIGURE 13-7 Magnetic resonance imaging (MRI) report, run-on block format.

report. The date in the heading is followed by the number and type of views taken and any special circumstances that could affect the examination: for example, whether the patient is fasting for a bowel study. Views obtained in addition to what is usual for a given study should be noted. Documentation should also include the quality of the study (*clear* or *blurry*), positive findings *(abnormal)*, negative findings *(normal)*, incidental findings in other areas of the film, the radiologist's impression or interpretation and diagnosis, recommendations for additional studies or treatment, and the signature of the radiologist. Several x-ray examinations can be described in the same report. Radiology reports should be incorporated into the patient's medical record for use if the physician needs to prove that the study was medically necessary. Radiology examinations must be documented in sufficient detail to justify reimbursement.

College Grove Hospital
4567 City College Avenue
Canyon Rim, XY 12345

RADIATION THERAPY CONSULTATION

Name: Theodore V. Valdez
Room #499
MR#380780

Requested by: John L. Morris, MD

Date: 6/15/20XX

HISTORY OF PRESENT MEDICAL ILLNESS: This is a 72-year-old who underwent decompressive laminectomy and Harrington rod placement in 2004 for angiosarcoma. Postoperative radiation therapy at St. Mary's Hospital: 4025 cGy[1] in 23 fractions (175 cGy), 4 treatments per week, 2 to 1 PA to AP portals measuring 13 x 9 cm at 100 SSD on 8 Mv Linac, 5 HVL cord block at 3000 cGy. Dr Davis estimates coverage T2 to T8. Myelogram and CT scan negative 2 years ago. However, developed cough and hemoptysis in past month. Chest x-ray and CT: Right perihilar mass extending into mediastinum with multiple central and 1 anterior mediastinal mass with postobstructive infiltrate, bilateral pleural effusion. Bronchoscopy: 75% narrowing right upper lobe orifice to subsegments, 50% narrowing right lower lobe orifice. Bleeding at right upper lobe orifice. Draining right pleural effusion and sclerodesis with negative cytology. Preliminary tissue diagnosis from right paratracheal area and mediastinoscopy: Probable angiosarcoma.

PAST MEDICAL HISTORY: Hypertension.

SOCIAL HISTORY: 50-year tobacco habit.

PHYSICAL EXAMINATION: General: Well-developed male in no acute distress. No palpable adenopathy. Lungs: Clear. Heart: Regular rate and rhythm. Abdomen: Unremarkable. Extremities: Without circulatory collapse or edema. Neurologic: Without focal deficit.

ASSESSMENT: Recurrent metastatic angiosarcoma with postobstructive pneumonitis and hemoptysis.

PLAN: 4000 cGy[1] to symptom-producing mediastinal disease. Initial 1000 cGy at 200 cGy fractions, then oblique off previously irradiated spinal cord and boost with 250 cGy fractions. No plans for chemotherapy. Discussed radiation therapy procedures, risks, and alternatives with patient, emphasizing possible long-term risks to spinal cord, lung, and heart as well as increased potential for morbidity resulting from prior irradiation. He agrees with treatment as outlined.

Sincerely

Barry T. Goldstein, MD
Radiology Medical Group, Inc.

trn
D: 061151200X
T: 06116/200X

FIGURE 13-8 Radiotherapy report, run-on modified block format.

Some of the types of radiology reports dictated are the following:

aortogram
arteriogram
arthrogram
barium enema
bronchogram
cardioangiogram
cholangiogram
cholecystogram
cineradiogram
computed tomogram (CT scan)
cystogram
echogram
encephalogram
esophagram
esophagogram
fluoroscopy (chest, colon, gallbladder, and stomach)
hysterosalpingogram
intravenous cholangiogram (IVC)
intravenous pyelogram (IVP)
laminagram
lymphangiogram
magnetic resonance imaging (MRI)
myelogram, spinal
nephrotomogram
nuclear magnetic resonance (NMR) study
pneumoencephalogram
retrograde pyelogram (RP)
scan (blood and heart, bone, full body, brain, liver, lung, spleen, and thyroid)
sialogram

Telephone
212.555.1247

Fax
212.555.2345

COLLEGE PARK HOSPITAL AND MEDICAL CENTER
555 LAKE VIEW DRIVE
BAY VILLAGE, OH 44140

June 15, 20XX

John F. Millstone, MD
5302 Main Street
Bay Village, OH 44151

Re: Waltrudis M. Tubbman

Dear Dr Millstone:

This 91-year-old woman was seen at your request. The patient was admitted to the hospital yesterday because of chills, fever, and abdominal and back pain.

The history has been reviewed. A prominent feature of the history is the presence of intermittent, severe, shaking chills for 4 days with associated left lower back pain, left lower quadrant abdominal pain, and fever to as high as 103 or 104 degrees. The patient has had hypertension for a number of years and has been managed quite well with Catapres 0.3 mg twice a day.

On examination, her temperature at this time is 100.6 degrees. The pulse is 110 and regular. Blood pressure is *190/100*. The patient has partial bilateral iridectomies, the result of previous cataract surgery. Otherwise, the head and neck are not remarkable. Lung fields are clear throughout. The heart reveals a regular tachycardia; heart sounds are of good quality, no murmurs heard, and there is no gallop rhythm present. The abdomen is soft. There is no spasm or guarding. A well-healed surgical scar is present in the right flank area. There is considerable tenderness in the left lower quadrant of the left mid abdomen, but, as noted, there is no spasm or guarding present. Bowel sounds are present. Peristaltic rushes are noted, and the bowel sounds are slightly high-pitched in character. The extremities are unremarkable.

Diagnosis: I believe the patient has acute diverticulitis. She may have some irritation of the left ureter in view of the findings on the urinalyses. She appears to be responding to therapy at this time in that her temperature is coming down, and also there has been a slight reduction in the leukocytosis from yesterday. I agree with the present program of therapy, and the only suggestion would be to possibly increase the dose of ampicillin to 500 mg every 8 hours, rather than the 250 mg q.8 h. that she is now receiving.

Thank you for asking me to see this patient in consultation.

Sincerely,

Harold B. Cooper, MD

wpd

FIGURE 13-9 Consultation report, letter form in modified block format.

single-photon emission computed tomography (SPECT) (heart and brain)
sonogram
stereoscopy
thermogram
tomogram
ultrasonogram (bile ducts, gallbladder, kidneys, liver, ovaries, and uterus)
upper and lower gastrointestinal (GI) series
venogram
ventriculogram

CONSULTATION REPORTS

Often, an attending physician seeks the advice and opinion of a consulting physician. The consultant dictates a report (Figure 13-9) that will be incorporated into the patient's hospital record. The physician could see the patient in consultation in the office, emergency room, or hospital; then a report is dictated and sent to the referring physician. Sometimes, a consultation associated with decisions relating to surgical intervention is transcribed STAT. The report may contain the present history, past history, x-ray and laboratory studies, physical examination, and impression and comments on findings, prognosis, and future course of treatment recommended. It can be dictated in letter form or report form, with content and headings similar to an H&P report.

Refer to Appendix C on Evolve for examples of consultation reports generated by hospitals and emergency departments.

AUTOPSY PROTOCOLS

When a patient dies in the hospital or within 24 hours of discharge from the hospital, the next of kin can request an autopsy or postmortem examination of the body to determine the exact cause of death. The complete protocol should be made part of the record within 90 days after death. Through autopsies, much knowledge has been gained that assists in the diagnosis and treatment of disease. Visual and microscopic examinations are done on every organ and related structure. When an organ is removed from a cadaver for the purpose of donation, there should be an autopsy report that includes a description of the technique used to remove and prepare or

preserve the donated organ. All states have laws that govern autopsies. When someone dies unattended or if there is suspicion of a crime (e.g., violent death, unusual death, child abuse, self-induced or criminal abortion, homicide, suicide, poisoning, drowning, fire, hanging, stabbing, exposure, starvation), an autopsy can be ordered by the court, or it can become the responsibility of the coroner's office to determine the cause of death. Professionals associated with the coroner's or medical examiner's office include the pathologist, forensic pathologist, forensic dentist, chemist, toxicologist, anesthesiologist, radiologist, odontologist, psychiatrist, and psychologist.

The written record of an autopsy is generally referred to as an *autopsy protocol*. In pathology, there are

PITMAN COUNTY
OFFICE OF THE MEDICAL EXAMINER
AUTOPSY PROTOCOL

Bethany, Patricia Marie   June 21, 20XX

This is an autopsy on a prematurely born female infant weighing 1.25 kg. The body measures 39 cm in length. The body has not been embalmed prior to this examination.

EXTERNAL EXAMINATION: The head, neck and chest are symmetrical. The abdomen is soft. The external genitalia are normal female. The extremities are symmetrical and show no evidence of developmental abnormality.

INTERNAL EXAMINATION
ABDOMINAL CAVITY: The abdominal cavity is opened, and the liver is enlarged, extending 4 cm below the costal margin in the right midclavicular line. The spleen appears enlarged. The intestinal coils are freely dispersed and contain gaseous fluid. All other organs are in normal position.

PLEURAL CAVITIES: The pleural cavities are opened, revealing the left lung to be collapsed and lying in the left pleural cavity. The right lung is partially expanded, and the pleura is smooth and glistening in both pleural cavities.

MEDIASTINUM: The mediastinum contains a moderate amount of thymic tissue.

PERICARDIAL SAC: The pericardial sac is opened and contains a few cubic centimeters of serous fluid. The heart is normal in position and appears to be average in size.

HEART: The heart weighs approximately 10 g. Thorough search of the heart fails to show any evidence of congenital abnormality. The foramen ovale has a thin membrane over the surface. The ductus arteriosus is noted and patent. There is no ventricular septal defect. All valves are competent. There is no rotation of the heart. The pulmonary artery is noted and appears normal. A few subendocardial and subepicardial petechiae and ecchymoses are noted.

LUNGS: The lungs weigh together 33 g. The left lung and the right lung sink in water, then slowly rise to the surface. The lungs are subcrepitant and atelectatic. (This is particularly noted in the left lung.) The bronchi contain a small amount of frothy mucus. The cut surfaces of the lungs are beefy and atelectatic. There are no cysts or tumors. The findings are consistent with hyaline membrane disease and pulmonary atelectasis.

LIVER: The liver weighs approximately 75 g. The liver appears enlarged and is reddish-brown and soft. The cut surface is reddish-brown and soft. There is no gross evidence of bile duct blockage. The gallbladder, cystic duct, and common bile duct are not remarkable.

(continued)

FIGURE 13-10 Autopsy protocol, modified block run-on block format.

five forms: the narrative (in story form), the numerical form (by the numbers), the pictorial form (hand drawings or anatomic forms), protocols based on sentence completion and multiple-choice selection, and problem-oriented protocols (a supplement to the Problem-Oriented Medical Record System). A numerical format is an orderly description of all autopsy findings and tends to prevent omission of minor details that can be forgotten during narration. Numerical format is therefore usually a longer protocol and requires more time to complete.

Many hospital autopsy protocols (Figure 13-10) contain the clinical history, which is a brief resumé of the patient's medical history and course in the hospital before death. It includes the pathologic diagnosis made

at autopsy, a report of the final summary, and the gross anatomy findings (visual examination of the organs of the body before any tissues are removed for preparation and examination). There is also a microscopic examination (an examination of the particular organs through the microscope). An epicrisis or final pathologic diagnosis is given at the end of the protocol. The epicrisis is a critical analysis (actual finding) or discussion of the cause of disease after its termination.

In forensic pathology, an autopsy protocol may be organized under the following general guidelines:

1. External description
2. Evidence of injury
   a. External
   b. Internal

Bethany, Patricia Marie
Autopsy Protocol, Page 2
June 21, 20XX

INTERNAL EXAMINATION continued

PANCREAS: The pancreas appears average in size, weighing approximately 1.5 g. The pancreas is yellowish-white and soft on the cut surface. There is no gross evidence of cystic disease.

SPLEEN: The spleen weighs approximately 4 g and is bluish purple. The spleen on cut surface is reddish-brown and soft.

ADRENAL GLANDS: The adrenal glands weigh together approximately 4.5 g. The adrenal glands are soft and tan, and the cortical portion is distinct from the medullary portion. There is no gross evidence of hemorrhage, cysts, or tumors. Both adrenals are similar.

KIDNEYS: The kidneys weigh together approximately 13 g. The capsule strips with ease, leaving a faint fetal lobulation and a reddish-brown soft surface. The cut surface shows the cortex and medulla, both of which are distinct and in average proportions. The parenchyma is reddish-brown, moist and soft. Both kidneys are similar in appearance and consistency. The ureters are not remarkable.

URINARY BLADDER, UTERUS, TUBES, AND OVARIES: These organs are grossly not remarkable.

GASTROINTESTINAL TRACT: The esophagus is examined as well as the stomach. There is no evidence of reduplication, ulcer, or tumor. The small and large bowel are not remarkable.

BRAIN: The brain weighs approximately 230 g. The brain is slightly edematous. A few petechiae are observed. On sectioning the brain anterior to posterior, the brain tissue is soft and somewhat edematous. The fluid in the ventricles is clear and watery. The cerebellum and cerebrum are symmetrical and grossly not remarkable. There is no gross evidence of hemorrhage or tumor.

SKELETAL SYSTEM: Not remarkable.

GROSS ANATOMICAL DIAGNOSES
1. Prematurity, 1.25 kg.
2. Pulmonary atelectasis.
3. Hyaline membrane disease.

STEPHEN M. CHOI, MD, CME
sw
D: June 21, 20XX   0700
T: June 21, 20XX   1350

FIGURE 13-10, cont'd

3. Systems and organs (cavities and organs)
4. Special dissections and examinations
5. Brain (and other organs) after fixation
6. Microscopic examination
7. Findings (diagnoses), factual and interpretative
8. Opinion or summary (conclusion), interpretative and opinion
9. Signature

Some autopsy procedures used for transcription protocols are not necessarily seen in other types of healthcare documentation. Because autopsy records can be entered into a court of law to relate information about the cause of death, clarity is essential so that interpretation of the typed material is accurately understood. Because of this requirement, more words tend to be spelled out, and abbreviations are kept to a minimum. Many states require that military time be used when documenting the time a body is brought in for autopsy (e.g., 1400 hours). Ciphers are used in stating nonmilitary time (e.g., 9:00 a.m.). Units of measurement are spelled out, such as pounds, inches, and grams. Quotation marks are never used to indicate inches but are used when indicating a marking on the body (e.g., tattoo device of the words "J.J. Tramp"). Temperature is typed "88 degrees Fahrenheit." Numbers can be typed as "2 fresh punctures" or "2 (two) stab wounds."

Numbers can be typed numerically and then spelled out in parentheses when clarity is emphasized. Metric terms are given as abbreviations (e.g., 0.5 cm, 200 mL, 3 × 3 mm).

Forensic dentists work closely with forensic pathologists. They describe bite marks by size, shape, and location. They swab for saliva to determine blood type. They make impressions or molds of the mark, and then photograph and make impressions of the suspect's dentition. When two medical examiners are involved, the reference initials of both at the closing of the protocol must be shown (e.g., MB:DVW:mod). Only general guidelines for typing protocols are stated here. Each county has different practices and must meet various legal requirements.

MEDICOLEGAL REPORTS

Medicolegal reports originate from medical offices and hospitals. When they originate from the latter, they usually come from the medical records department, in which personnel make copies or abstracts of record entries rather than transcribing them (Figure 13-11). The prudent physician responds to a request for medical information with a prompt and complete report and, in doing so, assists his or her patient in supporting claims for damages (probably including the physician's bill),

facilitates the attorney's representation of a client, and can often spare a trip to court. Usually, a report of this type involves an accident case or a workers' compensation case. The report is a legal document and is admissible as evidence in a court of law. Sometimes, the attorney abstracts data from the report and incorporates the information into a formal document presented to the physician for signature and subsequent notarization. Accuracy is essential.

The properly prepared medicolegal report follows a familiar format and is typed on the physician's letterhead stationery.

Patient Identification

The patient must be identified in the first paragraph. The patient's name, age or date of birth (or both), and address should be included. If the patient is a child, the names of the parents are noted with the patient identified as the "son of" or "daughter of" the parents.

Date of Accident or Work-Related Injury

The date of the accident or injury must be noted, including the time of day, if known. (The physician should check the date of the accident given by the patient's attorney against that in the medical record. If the dates do not agree, the patient must be contacted to clarify the discrepancy.)

History

The history of the accident, injury, or work-related illness is described. Use the patient's own words, including quotation marks whenever possible. Be as detailed and complete as possible, listing all the facts.

Present Complaints

The patient's present complaints at the time of the first visit are recorded. (Sometimes these are referred to as *subjective complaints.*)

Past History

The past history should be described along with any preexisting defects or injuries that could have a bearing on the present problem.

Physical Findings

Physical findings on examination are recorded in detail. (These are sometimes referred to as *objective findings.*)

Laboratory or X-Ray Findings

Laboratory or x-ray findings are included in the report. In some instances, photocopies of x-ray, electrocardiograph, or operative reports are made available.

CLARENCE F. STONES, MD
3700 LILAC LANE
GRANDVIEW, XX 00060

October 20, 20XX

Aetna Casualty and Surety Company
3200 Roosevelt Boulevard
GrandView, XX 03030

Dear Madam or Sir:

RE: Injured: Howard P. Winston
        Date of Injury: July 27, 20XX
        Employer: College Chemistry Company
        Case No.: 450-33-0821

EXAMINATION AND REPORT

HISTORY: This 43-year-old white male was working with a chemical
                      pump. It slipped and fell forward. He overcorrected and
fell. The pump fell on the patient, striking him in the occiput area. The approximate weight of the
pump was 325 pounds and was rolled off by a friend. The patient was knocked unconscious. He
attended a meeting the following day in Round Valley. The pain occurred a day later in Round
Valley. Then 3 days later, the pain was intense in the right shoulder and elbow. He went to Dr.
John Garrett for physiotherapy. The left side then began to give him trouble also. He had a
pressure type of pain in the left elbow, which was relieved by codeine. He entered College
Hospital in GrandView under Dr. Garrett's service. The right leg, and later the right thigh, began
getting numb. A myelogram was followed by fusion at C5-6 and C6-7. He wore a brace for 6
months. He still has right shoulder pain and neck pain with radiation into the right thumb and right
mastoid. In June 200X, he was admitted to Community Hospital. The left eye began drooping,
and there was no pupil dilatation. He was improved 1 week later. A myelogram and brain scan
were performed. There was pain on the left side, with pain into the rectum with spasms. He states
that he fell several times. The surgery was postponed because of the eyes and the sudden loss
of equilibrium.

FAMILY HISTORY: The father died of burns in a fire in 1990. The mother died of kidney
                      disease at age 82. He has two brothers and one sister, living and well.
He is widowed. His wife had cancer of the uterus. He has four children, alive and well. There is no
history of diabetes and no accidents.

ALLERGIES: PENICILLIN AND TETANUS.

PHYSICAL EXAMINATION

GENERAL: Blood pressure *122/78*; pulse 84 and regular. The patient is cooperative
                      and oriented to time and place.

(continued)

FIGURE 13-11 Medicolegal report, indented block format with mixed punctuation.

Consultation notes also can be photocopied and submitted with the medicolegal report.

Diagnosis

The diagnosis (or diagnoses in the case of multiple injuries) should be detailed.

Prescribed Therapy

Prescribed therapy must be described in detail. Each visit to the office must be listed, including any physical therapy treatments or medications prescribed.

Patient's Disability

Outline the patient's disability, describing work restrictions and including the dates of total or partial disability. The date on which the patient is permitted to return to work is given.

Prognosis

The prognosis is of paramount importance to the attorney and thus to the patient. The settlement can depend on the physician's estimate of continued pain and whether there will be future permanent disability.

Howard P. Winston
Page 2
October 20, 20XX

PHYSICAL EXAMINATION (continued)

HEENT: Head: Normal size and shape; no facial asymmetry. He
                    shows no evidence of elevated intracranial pressure.
Extraocular muscles intact. Pupils are equal and react briskly to light. At first, one gets the
impression that there might be a Horner syndrome on the left side because of inconstant ptosis of
the right eyelid, but this is not truly present.

NEUROLOGICAL EXAM: The patient walks with sparing of the left leg. There is no true
                    paralysis present.

REFLEXES: The right biceps and triceps are slightly reduced on the left side but
                    are present.

SENSORY: There is evidence of patchy hyperesthesia in the right upper
                    extremity but following no particular dermatomal pattern.

CEREBELLAR FUNCTION: Intact. Lower cranial nerves within normal limits. There were no
                     pathological reflexes elicited.

The remaining exam was deferred.

OPINION AND COMMENT: The patient continues to have slight dysfunction, principally in
                     left lower extremity and right upper extremity. It would seem to me
that the pupillary abnormality, which he experienced in June of 20XX, merits some investigation,
including arteriography. For his cervical disk problems, I would think that conservative treatment
is warranted.

                                        Sincerely,

                                        Clarence F. Stones, MD

SW

FIGURE 13-11, cont'd

Physician's Statement

The physician's statement of fees for services rendered is an integral part of the report to an attorney. The statement should be itemized by date and service, making sure the statement correlates in detail with the dates of treatment mentioned in the report. Preparation of a report for an attorney is time consuming, and the physician is entitled to charge a fee. Documents requiring extensive research of hospital records and consultants' reports merit higher fees.

Although many cases are settled out of court, the few that go to trial justify painstaking care in preparation of the medical report. Remember that the value of a detailed document cannot be overemphasized (especially considering that some physicians are asked to testify in a trial years after a patient's injury).

PSYCHIATRIC REPORTS

Psychiatry is one of the specialties of clinical medicine. It is a diverse field, and the language involves abnormal psychology, human behavior, and treatment terminology. Patients are referred to as *clients*. In a hospital setting, clients include mentally deficient, mentally impaired, and developmentally disabled persons, formerly referred to as *mentally retarded*.

For the mentally deficient client, an admission note could include a presentation of the problem stating the vital signs, current medications, allergies, medication taken in the previous 4 hours, present illness, psychological history, mental status examination, physical status examination, and a provisional diagnosis. Additional reports about the mentally disabled client could include a psychiatric evaluation, psychological evaluation, social history evaluation, rehabilitation therapy evaluation, discharge summary, and treatment planning conference. The conference is a program to establish the goals of treatment and track the progress that the client is making while under the treatment, with the ultimate goal of the client being placed back into society as a fully functional person.

Reports for a developmentally disabled client might include a medical history, review of systems, release summary, and clinical record documentation system, which is equivalent to a treatment planning conference for a mentally deficient client. These reports are more detailed because these clients can be so low functioning that even the most basic self-care skills cannot be performed on admission. Facility staff members attempt to teach these skills with attainment of the highest potential of each client as a goal.

A report dictated by a clinical psychologist would not necessarily contain a physical examination of the body systems or a list of the medications, but it would describe motor skill abilities. The main heading could be *Psychologic Evaluation,* and subheadings could be given as follows: *Purpose of the Report, Psychosocial History, Results of the Psychological Assessment, Mental Status Examination, Test Results, Impressions, Diagnosis,* and *Recommendations.*

Because so many clients have legal problems (divorce, marriage, adoption, negligence, physical abuse, disability, and so on), legal terminology is widely used. Some clients are seen for chemical abuse, and drugs could be referred to by slang or street terms; often, these terms are unknown by the novice MT. These terms change from day to day, and the list is constantly expanding. Most MTs prepare lists of these slang terms for reference to assist in typing up the reports. Many of the words encountered in psychiatric reports do not appear in a standard English dictionary or a medical dictionary, and so the use of special reference books will assist you. The *Diagnostic and Statistical Manual of Mental Disorders, Fourth Edition, Revised* (DSM-IV-R) is used for psychiatric diagnoses for the mentally disabled. This is an excellent reference book for the MT because all mental diagnoses are given with their code numbers. However, for developmentally disabled clients, the *International Classification of Diseases, 10th Edition, Clinical Modification* (ICD-10-CM) code numbers and the etiology are used. If the psychiatrist wishes, the DSM-IV-R is also used for the diagnosis. Refer to Figure 13-12 to see how the diagnoses and code numbers might be typed.

Psychiatric records often have stricter confidentiality laws governing them and are usually locked down with more stringent access. Generally, only personnel within the psychiatric unit have access to these records. Audits can be run on any electronic medical record, but because of the sensitivity of psychiatric records, audits are run more routinely. Because reports containing information about a person's mental stability are confidential, sometimes the information contained in the report is not divulged even to the client. To obtain medical information, the signatures of the physician and the client are required on a special release-of-information form. If the client is developmentally disabled, signatures of the physician and the guardian are needed. If authorized in writing by the client or guardian and by the psychiatrist in charge of the case, a copy of the report is sent to the referring medical practitioner or medical facility responsible for followup care of the patient. Psychiatric information can be sent to a placement facility if a client is to live in the community in a residential facility. This information gives the receiving facility data regarding treatment and medication. The court system can subpoena the medical records. See Appendix C on Evolve for a complete psychiatric evaluation macro.

Brief Review of Report Format Styles

BASIC BLOCK FORMAT OR MODIFIED BLOCK RUN-ON FORMAT

Statistical Data:	As determined by the facility.
	Aligned on top or bottom of page.
Margins and Spacing:	Double-space or single-space between topics.
	Single-spaced data.
	Margins narrow for entire document.
Title:	Centered on the page or flush with left margin.
Main Topic Titles:	Begun flush with left margin.
	Full capital letters.
	On a line alone or introducing data on same line.
Subtopics:	Full capital letters or combination
	Begun flush with left margin.
Data:	Begun on same line as topic or subtopic.
	or
	Begun on left margin.
Close:	As determined by facility.
	Dictator's name and signature area.
	MT's initials or other form of identification.
	Date and time of dictation.
	Date and time of transcription.

See Chapter 12 for more details.

State of California—Health and Welfare Agency	Department of Mental Health

GUIDELINES	Date of Report: 11-09-0X Dictated: 11-09-0X Transcribed: 11-09-0X **PSYCHIATRIC EVALUATION** **Unit 99**

A. PSYCHIATRIC HISTORY
1. Identification data
2. Source of information
3. Chief complaint
4. History of present illness (focus on recent illness, and include emotional behavior)
5. History of past psychiatric episodes
6. Relevant medical/ surgical/trauma/ medication history
7. Developmental history (if applicable)
8. Educational/Vocational
9. Relevant family history
10. Relevant social history

B. MENTAL STATUS EXAM
11. Attitude/Cooperation
12. General appearance (include speech)
13. Motor activity
14. Orientation
15. Mood and affect
16. Mental content
17. Memory
18. Fund of general knowledge
19. Cognition and comprehension
20. Abstraction ability
21. Counting and calculating
22. Judgement
23. Insight regarding illness
24. Patient strengths
25. Suicide, homicide, dangerousness

C. SUMMARY OF PSYCHIATRIC ASSESSMENT
26. Narrative summary (including Risk Potential)
27. Diagnosis (DSM III R)
28. Preliminary Treatment Plan
29. Prognosis
30. Signature and Title

PSYCHIATRIC HISTORY

1. This 17-year-old, single, Hispanic male patient was admitted to Greenvale Hospital on November 8, 20XX, on a temporary conservatorship 5353 from Pitman County. His birth date is September 24, 19XX. There is no religious reference. His mother is Mary Sanchez. Her address is 300 East Date Street, Woodland Hills, XY 12345. Telephone (555) 999-9999.

2. Information obtained by interviewing the patient and reviewing the accompanying papers from Greenvale Center. The patient speaks only Spanish. The interview had to be done through an interpreter. His information is not very reliable.

3. "I don't know why they sent me here."

4. Pedro was admitted to Greenvale Medical Center on August 26, 200X, because of bizarre behavior for 5 days. According to the report, 5 days prior to admission, he smoked marijuana dipped in PCP. He also smoked cocaine. He demonstrated bizarre behavior such as running nude in the streets, sticking his fingers into light sockets and receiving electric shocks, crawling under a car and trying to set it on fire. He was not sleeping. He laughed and cried inappropriately. He broke a restraint in the hospital. The drug screening test 1 on August 26, 20XX, was positive for cocaine and negative for PCP and other drugs. Peabody test in Spanish revealed his IQ was about 76. Beery development test of visual motor integration did not suggest organicity. He was treated with Haldol and discharged to his mother on September 22, 20XX; however, he was readmitted to Greenvale Medical Center Center on September 24, 20XX, on a 5150. His mother stated that after discharge from the hospital, he was fearful and childish. He presented bizarre behavior such as collecting household articles, painting the walls, attempting to play with medicine bottles, refusing to eat or sleep, walking around the house nude, collecting piles of objects in his room, attempting suicide by jumping off an apartment building. He laughed and cried inappropriately. His mother stated that he did not take street drugs, and he took only Haldol and Cogentin. However, on one occasion, he went to the store without supervision. At the Greenvale Medical Center, he was confused, disorganized, and disoriented. It was difficult for him to attend to a conversation or to concentrate. He was not able to function in school. He needs close supervision and care. He had been in physical restraints many times because of assaultive behavior. He also banged the walls and screamed. He was treated with Haldol 10 mg t.i.d. A long-term hospitalization was...

SANCHEZ, Pedro J. 999999-9 V.99   ☐ Continued

EVALUATION REPORT **PSYCHIATRIC** Confidential Client/Patient Information See W & I Code Section 5328 MH 5702 (Revised 7/87) CRDM Reference 2410	

FIGURE 13-12 Pages 1 and 4 of a psychiatric evaluation, basic block format. Note the diagnoses and code numbers at the end of the report: *Axis I:* substance abuse and other treatable conditions; *Axis II:* psychological disorders; *Axis III;* medical conditions; *Axis IV:* stressors; *Axis V:* global assessment of functioning (0-100). *GAF* means Global Assessment of Functioning Scale.

State of California—Health and Welfare Agency

Department of Mental Health

Date of Report: 11-09-0X
Dictated: 11-09-0X
Transcribed: 11-09-0X

Unit 99 -- PSYCHIATRIC EVALUATION

(Continued)

26.   Pedro's father deserted the family when Pedro was 11 years old. Around
        that time, he stopped going to school after finishing 6th grade. The reason
        for that was not clear. He lived with his grandmother after his mother left
        Honduras 4 years ago. About 8 months ago, he came to the United States
        to live with his mother because his grandmother was unable to handle him.
        He had been using cocaine and PCP for 6 or 7 months. It was felt that his
        first hospitalization at Greenvale Medical Center was due to PCP, Organic
        Mental Disorder. At this time, he appears retarded with residual
        symptoms of psychosis such as flat and inappropriate affect, loose associations,
        poverty of thoughts, no intention to go to school; and he needs constant
        supervision for daily living activities.

27.   Axis I: 298.9   Psychotic Disorder, NOS.
                           (Rule out 292.90 PCP, Organic Mental Disorder.)
                           306.90 Psychoactive Substance Abuse, NOS.
        Axis II: V71.09 No diagnosis.
                           (Rule out Mental Retardation.)
        Axis III: No somatic disorder.
        Axis IV: Discord with classmates.
        Axis V: GAF on admission 26; highest GAF last year unknown.

28.   Structured environment, special educational program, unit milieu, individual
        therapy, group therapy, and chemotherapy.

29.   Guarded.

30.

                    _____
                    Dan W. Stewart, MD

jrw

Page 4 SANCHEZ, Pedro J. 999999-9 U.99   ☐ Continued

CONTINUATION PAGE

☒ Assessment (Specify: __Psychiatric_____)
☐ Team Conference (Specify: _____)
☐ Consultation (Specify: _____)
☐ Other (Specify _____)

Confidential Client/Patient Information
See W & I Code Section 5378

MH 5705

FIGURE 13-12, cont'd

13-1 SELF-STUDY

DIRECTIONS: Retype the following data into discharge summary outline by using the basic block format. Set margins at 0.5. Pay careful attention to punctuation and capitalization. Set up the patient's name and other statistical data as you desire. Examine the discharge summaries in Appendix C on Evolve to get an idea of the variety of style options. Note topic changes and proper mechanics. The location of the headings for admitting diagnosis and discharge diagnosis can vary—occurring at the beginning of the report, in the natural order of dictation (as seen in Figure 13-1), or at the end of the report—as specified by the individual facility.

The patient is Marcia M. Bacon. The dictating physician is Henry R. Knowles, MD. The summary was dictated on May 10 and transcribed on May 11. The patient's hospital ID number is 52-01-96. The patient's room number is 248-C. The date of hospital admission was May 7, 20XX, and she was discharged on May 9, 20XX. Admission diagnosis: Torn medial meniscus, left knee. Discharge diagnosis: Torn medial meniscus, left knee; chondromalacia of the medial femoral condyle. History of present illness: The patient injured her left knee on April 11, 20XX, while playing tennis. She subsequently had difficulty with persistent effusion and pain in the left knee. An arthrogram prior to admission revealed a tear of the medial meniscus. Physical examination: absence of tenderness to palpation of any of the joint structures. There was approximately 30-55 mL of fluid within the joint. Range of motion was full. Laboratory data: admission hemoglobin was 15.9, hematocrit 47%, with a white count of 7400 with normal differential. Urinalysis was within normal limits. Chem panel 19 showed an elevated cholesterol of 379 mg%. Chest x-ray was reported as negative. Treatment and hospital course: The patient was taken to the operating room on the same day as admission, at which time she underwent arthroscopy. This revealed that she had a tear of the medial meniscus. Arthrotomy was performed, with medial meniscectomy. A chondral fracture was noted in the medial femoral condyle, measuring approximately 5 mm in greatest diameter. The edges of this were sheathed. Postoperatively, the patient's course was benign. There was no significant temperature elevation. She became ambulatory with crutches on the first postoperative day with no difficulty with straight leg raising. Disposition: The patient is being discharged home ambulatory with crutches and an exercise program. She is to be seen in the office in one week for suture removal. Condition at the time of discharge: Improved. Complications: None. Medications: None.

See Appendix A, p. 460, for one version of a transcript of this assignment.

13-2 PRACTICE TEST

DIRECTIONS: Retype the following data into an operative report by using the run-on block format and no variations. Set a 0.5 margin on right and left. Set up the patient's name and other statistical data as you desire. Pay attention to proper mechanics and capitalization. Date the report January 4, 20XX. See p. 306 for the run-on format.

The patient's name is John P. Dwight, and his hospital ID number is 86-30-21. The surgeon is Felix A. Konig. The patient's room number is 582-B. The preoperative and postoperative diagnosis is: otosclerosis, left ear. The operation is a left stapedectomy. The findings, otosclerosis, footplate. Under local anesthesia, the ear was prepared and draped in the usual manner. The ear was injected with two percent Xylocaine and one to six thousand epinephrine. A stapes-type flap was elevated from the posterosuperior canal wall, and the bony overhang was removed with the stapes curet. The chorda tympani nerve was removed from the field. The incudostapedial joint was separated. The stapes tendon was cut. The superstructure was removed. The mucous membrane was reflected from the ear, stapes, and the facial nerve promontory. The footplate was then reamed with small picks and hooks. A flattened piece of Gelfoam was placed over the oval window, and a five millimeter wire loop prosthesis was inserted and crimped in the incus. The drum was reflected, and a small umbilical tape was placed in the ear canal. The patient tolerated the procedure well.

13-3 PRACTICE TEST

DIRECTIONS: Retype the following data into a pathology report by using run-on block format. Date the report June 6, 20XX. See p. 306 for run-on format.

The patient's name is Joan Alice Jayne, and her hospital ID number is 72-11-03. The referring physician is John A. Myhre, MD, and the pathologist is James T. Rodgers, MD. The date the specimen was removed was June 6, 20XX. The patient's room number is 453-A. Pathology number is 532009. Specimen(s): The specimen consists of a four point five centimeter in diameter nodule of fibro-fatty tissue removed from the right breast at biopsy and enclosing a central, firm, sharply demarcated nodule one centimeter in diameter. Surrounding breast parenchyma reveals dilated ductules (microcystic disease). Frozen section impression: Myxoid fibroadenoma of breast. Microscopic and diagnosis: Myxoid fibroadenoma occurring in right parenchyma, the site of microcystic disease of right breast.

13-4 SELF-STUDY

DIRECTIONS: Retype the following data into a radiology report by using the tabulated block format. Remember to double-space between topics as done in full block format. Date the report June 8, current year. See p. 304 for modified block format.

The patient's name is Donna Mae Weeser. Her x-ray number is 16-A2, and her hospital number is 52-80-44. This patient is age 46. The referring physician is George B. Bancroft, MD, and the radiologist is Clayton M. Markham, MD. The examination is mammography, right and left breasts. There are retromammary prosthetic devices in position. The anterior parenchyma is somewhat compressed. There is no evidence of neoplastic calcification or skin thickening demonstrated. No dominant masses are noted within the anteriorly displaced parenchyma. No increased vascularity is evident. Impression: mammography right and left breasts shows the presence of retromammary prosthetic devices in position. The demonstrated tissue appears within normal limits.

See Appendix A, p. 461, for one version of a transcript of this assignment.

13-5 PRACTICE TEST

DIRECTIONS: Retype the following material into a consultation report. Use basic block format, and the current date. Watch for proper topic changes, placement, and mechanics. See Figure C-40, in Appendix C on Evolve, for a possible layout.

The patient's name is Hazel R. Plunkett. This is for Glen M. Hiranuma, MD and is written by Margo A. Wilkins, MD. The reason for the for neurological consultation is for evaluation and treatment of chronic and recurrent headaches. In the past, the patient has had episodes of probably typical migraine occurring perhaps six or eight times in her life. She remembers that her mother had a similar complaint. This would begin with loss in the field of vision; and then, approximately fifteen minutes thereafter, she would have a relatively typical, unilateral throbbing pain of a significant degree which would often incapacitate her. These headaches disappeared many years ago and have never returned. However, for the last eight years approximately, the patient has had recurrent daily headaches, always right-sided, with associated pain beginning in the back of the neck with stiffness of the right side of the neck, radiating forward over the vertex to the right orbit, the nose, and the jaw. She also notes some pain in the right trapezius area. The pain tends to appear from 10 a.m. to noon, when she will take a Fiorinal, and often after she goes to sleep at night (at about 12:30 a.m.). She controls this pain by taking Fiorinal, one to four a day, and Elavil, 75 mg at bedtime. She estimates that the headaches occur approximately twice daily, are relatively short-lived but occasionally last a full day. The pain is dull and heavy, not throbbing, and worse at some times than at others. On examination she was a quiet woman, not in acute distress, and somewhat dour; but she gave a careful and concise history. Her gait and station were normal. The head functions were basically intact. The fundi showed only modest arteriosclerotic changes. The temporal arteries were normal. Facial motility and sensation was normal. There was a significant right carotid bruit present which was persistent and which could be heard all along the course of the right carotid artery. It was not transmitted from the neck. There were moderate pain and tenderness at the insertion of the great muscles of the neck and the occiput, and palpation over this area consistently reproduced the patient's symptoms. She also had a persistent area of tenderness in the right trapezius muscle. Otherwise, power, size, and symmetry of the arms and legs were essentially normal. The deep tendon reflexes were brisk. There were no long tract or focal signs, and sensation was intact.

Impression: 1. Muscle contraction headaches, chronic. 2. Localized myositis, right side of neck, right shoulder girdle. 3. Right carotid bruit, silent, asymptomatic. Comment: The findings were discussed in detail with the patient but no neurological studies were done. I suggested simple measures of physical therapy to the neck including the use of heat, hot packs, and massage and advised also that she purchase a cervical pillow on which to rest during the day. Motrin, 400 mg twice daily and Lioresal 20 mg at night were suggested in an attempt to provide antiinflammatory and muscle relaxant properties. It may also be necessary to inject these tender areas which are quite well localized. This can be determined after 30 to 60 days on the treatment regimen outlined above. The patient also has what seems to be a silent right carotid bruit. Certainly she is without symptoms. This should be brought to the attention of those who are caring for her, so that if transient ischemic attacks appear in the future, appropriate steps can be taken. I do not think that the right carotid bruit has anything to do with the patient's headaches, which are not vascular, and certainly there is no sign of cranial arteritis.

13-6 REVIEW TEST

DIRECTIONS: Retype the following material into a hospital autopsy protocol by using the basic block format. Set up the patient's name and other statistical data as you desire. Use a current date and correct punctuation. The dictator is Dr Susan R. Foster, chief pathologist. See p. 302 for block format. Note that the main topic and subtopics vary from those shown in Figure 13-10.

I performed an autopsy on the body of Phyllis B. Dexter, Patient No. 65-43-90, at the College Hospital. Clinical Diagnosis: Congenital heart defect.

General Examination: The body is that of a well developed and well nourished newborn female infant, having been embalmed prior to examination through a thoracic incision and cannulization of the heart. The recorded birth weight is 7 pounds 2 ounces. Thorax opened: Considerable blood is present around the heart incident to the embalming procedure, and two incisions in the cardiac muscle are evident but the valves and great vessels do not appear to have been injured by the embalming procedure. Examination discloses a massive heart lying transversely in the midanterior thorax, the distended right ventricle exceeding in volume the ventricular mass. Examination discloses no enlargement of the ductus arteriosus or any significant deviation of the size of the great vessels. On exploration of the heart there is found to be a completely imperforate pulmonary artery at the level of the pulmonary valve, all 3 cusps of which appear to be adequately formed but fused by scar tissue slightly proximal to the free margins of the cusps. It is impossible to probe the existence of any opening in this area. The right heart is markedly hypertrophic, approximating three times the muscle mass of the normal infant heart. There is no evidence of an interventricular defect. There is a sacculation adjacent to the valve of the inferior vena cava as it enters the inferior right auricle and in the dome of this sacculated area the foramen ovale is demonstrated. The foramen is unusually small in diameter (estimated to be no more than 4 mm in diameter) and this is covered by a plica. It would appear that the pressure of the distended right auricle would further compromise the capacity of the foramen to transmit blood. In the absence of any interventricular defect, this would be the only way that blood could get from the right to the left side of the heart. The lungs are heavy and poorly serrated and the bronchial tree contains some yellowish fluid which, in the absence of feeding by mouth, must be assumed to be aspirated vernix. Abdomen Opened: The stomach contains some bloody mucus but no evidence of formula. The liver and abdominal viscera appear entirely negative throughout. Head: Not opened. Cause of Death on Gross Findings: Massive chylous pericardial effusion, etiology not established but presumptively related to defect in formation of thoracic duct tissue. Microscopic: Sections of the thymus gland revealed a generally normal histological architecture for the thymus of the newborn, epithelial elements still being distributed through the lymphoid tissues. Certainly no tumor is present in the thymic tissue. The pulmonary tissues are poorly expanded although the bronchi appear open. There are a general vascular congestion of pulmonary tissue and some apparent extravasation of blood into the poorly expanded alveoli. In addition, there are deposits of hyaline material on the surfaces of some of the air spaces that would indicate the existence of hyaline membrane disease. The liver shows marked congestion and a rather active hematopoiesis. The heart muscle is not remarkable and the epicardial surface does not appear thickened or unusual. The kidney tissue exhibits some punctate hemorrhages in the parenchyma consistent with anoxia. Microscopic Diagnosis: Renal hemorrhages incident to anoxia.

13-7 REVIEW TEST

DIRECTIONS: Retype the following data into an industrial accident report form and prepare an envelope. Use letterhead stationery. Use full block format, mixed punctuation, (see Chapter 6) and the current date. Watch for proper paragraphing, placement, punctuation, and mechanics.

The letter concerns the patient George R. Champion and was dictated by Dr James C. Taylor of 4532 Saint Charles Avenue, New Orleans, LA 70118. It is to be sent to an attorney, Ralph J. Claborne of 165 Colette, Suite A-1, New Orleans, LA 70120. Use a current date.

Dear Mr Claborne. My patient Mr George R. Champion was seen on September 14, 20XX. History of injury: Mr Champion was hit on the back of the head by a lettuce crate in April of 20XX. He saw stars but was not knocked unconscious. Present complaints: The patient says he can see for an instant then the left eye blurs and also itches. He has had this problem since his accident in April 20XX. When he is working and turns to the left he cannot see things out of that side since they are fuzzy. He can look at an object to the left and five seconds later it is gone. Physical examination: Visual acuity uncorrected: right eye, 20/80; left eye, 20/40. Manifest refraction: right eye, +1.75D = 20/30 Jaeger 1; left eye, +2.50 = 20/30 Jaeger 1. Visual field: full centrally. Motility: Near point of convergence = 8 cm; Near point of accommodation = 3.5D. Prism cover test: Distance = no shift; Near = 8 prism diopters exophoria. Cycloplegic refraction: right eye = +2.50 + 0.50 × 30 = 20/25 − 2; left eye = +3.25 + 0.75 × 125 = 20/20 − 1. Slit-lamp examination revealed abnormal cornea, conjunctiva, iris and lens. Ocular tension was 11 mmHg both eyes by applanation. Retinal examination revealed a normal optic disc, macula, vessels and periphery with direct and indirect ophthalmoscopy. Diagnosis: Compound hyperopic astigmatism with early presbyopia. Comments: I feel that this patient's focusing reserve was suddenly decreased by his accident when he was hit on the head. His basic problem of farsightedness coupled with a general weakness after the accident overcame his focusing reserve and caused his symptoms. I feel that glasses of the proper strength will enable him to see and focus. His problem of poor convergence and exophoria at near were also brought into prominence by the weakness he had after the accident. His age (38) means that he would have had symptoms within the next five or seven years due to his farsightedness. Recommended treatment: Glasses to be worn all the time. Eye exercises for convergence problem if the glasses do not relieve his symptoms. Disability: The condition is now stationary and permanent; and with the proper glasses, he should be able to resume his normal work load. Very truly yours.

13-8 REVIEW TEST

DIRECTIONS: Retype the following data into a psychiatric report form. Use letterhead stationery. Use full block mixed punctuation, and the current date. Watch for proper paragraphing, punctuation, placement, and mechanics.

The letter concerns the patient Tu Anh Dao and was dictated by Dr Stephen B. Salazar of 5028 South Broadway, Exeter, NH 03833. It is to be sent to Department of Social Services Disability Evaluation Unit, 15 Kenneth Street, Exeter, NH 03833. Head this report Psychiatric Social Survey.

Presenting Problem: This 29-year-old Vietnamese male was seen today at the request of the Department of Social Services Disability Evaluation Unit. Questions regarding mental status appearance simple repetitive tasks interests and daily activities and ability to relate and interact with public and coworkers were raised. The interview was conducted in the living room of the home in which he lives and has lived for the last three or four years. The claimant resides in this home with his mother and his 11-year-old younger sister. His mother and an interpreter were present in the room during the interview. The interview lasted one hour. The claimant was very quiet and at some points hardly audible. He declined to answer questions quite often during the interview. Several times during the interview the mother interrupted and gave answers to him. He seemed to show some pressure of speech and memory difficulties during the interview. History: The history revealed that Mr Dao was born in Hanoi Vietnam where he went to school up to the eighth grade. At the eighth grade he dropped out and began to farm doing rice farming. At age 26 he moved to Exeter. After arriving in Exeter he worked in a restaurant which he cannot name as a dishwasher for two or three months but he quit because the job in the first place was part time and temporary. He then worked for two years as a gardener and quit this job because of health problems he was always feeling sick. He also worked for one or two months as a carpenter but he quit because he did not have the money to buy the tools. In 2005 he was admitted to College Hospital where he had surgery and was in the hospital for one or two months during the winter of the year. He claims that the surgery was neurological although it could have been rather than on the brain an inner ear surgery due to vertigo and tinnitus problems. There is no history of any other hospitalizations. The claimant is the oldest son of five children he has two sisters and two brothers they are all living in the United States. Environment: The claimant has lived in his present house for one and a half years with his mother and his 11-year-old sister. He states that he wakes at 8 or 9 am. He walks around in the yard for awhile and then he eats breakfast he does not eat lunch but does eat dinner. He said that during this time his appetite is good and he eats because he is hungry. Once a week he leaves the house to see a doctor who checks for the surgery and his neurological problems. He states that he had a ringing in the left ear which was partially a result of the surgery. He has not done any kind of work since the head surgery and he has not done anything around the house. He reports difficulty with memory. He rarely does anything with friends except when they come over to visit him and only leaves the house to walk around the yard or go to the doctor appointments. He is able to dress himself and bathe himself but does not do any chores of any kind around the house. He states that his mother cooks for him and he has never cooked for himself and he does not do anything around the yard either. His grooming showed him to be wearing a shirt slacks with no shoes or socks and he was clean shaven his hair styled and neatly brushed. He reports going to bed around 1 or 2 am. Most of his day is spent listening to the radio and watching television. While showing that he could ambulate he had significant difficulty walking on his toes; he was unable to do this but he was able to walk on his heels and his gait appeared to be normal. There was no significant psychomotor retardation noted. Mental status: The mental status reveals a 29-year-old Vietnamese male who appears to be of average height and weight. He denied any paranoid ideations or auditory or visual hallucinations. He was oriented to time place and date and he was able to do 1 to 20 forward and backwards without any difficulty. He refused to do serial 7s although he was able to subtract 7 from 10 correctly. He showed difficulty with memory although he could remember that he had lived in the house that he lives in now for the last year and a half. He denied any headaches or visual difficulties or aura that might indicate seizure activity. He did have an affect of sadness and depression. When asked what he would change about himself he stated that he would change his bad health to good health. He has no goals at the present time. He is on no medication at the present time and he does not have a history of drug or alcohol use or abuse. He denied sleep or appetite problems or crying. There does appear to be some anhedonia. Medications: The claimant is taking no medications at the present time. Provisional Diagnosis: Axis I. Transient situational depression due to surgery mild to moderate. Axis II. Rule out organic brain syndrome. Observations and recommendations: Because there were no medical reports sent with this individual it would be recommended that there be a review to see if there actually was a surgery at College Hospital and what was the purpose of the surgery and what an update may be on his neurological function. In fact I would recommend a neurological evaluation to see if the depression emanates from the surgery itself or from some emotional disturbance. There is no indication that Mr Dao could handle his own funds and it is recommended that a payee be appointed if he is approved for disability. Thank you for the consultation. Very truly yours

13-9 FINAL REVIEW

DIRECTIONS: Examine the figures for operative reports in this chapter and Appendix C on Evolve. Make a list of the following subjects on separate sheet of paper, and insert all of the words you find under each topic subject:

► Position of patient
► Instruments and tools used
► Type of anesthesia and material
► Suture materials
► Procedures performed

EXAMPLE

Position of patient

    Supine

    Prone jackknife

Instruments and tools used

    Scissors

    Bovie clamp

Type of anesthesia and material

    0.5% Marcaine

    Bupivacaine

Suture materials

    4-0 Prolene

    2-0 chromic

Procedures performed

    Excisional biopsy

    Hemorrhoidectomy

13

CHAPTER

CHAPTER 14

Writing Business Documents: Email, Memos, Agendas, Minutes, and Policies

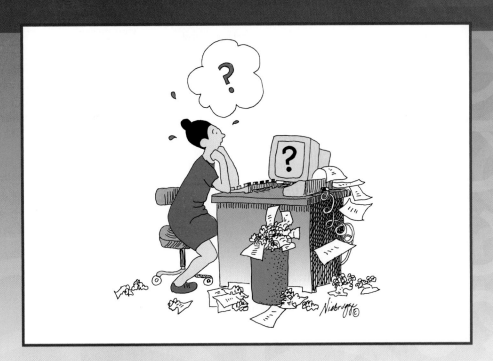

OBJECTIVES

After reading this chapter and completing the exercises, you should be able to

1. Discuss the importance of being able to compose business documents and reports.
2. Recognize the rules for writing clear and concise business documents.
3. Compose a business email and a business memo.
4. Recognize and use rules for writing email messages and memos.
5. Consider sensitive issues in sending email messages and practice email etiquette.
6. Explain the problems that may arise when sending medical records as email attachments.
7. Discuss the importance of maintaining confidentiality in writing and storing email messages.
8. Type an agenda for a meeting.
9. Record, prepare, and type minutes for a meeting in correct format.
10. Prepare a hospital policy document in typical format.

INTRODUCTION

This chapter explains in detail the format for reports other than medical reports regarding patient care. (Refer to Chapter 12 for information on preparing a history and physical (H&P) and to Chapter 13 for preparing miscellaneous medical reports.) You will learn how to set up, prepare, and type business email documents, hospital policies and protocols, memos, and meeting agendas and how to record and type minutes for a meeting.

Formats enhance written communication; however, the most important aspects of composing such documents are the readability and effectiveness of the communication.

COMPOSITION GUIDELINES

Writing Sentences

Good business writing is clear, concise, correct, complete, and considerate. If the basic element used to convey meaning—the sentence—is unclear, the entire message may be difficult to understand. Good sentence structure requires application of all rules of English grammar and avoidance of certain particularly common errors.

Be sure you have studied Chapter 10 and have completed the exercises and reviewed any problem areas. You can always refer to Chapter 10 to check any problems you may encounter. Even though Chapter 10 addresses the issue of grammar as if you were making sure someone else's words were used correctly, the same directives apply to you as the writer. Material should be specific and organized free of ambiguities and generalities. The following is a simple review with a few additional hints to help you compose. Begin by examining some problems to avoid.

Sentence Fragments

A sentence is a group of words that expresses a complete thought and must contain a subject (usually a noun) and a predicate (usually a verb). Any combination of words that does not fulfill these conditions is not a sentence and should be avoided in good business English.

Run-on Sentences

When two sentences are run together without any connecting word (e.g., *although, therefore,* or *and*) or punctuation (a semicolon, dash, or colon) to divide them, they can be difficult to understand.

EXAMPLE

Dr Broughton is out of town, therefore I am replying to your memo. (incorrect)

Each phrase could stand alone as a separate sentence. Therefore, the phrases should be separated by a word or by some form of punctuation stronger than a comma. The example could be corrected in any of the following ways:

Dr Broughton is out of town; therefore, I am replying to your memo.

Dr Broughton is out of town. Therefore, I am replying to your memo.

Because Dr Broughton is out of town, I am replying to your memo.

Parallel Structure

Always express coordinate elements within a sentence or within a list in similar grammatical forms. Match nouns with nouns, infinitives with infinitives, verbs with verbs, adjectives with adjectives, and so on.

EXAMPLE

Learning to write is a challenge and interesting.

Here, writing is described with a noun *(challenge)* and an adjective *(interesting)*. It would be better to use two adjectives and change the sentence to read as follows:

Learning to write is challenging and interesting.

Examine the lack of coordinate elements in the following examples.

EXAMPLES

The three purposes of this study:

To enhance communication between members of the team.

So that we can provide a retrospective study of care.

To be able to strengthen the team leader's role.

IMPROVED

The following are examples of the purpose of this study:

To enhance communication between members of the team,

To provide a retrospective study of care, and

To strengthen the team leader's role.

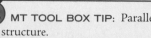 MT TOOL BOX TIP: Parallel lists—a tool for good structure.

Dangling Constructions

The most awkward and sometimes embarrassing errors in writing often result from poor sentence construction. Sometimes, certain kinds of phrases and clauses, usually occurring at the beginning of a sentence, do not agree logically with the subject. These constructions are referred to as "dangling."

To correct a dangling construction, make the subject of the sentence the *doer* of the action expressed in the troublesome phrase or clause. If that step is not at all feasible, rework your sentence completely to make it logical. Examine these "danglers" and a possible restructure of the sentence.

EXAMPLE

Having met his wife's aunt, a family dinner was planned.

IMPROVED

A family dinner was planned to celebrate meeting his wife's aunt.

EXAMPLE

Leaving the building, the door caught my coat.

IMPROVED

The door caught my coat as I left the building.

Unnecessary or Repetitious Words

Eliminate unnecessary phrases and useless words without sacrificing meaning. Strive to be simple and direct.

Wordy	Concise
I have taken the liberty of writing at the present time	I am writing now
In view of the fact that	Because
Additional reports will be issued from time to time in the future	Additional reports will be issued periodically
It is the hope of the undersigned	I hope

Notice the unnecessary phrases and useless words italicized in the following examples:

Give this memo your prompt *and speedy* attention

Your email arrived *in this office*

We will have a meeting *coming up*

We will convert *over* to

my *personal* opinion

my *actual* experience

adequate *enough*

combine *together*

each *individual* transcriptionist

eliminate *altogether*

sum *total*

filled to *capacity*

future plans

true fact

Substitute the words in the right column below for those in the left column.

Avoid	Use
converse	talk
is fully cognizant of	knows
the writer	I
relative to	about
in regard to	about
in connection with	about
will you be so kind as to	please
are in need of	need
in the amount of	for
in the event that	if
under date of	on
in the near future	soon
a substantial segment	many
interrogate	question
due to the circumstance	because
during the course of	during
at the present time	now
at this point in time	now
despite the fact that	although
due to the fact that	because
on account of	because

Avoid the use of *up* when it adds no meaning to the verb.

EXAMPLES

We have to finish *up* this dictation before we leave this evening.

I was asked to head *up* the committee.

14-1 SELF-STUDY

DIRECTIONS: Recast the following sentences to avoid run-on structure. Type your answers to these problems and those that follow on a separate piece of paper. Check your answers in Appendix A, p. 461.

1. Please recheck this, it is your responsibility.
2. Remodeling is taking place in the emergency room, therefore reroute all patient traffic to Ward B until further notice.
3. The new chief of staff will take over the first of next month, furthermore many new physicians will be added to the active staff roster.

Rewrite the following to maintain parallel structure.

4. To be accurate and meet your production level is important here.
5. Pull the patient's record, notifying the doctor of the emergency, then give the record to the doctor and be sure to relate any information you have received.
6. Please observe the following:
   a. Enter your department number on each requisition.
   b. Use the preprinted requisitions.
   c. If the preprinted requisition is not available for the record you require, refer to the patient register.
7. Please include these in the list for duties of the custodian of records:
   a. to keep minimum turnaround time
   b. corrections must be made in the proper way
   c. be sure the records are signed or initialed
   d. do not let unauthorized persons see the records without a release

Eliminate the dangling construction in the following sentences:

8. I saw many new flowers jogging through the parking lot.
9. While on vacation, my dog stayed at my mother's house.
10. Her first and only child was born at age 44.
11. The record was finally returned floating through the department.

Strike through the unnecessary words that take up space and add nothing to the ideas expressed. (You may write directly on the page or type your answer on a separate sheet.)

12. Mrs Benson just recovered from an attack of pneumonia.
13. Your memo arrived at a time when Dr Berry was on vacation.
14. The water is for drinking purposes only.
15. We will return the equipment at a later date.
16. We are now engaged in building a new medical wing.
17. The report describes the patient's medical records during the period from May 2000 to May 2001.
18. The operative procedure lasted up to 8 hours in duration.
19. The new printer is smaller in size.
20. The patient's disability will last a period of 4 weeks.

Correct the grammar in the final sentences by adding, eliminating, or changing parts of the sentences.

21. I feel the nursing personnel as well as pulmonary medicine staff will benefit from the information and instructions.
22. The Advisory Committee and Management Department would like to express their thanks for the time you gave to present the material to us.
23. For this reason, that the medical record might be the physician's only witness in court, that record must be completely accurate.
24. By writing one, learns to write.

Planning and Writing Paragraphs

A good way to form paragraphs is to strive for a one- or two-paragraph memo or email. These documents are brief and require only a few paragraphs. If a document has more than two paragraphs, it might not be poorly constructed, but it probably does need to be tightened up. However, check the document to see whether anything is lacking. (Often, the missing element is the personal touch—the extra element that communicates feeling to the reader.) Concentrate on informing your readers, not on trying to impress them.

Therefore, a document should have two characteristics: one subject and two aspects—feeling and thinking.

Start by taking out excess verbiage. One fault of poor writing is complexity. Often this fault is caused by burying the main idea deep in dates of prior correspondence, invoice numbers, identification numbers, and so on. The cure for this problem is simple: Use a subject line. This step lets you make your point immediately in the main part of the documents. It allows you to make your point early, clearly, and concisely.

Another frequent cause of complexity is trying to cover more than one subject in one document. The remedy for this fault is to write two documents. If this remedy is inconvenient, write one document as if it were two, and use a final paragraph to sum up the substance of both subjects.

Your paragraphs should be concise and courteous. Try this method: In your opening paragraph, state the problem or make the point; in your second paragraph, elaborate or provide detail and sum up or state what has to be done.

OPENING TOPIC

Write a topic sentence that states the main idea to be developed. Place the topic sentence at or near the beginning of the document. Concentrate on the purpose for writing about this subject and on the expected outcome.

TRANSITIONS

Use connective phrases, such as *however, therefore, nevertheless, for this reason, in fact, in contrast,* and so on, to achieve transitions within or between paragraphs. You do not want an abrupt change in shifting to the next sentence or the next paragraph.

SECOND PARAGRAPH

Give details in sequence (chronological or locational), or use enumerations such as *first, second, third,* and so on. Remember that this paragraph elaborates and provides all the necessary details for the reader.

FINAL SENTENCE

In the final sentence, state clearly the results, reaction, action, or desired attitude. If you outlined your document first, this sentence will coincide with that part of the outline.

Beginning to Write

▶ Make an outline. Decide if your outline is chronological or by order of importance. The first paragraph has all the key points. Flesh this paragraph out and go into detail as you go along.
▶ Begin by saying what you want to say. Be concise, yet complete, and courteous.
▶ Use simple declarative sentences.
▶ Avoid trite openings.

NOT: In reference to your correspondence of July 14 informing me…
BUT: Thank you for reminding me…

▶ In writing for another person, use an impersonal tone, place the other's name foremost, or use passive voice.

NOT: I am glad to inform you that the results of your tests…

BUT: This letter is to inform you that the results of your tests…

OR: Dr Berry asked me to inform you…

NOT: I submitted the report on…
BUT: The report was submitted on…

In passive voice, the subject is acted upon; the person or thing performing the action is the object of the sentence. This construction can become awkward, weak, wordy, and unclear. It lacks the strength and precision of active voice. Therefore, we avoid using the passive-voice verb construction, as illustrated in the preceding example.

EXCEPTION: The reason outlined above.

A good balance of active and passive voice can be pleasant but will depend on where you want to place your emphasis in writing.

NOT: The surgery was performed by Dr Augustus. *(Passive)*
BUT: Dr Augustus performed the surgery. *(Active)*

NOT: He was released for return to his regular employment by Dr Berry. *(Passive)*
BUT: Dr Berry released him for regular employment. *(Active)*

Notice in the preceding example of passive voice that it not only takes longer to say what you want to say but also could appear that Dr Berry is the employer.

▶ Use a positive approach. Discuss what can be done instead of what cannot.

NOT: We are unable to permit you to use the auditorium for the conference on the date you requested.
BUT: We will be pleased to accommodate your conference in the auditorium on the following dates…

▶ Avoid words that antagonize, such as overlooked, failure, neglected, forgot, careless, and mistake.

NOT: We do not understand your failure to complete the dictation on schedule.
BUT: We are certain that your problem with incomplete dictation is due to some unavoidable circumstance or a misunderstanding of the schedule.

▶ Use a subject line on memos and emails. This device lets you make your point immediately in the main part of the document.

Body of the Document

▶ Use simple, natural language similar to that of your everyday conversation. Avoid unnecessary words and phrases; insert them solely for cadence and balance (see p. 367).

14

CHAPTER

- Be sure you tell the reader all he or she needs to know in order to act or respond. You must remember to support your theme, and any secondary ideas should be related to the main one. Point the recipient toward a required action or attitude.
- Use courteous language: *please, thank you, I appreciate.*
- Use short and interesting sentences; vary the construction of your sentences.
- Avoid favorite words or expressions, and be sure that you are not "cute" or flip.

  NOT: I *certainly* am relieved that you will be able to take over the graveyard shift, and I *certainly* appreciate your *stepping up to the plate* and getting back to me so quickly…
  BUT: I am relieved that you will be able to take over the graveyard shift, and I appreciate your quick response.

- Do not confuse the reader with abrupt moves from one idea to the next.
- Use words your reader will understand, and avoid using unnecessary technical terms or abbreviations.
- Avoid "dummy" subjects.

  NOT: It is believed that surgery may solve this problem…
  BUT: Surgery may solve this problem…

Closing of the Document

- Acknowledge a favor if there was one.

  ### EXAMPLE
  Thank you for the invitation to participate.

- Make an appropriate apology if necessary.

  ### EXAMPLE
  We are sorry for any inconvenience this delay may have caused.

However, do not "overapologize" or pass the blame to someone else.

  NOT: I do not know how I could have made such an awful mistake, and I promise I will never let it happen again.
  BUT: I am sorry that my negligence inconvenienced you.

- Create a feeling of cooperation and good will.

  ### EXAMPLE
  We look forward to your presentation at our conference.

- Avoid the "-ing" endings.

  NOT: Hoping to hear from you
  Trusting this will give you time
  Thanking you in advance
  Looking forward to meeting you
  BUT: We hope to be hearing from you
  We trust this will give you time
  Thank you in advance
  We look forward to meeting you

WRITING MEMORANDA

The purpose of the memo (*memorandum;* plural, *memos* or *memoranda*) is to quickly and economically send a communication to one or more people within the office, company, department, or hospital. A memo conveys a very formal, a casual or informal, or an impersonal impression. Usually, courtesy titles are not used for the addressees or the writer; the use of first names or initials is acceptable. Decide whether the memo dictates a formal or informal approach, and treat the use of names accordingly. Memos can be of one type or a combination of several types: *informative,* providing facts and explanations; *directive,* containing step-by-step instructions with explanations; or *administrative,* stating policy or official opinion or judgment on a topic. Memos provide permanent or temporary records. Avoid writing memos about a confidential matter or delicate subject.

 MT TOOL BOX TIP: Proper formats for letters are important tools.

General Format

A special format is used for writing memos; it is similar to that used in writing business email. Composing a memo is very much like composing a letter. First, determine what you want to say and why you are saying it. Second, think of your reader. Design the memo in such a way that the information you want to communicate is easy to absorb and in such a form that the reader will be able to use the information easily. As in all business writing, the message should be clear, concise, correct, considerate, and complete.

Preprinted and Computer-Formatted Macros

Some businesses prefer to have preprinted forms or computerized formats to simplify and standardize the treatment of the information. Your word processing software has a sample template for you to use or modify. You can make your own template or macro if you write memos frequently. The current date is automatically inserted, and various type fonts and sizes are provided to add interest to the appearance.

Typed Format

When using plain paper, type the appropriate headings. Use the hanging indent feature to vertically align the columns based on the longest guide word in each column or set tab stops two or three spaces after the longest guide word in each column so that the information is vertically aligned. This format is preferred

---

MEMORANDUM

DATE: September 22, 20XX

TO: Andrea M. Abbott
                 Kirsten H. Andrews
                 Katelyn P. Delaney

FROM: Susanne Woodnow, MD

SUBJECT: Speech recognition software.

We have finally made the decision to implement the speech recognition software that was demonstrated to our department last month. We will be able to take applications from those medical transcriptionists who would like to begin the training program for the software application immediately.   The first training program will be able to accept 5 students with 5 additional students each following Monday until everyone who wishes to apply has been trained.   Training will begin on October 15 at 8 a.m. Training consists of three 2-hour classes.

Please notify all MTs in your section of this opportunity. Those whose work hours conflict with training times should also apply, and we will schedule special classes for them.

All classroom time will be compensated at the usual hourly rate.

tra

FIGURE 14-1 Example of a memorandum, vertical style.

when additional space is required for the list of the persons receiving the memo.

The following elements are used in setting up the format for the memo, with an explanation for each. The first four headings are typed on the actual memorandum. (Figure 14-1 depicts the memo format.) Preprinted forms, made of less expensive paper than letter stationery, are usually available, but if not, use plain paper and type in the headings. Use wide (1¼ inch) top and side margins. You can use boldface for your headings.

Date: Date of origination.

To: A list of the persons or departments for routing the memo. When you send a memo to individuals who are on the same level (e.g., all MTs), list the names in alphabetical order. If a memo is being sent to individuals on various professional levels, list the names by rank. Indicate distribution by writing *please route* on a single copy of the memo with names listed or by making a copy for each person or department.

From: Writer or speaker. The originator usually does not sign the memo but may initial it next to his or her name or at the bottom of the memo.

Subject: The subject line appears in the heading and tells the reader what the memo is about; thus, the reader can get right to the main point. The accuracy of the subject line is extremely important.

Headings can be vertical or horizontal, depending on the employer's or typist's preference. The order in which the four headings are listed can vary, but the subject heading is always the last in the lineup.

VERTICAL

Format a vertical-style memo as follows:

DATE:
TO:
FROM:
SUBJECT:

▶ Type the headings flush with the left margin.
▶ Use full capital letters, followed by a colon.
▶ Type the memo 2 inches from the top of the paper.
▶ Double-space between headings.
▶ Tab twice to clear the outline words and fill in the headings.
▶ Begin the body of the memo three line spaces after the last heading.
▶ Single-space the body of the memo.
▶ Double-space between paragraphs.
▶ Use full block format.

Figure 14-1 is a sample of the vertical-style memo.

HORIZONTAL

TO: DATE:

FROM: SUBJECT:

Format a horizontal-style memo as follows:

▶ Type the first two headings flush with the left margin.

▶ Double-space between the headings.

▶ Tab twice to fill in the name or names of the recipient or recipients of the memo.

▶ Repeat tab to fill in the name of the author.

▶ Type *DATE* and *SUBJECT* to the right of the center of the page.

▶ Use two tabs to begin typing the date from the first letter of *DATE*.

▶ Use two tabs to fill in the name of the subject from the first letter of *SUBJECT*.

▶ Begin the body of the memo three line spaces after the last heading, and complete as described for the vertical style.

You can see that this format is not as easy to follow as the more popular vertical style and could be inappropriate if the subject line is lengthy.

If you frequently use email to send memos, you need only insert the names of the recipients with their email addresses and the subject, because the date and your name will appear as a regular part of the email message. More email guidelines are given at the end of these memo-formatting guidelines.

Closing Elements

The memo is completed with the typist's initials two line spaces after the last line of the body of the memo. It is not necessary to type the author's initials, but the typist should do so if it is the custom in the organization. A typed signature line is not used, and the author/dictator does not sign the memo. (There is a trend toward omitting the *from* line in favor of a typed signature at the close of the memo. If you choose this less formal approach, the author can initial or sign the memo here.) Even though the memo is not signed by the author, it should always be submitted to him or her for approval before it is distributed. Some writers initial their memo after their name on the *from* line. Reference initials, enclosures, and copy notations should be handled exactly as they are in a letter, in the following order, one or two line spaces below one another and beginning two line spaces below the closing:

▶ Reference initials

▶ Enclosure line

▶ Copy notation

▶ Postscript

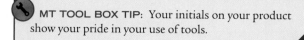

MT TOOL BOX TIP: Your initials on your product show your pride in your use of tools.

Continuations

Avoid lengthy memos, but if the memo must continue to an additional page or pages, begin typing 1 inch from the top of the page and type your headings: name of the addressee, date, and page number. After three line spaces, continue with the body of the memo. Memos should deal with a single subject; therefore, be alert when confronted with a lengthy memo. It could be necessary to formulate an additional memo with a new subject line.

GETTING STARTED WRITING

One of the major hurdles in writing is getting through the agonizing stage of deciding what to say and getting started. Some authors, expecting to produce simultaneously a well-planned, well-written, and polished document, try in vain to organize their thoughts and compose while sitting in front of their computer.

Be realistic. Organize your thoughts on scratch paper before you begin. Plan carefully. The extra steps you take to make a rough draft of your thoughts are not wasted because you will have the document more than half-written before you actually start to compose it.

Practice with a memo, but the guidelines pertain to other documents as well.

Make an outline to cover the following points:

1. Why: Formulate a clear idea of the reason for the message. Clearly state your purpose for writing.

2. Who: Know the audience to whom you are writing and how that audience should be approached.

3. What: List all information to be conveyed. List the secondary or supporting topics that go with the central idea. Be careful about details.

4. Reaction: Describe how you expect the recipient to react, your desired action, attitude, or result.

Using your outline, list exactly what you want to say; be clear, concise, coherent, and specific. Choose strong, precise words; place your words correctly; and plan your sentences well. Writing is more precise and a bit more formal than the spoken word, and you need to keep that difference in mind. Remember that you want to convey a particular message without confusion or excess verbiage. A concise document, be it a staff memo or an email, avoids anything that the reader already knows. However, sometimes it is necessary to "remind" the reader of certain things before continuing with new information.

Composing Example

When you know exactly what you need to say, you must organize your material in an orderly manner and learn how to express yourself well. See how this plan works with the following outline:

1. Why: The staff lounge is inadequate and is disorganized.
2. Who: Hospital remodeling committee.
3. What: Can this area be expanded, remodeled, or reorganized?
4. Plus: Are there any other underutilized areas that can be converted into a staff lounge either as a second lounge or a larger lounge?
5. Reaction: The remodeling committee will place the physician's request on the agenda for the next meeting.

Here is a memo that follows this outline:

DATE: Today
TO: Remodeling Committee
FROM: David R. Blankenship, MD, Chairman, Housekeeping Committee
SUBJECT: Staff lounge for 3B

The staff lounge on 3B is inadequate and disorganized.

▶ There is not enough storage area in either refrigerator for lunch bags and break items.
▶ There are not enough tables and chairs to accommodate the personnel who use the lounge from 6 a.m. until 4 p.m. (There are 2 large round tables, 11 table chairs, 4 lounge chairs, and 1 coffee table.)
▶ There are not enough hooks for staff to hang up jackets, lab coats, and so on. (There are 6 wall hooks and 1 hat rack with 4 arms.)
▶ There are not enough refuse bins to contain debris. (There are two 30-gallon bins.) (Housekeeping has to return to clean this area outside of normal cleanup duties.)

I am requesting a larger area be established for the 3B staff lounge, with an additional refrigerator, chairs, tables, refuse containers, and storage lockers. If a larger area is not possible, please consider an additional staff lounge to accommodate our staff on 3B. Please give this situation high priority and place this problem on your agenda of the next meeting of the Remodeling Committee.

    Thank you.

Here is how the preceding memo came to be written: Dr Blankenship came to the transcription department and asked for help. He said he had run into "Bob" (the head of the hospital remodeling committee) in the elevator and told him that there were major problems with the staff lounge on our floor. Bob said, "Put it in writing, and I'll put it on the agenda when we meet next week." Dr Blankenship asked you to send Bob a memo about the problems (which he briefly outlined) so that it would be on their agenda. Do you think that the writer of this memo has adequately responded to Dr Blankenship's request?

Review of Your Document

Finally, reread the document and see whether it covers clearly and exactly what you want to say. Did you follow your outline and include all elements from your outline? It is often a good idea to put aside something that was particularly difficult to compose and complete some other chore. When you come back to the document, you could find some changes to be made, or you could be satisfied with it. Now make sure you have followed your outline and have omitted nothing. Read your document as if you were the person receiving it. Do you have any questions? No. (Good!) Yes. (Rewrite!)

▶ Be sure you have written clear, correctly worded sentences.
▶ Be sure that your grammar, spelling, and punctuation are accurate.
▶ Scrutinize the document for clarity, content, and tone.
▶ Review your plan and check that your plan is complete.
▶ Be prepared to revise, rewrite, and eliminate redundant phrases; change the positions of sentences; and correct the grammar.
▶ Seek criticism and accept it gracefully.

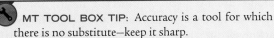

MT TOOL BOX TIP: Accuracy is a tool for which there is no substitute—keep it sharp.

ELECTRONIC MAIL

Electronic mail (also called *email* or *e-mail*) is the process of sending, receiving, storing, and forwarding medical records, messages and other forms of electronic communication (e.g., newsletters, photos, attachments, and reports) over computer networks and the Internet. Time and money are saved by using this system of sending and receiving communications. You can set the importance level of your documents by selecting the priority level from your email menu. When sending email, it is important to follow the Health Insurance Portability and Accountability Act of 1996 (HIPAA) regulations (see Chapter 1) and etiquette guidelines. When sending email memos and other business email, remember that your recipient could receive hundreds of messages every day. Keep a few courtesies in mind when composing this special correspondence.

Attachments

▶ Add a cover note when sending an attached file, so the receiver will know to look for it.
▶ Avoid attachment problems by copying the text and pasting it into the body of your message.
▶ Don't forward large files without compressing them.

Confidentiality

- Observe confidentiality issues in both sending and receiving email messages.
- Don't send a message that you do not want made public. Some courts have ruled that a company's email is company property, and employers are allowed access to their employees' email files.
- Use password protection, encryption, and authentication in transmission of patients' records. Data security must be ensured. When protected health information is sent via email, the email itself must be encrypted. This encryption is accomplished by using a pair of individual electronic "keys." One key is public and the other is private. The public key does not need to be protected and can be publicly published. It can be used by any sender to encrypt the email; only the private key, which must be protected, can decrypt the email. For example, if you want to email sensitive information to another medical facility, you would use their published public key to encrypt the document. Upon receipt, the receiving office would use their private key to open the document for viewing. Private keys are protected by a physical device (key card) and/or password.
- Don't use or disclose protected health information without a signed consent form. (Patients must acknowledge they understand the risks of email information.)
- Don't use patient identifiers in the subject field.
- Insert a notice macro at the end of your email communication such as the following:
  "This email may contain confidential and privileged material for the sole use of the intended recipient. Any review or distribution by others is strictly prohibited. If you are not the intended recipient, please contact the sender and delete all copies."

Content

- Insert a meaningful, detailed, and straightforward subject line. Many people use the subject line as a filing system and depend on it to locate key information later. Update the subject line when you send a reply.
- Write your message with the same tone and style as those used for a business letter or memo.
- Use an informal greeting comparable to that used for a postcard.
- Choose words carefully when expressing emotion or describing feeling. These comments can be misinterpreted because the receiver cannot see the body language or hear the tone of voice.
- Number requests when you have more than one.
- Use bullets to emphasize action items.

- Do not incorporate fancy fonts; they could be received as confusing characters.
- Retain portions of an original message so the recipient can see what is referred to.
- Snip (delete) text by inserting <snip> or <SNIP> where you have eliminated extraneous portions of the original message, retaining only relevant text.
- Avoid writing complicated and detailed information; a telephone call could be a better choice with email used as a follow up or recap.
- Be careful to address the email correctly so it reaches the correct destination There are no spaces in email addresses, and the exact configuration, with uppercase and lowercase letters, numbers, the @ symbol, and domain tag, must be given.

EXAMPLE

griffs@aol.com

- End each message with a signature file of about four lines. This file should contain your name, email address, and telephone and fax numbers.
- Use only essential punctuation.
- Do not use tabs or make columns; these elements can change during electronic transmission. The recipient generally receives the message restructured, and these odd arrangements make the message difficult to read.
- Check spelling, grammar, and accuracy.
- Do not put anything in an email that you would not want to "see on the front page of the newspaper."
- Remember that emails can be forwarded to others without your knowledge or consent.

Copies

- Retain copies of your messages for a specific period so you can refer to them if necessary. Some systems allow you to organize messages into files.
- Print and file messages when a paper record is needed.

Distribution Lists

- Include all individuals who have a legitimate need to receive the information when you distribute an email message. Send copies only to those who need to know.
- Suppress and blind copy (BCC) distribution lists when you send a document to a large group of recipients, both to cut down on the length of the document and to guard the name and address privacy of the recipients.
- Send the message only to those persons directly concerned with the message. Because it is very easy to send copies to many different recipients, many messages sent simply add to the accumulation of clutter.

Etiquette

▶ Do not write anything racially or sexually offensive or sarcastic or use language that could be considered off-color.

▶ Use proper grammar and spelling. Remember that your correspondence reflects your professionalism.

▶ Do not forward jokes, junk mail, or advertising in a business setting.

▶ Do not gossip or send remarks about other individuals or discuss proprietary information.

▶ Do not write about bad news or delicate issues that would be better dealt with in person.

▶ Do not send chain letters.

▶ Do not respond immediately to any message that upsets you.

▶ Follow policies instituted by the employer on use of email for personal correspondence.

▶ Inquire about the company's policy for subscribing to news groups or lists.

▶ Follow company guidelines for retaining and deleting messages.

▶ Respond promptly to any message you have received. If you are unable to give a compete response, at least acknowledge receipt and let the sender know when you will respond in full.

▶ Check your mailbox frequently—at least twice a day.

▶ Respect the sensitivity level that the sender has applied to the communication.

▶ Do not forward personal mail unless you have the original sender's permission to do so.

▶ Credit the individual if you are quoting someone in the message.

▶ Do not send messages to those in your employ pointing out errors or shortcomings.

▶ Use "automatic reply" to notify the sender of your targeted return date when you are unable to respond to your email on a regular basis.

▶ Do not capitalize full words. Doing so implies that you are shouting at the recipient. Instead, put asterisks around sentences or phrases that you want to emphasize.

EXAMPLE

Please telephone me immediately!

▶ Keep messages short.

▶ Do not use email to avoid speaking directly to someone.

Response

▶ Establish rules for responding to email by return email or telephone. This practice keeps you from waiting for a reply that simply never comes or arrives too late for the business at hand.

▶ Do not rule out using the telephone instead of email to respond to an email message. You might be surprised to find that your task suddenly became easier.

▶ Change the subject line to reflect a change in the focus of the message.

▶ Return to using the telephone instead of email if it is not necessary to have something in writing and you are corresponding with a single person. The main asset of email correspondence is that you can write when it is convenient for you and your recipients can read when it is convenient for them. However, if something needs to be taken care of immediately, don't depend on your email to do it.

 14-2 SELF-STUDY

DIRECTIONS: Compose the following two email documents for your signature at the direction of one of the staff physicians. Check your answers in Appendix A, p. 462.

1. William A. Berry, MD, has asked you to write the following email for your signature. Dr Berry has made arrangements for one of his patients, Mr Ray Littlefield (email address rlittle@home.net), to see another physician, Paul R. Vecchione, in consultation.
   ▶ Make your outline first.
   ▶ Compose your document by following the appropriate rules.
   ▶ Use today's date and then invent the necessary information to write Mr Littlefield, who knows that these arrangements were to be made.

2. Dr Berry has agreed to address the high school Parent-Teacher Association (PTA) in the community about the increased use of alcohol by young adults. Compose an email to the program chairperson; invent the necessary data. Part of Dr Berry's presentation will be the screening of a 20-minute film titled "More Than a Few Beers." He will be prepared for a question-and-answer period to follow his presentation.

- ▶ Make your outline first.
- ▶ Compose your document by following the appropriate rules.
- ▶ Use today's date. You can invent the necessary information to write the program chairperson.

NOTE: Often students ask why one cannot simply use the telephone and call the firm or person involved to take care of the business. The answer is simple: You need the "conversation" in writing; you frequently need a transcript of exactly what was "said."

TYPING HOSPITAL PROTOCOLS AND REPORTS

Hospital protocols are also known as hospital reports or hospital policies. Each hospital department or division has specific policies and procedures. Because each institution has variances, only general guidelines on format, headings, and subheadings are given here. Hospital protocols have individual headings for the topics and titles. These vary, just as the nature of the report varies. See Appendix C on Evolve for a hospital nursing policy and for an administrative policy concerning medical records. The originator of a report may or may not formulate the title; so the title of each section is abstracted from the main idea and expressed in that section. The hospital or institution usually has a special format, and often special paper or a word processing template, for typing these documents.

> 🔧 **MT TOOL BOX TIP:** Accept that policies, rules and procedures keep your tools in perfect working order.

Headings and Outline

The format follows outline form and is in full block, modified block, or indented style. If there is more than one paragraph under a specific title, construct paragraphs just as you would in a full block letter: double-space and begin the new paragraph flush with the left margin. A policy report should be headed with the title of the policy and its identifying number. Headings should be consistent throughout the report and should follow simple guidelines:

1. Title: centered on the page and typed in full capital letters. It may be underlined or typed in boldface if you desire.
2. Main topic titles: full capital letters, underlined.
3. Subtopic titles: full capital letters, not underlined.
4. Minor topic titles: uppercase and lowercase letters, underlined.
5. Page one: If the protocol is for a department in the hospital, such as the emergency department, the page could be shown as ED-1; imaging department may be shown as ID-1, and so on.

Lists

The following rules apply to using lists in memos, reports, minutes, or policies.

1. Lists can be introduced with serial numbers or letters of the alphabet followed by a period or parentheses. Bullets (●) are also appropriate substitutes for numbers or letters.
2. Lists are typed in block format under the beginning of each line, and typing is not flush with the number, letter, or bullet; instead, it is indented and

FIGURE 14-2 Sample format for a hospital procedure or policy. (From Diehl MO: *Medical Transcription Guide: Do's and Don'ts,* ed 3, Philadelphia, 2004, Saunders.)

blocked with the first line of text following the number, letter, or bullet.

3. Lists do not need to be complete sentences but should be terminated with periods.

4. Lists should have parallel construction (see p. 386) and be grammatically consistent.

Multipage Reports

If hospital documents continue past one page, type the word *continued* at the bottom of the completed page. The subsequent page or pages begin 1 inch from the top of the page with the title of the document, the page number (the second page might be shown as ED-2 for emergency department, ID-2 for imaging department, and so on), and any other important data (e.g., the policy number).

Closing Format

Figures 14-2 and 14-3 illustrate sample closing formats for reports or policies. Figure 14-3 is typed in the full block format. Every report or policy should include the name or initials of persons involved in its preparation and transcription. Hospital protocols or policies are approved by hospital committees and are reviewed and revised from time to time.

Wood Creek Medical Center
50 South Main Street
Wood Creek, XY 12345

MEDICAL RECORD PROCEDURES

SUBPOENAS
Medical records shall only be removed from the hospital jurisdiction in accordance with court order, subpoena, statute, or approval of the hospital administrator. Only those individuals specifically authorized by the director of medical records may accept subpoenas for medical records.

Unless specifically authorized by the administrator, no subpoena will be accepted by medical record personnel for cases in which the hospital is a party to the action. These subpoenas must be served upon the administrator or his or her designee in the case of his or her absence. The subpoenaed medical records will be given to the administrator to be placed in a controlled environment.

If it appears necessary to remove medical records from the jurisdiction of the hospital, as under court order, subpoena, or statute, an effort will be made to ascertain if it would be acceptable to send copies of the record rather than the original medical record.

CONTINUING EDUCATION AND INSERVICE TRAINING
Medical record department personnel shall be encouraged to participate in educational programs, professional associations, organizational meetings, and pertinent correspondence courses related to their duties. Educational achievement shall be documented.

FILING OF INCOMPLETE MEDICAL RECORDS
Except on order of the medical record committee, no medical record shall be filed until it is complete.

LIST OF COMMONLY USED ABBREVIATIONS, ACRONYMS, AND SYMBOLS
A list of approved abbreviations, acronyms, and symbols for use in the medical record will be maintained in the medical record department. The list shall be approved by the medical staff.

MICROFILMING MEDICAL RECORDS
Charts will be microfilmed after a reasonable time depending on the filing space available for completed medical records. The microfilming will be done by the medical record microfilm clerk. Records will be screened before they are microfilmed to ensure accurate patient identification. Each processed microfilm roll will be reviewed before the destruction of the original records to ensure readability of the film.

Approved_____   Policy Number 90-100

Effective date: June 1, 20XX   Revised:

Reviewed: Revised:

Reviewed:

FIGURE 14-3 Example of a page from a hospital policy and procedure manual, illustrating full block format. Wording and content of hospital policies and procedures vary from institution to institution.

AGENDA

An agenda is prepared before a meeting and establishes the order of business of the meeting and the items to be discussed or the plan of activities. It is mailed to the meeting participants before the meeting or distributed as the meeting begins. The secretary of the organization or committee can use a copy to assist in taking notes and preparing the minutes.

The format of the agenda should be functional and easy to read. These goals are achieved by using such layout techniques as centered headings, columnar lists for agenda items, and white space between items. The agenda should be typed, double-spaced, and, if possible, kept to one page. Roman numerals are often used to number the items. The following information may be included in a formal agenda:

1. Name, date, and time of the meeting (centered on the page).
2. Location of the meeting.
3. Call to order.
4. Roll call and/or introduction of members and/or board of directors.
5. Introduction of guests and/or new members.
6. Reading and approval of the minutes of the previous meeting.
7. Officers' reports. This heading is for a main topic; the individual reports are listed as subtopics.
8. Committee reports. This heading is for a main topic; the individual committee reports are listed as subtopics.
9. Old business. Unfinished business from the previous meeting is included. Old business is a main topic. The individual topics constituting old business are listed as subtopics.
10. New business. New business is a main topic. The individual presentations (when known) constituting new business are listed as subtopics. Additional space is allowed at this point so that new topics can be added shortly before the meeting (at the president's discretion) or during the meeting.
11. Announcements. Announcements often include when and where the next meeting will be held.
12. Adjournment.

Figure 14-4 provides a sample informal agenda, and Figure 14-5 provides a sample formal agenda.

Team Medical Management Program Agenda

May 9

☐ Call to order
☐ Roll call
☐ Approval of minutes of last meeting
☐ Reports of officers
☐ Reports of committees
☐ Old Business
  • Attendance
  • Changes in meeting time/day
  • Special project funding
☐ New Business
  • Health Fair
  • Treadmill
  • Vacation schedules
☐ Announcements
☐ Adjournment

FIGURE 14-4 Example of an informal agenda with squares and bullets introducing subheadings.

AGENDA

TEAM MEDICAL MANAGEMENT PROGRAM

May 9, 20XX

I. Call to Order

II. Roll Call and introduction of guests
James Morgan, MD, representative from Wood Creek Hospital

III. Approval of Minutes of April 14, 20XX

IV. Officers' Reports: Treasurer's report

V. Committees

1. Bylaws Committee
2. Membership Committee
3. Nominating Committee
4. Credentials Committee

VI. Old Business

1. Attendance
2. Proposed changes in meeting time or day
3. Special project funding

VII. New Business

1. Health Fair (Dr Dunn)
2. Evaluation of treadmill (Dr Patton)
3. Discussion of 20XX vacation schedules (Dr Majur)

VIII. Announcements

Position open at Desert View Community. See Ron Miller.

Next meeting: Wednesday, June 18, 20XX, 3 p.m., Board Room (subject to approval today)

IX. Adjournment

FIGURE 14-5 Example of a formal agenda.

 14-3 SELF-STUDY

DIRECTIONS: Referring to Figure 14-6, use that format, with Roman numerals, and type an agenda that might have been prepared before this meeting took place.

See Appendix A, p. 463, after you have completed the exercise.

MINUTES

Minutes (Figure 14-6) are the notes taken or a brief summary of what was discussed and decided upon at a meeting. Minutes become the official documentation when approved by the members of the organization. A standardized form can be used to fill in information as the meeting is conducted. Basically, this form corresponds to the items in the agenda for the meeting. Minutes are usually taken by the recording secretary,

---

Desert View Hospital   Mirage, Arizona

SAFETY COMMITTEE MINUTES

DATE
A meeting of the Safety Committee was called to order at 2:05 p.m. on August 22, 20XX, in the Board Room.

MEMBERS PRESENT
Jack Herzog, Terri Peters, Bobbi Lee, Rita Hardin, Bob Duncan, Roland Wolf, Joan Yubetta, Carolyn Rath, Pam Hollingsworth, and Dave Leithoff.

MEMBERS ABSENT
Absent and excused were Peter Hulbert, Nary Harreld, and Carolyn Germano.

MINUTES
The minutes of the previous meeting were read. Bobbi Lee's name was added to the list of members present for the July 26 Safety Committee Meeting. The minutes were then approved as corrected.

ROTATION OF MEMBERSHIP
A discussion was held concerning rotation of membership. It was suggested that Doreen Black be admitted as a member of the committee. It was also suggested that each member take turns inviting one guest, with Bob Duncan bringing the first guest. Jack Herzog will contact the departments not represented at the Safety Committee.

ELECTRICAL SAFETY PROGRAM
Joan Yubetta suggested that an electrical safety program be started. Rita Hardin reported that electrical cords are not being taped down.

FIRE DRILLS
Dave Leithoff reported that there had been no fire drill for over a month and suggested that there should be one by the end of September.

FIRST AID
Terri Peters reported a total of 36 injuries for the month of August. Back injuries were down to 5 for August. There were 7 falls, 3 cuts, and 1 foreign body. It was suggested by Bob Duncan and Terri Peters that a form be designed for reporting scratches, puncture wounds, and so on.

BEVERAGE SPILLING
It was suggested that Bobbi Lee put an article in the *Capsule* on the spilling of beverages. It was further suggested that spill stations be set up in key places in the hospital. Bob Duncan will bring this up in the cabinet meeting.

ADJOURNMENT
There being no further business, the meeting was adjourned at 4:15 p.m. by Bob Duncan, Chairperson.

Dave Leithoff, CMT, Recording Secretary

FIGURE 14-6 Example of minutes, full block style.

although anyone attending the meeting may take minutes. It is helpful to have the minutes of the previous meeting, a list of the membership, committee lists and descriptions, a copy of bylaws that the organization has adopted to govern its meetings, and the agenda for the meeting. The detail with which the notes are taken (or recorded) is determined by the organization and the business conducted. Depending on the policy of the organization, discussions are summarized and speakers are cited. With experience, you will learn what to record verbatim, what to paraphrase, and what to omit from the record. Format is flexible but can be done as follows.

Title

The heading is usually centered on the page and typed in full capital letters. Underlining is optional.

Date, Time, and Place

Date, time, and place of the meeting are part of the heading or part of the report itself. The presiding officer is identified with the *call to order* or adjournment notation.

Names of the Members

Names of the members present, as well as members absent, may be listed in the minutes. If roll is taken, that sheet may be attached to the minutes. The names are usually listed in alphabetical order. The names are listed with appropriate titles and other identifying information of any *ex officio* members or guests in attendance.

Format

The format should be consistent from meeting to meeting and secretary to secretary. The events should be reported in the order in which they occurred during the meeting. Outline format should be followed with the full block, modified block, or indented style. The titles of the sections follow those of the agenda used at the meeting itself. Roman numerals are often used to introduce the titles of each section. In general, headings (with or without numbers) should be typed flush with the left margin. The material under the headings is single-spaced, and double-spacing is used between headings. The headings are typed either in full capital letters and underlined or with just the initial letter of the main words capitalized and the entire heading underlined.

The following items should be included: approval of minutes of the previous meeting; records of all officer and committee reports; records of all motions, seconds, and so on; action on any unfinished business; record of new business; announcements, including the date, time, and place of the next meeting; and the time of adjournment.

If the minutes are longer than one page, type the word *continued* at the bottom of each completed page. The subsequent page or pages begin 1 inch from the top of the page with the title of the minutes, the page number, and any other important data.

Lists

Lists follow the same guidelines as described in the previous section, "Typing Hospital Protocols and Reports."

Closing

Use the salutation *Respectfully submitted,* followed by a triple space and the originator's name, to close the minutes, or just leave a triple space, type in a blank line, and type the originator's name under the line. The typist identifies the preparation of the document with a two- or three-letter identification (i.e., initials) and a double space at the end, flush with the left margin.

Distribution

The minutes should be typed as soon as possible after the meeting, and a copy should be distributed to all members (those present at the meeting and those absent) unless it is the custom to read the minutes at the following meeting. Some committees or organizations have a special distribution list that includes anyone who needs to be aware of the proceedings. At the next meeting, the minutes are read aloud or distributed to the members and amended if necessary, either on the page or, if lengthy, typed separately and attached as an addendum.

OUTLINES

Outlines are traditionally set up as shown in Figure 14-7. Remember that you must have at least two divisions or subdivisions in each set; otherwise, a set cannot be made. Roman numerals, Arabic numerals, and letters of the alphabet are used to identify different heading levels. A period and a double space follow each number or letter of the alphabet except on the levels at which the parentheses are used; in that case, you double-space after the closing parenthesis. The outlines are indented so that successive levels are obvious. Leave space to backspace from the main topics to accommodate the width of the Roman numerals. It is helpful to set the decimal tab to align these numerals properly.

14

CHAPTER

TITLE CENTERED AND TYPED IN FULL CAPS

I. Main Topic (first item) (Capitalize the first letter of each important word.)
   A. Secondary heading (Capitalize the first letter and any
   B. ...   proper nouns here and at all
   C. ...   other levels.)
   D. ...
       1. Third-level heading
       2. ...
       3. ...
       4. ...
          a. Fourth-level heading
          b. ...
            (1) Fifth-level heading
            (2). ...
            (3) . ...
              (a) Sixth-level heading
              (b) . ...
II. Main Topic (second item) (You will have to backspace once
   A. . . .   to allow for the roman numeral
   B. . . .   for balance.)
   C. ...
       1. ...
       2. ...
   D. ...
       1. ...
       2. ...
       3. ...
III. Main Topic (third item) (You will have to backspace twice on
              this line for balance.)

The major headings and subdivisions may be a single word or phrase;
long phrases or clauses; complete sentences; or any combination of
sentences, phrases, and single words.

Indent as follows:
   Align roman numerals to the left margin.
   Set tab stops for four-space indent under each topic.
   Begin the second line of an item directly under the first letter of that line.

Spacing is as follows:
   Triple space after title.
   Double-space before and after each main topic.
   Single-space subdivision items.
   Double-space throughout very brief outline.

FIGURE 14-7 Outline mechanics.

REFERENCE MATERIALS

Many kinds of reference materials are available to assist you in writing. A good dictionary, a punctuation and grammar book, a style manual, and a thesaurus should be in your desk library. Your software program should provide you with both a dictionary and a thesaurus under the Tools menu. All of these except the thesaurus have been discussed in previous chapters; the thesaurus is discussed now.

Thesaurus means "treasury" in Greek, and it can be a real treasure for you. A dictionary is used to find the meaning of a word, and a thesaurus is used to find an alternative word to express the same idea (synonym). Or you could have a negative idea that you want to make positive; the thesaurus also contains antonyms, which are words that mean the opposite of your target word.

Every synonym listed is not an exact substitute for the word you might want, however, and you must ensure that the word not only fits the context of the sentence but also is a word that you would use comfortably.

For example, if you decide that you want to use another word for *stolen* in the sentence *My jacket was stolen,* you look for *steal* in the thesaurus. There you find many synonyms, but not all are applicable to *stolen* as expressed in the sentence: The jacket could not have been *robbed, abducted, embezzled, purloined, plundered, swindled,* or *plagiarized.* Furthermore, the slang expressions *pinched, carried off,* and *ripped off* might even carry an additional meaning that you do not intend. However, you also find the word *taken; taken* fits what you want to say and you are comfortable with it.

Some thesauruses are arranged alphabetically, like a dictionary; in others, you have to look up the "idea" of the word and use cross-references. Definitions usually are not given. You will need to explore your thesaurus to see how it is organized. Most computer software programs contain an alphabetic-style thesaurus. (Some of these are in combination with a spell-check program or under the Tools menu.) When composing a document, you can instantly bring up a list of substitute words for the particular word for which you need a choice. However, sometimes a book list is faster and more helpful.

 MT TOOL BOX TIP: Reference books = huge tools.

 ## 14-4 SELF-STUDY

DIRECTIONS: You need your computer or reference book thesaurus for this assignment. This assignment is to help you become familiar with using a thesaurus as a reference source for achieving variety in word usage.

Using a thesaurus as a reference, type three to five words that can be substituted for each of the following overused words:

1. know
2. awful
3. tell
4. nice
5. think

See Appendix A, p. 463, for possible responses.

 ## 14-5 REVIEW TEST

DIRECTIONS: As you can see from Self-Study 14-4, the word choices are very broad but can become very limiting when they are to be substituted for other words and made to fit into the context of a complete thought. In the following exercises, more than one word in each exercise needs a substitute, and you need to be sure that each substitute word fits the context of what you want to say. Often, it is necessary to change other words in the sentence to make the new word fit properly. Retype each of the following sentences, substituting your alternative word or words for those in italics. *You should write two complete sentences for each of the first two target sentences.* You may adjust each sentence to fit your needs.

EXAMPLE

How much did you *get* from that *game* you *played?*

Possible rewrites:

How much did you *obtain* from that *contest* you *entered?*

How much did you *receive* from that *match* you *made?*

1. She *needs* to ask the *supervisor* for a *change* in her work schedule.
2. It is difficult to *know* how to edit some *incorrect* dictation.
3. Please *arrange* for your *transcription* to be faxed on time.
4. Please *excuse* my *delay* in *answering* your request.
5. It gives me *great pleasure* to welcome you.
6. We, as a *rule,* do not *employ inexperienced* transcriptionists.

14

CHAPTER

14-6 PRACTICE TEST

DIRECTIONS: The following text is from a section of the hospital's cardiovascular laboratory procedure manual. Type an outline in correct full block format with careful attention to main headings, subheadings, and additional heading levels. Refer to Figure 14-3. Begin by typing page CV-15; the second page is CV-16. The document is titled *Holter Monitor*. At the end of the procedure, put in the approved signature line; the effective date is the current date. The policy number is 90-202.

Objective: To obtain a magnetic tape record of a patient's electrocardiographic activity over a 24-hour period. Equipment: 1. Holter monitor. 2. Battery. 3. Tape. 4. Patient cable. 5. Universal cable. 6. ECG machine. 7. ECG electrodes. 8. 2 x 2 pads, alcohol, and Redux paste. 9. Transpore tape. 10. Patient diary. 11. Shaving prep kit. Procedure: 1. Verify the physician's order by checking the medical chart. 2. Assemble all equipment and bring to the patient's bedside. 3. Introduce yourself to the patient and thoroughly explain what you are about to do. 4. Verify the patient's identity by checking the patient's ID bracelet. 5. Have the patient remove all clothing covering his or her chest. 6. Locate the necessary anatomical landmarks and prepare the five areas as follows: a. Shave all hair. b. Cleanse the area with alcohol. c. Scrub the cleansed area with Redux paste. d. Remove the Redux paste with alcohol. 7. Attach the electrodes to the patient's chest: a. 2nd rib space on the right side of the sternum. b. 2nd rib space on the left side of the sternum. c. Over the xiphoid process. d. Right V4—Right midclavicular at the 5th intercostal space. e. Left V4—Left midclavicular at the 5th intercostal space. 8. Attach the electrode cables to the patient: a. White—right arm. b. Brown—left arm. c. Black—V1. d. Green—right leg. e. Red—left leg. 9. Tape the electrode cables in a loop on the patient's abdomen, allowing the cable to hang free. 10. Place a tape in the Holter monitor unit. 11. Place a battery in the Holter monitor unit. 12. Attach the recorder to the belt or shoulder strap (patient's preference). 13. Plug Universal cable into recorder. 14. Connect RA, LA, RL, LL, and V1 from ECG machine to Universal cable. 15. Connect patient cable to recorder. 16. Run a short strip on the ECG machine to verify the quality of the tracing (L1, L2, L3, AVR, AVL, AVF, and V1). 17. Disconnect Universal cable from recorder unit. 18. Set time on recorder and start Holter monitor. 19. Record starting time in the patient diary and explain the importance of the diary to the patient. 20. If the patient is an outpatient, remind him or her of the importance of returning in 24 hours. 21. After 24 hours, record ending time in the patient's diary. 22. Remove the cable from the recorder. 23. Remove the cable and electrodes from the patient. 24. Prepare the tape for scanning. Care of Equipment: 1. Exercise caution when handling unit to avoid dropping. 2. Instruct patient not to bathe, shower, or go swimming while the unit is attached. 3. Clean recording heads and capstan with alcohol after each patient use. Important Points: 1. Proper preparation of the patient's chest is important for a good recording. 2. Run a short strip with the ECG machine to ensure that the electrodes are placed correctly. 3. Make sure the patient thoroughly understands the importance of the diary.

14-7 REVIEW TEST

DIRECTIONS: Please select the letter that identifies the words or sentence that answers or completes the sentence. Write the identifying letter in the blank provided.

1. A run-on sentence _____
    a. is fragmentary.
    b. has a nonessential appositive.
    c. has two or more independent clauses.
    d. is not punctuated or is done so incorrectly.

2. Which of the following best defines the term *synonym?* _____
    a. The name of a person prominent in medicine.
    b. A word that means same as another.
    c. A word that sounds like another word.
    d. A phrase that uses *like* or *as* in a comparison.

3. Which word is the antonym for *backward?* _____
    a. forward
    b. foreword
    c. delayed
    d. inverted

4. *Parallel construction* means that lists are formed from _____
    a. equal-length phrases or clauses.
    b. word sets in which all the items are the same grammatical form (all nouns, all verbs, all infinitive phrases).
    c. words that describe the progression of a set of instructions or steps.
    d. two or more independent clauses.

5. *Dangling construction* in a sentence means that _____
    a. active voice is used most often.
    b. passive voice is used more often.
    c. there is no clear antecedent for a phrase or clause in the sentence.
    d. certain words are repeated and overused in the sentence.

14

CHAPTER

WE HOPE YOU HAVE NOT BEEN USING THESE RULES*

1. Make sure each pronoun agrees with their antecedent.
2. Just between you and I, case is important.
3. Verbs has to agree with their subjects.
4. Watch out for irregular verbs which have crope into English.
5. Don't use no double negatives.
6. A writer must not shift your point of view.
7. When dangling, don't use participles.
8. Join clauses good like a conjunction should.
9. Don't write a run-on sentence you got to punctuate it.
10. About sentence fragments.
11. In letters reports and articles use commas to separate items in a series.
12. Don't use commas, which are not necessary.
13. Its important to use apostrophe's correctly.
14. Check to see if you have any words out.
15. Don't abbrev.
16. In the case of a letter, check it in terms of jargon.
17. As far as incomplete constructions, they are wrong.
18. About repetition, the repetition of a word might be real effective repetition—take, for instance, the repetition of words in Lincoln's Gettysburg Address.
19. In my opinion, I think that an author when he is writing should not get into the habit of making use of too many unnecessary words that he does not really need in order to put his message across.
20. Last but not least, lay off clichés.

*With permission of *The Reader's Digest*, March 1963, "Pardon, Your Slip Is Showing."

14

CHAPTER

Making the Transition from MT to Speech Recognition Editor

OBJECTIVES

After reading this chapter and completing the exercises, you should be able to

1. Demonstrate the use of critical thinking skills in problem solving.
2. Name some of the skillsets used in critical thinking.
3. List the three competency levels of a medical transcriptionist.
4. State why and how quality editing will improve your transcription results.
5. Name some of the attributes of a skilled quality assurance editor.
6. Name some of the attributes of a skilled speech recognition editor.
7. Demonstrate the ability to detect errors in speech recognition dictation/transcripts.
8. Discuss the transition from medical transcriptionist to speech recognition editor.
9. Practice using keyboard shortcut keys.

Note from the Author

Imagine my surprise many years ago when I sent one of my students to a local transcription company to complete an internship program and the director told me that the student would begin as a quality assurance editor. I had to immediately remind the director that this was a beginning student with just 3 semesters of education and practice. She replied, "I begin all our new hires in quality assurance before I move them on to MT. In this way they appreciate what QA does and they learn a lot more about transcription for our company than they would on a single account." She went on to tell me that the documents all beginners labored over, including my students, were followed up by regular QA staff. In other words, this edit was not the final one by any means. These QA beginners on trial had to learn the style of the company, practice research, develop acute listening skills, learn how to fill in blanks left by the MT, be prepared to go over and over the transcript, compare the document they were working with to similar transcripts, and so on before giving up and bringing it to her. They had to find spelling errors, capitalization errors—well you know what they were looking for. My question was did they ever find anything?

I was also concerned that my student would become intimidated and discouraged. Wrong. She loved it and said she learned more in a week than she had all semester with me. Well, that is what I got for asking.

INTRODUCTION

This chapter does *not* contain the tools and information to make you a quality assurance editor. What this chapter does contain is the information you need to appreciate the functions of the QA process and prepare you to eventually make the transition into this field after many years as a medical transcriptionist (MT).

The emphasis of the chapter is to prepare you to edit speech recognition documents after you have met the criteria for that function. One must always plan ahead, and it is not too early for you to plan for the transition into editing speech recognition documents.

MEDICAL TRANSCRIPTIONIST TERMINOLOGY

Hay Management Consultants, an independent human resources consulting firm, carried out an independent study of the MT profession and identified three distinct professional levels for MTs. It is important to review them here. (Professional Level 1 was introduced to you in Chapter 1.)

Professional Level 1

Position Summary: Medical language specialist who transcribes dictation by physicians and other healthcare providers in order to document patient care. The incumbent will likely need assistance to interpret dictation that is unclear or inconsistent or need to make use of professional reference materials.

Nature of Work: An incumbent in this position is given assignments that are matched to his or her developing skill level, with the intention of increasing the depth and/or breadth of exposure or the nature of the work performed (type of report or correspondence,

medical specialty, originator) is repetitive or patterned, not requiring extensive depth and/or breadth of experience.

KNOWLEDGE, SKILLS, AND ABILITIES

▶ Basic knowledge of medical terminology, anatomy and physiology, disease processes, signs and symptoms, medications, and laboratory values. Knowledge of specialty (or specialties) as appropriate.
▶ Knowledge of medical transcription guidelines and practices.
▶ Proven skills in English usage, grammar, punctuation, style, and editing.
▶ Ability to use designated professional reference materials.
▶ Ability to operate word processing equipment, dictation and transcription equipment, and other equipment as specified.
▶ Ability to work under pressure with time constraints.
▶ Ability to concentrate.
▶ Excellent listening skills.
▶ Excellent eye, hand, and auditory coordination.
▶ Ability to understand and apply relevant legal concepts (e.g., confidentiality).

Professional Level 2

Position Summary: Medical language specialist who transcribes and interprets dictation by physicians and other healthcare providers in order to document patient care. The position is also routinely involved in research of questions and in the education of others involved with patient care documentation.

Nature of Work: An incumbent in this position is given assignments that require a seasoned depth of knowledge in a medical specialty (or specialties). Or the incumbent is regularly given assignments that vary in report or correspondence type, originator, and specialty. Incumbents at this level are able to resolve nonroutine problems independently or to assist in resolving complex or highly unusual problems.

KNOWLEDGE, SKILLS, AND ABILITIES

▶ Seasoned knowledge of medical terminology, anatomy and physiology, disease processes, signs and symptoms, medications, and laboratory values. In-depth or broad knowledge of a specialty (or specialties) as appropriate.
▶ Knowledge of medical transcription guidelines and practices.
▶ Excellent skills in English usage, grammar, punctuation, and style.
▶ Ability to use an extensive array of professional reference materials.
▶ Ability to operate word processing equipment, dictation and transcription equipment, and other equipment as specified and to troubleshoot as necessary.
▶ Ability to work independently with minimal or no supervision.
▶ Ability to work under pressure with time constraints.
▶ Ability to concentrate.
▶ Excellent listening skills.
▶ Excellent eye, hand, and auditory coordination.
▶ Proven business skills (scheduling work, purchasing, client relations, billing).
▶ Ability to understand and apply relevant legal concepts (e.g., confidentiality).
▶ Certified medical transcriptionist (CMT) status preferred.

Professional Level 3

Position Summary: Medical language specialist whose expert depth and breadth of professional experiences enables him or her to serve as a medical language resource to originators, coworkers, other healthcare providers, and/or students on a regular basis.

Nature of Work: An incumbent in this position routinely researches and resolves complex questions related to health information or related documentation and/or is involved in the formal teaching of those entering the profession or continuing their education in the profession and/or regularly uses extensive experience to interpret dictation that others are unable to clarify. Actual transcription of dictation is performed only occasionally, because efforts are usually focused on other categories of work.

KNOWLEDGE, SKILLS, AND ABILITIES

▶ Expert knowledge of medical terminology, anatomy and physiology, disease processes, signs and symptoms, medications, and laboratory values. In-depth or broad knowledge of a specialty (or specialties).

▶ In-depth knowledge of medical transcription guidelines and practices.
▶ Excellent skills in English usage, grammar, punctuation, and style.
▶ Ability to use a vast array of professional reference materials, often in innovative ways.
▶ Ability to educate others (one-on-one or group)
▶ Excellent written and oral communication skills.
▶ Ability to operate word processing equipment, dictation and transcription equipment, and other equipment as specified and to troubleshoot as necessary.
▶ Proven business skills (scheduling work, purchasing, client relations, billing)
▶ Ability to understand and apply relevant legal concepts (e.g., confidentiality).
▶ CMT status preferred.

MEDICAL DOCUMENT QUALITY EDITOR TERMINOLOGY

QA editors must have all the professional level 3 knowledge, skills, and abilities outlined previously. Additionally, the QA editor is both an educator and a highly trained professional with interpretive judgment and critical thinking skills. A QA editor must have years of experience in transcription. There is no equipment to assist in thinking critically. You must acquire this skill.

▶ Retrospective editors review reports after the documents have been signed.
▶ Concurrent QA editors review documents before signature by originator. These reviewers should complete the review within 24 hours and should include the corrected text with references. (The MT should be able to challenge a review.)

The QA editor must be able to:

▶ Accurately evaluate the context of medical documents to determine if something is, in fact, an error.
▶ Compare the transcript with the voice dictation (not merely proofreading).
▶ Identify and correct errors and inadequacies within a document.
▶ Evaluate error patterns.
▶ Emphasize the prevention of errors.
▶ Cite references for all corrections.
▶ Provide statistical reports.
▶ Provide policies and procedures for training both originators and MTs.
▶ Review random reports for MTs and originators.
▶ Maintain consistent subjective judgment.
▶ Have mentoring skills.
▶ Institute education techniques to improve quality.

Editors should preferably review transcripts at the time of completion of the document because this is the best time to review problems and to praise success. Retrospective editing is done when turnaround time is not

Job Title: Quality Assurance Editor FLSA Status: Non-Exempt	Reports to: Transcription Manager Date Approved: 07/17/20XX

Summary Statement: This job description is not intended and should not be construed to be an exhaustive list of all responsibilities, skills, efforts, or working conditions associated with the job. It is intended to be a reflection of those principal job elements essential for recruitment and selection, for making fair job evaluations, and for establishing performance standards. The incumbent shall perform all other functions and/or be cross-trained as shall be determined at the sole discretion of management, who has the right to amend, modify, or terminate this job in part or in whole.

JOB DESCRIPTION

PURPOSE: Concurrent quality review of documents transcribed by team MTs.

PRIMARY FUNCTIONS – JOB DUTIES: Qualified individuals must have the ability — with or without reasonable accommodation — to perform the following duties:

1. QUALITY
    *   Fills in blanks, answers questions, verifies demographics, and performs any other functions as necessary to complete transcribed document to upload status.
    *   Maintains quality and productivity standards per company requirements.
    *   Researches and resolves complex questions related to demographic information or related documentation.
    *   Regularly uses experience to interpret dictation that others are unable to clarify.
    *   Works closely with the Transcription Manager and Lead MT to assure coverage, communication, timeliness, and quality standards are addressed consistently.
    *   Assists as necessary to resolve non-routine problems independently or to assist in resolving complex or highly unusual problems.

2. COMMUNICATION: Answers MT questions regarding site specifics, formats, style, and terminology as necessary for document completion. Provides ongoing professional feedback to MTs to build confidence and assist in professional growth. Maintains confidentiality and privacy in all responsibilities.

3. TRAINING: Assists with training of new hires and seasoned MTs regarding quality issues. Develops site notes for MT referencing.

4. TECHNICAL: Ensures personal proficiency in systems and processes, including basic troubleshooting, trouble ticket, and problem resolution.

5. TRANSCRIPTION: Transcribes as necessary. Transcribes all types of dictated reports, including but not limited to history and physicals, consultations, operative reports, discharge summaries, emergency room reports, radiology, cardiology, and progress notes. Transcribes half of scheduled hours per day on production pay.

JOB REQUIREMENTS

*   Five years' experience in acute care transcription.
*   Appropriate education in medical transcription; certified medical transcriptionist (CMT) within one year of hire.
*   Seasoned knowledge of medical terminology, anatomy and physiology, disease processes, signs and symptoms, medications, and laboratory values. In-depth or broad knowledge of radiology or other specialities as appropriate.
*   In-depth knowledge of transcription guidelines and practices.
*   Ability to use an array of professional reference materials.
*   Knowledge of medical transcription practices and relevant legal concepts, including but not limited to HIPAA privacy and confidentiality.
*   Ability to work independently with minimal or no supervision.
*   Ability to concentrate with excellent listening skills.
*   Excellence in English usage, grammar, punctuation, and style.

FIGURE 15-1 A copy of a job description and job requirements from a national transcription organization.

vital, so the editor must select random samples of documents with voice files and save the files so they will not be purged. Reviews must be thorough and fair, consistent, and not punitive. Consideration must be given to the document author and to errors due to poor grammar, diction, sound quality, and accent as well as content errors. The evaluation must be perceived as an opportunity for training.

Additionally, editors must be able to tactfully approach the document **originators** to resolve difficult questions and flagged reports. The editors must discuss potential risk management issues or breach of confidentially or HIPAA privacy.

See Figure 15-1 for a national transcription company's job description and job requirements for Quality Assurance Editor.

SPEECH-RECOGNIZED DRAFT EDITING

"Back end" speech recognition (BESR) refers to the process by which the author dictates into a digital dictation system in which the voice is routed through a speech recognition (SR) engine and the recognized draft document is routed, along with the original voice file, to the speech recognition editor who verifies the accuracy of the draft and finalizes the report. Speech recognition brings efficiency to the transcription process. It can dramatically improve the productivity and value of the medical language specialist. The editor works with SR technology to produce a complete and accurate document. MTs have to work differently, but SR makes them much more productive if they embrace the technology.

The switch from the skill set used in transcribing to editing SR documents is not easy. MTs are used to looking at their document as they transcribe, correcting and editing as they go along. The SR editor may be looking at a variety of errors and may not be able to see them. A person can be fooled into thinking that what is on the screen and simultaneously heard on the audio is correct because the brain will translate the data into something that makes perfect sense. There is a tendency to see what you expect to see rather than

what is really there. Therefore the SR editor has to be extra careful and extra alert to avoid making this mistake. Not only can the speech engine make an error but the dictator can also make an error. One must overcome the power of suggestion, pay careful attention to details, and spot tiny errors to produce a quality document (Figure 15-2). These are not tiny errors but this example gives you an idea how easy it can be to skip over tiny errors.

To qualify to even attempt transcribing/editing a document that has been dictated by using SR technology, you must have attained all the requirements listed previously as a level 1 medical language specialist. Here is a quick review of those skills.

KNOWLEDGE, SKILLS, AND ABILITIES

▶ Basic knowledge of medical terminology, anatomy and physiology, disease processes, signs and symptoms, medications, and laboratory values.
▶ Knowledge of specialty (or specialties) as appropriate.
▶ Knowledge of medical transcription guidelines and practices.
▶ Proven skills in English usage, grammar, punctuation, style, and editing.
▶ Ability to use designated professional reference materials.
▶ Ability to operate word processing equipment, dictation and transcription equipment, and other equipment as specified.
▶ Ability to work under pressure with time constraints.
▶ Ability to concentrate.
▶ Excellent listening skills.
▶ Excellent eye, hand, and auditory coordination.
▶ Ability to understand and apply relevant legal concepts (e.g., confidentiality).

Additionally the SR editor must be able to recognize, interpret, and evaluate inconsistencies, discrepancies, and inaccuracies in medical text drafts and to clarify, flag, or report the problems as needed. The SR editor must have an understanding of medicolegal responsibilities to ensure compliance with local, state, and federal standards and must be able to multitask. The editor must be able to work under pressure with time constraints and must be able to work independently

Cna yuo raed tihs? I cdnuolt blveiee taht I cluod aulaclty uesdnatnrd waht I was rdanieg. The phaonmneal pweor of the hmuan mnid, aoccdrnig to rscheearch, it dseno't mtaetr in waht oerdr the ltteres in a wrod are, the olny iproamtnt tihng is taht the frsit and lsat ltteer be in the rghit pclae. The rset can be a taotl mses and you can sitll raed it whotuit a pboerlm. Tihs is bcuseae the huamn mnid deos not raed ervey lteter by istlef, but the wrod as a wlohe.

Azanmig huh? I awlyas tghuhot slpeling was ipmorantt!

FIGURE 15-2 Illustration of "misspelling" your eye will accept and understand.

with minimal or no supervision. Quality standards are exactly the same regardless of method of production.

Participation in continuing education and a desire to keep up-to-date and to learn the latest technology advancements and trends are important for a candidate in this role. Finally, the editor must have a thorough knowledge of medical transcription guidelines and practices.

Learning to edit an SR document means you are the editor now. You are not reviewing someone else's transcript; you are editing a "rough draft" that exists on the screen and is accompanied by the dictation. The draft is filled with words, numbers, abbreviations, and so on that are suggested by what was said, and coordinating all of this is not easy. One would think that the job is mostly done; well, it is mostly done, but what sort of document is it? How is it done? Is it correct and complete? The editor is handicapped by seeing something that "fits," so errors are easily overlooked. (In your own writing, have you ever typed a homonym for the word you actually wanted and were startled to find the mistake when you returned to proofread? You wondered how you could do that. You knew exactly what word you wanted, but your brain was perfectly happy to give you an excellent substitute, but not the right substitute—in fact, not excellent at all.) Your mind works differently during editing than it does during transcribing. When you transcribe, you determine whether what the dictator says makes sense. When you are listening/editing, you are trying to decide whether what was said matches what is on the screen. When you are looking at an SR draft and listening to the speech that accompanies it, you must not only look and listen but also interpret the meaning of what is actually on the page. What the dictator actually meant might not be what is on the page. How can you learn to do this? How do you prepare? Like much you have been learning, this skill comes with time, with practice, with work developing your critical thinking skills, with becoming a word detective, and with a keen desire to learn to make the process work. Think of editing as a puzzle with pieces missing, but all the pieces "seem" to be there.

For example, your eyes can easily skip past a missing word; because you know the word should be there, your brain just lets you proceed on your way and you never miss the word at all. To edit SR, you must train your brain to not let you see something or accept something that is not there. You have to make a whole, complete piece out of the document before your eyes.

Context becomes vital. All the words are there, the sentence is complete, but there could be flaws in the outcome.

When you read, you don't read every single letter in every word or every word in every single sentence. You have learned to recognize patterns of words. If you read, "We heard musical notes and realized it was the ice cream t ." The final word you "see" is going to be *truck*, not *train*, *trolley*, or *tank*. If one of those words were there, you would probably ignore it. Human perception is economical. You notice some things but not others. The better you read, the better you skim; details are overlooked. Words are viewed, recognized quickly, and placed appropriately and accurately in context. When you edit, the word *skim* cannot be in your vocabulary. Details cannot be overlooked.

EXAMPLES

Problem A:

Transcribed on the screen:

He was seen by Dr. David in the emergency department who felt that he did not need a minister but did recommend followup and lithotripsy.

Dictated:

He was seen by Dr. David in the emergency department who felt that he did not need admission but did recommend followup and lithotripsy.

Now ask yourself this question when you see what was transcribed in Problem A: What does seeing a minister have to do with having a followup lithotripsy? So, your thinking directs you to listen again and you discover the dictated word was actually *admission*.

Problem B:

Transcribed on the screen (in reference to a patient's brain scan):

The patient has intrarenal hemorrhage.

Dictated:

The patient has intracranial hemorrhage.

In Problem B you are aware that the patient's brain is being discussed, not his/her kidneys. This knowledge helps you correct the transcript.

Problem C:

Transcribed on the screen:

No oral intravenous contrast.

Dictated:

No oral or intravenous contrast.

In problem C you are alert to the fact that contrast material cannot be both oral and intravenous. Thus you find the tiny, but important, missing word *or*.

Problem D:

Transcribed on the screen:

...showed ST changes on the echocardiogram

Dictated:

...showed ST changes on the echocardiogram

You know that this was a slip from the dictator because *echocardiograms* do not measure ST elements; *electrocardiogram* is the word intended.

Problem E:

You open your dictation and the patient's demographic data pop into view as follows:

NAME: Johnson, Irma Lucille   DOB 2-17-2011
MRN: 98360632   Visit #: 00096543
ACC #: 302-40-8392   ADM MD: David
                                        Markton
EXAM: PET LUNG STAGING

Remembering that this first part of the document is critical to patient safety and then knowing that you need to make certain that you have the correct data for the patient, you become alert to the fact that this patient is a toddler with a name from the previous century. Further checking reveals the incorrect DOB. Always double-check the account numbers, medical record number, and other data as well, because the year date might not be the only error.

Common expressions can cause problems because they are so routine that the dictator rushes through them, leaving the document with the wrong word set and no clue to the correct one. Maybe there are clues. You need to learn to look for clues as you did in Problem E.

Problem F:

This is a longer narrative, a typical segment to work with.

Transcribed on the screen:

Plan: The patient will be discharged home and took her sister to follow with her primary care doctor within the next week. The patient to return to emergency department sooner for numerous complaints. The patient instructed for 12 Percocet 12 by me to take as needed for pain and spasm.

Please look it over and work with it before you look at the actual corrected transcript below.

PLAN:

1. The patient will be discharged home.

2. The patient is instructed to follow with her primary care doctor within the next week.

3. The patient **is instructed** to return to the emergency department sooner **for any new or worsening** complaints.

4. The patient **was given a prescription** for 12 Percocet **and told** to take as needed for pain and spasm.

GUIDELINES

To help you obtain some details quickly, you will need some guidelines to help you improve your productivity and turnaround time (TAT). One such set of guidelines is facility-specific guidelines, coming from the place your document originated.

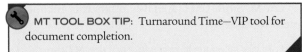 MT TOOL BOX TIP: Turnaround Time—VIP tool for document completion.

Demographic Data

Demographic data includes a list of names, addresses (including email), fax numbers, credentials for all healthcare providers, including physician dictators, chiropractors, osteopaths, nurse practitioners, assistants, therapists, and technicians. The names and addresses of local hospitals, clinics, imaging centers, outpatient surgery centers, healthcare providers, university medical training centers, sanatoriums, nursing homes, and pharmacies also should be available, preferably in a database.

Facility Specifics

Guidelines include lists of regional slang and jargon along with commonly used abbreviations. Have a review bank of documents with the patient identifiers removed to aid the editor in style preferences. Providers dictate their most common phrases and procedures, and the editor can become familiar with terms, instruments, drugs, formats, style, and so on. This information can be helpful when words are slurred.

Format and File Type

Documents (as described previously) provide clues to favorite formats as well. Having a bank of document types is valuable and can save research time. There should be a specified or preferred format for each job type, for example, H&P, operative report, SOAP note, office progress note, medicolegal narrative, consultation, discharge summary, and so on. The general length of each document should be included.

 MT TOOL BOX TIP: Practice good file maintenance from the beginning (e.g., the first document you save).

CRITICAL THINKING

New MTs are often better at editing BESR because their lack of experience makes them more careful, and they don't anticipate wording that might not be there. Knowledge of content, therefore, can become an impediment. Critical thinking requires you to:

▶ Gather facts.
▶ Evaluate the information gathered.
▶ Think with an open mind.
▶ Understand what you hear.
▶ Engage others in solutions.
▶ Analyze.
▶ Use common sense.
▶ Use all reference aids available.

15

CHAPTER

Lea M. Sims, CMT, AHDI-F, offers this encouragement to students:

I can give no greater piece of advice to a new MT than this: Do not hide from difficult dictators, be they speed demons or ESL. They are the greatest training you will ever get and learning from them will fine-tune your ear like nothing else. Being able to transcribe the most difficult work will tremendously impact your long-term employability and marketability in this industry.

| Received: | Sat Oct 10 20:51:56 CDT 2009 |
| Due: | Mon Oct 12 20:51:56 CDT 2009 |

| Patient | Templates | Macros | Distribution | Comment |
| Transcriptions | Labels | Feedback | | |

For MT   For Dictator

This feedback is intended for the MT

- [ ] Addresses
- [ ] Anatomy & Physiology
- [ ] Creative Transcription
- [ ] Delete this transcription
- [ ] Drug Names
- [ ] Format/Template
- [ ] Laboratory Tests & Results
- [ ] Macro Missing/Bad
- [ ] Medical Equipment & Tools
- [ ] Medical Procedure or Diagnosis Terms
- [ ] Patient Demographics
- [ ] People
- [ ] Places
- [ ] Punctuation
- [ ] Spelling

Comment:

Screenshot of feedback from editor to MT. (Courtesy M*Modal, Pittsburgh, Pennsylvania.)

15-1 PRACTICE TEST

DIRECTIONS: In the following examples, see if any part of the recognized dictation alerts you to look more closely. Circle the problem and then write the correction and/or comment on the blank provided. Some examples do not contain a problem so just write "none" on the blank. Indicate any correction as necessary to make the document accurate and complete. You have done these sorts of things in self-studies many times before. This set is not that much different.

1. The patient wears a hearing aide in the left ear.
   Errors and corrections if any:

   _____

   _____

2. A small nodule was removed measuring a centimeter in diameter.
   Errors and corrections if any:

   _____

   _____

3. There were 2 foci of activity at L3 and left iliac bone suspicious for metastases.
   Errors and corrections if any:

   _____

   _____

4. The patient, who has a 2-pack-a-day cigarette habit, has been unable to quite smoking.
   Errors and corrections if any:

   _____

   _____

5. The biopsy came back basil cell carcinoma.
   List your thoughts about this expression:

   _____

   _____

   Errors and corrections if any:

   _____

   _____

6. He experienced sensor and neural hearing loss.
   Errors and corrections if any:

   _____

   _____

7. The patient currently has one warm, soft stool per day.
   Errors and corrections if any:

   _____

   _____

8. During surgery, he required two units of patched red blood cells.
   Errors and corrections if any:

   _____

   _____

9. Weber test lateralized to the left; difference test was equal; air conduction greater than bone conduction
   bilaterally.
   Errors and corrections if any:

   _____

   _____

10. When this baby was born, there was obvious deformity of the (left foot, excuse me, I meant the right foot),
    which has not been corrected itself.
    Errors and corrections if any:

    _____

    _____

11. I gave her a prescription for APC with codeine 1 p.o. q.6 h. p.r.n. pain, #15. This is not refillable.
    Errors and corrections if any:

    _____

    _____

12. HEENT: R. sclera hemorrhoid.
    Errors and corrections if any:

    _____

    _____

15

CHAPTER

13. IMPRESSION
   1. Probable 6.0-mm midsigmoid polyp on a stock, unchanged.
   2. Diverticulosis, moderate; otherwise normal barium enema.
   Errors and corrections if any:

   _____

   _____

14. Fundus evaluation revealed both disks to have a 3 to 4+ pallor. There was no definite arterial or narrowing, and the maculae appeared normal bilaterally.
   Errors and corrections if any:

   _____

   _____

15. She has a short upper lip visa vie the lower lip.
   Errors and corrections if any:

   _____

   _____

16. She remained dependent on some degree of pressure support.
   Errors and corrections if any:

   _____

   _____

17. At this point in time, I feel that the patient is gravely disabled, that he cannot provide food, shelter, or clothing for himself nor make decisions in regards to his medical or financial affairs in his best interest.
   Errors and corrections if any:

   _____

   _____

18. The patient has a normal testicular examination; his testicles are distended bilaterally.
   Errors and corrections if any:

   _____

   _____

19. The patient also complains of lightheadedness and flushing when rising too quickly or bending forward to quickly.
   Errors and corrections if any:

   _____

   _____

20. Pain management: Tylenol 650 mg p.o. q.6 hours p.r.n. pain.
   Errors and corrections if any:

   _____

   _____

21. The patient received a 5000-unit bonus of IV heparin.
   Errors and corrections if any:

   _____

   _____

22. Her extraocular eye movements are full and conjugate.
    Errors and corrections if any:

    _____

    _____

23. We need to determine if she has a protein essences.
    Errors and corrections if any:

    _____

    _____

24. The patient lives with her frail has been at home.
    Errors and corrections if any:

    _____

    _____

25. This 54-year-old homeless Asthenic lady was again admitted experiencing a seizure in a liquor store.
    Errors and corrections if any:

    _____

    _____

15-2 PRACTICE TEST

DIRECTIONS: In the following problems, make any correction necessary to make the snippet accurate and complete. Some snippets do not contain an error. Find the error or errors in the problem, if any, and describe what must be done to correct it/them. Some of the problems are longer than those you have previously worked with. Since the voice file is not provided, you have a disadvantage because you will be examining just the printed results. Circle the error or write out the problem and describe what must be done to make the transcript correct. Make comments as necessary to explain your rationale.

1. The patient has no really significant chronic medical problems except for the following: history of chronic obstructive pulmonary disease, diabetes, hypercholesterolemia, hypertension, atrial fibrillation, myocardial infarction in 2007, and abdominal aortic aneurysm.
   Errors and corrections if any:

   _____

   _____

2. FINDINGS: The lung bases are clear. There are no focal lesions in the liver or spleen. The pancreas, adrenal glands, and right kidney are unremarkable. There is mild left hydronephrosis. Obstruction appears to be due to at least and possibly 2 small stones at the left ureterovesical junction.
   Errors and corrections if any:

   _____

   _____

3. After sharp debridement and the Microscaffold collagen antibacterial silver dressing, the periwound erythema was significantly decreased and full closure was noted within 6 weeks.
   Errors and corrections if any:

   _____

   _____

4. Findings: There is a vivid FDG uptake in the left upper lobe mass. The abnormal activity extends to involve a large area of the left lower lobe, the left hilum, and extensive mediastinal involvement.
   Errors and corrections if any:

   _____

   _____

5. Discharge Death Diagnoses: Persistent refractory and vasodilatory sepsis, initially due to beta hemolytic streptococcus fascilitis with septicemia.
   Errors and corrections if any:

   _____

   _____

6. GU: Normal testes, cords, epididymis.
   Errors and corrections if any:

   _____

   _____

7. Mild stiffness in swing phase on the left with a strongly positive rectus test. Valgus alignment of the left foot, accompanied by subluxation of the peroneus brevis tendon.
   Errors and corrections if any:

   _____

   _____

8. HPI: Patient presents today for followup PE: Her nasal cavity is well healed. Ostiomeatal complexes are open and patent.
   Impression: 1. She is overall doing well.
   Disposition: 1. We will follow her up PRN.
   Errors and corrections if any:

   _____

   _____

9. I would add, as a final note, that the "take home message" for me, with respect to the management of this patient, is that regardless of the level of experience on the part of the surgeon or the extent of the workup involving a pain complaint, it is probably never a good idea to suggest to a patient that psychiatric intervention might be appropriate or helpful. Certain individuals will never take this as a constructive suggestion and it may only serve to make them mad or even hostile.
   Errors and corrections if any:

   _____

   _____

10. The patient is a 54-year-old male with diabetes, hypertension, and an extensive cardiac history including status post CABG.
    Errors and corrections if any:

    _____

    _____

11. There is a large mass in the left upper lobe measuring approximately 6.0 X 5.1 X 5.6 cm in maximum AP, transverse, and craniocaudal dimensions, respectively.
    Errors and corrections if any:

    _____

    _____

12. Impression: Traumatic abrasions of left external auditory canal and tympanic membrane.
    Treatment: Patient given a prescription of Cortisporin Otic 3 drops q.i.d. in the right ear, #10 cc. Also given a prescription for audiogram to be done at University Speech and Hearing Center. Patient is to be rechecked after the audiogram.
    Errors and corrections if any:

    _____

    _____

13. She has been started on Atromid-S 500 mg b.i.d. initially. I have been informed that this is not covered by Medicaid, and a treatment authorization is difficult to obtain, even with patients with lipid abnormalities as significant as hers.
    Errors and corrections if any:

    _____

    _____

14. Physical examination showed findings consistent with a chronic vasomotor rhinitis, and I have placed him on ampicillin 250 mg 1 q.i.d. and on Dimetapp Extentabs 1 b.i.d. and on prednisone 5 mg, starting off with 40 mg/day, decreasing down to 5 mg over a 12-day period. I will be rechecking him in 10 days. When he is sufficiently recovered, he will be referred back to your office for continuation of your care.
    Errors and corrections if any:

    _____

    _____

15. An endometrial biopsy was done, and the uterus measured 9 cm in depth, which represents a slight enlargement. A large amount of hyperplastic-appearing tissue was obtained on the biopsy. As you know from your copy of the biopsy report, she does have a grade III cystic endometrial hyperplasia with focal adenomatous hyperplasia.
    Errors and corrections if any:

    _____

    _____

16. 2/27/XX: No seizures since December last year. He remains on Dilantin 100 mg with Phenobarbital 15 mg 1 q.i.d. Neurologic exam and blood pressure normal. He took medications this morning. Will obtain an EEG. Prescription for Dilantin and phenobarbital were called in to Round Valley Pharmacy.
    Errors and corrections if any:

    _____

    _____

17. EXAMINATION: Well-developed, well-nourished white female. There is no CVA tenderness. There is some suprapubic tenderness. Pelvic and rectal examinations reveal several small, vesicular, tender lesions on the upper vulva bilaterally, grossly consistent with herpes. There are a few enlarged tender nodes in the right inguinal area. The vagina has a fair amount of discharge. The cervix is clean and somewhat tender. The uterus is anteflexed and slightly tender. The adnexa are within normal limits. The bladder and urethra are quite tender.
    IMPRESSION: 1) Herpes progenitalis. 2) Vaginitis. 3) Cystitis.
    Errors and corrections if any:

    _____

    _____

15

CHAPTER

18. The patient has been concerned because of the increased redundancy of skin of the upper and lower lids, formation of jowls, and the dropping of skin beneath the chin in the neck area. She is also concerned somewhat about some small wrinkles around her mouth.
Errors and corrections if any:

_____

_____

19. Since her discharge from the hospital, the patient has continued to do well. She has had no further episodes of palpations. She has only required occasional Valium. She did not drink for several days but now is starting to drink again but is limiting herself to one drink per day.
Errors and corrections if any:

_____

_____

20. Patient returns for followup visit and since last seen has continued to do well. Her appetite is improved. Her diarrhea has improved with the Metamucil, and she has gained approx 5 lbs. Her repeat UA is improved with 3-5 wbc's; urine culture with no growth. She is to continue with Metamucil 1 pack t.i.d. and return in 2 month's time.
Errors and corrections if any:

_____

_____

21. CHIEF COMPLAINT
The patient is a 28-year-old female secretary for Center City Chemical. She complains that while she was delivering a message to the loading dock area yesterday afternoon, at approximately 3:30 p.m., a palate slipped and a splinter of one of the palates went into her right ear.
Errors and corrections if any:

_____

_____

22. CHEST: Breasts: Normal male. Lungs: Clear to P&A. Heart: No jugular venous distension. S1 and S2 are normal. There is a 1-2/6 systolic ejection murmur at the left upper sternal border. There is mild tenderness in the left upper quadrant. No obvious hepatosplenomegaly. Bowel sounds are normal. GU: Normal circumcised male. No testicular masses or tenderness. RECTAL: No masses; no tenderness.
Errors and corrections if any:

_____

_____

23. PHYSICAL EXAMINATION
Temperature 102 degrees F. Pulse 100. Respiration rate 75. Weight 15 pounds. Anterior fontanelle was slightly bulging. Throat was hyperemic; no exudate. Neck was rigid and stiff. Chest showed slight intercostal retractions. Lungs revealed bilateral rhonchi. No rales heard. Abdomen showed no organomegaly. Umbilical hernia present. Extremities were slightly hypertonic. Neurological exam showed positive Kernig, positive Brudzinski, and positive Babinski signs. DTRs were normal.
LABORATORY DATA
At admission: White blood cells 17,000, with 31% polys, 63% lymphs, hematocrit 16, hemoglobin 5. Post transfusion to discharge: Hematocrit 27 to 34. Urine at admission: Protein 1+ and casts present. After hydration, urine always normal.
Errors and corrections if any:

_____

_____

CHAPTER 15

24. Operative Report
PREOPERATIVE DIAGNOSIS
Suspect ruptured bladder and urethral transection.
POSTOPERATIVE DIAGNOSIS
Traumatic cystotomy (anterior vesical wall) and urethral transection (bulbomembranous junction).
OPERATION
1. Closure of bladder perforation.
2. Cystostomy.
3. Reapposition of urethral transection.
FINDINGS
A 3 to 4 cm long perforation was found in the anterior bladder wall just above the vesicoprostatic junction. The incision was extended superiorly, and the rest of the bladder wall was examined from the inside. No other lacerations were found. A #5 ureteral catheter was passed without difficulty into the left renal pelvis. The catheter irrigated without difficulty. The urethra was thus demonstrated to be intact. The catheter was removed.
Errors and corrections if any:

_____

_____

25. A running 2-0 chromic catgut suture was used to ligate the internal hemorrhoidal pedicle, and then the dentate line was approximated with interrupted sutures of 2-0 chromic, closing the wounds with running 2-0 chromic catgut suture after obtaining hemostasis and removing secondary hemorrhoidal groves from under the skin flaps.
Errors and corrections if any:

_____

_____

26. LABORATORY
Portable chest x-ray reveals normal heart size and contour. The lung fields are clear. Endotracheal tube is in place. The right subclavian CVP line is seen and is in good position in the superior vena cava. Arterial blood gases on 35% oxygen with a ventilator rate of 6, pH 7.38, pO2 153, pCO2 46.
Errors and corrections if any:

_____

_____

27. The x-rays showed no evidence of facture luckily, but they did show quite a bit of discomfort.
Errors and corrections if any:

_____

_____

28. Type II diabetes mellitus, not well controlled according to her home glucose readings.
Errors and corrections if any:

_____

_____

29. This 18-year-old female presented with a dehisced C-section incision. Among her complications is that the child did not survive. She developed pancreatitis with ascites and the incision was the portal for drainage. She developed pseudomonas and S. epidermis in the incision. The wound measured 16 cm X 4 cm X 4 cm and silver alginate/CMC with NPWT initiated.
Errors and corrections if any:

_____

_____

30. You have this problem:

You think the dictator mispronounces a word and you don't know if it is the word on the screen or not.
Perhaps you have never heard of the word and do not really understand it. What do you do?

_____

_____

 MT TOOL BOX TIP: Taking frequent breaks when you are studying and working is a tool for health.

SPEECH RECOGNIZED DRAFT EDITING SKILLS

To increase productivity when editing SR documents, it is helpful if you avoid using the mouse to carry out computer functions. You lose time whenever your hands leave the keyboard to use the mouse and then have to be repositioned on the keyboard to resume typing. Learn to use the shortcut keys on the keyboard. If you have already learned to produce documents in this manner, you will be one step ahead. If you have been relying on the mouse and pull-down menus, now is the time to learn these keyboard commands and shortcuts. See Table 15-1 for a list of Windows shortcuts. There are many shortcut keys available in Word. Here's a tip for memorizing the shortcut keys: Choose 3 or 4 shortcuts you want to memorize. Write them on a sticky note and place the note on your computer monitor. Every few days, as you memorize these keystrokes, replace your sticky note with another list of 3 or 4 keystrokes. Other shortcuts could be available to the editor depending on the SR platform used by the company.

LETTING GO

The final skill you need to use could be the most difficult of all because you have been learning to be meticulous in your editing of documents. Some customers (hospital, clinic, etc.) do not want to pay for, and they are not interested in having, an attractive document or one that is "easier to read." The hardest thing for an experienced MT to adjust to is "letting it go" when the desire to edit something that is not exactly right but has no bearing on content appears in the SR document. Make as few changes as possible to recognized text and edit only when the errors change or influence the meaning of the dictation. A barrier to your success may be your inability to forgo cosmetics and to just concentrate on content.

Your progress could be impeded by making a document more readable when making it accurate is your primary function.

EXAMPLE

SR document:

Impression: pulmonary edema probably precipitated by hypertension with resultant respiratory failure, hypertension, diabetes, probable aspiration, probable chronic obstructive pulmonary disease.

Your preferred transcript:

IMPRESSION

1. Pulmonary edema, probably precipitated by hypertension with resultant respiratory failure.

2. Hypertension.

3. Diabetes.

4. Probable aspiration.

5. Probable chronic obstructive pulmonary disease.

Actual completed and edited document:

Impression: pulmonary edema probably precipitated by hypertension with resultant respiratory failure, hypertension, diabetes, probable aspiration, probable chronic obstructive pulmonary disease.

There are no edits in this completed document. You can see why someone would be unwilling to pay for the time it took to change the SR document into your preferred transcript. Numeric lists, stacked formats, capitalized words, and proper punctuation simply may no longer be the client's preferred transcript.

EXAMPLE

SR document:

Ostiomeatal complexes are open and patent.

Your preferred transcript:

Ostiomeatal complexes are open.

Actual completed document:

Ostiomeatal complexes are open and patent.

(You probably would not take the time to delete the redundant expression that follows *open* for a client that does not want to pay for fine editing.)

15

CHAPTER

TABLE 15-1   Common Keyboard Commands to Increase Productivity*

WINDOWS SHORTCUTS:

Window key	Activate Start menu
Windows+E	Open Explorer (can do more than once)
Windows+D	Return to desktop

WORD SHORTCUTS:

Ctrl+A	Select **a**ll
Ctrl+B	**B**old text
Ctrl+C	**C**opy selected text or object
Ctrl+D	**D**efault
Ctrl+E	C**e**nter a paragraph
Ctrl+F	**F**ind text, formatting, and special items
Ctrl+Shift+F	**F**ind in email
Ctrl+G	**G**o to specific page
Ctrl+H	Replace text, specific formatting, and special items
Ctrl+I	**I**talicize text
Ctrl+J	**J**ustify a paragraph
Ctrl+K	Hyperlin**k**
Ctrl+L	**L**eft align a paragraph
Ctrl+M	Indent a paragraph from the left (**m**ove)
Ctrl+N	Create a new document
Ctrl+O	**O**pen a document
Ctrl+P	**P**rint
Ctrl+Q	Remove paragraph formatting
Ctrl+R	**R**ight align a paragraph
Ctrl+S	**S**ave a file
Ctrl+T	Create a hanging indent
Ctrl+Shift+M	Remove a paragraph indent from the left
Ctrl+Shift+T	Reduce a hanging indent
Ctrl+U	**U**nderline text
Ctrl+V	Paste selected text
Ctrl+W	Close a document
Ctrl+X	Cut selected text
Ctrl+Y	Redo the last action
Ctrl+Z	Undo the last action
Shift+Enter	Create a line break
Ctrl+Enter	Create a page break
Ctrl+Shift+Spacebar	Create a nonbreaking space
Ctrl+Shift+Hyphen	Create a nonbreaking hyphen
Ctrl+Equal Sign	Subscript formatting
Ctrl+Shift+Plus Sign	Superscript
Ctrl+Spacebar	Remove manual character formatting

WORD SHORTCUTS:

Ctrl+1	Single-space lines
Ctrl+2	Double-space lines
Ctrl+5	Set 1.5-line space
Ctrl+0	Add or remove one line space preceding a paragraph
Ctrl+F2	Print Preview
Ctrl+F10	Split screen
Alt+F3	Create an Auto Text entry
Alt+F4	Quit Word
Alt+F7	Find the next misspelling or grammatical error
Alt+Tab	Toggle between programs
Shift+F3	Change the case of letters
Shift+F5	Move to a previous revision
F7	Activate spellchecker
F8	Select word, select sentence, select paragraph
F12	Choose the Save As command
Alt+Ctrl+C	Insert copyright symbol
Alt+Ctrl+Period	Insert an ellipsis
Alt+Ctrl+R	Insert registered trademark symbol
Alt+Ctrl+T	Insert trademark symbol

MOVE THE INSERTION POINT:

Backspace	Delete one character to the left
Ctrl+Backspace	Delete one word to the left
Delete	Delete one character to the right
Ctrl+Delete	Delete one word to the right
Left Arrow	One character to the left
Right Arrow	One character to the right
Ctrl+Left Arrow	One word to the left
Ctrl+Right Arrow	One word to the right
Ctrl+Up Arrow	One paragraph up
Ctrl+Down Arrow	One paragraph down
Up Arrow	Up one line
Down Arrow	Down one line
End	To the end of a line
Home	To the beginning of a line
Page Up	Up one screen
Page Down	Down one screen
Ctrl+End	To the end of a document
Ctrl+Home	To the beginning of a document

*Keyboard commands to avoid the use of the mouse to carry out computer functions.

15

CHAPTER

15-3 TRANSCRIBING "BACK END" SPEECH RECOGNITION DOCUMENT PRACTICE

DIRECTIONS: On the Evolve website, you will find 10 real-life speech recognition documents with both voice files and screen files. Please transcribe the first two of these as your instructor directs. Do not practice the "Letting Go" method, but do your best to turn out a perfect transcript. It is probably not a good idea to try out the keyboard shortcuts at this point unless you are already familiar with them. You could have enough trouble with your transcripts without adding any additional steps to the process.

Patient's names are not used, of course, so just type XXX when the dictation makes a ding sound. Consult Appendix D in your textbook for place names and person's names that are used. Also note the format styles that are used in the keys and make sure to follow them.

Before you begin, you might consider increasing the zoom on your document. Just remember to return to the correct size when you are finished.

The answers to the first two files are provided for you to examine in Appendix A. Please avoid checking them until you have completed each one. After you have checked your transcript, relisten to the dictation and examine the key as you do so.

15-4 TRANSCRIBING SPEECH RECOGNITION REVIEW

DIRECTIONS: On the Evolve website, you will find 10 real-life SR documents with both voice files and screen files. You will have completed and checked the first 2 with the key. Please transcribe the last 8 as your instructor directs. Do not practice the "Letting Go" method, but do your best to turn out a perfect transcript. It is probably not a good idea to try out the keyboard shortcuts at this point unless you are already familiar with them. You could have enough trouble with your transcripts without adding any additional steps to the process.

Patient's names are not used, of course, so just type XXX when the dictation makes a ding sound. Consult Appendix D in your textbook for place names and person's names that are used. Also note the format styles that are used in the keys and make sure to follow them.

Before you begin, you might consider increasing the zoom on your document. Just remember to return the zoom to the correct size when you are finished. Your instructor will give you the keys to these as you complete them.

CHAPTER 16

Establishing Your Career and Applying for Transcription Positions

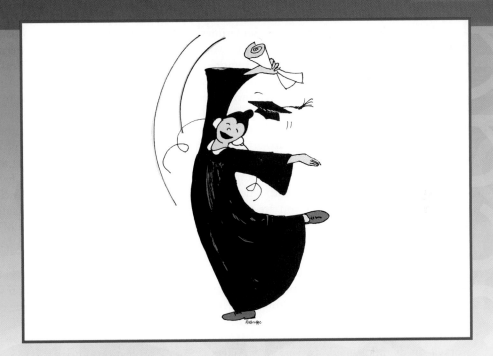

OBJECTIVES

After reading this chapter and completing the assignments, you will be able to

1. List prospective employers.
2. Identify your employment goals.
3. List the considerations for being a remote-based worker.
4. Identify marketing goals.
5. Compose a cover letter to accompany your resumé.
6. Prepare a resumé.
7. Research employment websites.
8. Identify temporary jobs in your locale.
9. Prepare for an interview.
10. Compose a thank-you note to follow up an interview.
11. Explain professionalism.

INTRODUCTION

At last, you think, here I am; I am finished with all of the studying, and now I can look for my first job.

Wait just a moment. Now is the time to stand back and see where you have been, how far you have come, and what exactly it is that you should do next. First, do not be too sure that you are ready for your first job. A lot of readiness has to do with exactly what it is that you want to do, and determining that goal is your first task now. What exactly is it that you think you can do, and what exactly do you want to do? Sometimes students think that because they really want to work out of their own homes, being part of the remote-based work force will be easy because they will have a single client, work by themselves, choose their own schedule, take as long as they want to complete a project, and so on. Some students think they will seek employment in a large institution where they can slip sort of unnoticed into the pool of other novices. Finally, others think, Good grief, am I ready, and who will want me?

Begin at the beginning. Start with where you have been before you look at where you are going or what you want to do. You have done a lot if you have finished the text, but you have, after all, studied only the basics, the background. A lot of how prepared you are to begin your career depends on how much actual transcribing you have done. Have you finished all of the Systems Unit Method (SUM) dictation (Health Professions Institute, 209-551-2112), the AHDI dictation (209-527-9620), and the dictation that accompanies this text? Have you worked on dictation made by foreign speakers (ESL, English as a second language); transcribed actual dictation from other sources, completed an externship for a transcription service or hospital? Have you participated in an apprenticeship or work-experience program?

If you have graduated from an AHDI-approved program and earned the RMT credential, you could qualify to participate in the Department of Labor Registered Apprenticeship Program. This program accepts recent transcription graduates and pairs them with employer-participants. The employer-participants provide on-the-job training. For details on this program, visit AHDI at www.ahdionline.org.

Those hours spent actually transcribing and developing an "ear" for this art are very important. Have you developed your research skills, or have you depended on others to help you out of tough dictation or, worse yet, looked at a key to the transcript? Have you transcribed only "canned" tapes (those produced by non-professionals reading documents)? Are you open to criticism both from yourself and from those who will view your work? Are you ready to learn how to use new equipment, work long hours (and not produce much), and not get any praise for what you do produce? What you need right now is this attitude: I will go anywhere, anytime, anyplace, and do anything for anybody for any amount of money...just to get started. That idea is the right idea. Now, you have decided that you *are* ready. You *do* have the skills in place. So exactly what is it that you want to do?

WORKING FROM HOME

The Remote-Based Work Site

One popular goal is working out of your home. Determine what you need to be successful in reaching this goal. You have already decided that you are prepared to be a professional medical transcriptionist (MT). The next decision you have to make concerns your client base. Are you going to begin searching for your own client or clients, or are you going to approach a transcription company, work for the company, and transcribe the work from your home office? These are two very different aspects of being an independent MT. If you decide that you want to develop your own client base, get prepared for that first client. If you want to set up your own home-based business, establishing a relationship with an experienced MT who has such a business is a good idea. It would be practical to complete an externship with this person and, hopefully, have that person as a mentor, working not only on your transcription skills but also on your entrepreneurial skills. How do you really provide excellent service to a client, earn money, be productive, and be happy?

One good thing about working at home in this profession is that it has been done, it is being done, and it can be done very successfully. You want a part of that success. In fact, medical transcription is probably one of the best professions to be in if you want to take advantage of telecommuting. Dictation can be accessed by phone line or over the Internet, and work can be transmitted electronically after it is transcribed. I am sure that you already have in mind, however, the many advantages of working out of your home office, and so it is not necessary to recite them. They will be as varied as you readers are varied. However, some other issues need to be examined realistically.

The Home-Based Entrepreneur

Because it is the goal of many students to work from home, the best way to get started is to establish exactly what it means to work from home legally, emotionally, financially, and practically.

Just a few ideas concerning working from home are given here. These ideas are simply to get you thinking about the commitment and to encourage you to plan carefully for this endeavor and explore it thoroughly if you decide that working from home is the route you want to take.

16 CHAPTER

Before you begin to develop your plans to work from home, it is a good idea to purchase the comprehensive reference *The Independent Medical Transcriptionist,* by Avila-Weil and Glaccum, 5th edition, from Rayve Productions Inc., (800) 852-4890, and read it thoroughly. This book will provide you with every necessary detail and will encourage you as well.

Terminology for Home-Based Workers

The Internal Revenue Service (IRS) uses three different terms to determine your work-from-home status. It is essential that you are clear about the category of your employment from the very first day, so that when it comes time to pay your taxes, there are no surprises. It is important that you consult with your accountant or attorney to help you determine whether you are an employee or an independent contractor. Here are just a few definitions to help you see the differences. There are tax advantages to working from home, but only an expert can advise you on what is tax deductible, what records need to be kept, what federal tax forms need to be used, and so on.

EMPLOYEE

An employee is someone who performs services for an employer who controls what the employee does and how the employee does it. It makes no difference whether the employee is telecommuting or on site. The employee receives a W2 form detailing earnings and withholdings. The employer withholds the employee's federal income tax, Social Security contributions, and Medicare contributions. The last two items equal 15.3% of an employee's income. (The employer pays half, or 7.65%, and the employee pays half.) According to IRS Publication 15A, anyone who performs services is an employee if an employer can control what is done and how it is done.

STATUTORY EMPLOYEE

Basically, a statutory employee is an independent contractor who is treated as an employee, but only the Social Security and Medicare contributions are withheld by the employer, with both parties paying half of these contributions. A statutory employee is responsible for paying his or her own federal income tax.

INDEPENDENT CONTRACTOR

An independent contractor must pay both the employee and the employer portions of the Social Security and Medicare contributions, or 15.3% of earned income. The good news is that the employee's half is deductible; the amount paid reduces taxable income the same way a business expense does. An independent contractor receives a 1099 form each year from each employer who has paid the contractor more than $600. The employer sends a copy of the form to the IRS. An independent contractor is required to pay quarterly estimated federal taxes. Estimated state and local taxes have to be reported quarterly as well.

Independent contractors are not covered by an employer's workers' compensation insurance, and they do not receive such benefits as medical insurance, unemployment compensation, contributions to retirement funds, or paid vacations. The independent contractor, not the employer, provides the tools and supplies needed to perform a job. An independent contractor can perform similar services for more than one client and can hire assistants or subcontractors. In addition, a contractor can terminate the relationship with an employer at any time with no penalty unless the contract between the worker and the employer states otherwise.

MARKETING YOURSELF

Use the following list to market yourself and your business:

▶ Write your marketing plan; decide whom you want to serve.
▶ Research to determine what rates are being charged, and decide what you will charge. Find out what employers will actually pay for your services. Do not sell yourself short; charge what you are worth.
▶ Prepare flyers (Figure 16-1), mailings, and brochures describing what services you will provide. Market yourself as a specialty service and in such a way that you stand out from your competition.
▶ Be prepared to discuss your productivity capacities and what you have done to increase your productivity.
▶ Keep your client base balanced. To protect yourself in times of shifting sources of transcription, try not to allow any one client to account for more than one third of your business.
▶ Talk with people about what you do.
▶ Be sure you can be reached. Set up voice mail for when you are unable to answer the phone, because voice mail picks up when you are on the phone.

THE HOME-BASED BUSINESS

Office Space

Your office must fit into the household environment. Define and separate your workspace from the family living space, and choose a location where you will be disturbed the least (e.g., partition off a section of the living room, dining room, or family room or convert or remodel the garage, attic, or basement). It is a challenge to get and keep a business and at the same

16
CHAPTER

A

800-123-4542

Post Office Box 19685

GrandView, CA 92000

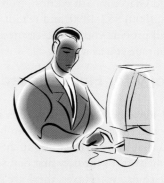

PDQ Transcription

A Medical Transcription Service

by

Peter Dean Qualen

B

Service Oriented
Professional • Accurate • Reliable

- *Customized to your practice*
- *Reasonable rates*
- *Latest technology used to prevent errors*
- *Free dictation pick-up and document drop-off*
- *48-hour turn around time*
- *Micro and standard-sized cassettes accepted*
- *Locally based and operated*

Strict Confidentiality

- *HIPAA Compliant*
- *Patient information is never shared*
- *Computers are password secured*
- *All files purged every 3 months**
  * Archive CD available upon request
- *Draft copies shredded on-site*

Please call for more information
800 – 123– 4542

FIGURE 16-1 Example of a business flyer. **A,** Side one. **B,** Side two.

time convince family and friends that you are actually working in the "home office" despite where you have set it up. Remember to set boundaries for outside callers as well.

Plan to have storage space and shelf space for files, reference books, and so on. Organize your workspace for control; determine which items you use daily, weekly, monthly, or yearly, and then place them accordingly. It is very important to have storage outside your office space in a remote location.

Equipment

Hire a computer/software expert to help you set up your business equipment correctly. Here are a few things to consider:

- Current, legally purchased operating system.
- High-speed Internet access.
- Comfortable, sturdy, ergonomically correct work station.
- Word expander.
- Comprehensive reference library.
- Private and professional telephone lines.
- Space for your desk and chair.
- Storage space for books, supplies, reference materials, telephone, computer, printer, scanner, fax, shredder, and other necessary materials and equipment.

Have a phone line installed for business calls and a fax machine. Make sure clients can reach you. Voice mail and other telephone aids will help you when you have to be away from your business. (Voice mail picks up calls so that clients never get a busy signal.)

Records and Finances

Keep track of everything that could possibly be considered a business expense, and keep receipts. Begin with a list of your training expenses, including books, gasoline, and registration fees. Your major expenses will be your computer, software, office furniture, and so on. Do not overlook courier fees, marketing, utilities, Internet fees, telephone, mileage and vehicle use, professional dues, reference books, subscriptions to professional journals, and supplies (such as stamps, paper, and ink).

Emotional Needs

An MT needs to address the reality of working from home and what it means to be self-employed. If you imagine that being self-employed basically means that you are your own boss, be realistic: The job is done the dictators' way. You need to be able to work with little or no one-on-one support (which can be found in an office setting). Do not neglect the importance of networking with other professionals. Join or set up a networking group that meets regularly, join organizations of other professional groups, and attend workshops.

Do not neglect the hobbies and friendships you had before you began your business. Make quality time for your family, and protect blocks of time dedicated to helping with homework, playing, going on excursions, and so on.

Professional Considerations and Work Ethics

Here are some additional considerations to remember when you decide to establish your own home-based business:

- Keep commitments and schedules. When you agree to a schedule, it is imperative that you keep it. Some at-home workers think some business rules do not apply just because they are not at the worksite.
- Maintain regular business hours. Set up a regular routine. (You can have whatever hours you want, but you need to be sure that you are available for your clients when you say you will be.)
- Take a home-based business seriously, and be realistic about the time it will take to get you established (at least 6 to 12 months).
- Be flexible.
- Be prompt and punctual. Meet all deadlines.
- Develop excellent phone and email manners (return and follow up all calls and emails promptly).
- Read professional journals.

Business

Be careful to attend to the nontranscription responsibilities to help you establish a secure business endeavor:

- Make a business plan and list what equipment and software you need.
- Seek out a support group made up of other home-based workers.
- Contact the U. S. Small Business Administration for advice (www.sba.gov). Click on "Tools" and type in "Assessment Tool" to take the quick Small Business Readiness Assessment Test.
- Arrange for start-up funds.
- Have written agreements with clients and vendors.
- Ask colleagues about contracts they use and their marketing strategy.
- Find a trustworthy mentor.
- Work for a while for someone who is established in the business you envision for yourself.
- Attend seminars on small businesses and marketing.
- Plan for vacation relief and assistance for overflow work.
- Make your business official.
- Determine what regulations apply to doing business in your area. It is important to obtain a copy of the laws and regulations of your community. Requirements for business licenses and regulations vary greatly.

16

CHAPTER

- Clarify any zoning restrictions that apply to having a home-based business.
- Make sure that you are aware of the tax laws relative to operating as an independent contractor.
- Take necessary legal steps to safeguard your business.
- Select a memorable name that fits your business.
- Customize a logo and use it on all business products, such as letterheads, flyers, and business cards.
- Register your business name.
- Consider errors and omissions insurance to cover you against claims that your service harmed someone.
- Be aware of the Health Insurance Portability and Accountability Act of 1996 (HIPAA) regulations that affect you and your work. (See Chapter 1 for guidelines.)
- Have an attorney, an accountant, and a computer specialist available for consultation.
- Establish a separate business bank account.
- Write contracts. Having a written contract helps ensure that you are taken seriously as a business. Spell out specifics, such as the service you are providing, when you will provide it, costs, and clients' obligation to pay.
- Bill immediately upon delivery, and act promptly on overdue accounts.
- Keep your regular job and use your new business as a sideline until you can rely on the new business for income.

Qualities

The following characteristics can help you achieve success in a home-based business:

- Be an effective time manager.
- Have the ability to sit quietly and stay focused.
- Do not be dismayed when you have to disregard unnecessary interruptions by your family.
- Accept constructive criticism.
- Be able to ask questions without feeling inadequate.
- Manage your time well and get to work on time. Set times and days when you will work.
- Plan and take scheduled breaks. (Try to break when work is interesting and inviting you to go forward. This trick helps you reestablish momentum when you return.)
- Make time for your personal life, and do not neglect your family and friends.
- Protect your free time as zealously as your work time, so that you have fun and avoid burnout.
- Look professional and be punctual when visiting a job site or a client.
- Be patient in getting your business up and running and making a profit.

Patricia Stettler, CMT, AHDI-F, and educator, sums up some of the considerations you need to remember in setting up a home-based business with this admonishment in the July 2005 issue of *Plexus*:

> No one can efficiently or effectively transcribe complex medical reports while doing anything else at the same time. This includes laundry, babysitting, and cooking dinner. The at-home MT must block out periods of time that can be devoted to transcription. Preferably these time blocks are at least two hours each so the MT has the opportunity to "get into the zone" where one is most productive. An MT is a professional, doing a highly skilled job that involves patient safety. If one wants to be treated as a professional, one needs to act like a professional.

Developing Clientele

Call local competitors and obtain information on the range of fees based on character count, line count, page count, visible black character (VBC) count, or hours worked so that you have an idea of what to charge as a fee for your work. Research your market area to see who will use your services in the community, such as physicians' offices (e.g., orthopedists, cardiologists), hospitals (e.g., medical record, pathology, or radiology departments), clinics, nurse practitioners, national companies, and so on. You can find work by substituting for MTs who are ill, on vacation, or overloaded. Other professionals in search of MTs are chief residents going into private practice, new physicians in town, a physician appointed to head an association, physicians who are changing offices or adding colleagues, visiting nurse associations, marriage and family counselors, clinical psychologists, and medical researchers. Send prospective clients a letter (Figure 16-2). Your major responsibility is to convince clients that your service is better than that of the competition. Stress dependability; efficient service; professional, prompt turnaround of quality work; a dedicated telephone line for incoming dictation; courier service (pickup and delivery); and so on. Misunderstandings about agreements can occur, so put everything in writing (Figure 16-3). If you change the terms of the agreement, write a letter outlining the new terms.

Professional Fees

Some self-employed MTs consider a standard page to be 30 single-spaced lines. First pages are counted as a whole page, even when the letter or report is half a page. The final page of the work is prorated: fewer than 15 lines is a half page, and more than 15 lines are considered a full page. The monthly statement to the client should consist of a detailed record of patients' names; dates of each report; and number of pages, number of lines, or hours, depending on how you structure your fees (Figure 16-4). You could establish

---

LETTERHEAD

Date

Client's Name
Address
City, State ZIP Code

Dear:

For eight years, I have worked as a medical transcriptionist for Adrianna's STAT Med Trans Service. I am now establishing my own business. Perhaps your office or hospital has an overload or your medical transcriptionist is planning a vacation. Maybe you have a manuscript you need typed for a medical journal or you need a personnel manual, grant proposal, or research paper prepared. You can be assured of the following:

- Consultation rendered at no charge.
- Accurate, complete, and speedy medical transcription. All work is proofread.
- Courier service (pick up and delivery available). Your transcripts will be delivered to you on the day and at the hour you specify.
- Low competitive rates.
- Premium pay for overtime work eliminated on in-house transcription.
- In-house office space and equipment requirements reduced or eliminated.
- Personal, professional, dependable service provided on a temporary "fill-in" basis.
- Service available 24 hours a day, 7 days a week, including holidays.
- Call-in dictation from any location available.
- Retyping of a report at no charge if you are not satisfied with the transcript.
- HIPAA-level confidentiality maintained and guaranteed.

My business equipment includes a scanner, PC, iMac, and secure fax, and I run Microsoft Word, Windows 7, and Excel. My transcription equipment is adaptable to digital, standard, and mini-cassettes.

Professional references will be supplied on request. I am a certified medical transcriptionist (CMT) and a member of the Association for Healthcare Documentation Integrity. I welcome the opportunity to speak with you personally about this new service in the near future. If you need my services immediately, please call and leave a message. Please keep my business card (enclosed) and telephone number on file in case you need my services in the future.

Sincerely,

FIGURE 16-2 Example of a letter outlining an MT's services for a prospective client.

a minimum charge. In trying to obtain a client, state the following:

> My charge is computed on a per-page level, because this is quicker for you to check and for me to compute. I am currently charging _____ cents a line on full, single-spaced pages. This method works out to $ _____ a full page for billing purposes.

To help you compute your charge, use a line-counter utility, such as Spellex AccuCount, created specifically to help MTs count lines or words. Consider using the visible black character (VBC) method to measure documents. This is the recommended standard and cannot be manipulated or inflated with unseen extra spaces, increased margin widths, tabs, increased font sizes,

or formatting codes. Establish a separate fee base for redoing a document because the client changes words, lines, or paragraphs or does other personal editing of the original.

Subcontracting

If someone who is self-employed gets too much work and asks you to complete some of the work, you are subcontracting. The self-employed MT will pay you a certain amount per line, per page, or per hour and will keep a percentage of the total amount billed the client. Payment should be made at the time of delivery of the work to the self-employed person, because you, the subcontractor, are not dealing directly with the client.

LETTERHEAD

DATE

Client's Name
Address
City, State ZIP code

Dear

This is to confirm my conversation with you yesterday regarding transcription of your medical reports.

I agree to deliver completed transcripts to your clinic within 24-36 hours after the dictation is picked up.

The rate is _____ cents per line, with a 60-character line count. Editing is $ ___/hour for client rewrite of the dictation. There is no charge for minor adjustments (1-3 words) to the transcript.

Please call me any time you need my service. I look forward to transcribing for the physicians in your clinic.

Sincerely yours,

Note: List as many specifics as you can. This example is minimal. For instance, you might wish to make the second paragraph specific by stating, "I agree to pick up dictation on Tuesday and deliver on Thursday."

FIGURE 16-3 Example of a letter outlining terms of an agreement. (Never make simple oral agreements.)

OPPORTUNITIES FOR EMPLOYMENT

First, tell everyone you know—friends, relatives, and professional contacts—that you are now available for work. Be aware of the hidden job market, hidden employment opportunities available to you through networking. These job openings are known to current employees of an organization and usually are reserved for word-of-mouth referrals. These jobs are not posted on websites or otherwise advertised. When you hear of a job through networking, you stand a much better chance of getting an interview because the person hiring will automatically evaluate your resume and do so more favorably because of the network referral.

Members of your professional organization, instructors, work-study mentors, employed MTs, and your personal physician are all good networking sources.

Always carry copies of your resume in case you meet someone you think can be of help in your search. (Remember, most jobs are not advertised.) In addition, provide your instructors or school placement office with your resume so that they will have it handy and be truly knowledgeable about your background if a prospective employer contacts them. School counselors can also give you leads on where to look for a job.

Make frequent visits to hospitals and large medical clinics and check the human resources bulletin board. Openings are often listed in this manner before they are publicized. When you visit a medical facility, let the

LETTERHEAD

Date

Client's Name
Address
City, State ZIP code

BILLING STATEMENT

Tapes	Patient's Name	Report* Code No.	Pickup Date	Delivery Date	Pages or Hours	Balance Due
1	Mary Brown	3	11-22-0X	11-23-0X	13.5 pages	
2	Sue Morse	4	11-22-0X	11-23-0X	4.0 pages	
3						
4						
5						
6						
TOTALS		2			17.5	$

RATE: $____ per full single-spaced page (equals ____ cents per line).

TERMS: *Terms should be stated on the billing statement, such as payable on delivery, net 30, net 15 days from invoice, end of month, payment due within 15 days of invoice, and so forth.*

*Report Code No.
1 = Chart note
2 = Consultation
3 = Discharge Summary
4 = History and Physical
5 = Letter
6 = Operative Report
7 = Other

FIGURE 16-4 Example of a billing statement.

staff members know you are looking for a position and would appreciate any leads. Leave your business card, resumé, and/or flyer with the office manager.

Go to the human resources department of local hospitals, medical clinics, transcription businesses, and word processing centers, and complete a job application to be filed in case an opening occurs in the future. Seek out the transcription department and speak to the person directly in charge of hiring. Many large institutions have job lines, and you can telephone and hear information about any openings for employment. The title and salary range are usually given.

Consult the telephone directory or medical society roster for sources, and make a blind mailing of your resumé to possible prospects. In the Yellow Pages of your telephone directory, physicians are listed under "Physicians and Surgeons," and typing services are generally listed under "Secretarial Services."

The state employment department could have a list of available jobs, and there is no charge for this service. If you use a professional employment agency, you must be prepared to pay a fee if the agency places you.

Join a chapter of the American Health Information Management Association or Association for Healthcare

Documentation Integrity. By attending meetings and receiving their professional magazines and bulletins, you could learn of a job opportunity. Contact the national headquarters of each association for further information about local chapters. Subscribe to *Advance,* a free online publication that includes important information about medical transcription and advertisements from medical transcription companies (www.advanceweb.com).

Association for Healthcare Documentation Integrity
100 Sycamore Avenue
Modesto, CA 95354
Telephone: 800-982-2182
Fax: 209-527-9633
www.ahdionline.org (click on "Resources")

American Health Information Management Association
233 North Michigan Avenue
Chicago, IL 60601
Telephone: 1-800-335-5535
www.AHIMA.org

Health Professions Institute
http://www.hpisum.com

Clinical Documentation Industry Association:
http://www.mtia.com

If you plan to work in Canada, contact the following resource:
Ontario Medical Secretaries' Association
150 Bloor Street West, Suite 900
Toronto ON, M5S 3C1
Telephone: 416-340-2935
Fax No.: 416-599-9309.
www.OMSA-hca.org

A good objective for a new MT wanting to telecommute is to find employment with a service. Large transcription services offer the best opportunities for employment, training, support, continuing education opportunities, and the quality assurance that a new MT needs. Many of the concerns just discussed do not apply to the employee of a transcription service, and that distinction is a plus for the beginner. Large organizations with training programs are, in fact, your best chance for getting a good start. They will train you to use their equipment with the voices of their speakers, with their formats, and under the direction of their quality control. *And*—this is a big *and*—employees who want to work at home often are able to do so with the approval and often the loan of equipment from the company. More and more large organizations are training and then releasing their employees to the environment that the employees prefer. Be sure to keep your expectations reasonable; it takes time and dedication to become skilled in this profession.

What if you are in that group of "Good grief, I think I am ready, but who will want me? I can't work at home alone; I don't want to be part of a large organization. I love doing this, but where do I belong?" Be open-minded and try whatever turns up. Consider how this last possibility works.

First, most jobs are not advertised. That fact is hard to understand sometimes, but it really works that way. Just as you are going to be telling everyone you know that you are now looking for a job as an MT, prospective employers are sending out the news that they are looking for an MT. In some instances, they do not get to the advertising stage because they know they do not need to. Their friends and employees begin to talk and to look, notices are posted, a blurb goes on the job lines, schools are called. When that method does not work, they finally place ads. One reason they have to place ads today: they are looking for you, and there are really not enough of you trained to fill all the positions. They have to be competitive to lure you in.

Before you go on to the next task of finding these openings and applying for them, consider the kinds of jobs available. Often students want to know just one simple thing: what is the easiest medical transcription job? It is understandable that you might feel the need to ease into this profession. It is acceptable that you are not ready to tackle everything, and your honesty is to be admired. To answer the question: a single voice, a single medical specialty is the easiest. If an excellent dictator is available, the job is easy. Even without an excellent dictator, however, you will be surprised at how fast you can become skilled with the one voice and the one specialty. Even transcription for a small facility with several voices and one specialty is not too difficult. Some people never look at this type of transcription as a stepping-stone to far more complicated transcription. Rather, they see it as a perfect match for their personality, and they never leave this comfortable environment. These jobs can be in the facility itself, or you can have this office as your client in a home-based business.

It is important for you to make a list now of your basic requirements for employment. This list is a real list: not something to just think about, but a written list. It should include the salary you hope to earn; where you would like to work; the hours, part time or full time; the medical specialties you think you would like and why; the new skills you would like to use; the old skills you would like to use; your short-range plans; your long-range plans; your strengths; and your weaknesses. Even though this list is just a dream sheet, it gives you focus, and it is fun when you look back and see whether any or how many of these goals were achieved.

Electronic Job Search

There are a few ways to approach the use of computer technology to find a job. One method is to subscribe to an online computer service. These services have bulletin boards for subscribers interested in medical transcription, and you can post a notice or resumé. Discard traditional resumé-writing techniques (action verbs) and focus on action words (nouns), such as "transcriptionist" and "manager." Use labels or key words, such as "education," "experience," "skills," "knowledge," and "abilities." Avoid decorative or uncommon typefaces; do not use underlining. Minimize the use of abbreviations except for CMT and RMT (certified medical transcriptionist and registered medical transcriptionist). For an electronic resumé, forget the one-page rule; use three or four pages.

A book on electronic job searching is *Guide to Internet Job Searching 2008-2009,* by Margaret Dikel and Frances Roehm (McGraw-Hill, 2008).

Other websites you might consider using are:

job-hunt.org
careerjournal.com
quintcareers.com
monster.com
mtjobs.com
jobcentral.com

Program your computer to alert you about postings from news sources that you specify. Both Yahoo and Google will send you free email alerts when the topics you have identified appear online. You specify how often and when you want to receive alerts on your target topics. Be very specific in the key words for the target topics you select because alerts will come from published text, headlines, summaries, organizational names, and so on. You want your search base to be very narrow, for instance *medical transcription* in contrast to *transcription.*

Your Resumé

Now is the time to discuss the preparation for looking: the flyer for your home-based business or the resumé for the small facility or the large hospital or transcription service.

If you have an old resumé, update it by adding your new education, skills, and plans. You might like to read the information on resumé writing just to make sure that your resumé represents you. If you have never written a resumé before, it is often easier to begin with a work sheet. See Figures 16-5 and 16-6 for sample worksheets. Make copies of the worksheet for each job you have ever held, and then complete a worksheet for each of the jobs. By filling in a worksheet, you begin to gather the information you need to compile your resumé. Make a copy of Figure 16-6 to flesh out the data for the resumé. When these are complete, you have the background for

your resumé, and you can begin to compile it in the most attractive format you can. See Figures 16-7 and 16-8 for completed, attractive resumés.

A resumé is a personal statement about you and your work. There is no exact format to be followed, but usually a resumé is chronological or functional, or sometimes a combination of the two. A *chronological* resumé is arranged historically, stating recent experiences first, along with the dates and descriptive data for each job. A *functional* resumé highlights the qualifications or various duties that an individual can perform. The *combination* format emphasizes job skills, as well as dates and places of employment. The examples in this chapter give you a few suggestions for organization as well as format.

A one-page resumé is ample for a beginning transcriptionist, but someone in midcareer may require two or three pages. However, even if you have enough information for two or three pages, try to condense it to one page. Put references on a second page if you must. When you are not actively looking for a job, keep a few copies of a carefully prepared resumé on hand in case an opportunity arises unexpectedly.

Your resumé should be professionally reproduced on white or off-white bond paper. Handwritten resumés are never acceptable. Carefully check your resumé for spelling, punctuation, and typographical errors. Be sure that you have someone else proofread your resumé, that person could spot typographical errors and give you additional suggestions. Even one misspelled word or typographical error could discourage a prospective employer and negate your opportunity for an interview. Use wide, neat margins, and balance the information well to produce an attractive page. Because you need several copies of the resumé, have it reproduced on a copy machine that produces excellent photocopies, or have it printed professionally. Generate the resumé by a laser printer for a professional appearance of highest quality. Be prepared to fax your resumé with a cover letter. Have your cover letter prepared with a blank available for the name of the recipient and the telephone number. Keep an electronic version of both resumé and cover letter for those prospects who invite you to submit your resumé online. Consider putting your resumé on an Internet job bank. AlliedHealthCareers.com is one such site.

The title for your resumé can be *Resumé, Personal Data Sheet,* or *Biographical Sketch.* The body of the resumé should begin with your name, address, and telephone number. (Whenever you have a resumé under consideration, be sure that you have a professional-sounding message on your answering machine. "Cute" messages and children's voices are inappropriate at this time.) The Civil Rights Act of 1964 allows you to exclude your age, birth date, marital status, height, weight, and physical condition.

The second major subject of your resumé should be your educational background. Include the high

WORK EXPERIENCE

Job Title: _____

Company Name:_____

City, State:_____Phone:_____

When Employed: from_____ to _____

Supervisor's name:_____Title:_____

The major job duties/responsibilities: _____

_____

_____

Special awards, assignments, or accomplishments in this job:_____

_____

_____

Use action verbs when you can to describe your major job duties and responsibilities (reorganized, supervised, scheduled, maintained, created, designed, improved, developed, trained, established, planned, organized.)

EXTERNSHIP EXPERIENCE

Type of site:_____ Hours completed:_____

Transcription accomplished:_____

FIGURE 16-5 Worksheet for writing a resumé. Make a copy for each job you have ever held, and fill in the top part for each job.

school, college, and any business school that you may have attended. If you received any awards or scholastic honors, these should also be included. Be sure to highlight and carefully explain your medical transcription training.

After listing your education, list your work experience. You can begin with your most recent place of employment and end with your first position, or you can use the reverse order. Include summer, full-time, part-time, and temporary jobs, as well as volunteer work, and be sure to list past job accomplishments. Describe *briefly* the duties that you had in each position. It is not necessary to state reasons why you left a job; this question can be asked during the interview or can appear on a job application form. Job-hopping or gaps of several months between jobs may be scrutinized; if you wish, this situation can be dealt with during an interview. References can be listed, or you could state, "References furnished upon request." Choose references from among former employers and teachers,

a family physician, or a friend who is a professional MT. Always ask permission to use the names of your references on your resume. Indicate what your relationship is or was with each reference: that is, former (or current) instructor, employer, supervisor, friend for however many years, and so on.

When you apply for a position as an MT, list your typing skills in words per minute and your transcription speed in lines or characters per hour. Remember to list all equipment and word processing programs you know how to use proficiently (word expanders, Excel, Windows, PowerPoint, Microsoft Word, etc.). State your membership in professional organizations, along with any offices or leadership positions you have held. Mentioning hobbies or special interests is optional because this material is irrelevant. However, if you are fluent in another language, be sure to list this information. You might insert a brief statement of career goals for the next 5 or 10 years. When you telephone a prospective employer, inquire whether the employer

SPECIAL SKILLS: Include skills such as computer program fluency, editing, drugs, disease processes, anatomy/physiology, medical terminology, word research, office equipment operation, second language fluency, and any other skills you feel support your job objective. Indicate level of proficiency.

_____

_____

_____

LICENSES/CERTIFICATES/CERTIFICATION: List all you have earned.

_____

_____

COURSES COMPLETED OR IN PROGRESS: List any special training or course work you have completed that is specific to your job objective.

_____

_____

_____

AFFILIATIONS: Professional, community, scholastic, or extracurricular organizations in which you have been actively involved. Indicate any offices held.

_____

_____

_____

AWARDS/HONORS: Awards, honors, or special recognition not previously listed elsewhere that you wish to include.

_____

_____

_____

REFERENCES: Furnished upon request. (This line is optional. Current rationale is that it is understood, and space might be better used.)
(Create a separate reference listing to provide prospective employers. Indicate relationship or title, such as "supervisor," "coworker," or "company owner.")

_____

_____

_____

FIGURE 16-6 Continuation of worksheet for writing a resumé. Copy and complete this worksheet before you begin to compose your resumé.

prefers the resumé faxed or mailed. In a competitive employment atmosphere where time is important, use every advantage possible.

Cover Letters

If you are sending your resumé to a prospective employer, an attractively and flawlessly typed letter of introduction or a cover letter is important. The letter should be composed for a specific job opening and should contain information not already in your resumé or information that you may want to highlight and bring to the interviewer's attention. Your letter should be more than a cover sheet for your resumé. You want the letter to set you apart from other applicants by providing a glimpse of your personality and your eagerness to work either in this career field or for a specific organization. Focus on just a few qualities that distinguish you most. Try to connect these qualities to the requirements of the position. For example, "I have a strong background in English grammar, and I understand the position is a trainee slot for your editing and quality control manager. I would like to discuss with you…" The letter should be addressed to an individual, whenever possible, and mailed with the resumé. Both letter and resumé should contain your name, address, and telephone number (Figure 16-9). Ask for an interview before you close your letter. Carefully proofread the letter for typographical errors and for errors in spelling, punctuation, and grammar.

Temporary Jobs

There are reasons to work temporarily or as a permanent part-time employee. It can be difficult to decide exactly where you want to work at first. You could need an income to meet monthly bills while you are waiting for a full-time position. As an MT, you can work for

Margaret Mary Mulvaney
7853 Golden Way Road, Wood Creek, XX 98765
(555) 654-2345

OBJECTIVE

Obtain a position as a medical transcription document editor

TECHNICAL SKILLS

- Type 75 wpm
- Shorthand 145 wpm
- Excel
- OpenOffice
- Microsoft Word
- Speech Recognition
- Access
- PowerPoint
- Outlook

HIGHLIGHT OF TRAITS

Conscientious   Productive   Creative   Flexible   Organized   Dedicated

PROFESSIONAL EXPERIENCE

Medical Transcriptionist – 5 years
    Transcribed a variety of acute care and general hospital reports

Executive Secretary –10 years
    Typed complex official documents, agreements, policy manuals
    Prepared conferences and board of directors meetings
    Prepared records, agendas, notices, minutes and resolutions of board of directors' meetings
    Assisted In preparation of budget and annual reports of organization
    Prepared official documents in accordance with licensing regulations
    Maintained filing systems
    Established record-keeping and comprehensive record of board of directors activities
    Assisted in editing a monthly newsletter; printed and arranged bulk mailing

Human Resources Secretary – 3 years
    Composed and typed correspondence
    Coordinated collection of information for schedules, census records, program changes
    Developed and maintained forms for agency-wide use
    Assisted in providing personnel services and routine policies and procedures

General Office
    Typed invoices and prepared monthly statements for accounts receivable
    Maintained personnel files, attendance and salary records
    Typed copy for advertisement

PROFESSIONAL EMPLOYMENT HISTORY

Physicians and Surgeons Acute Care   2008-present
Brown's Medical Transcription Service   2007-2008
Ove Arup & Partners, Johannesburg, South Africa   2001-2007
Manpower Int., Johannesburg, South Africa   1998-2001

EDUCATION

Secretary & Administrative Assistant – National University
Computers/Word Processing Medical Terminology, Transcription Skill Building – Lake View College
Advanced Medical Transcription – Lake View College

FIGURE 16-7 Example of an attractive resumé. The references are not shown; they were placed on a separate page.

various employers or for one particular office or hospital, doing overflow work. Depending on the need for MTs, many communities can use part-time MTs.

Usually you can find temporary or part-time work from the sources mentioned, or a company that places you can hire you. Some of these national companies are Kelly Services, TOP Services, and Ultimate Staffing Services. Some have branch offices in foreign countries.

Your community could have other local and regional temporary employment firms. Look in the Yellow Pages of your phone directory under the heading "Employment—Temporary." There are some advantages in applying to such a company: it will screen you, test your skills, place you into a job category or categories, and have incentive plans to encourage you to remain with it instead of taking a full-time job. Obtain a typing speed

---

Ralph Perez

13821 Casselberry Court, Solo Lake, XX 98765
(555) 676-3733

Objective   Obtain a position as a medical transcriptionist

Technical Skills   Type 65 wpm   Access   PowerPoint
                       Excel   OpenOffice   MS Word

Work History   **Medical Field Claims Examiner Company**
- Served as a technical resource for team members by answering medical claim questions and providing feedback to supervisor.
- Acted as supervisor in absence of supervisor.
- Provided customer service support.
- Reviewed and considered whether the treatment being rendered is consistent with the diagnosis submitted.
- Identified and referred all claims appearing to warrant further medical investigation (fraud investigation or dollar review) to the home office.

Radiology Outsource Specialists
- Transcribed radiology reports and distributed them to the providers.
- Made telephone contact with doctors, insurance personnel, and patients.
- Was responsible for scheduling patient visits for x-rays and imaging.

Education   2001 - 2004 Solo Lake Community College, AS degree awarded
- Medical Transcription (beginning and advanced)
- Medical Terminology Skill Building (advanced medical terminology)
- Work Experience - 570 hours
- Human Biology
- Business English and Communications
- College Keyboarding and Document Processing
- Microcomputer Word Processing
- Medical Office Management
- Medical Billing
- Study Skills and Time Management
- Speech Recognition Editing

Awards
- Vice Principal List
- Perfect Attendance
- Dean's List

References   Name   Name
                   Address   Address
                   Telephone Number   Telephone Number
                   Relationship   Relationship

FIGURE 16-8 Example of an attractive resumé. Suggestions are given for the display of references.

certificate while you are still in school to avoid taking a typing test under stress.

When you work as a "temp," rather than being isolated in one place, you can have the experience of working in many places and learn a variety of procedures. There is less chance that routine work will become boring or stale. Work schedules are flexible, and if you are called for a job and cannot report that day or week, you are not obliged to take the job. If a business has to cut costs, it tends to use temps rather than hire permanent employees to handle short-term increases in workload. Physicians whose offices are near resort areas could have to handle seasonal peak volumes of work and need temporary help. Temporary firms do not encourage it, but if an employer wants to hire you full time, there can be allowances in the contract for you to accept such a position.

Because medical transcription is a specialized technical position, a temp with medical transcribing skills can often command higher wages than other employees with similar skills. Workers' compensation insurance is provided through temporary agencies, but group health insurance is not. Fringe benefits are likely to be cash bonuses for long or exceptional service or for recruiting other employees to the temporary employment firm. Some firms offer their employees profit-sharing plans and paid vacations. If travel is an objective, you can obtain work through national and international firms and work out of any of their branches.

Your present address
City, State ZIP code
Your telephone number
Date of typing this letter

John Doe, MD or
Personnel Director
Street Address
City, State ZIP code

Dear Dr. Doe:

1st paragraph - Tell how you heard of the position. Tell why you are writing by naming the position, medical transcriptionist.

2nd paragraph - State one or two qualifications you consider to be of greatest interest to the doctor or hospital. Explain why you are interested in his or her practice, location, or type of work. If you have past experience or special training, be sure to mention it.

3rd paragraph - Refer the reader to the resumé or application form enclosed.

4th paragraph - End the letter by asking for an interview and suggesting a date and time or stating that you will call for an appointment. If this letter is to request further information about the job opening, enclose a self-addressed, stamped envelope as a courtesy. The closing statement should not be vague but should give the reader a specific action to take.

Sincerely,

(your handwritten signature)

Type your name

Enclosure

FIGURE 16-9 Example of a cover letter with hints for composition.

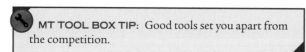

MT TOOL BOX TIP: Good tools set you apart from the competition.

INTERVIEW SKILLS

Prepare for the Interview

To prepare for an interview, find out as much as you can about the job and the organization involved. If the organization has a human resources development department, ask whether you can be permitted to read the job description for the position for which you are applying. Brush up on any technical jargon or terminology associated with the medical specialty of the physician. Be sure to use current document terminology, such as work types, turnaround time, speech recognition, electronic health record, line count, visible black character, and so on. If you visit an office for an application, you could be asked to remain for an interview; therefore, be prepared.

One way to prepare for an interview is by role-playing. You could be interviewed by one person or by a panel of people; therefore, be prepared for either event. Ask yourself questions in front of a mirror so that you will be prepared and will not stumble on the answers (or give a friend a list of questions to ask you). Use a tape recorder and then replay the tape to see how you sounded when you asked yourself the questions. Here are some questions for role-playing that can be of some help. See if you can answer them spontaneously and honestly.

EXAMPLE

Employer: If you are hired, how will you want me to assist you in your work?

Job candidate: I would expect you to help me learn your policies and procedures, and then I'd ask for help if I didn't understand something.

This type of answer would indicate to the employer a job candidate's ability to work independently and a willingness to seek advice when advice is needed.

Other possible questions or requests include the following:

▶ Tell me something about yourself.
▶ What question do you have for me?
▶ What is your major weakness?
▶ Why do you want to work for me? Or for us?
▶ What would really surprise me about you?
▶ What reading material would I find in your home?
▶ Why do you think you would like this job?
▶ What special qualifications do you have that make you feel you will be successful?
▶ What have you done that shows initiative and willingness to work?
▶ How did you earn money while you were going to school?
▶ Tell me a story about being placed in an ethical dilemma and what happened?
▶ How do you spend an 8-hour day?
▶ What is your favorite success story? Failure story?
▶ What salary do you expect?
▶ How did you obtain your last job, and why did you leave it?
▶ What does success mean to you?
▶ What type of person do you like to work for?
▶ How is your health? (Although it is illegal to ask this question, how would you respond to this type of question?)
▶ Share some stories about the two most influential people you know.
▶ What do you plan to be doing five years from now?
▶ Have you any plans to further your education?
▶ What should I have asked you that I haven't?

When you are asked a question, reply in a manner that will bring out your strong points and assets. Do not reply immediately; *think* carefully and be alert to the reply you know the interviewer wants to hear, but be aware of your handicaps and be ready to emphasize your best qualities. For example, if the interviewer notes that your typing speed is not high, you might emphasize that your accuracy is very high (if it is high). If you are short on practical experience, point out your excellent school record. An interview for a job is the one time when you may be completely frank about your qualifications without being considered a boaster or a braggart. Do not sell yourself short or make negative

statements about yourself. Do not discuss personal problems. Be enthusiastic and *ask* for the position if you want it.

Check out the website www.best-interview-strategies.com for additional interview hints.

The Interview

TELEPHONE INTERVIEW

Arrangements can be made to carry out a telephone interview and you need to prepare for this just as carefully as you prepare for a personal interview. Be ready and available when the call is expected. Remember that old truism: You never get a second chance to make a good first impression. Be sure that your children, pets, and other sources of interruptions are out of the house. Ask if you can use your speaker phone so that you can have your hands free, and be sure that no other telephones are capable of ringing through and distracting you. Have your resumé handy to refer to if necessary, even if the interviewer has received a fax or paper resumé from you. Prepare a worksheet on your computer and fill it in with answers to the questions you have prepared. Prepare questions just as you would for a personal interview. Type any pertinent information given by the interviewer. Follow up the interview with a thank you note (discussed following the "Personal Interview" section).

PERSONAL INTERVIEW

Arrive early for the interview to allow time for parking, finding the proper site, relaxing, and catching your breath. Bring a pen, a notepad, and your resumé. Dress carefully for the meeting. Remember all the truisms about "first impressions." Because you do not know the attitude of the interviewer, you should always be correctly attired. Dress appropriately in tailored attire for the occasion. All sorts of studies have been done on suitable dress style and color (Blue, with gray as a runner-up, is what many experts suggest.). Do not smoke or chew gum. Try to eliminate nervous habits, such as thumping your fingers on the table, wringing your hands, or clicking the lid on a pen. Do not take anyone with you to the interview. Be enthusiastic about a job prospect.

> 🔧 **MT TOOL BOX TIP:** You only have one chance to make a good first impression.

Make a checklist of questions on a notepad or on 3 x 5 cards so that you do not forget to ask the interviewer any questions you have about the position. After you are introduced to the interviewer, make a point to remember his or her name, and use the name in your conversation. Look the interviewer in the eye when answering questions; be careful not to avert your eyes. Maintaining eye contact implies sincerity.

Some jobs have fringe benefits about which you could have questions. Here are several pertinent ones. However, be careful not to appear too interested in benefits.

▶ What is the salary? (If the interviewer does not bring up salary, you are entitled to ask what he or she can offer. In general, you should wait with this question until after you have been offered the job.) Find out whether the position pays an hourly wage or pays by line count. Ask what the minimum line count is, how lines are counted, and whether there is a pay differential for lines past the minimum.

▶ Does the firm encourage or provide continuing education for its employees?

▶ Will the employer pay tuition for courses to further skills?

▶ What are the opportunities for advancement?

▶ What types of insurance plans are available? Does this facility contribute to them? Is group health insurance, a pension, or profit sharing available?

▶ What are the starting and quitting times?

▶ Is there an incentive pay program?

▶ Is overtime often required? If so, what is the pay for it?

▶ How long must a person be employed before paid vacation time is available?

▶ Are sick days given?

▶ Does the company have a cafeteria? How much time are employees allowed for lunch or coffee breaks?

▶ What kind of equipment is provided?

▶ How and when can an employee qualify for a raise?

▶ What is the ceiling salary in this job description?

▶ Are there any dress restrictions that employees must observe?

▶ Does the company pay for membership fees in professional organizations?

Many questions are considered discriminatory in a job interview. A prospective employer cannot ask about the following:

▶ Your age

▶ Date of birth

▶ Birthplace

▶ Ethnic background

▶ Religious beliefs

▶ Native language

▶ Maiden name

▶ Marital status

▶ Date of marriage

▶ Whether your spouse is employed

▶ How much your spouse earns

▶ The number of dependent children living with you

▶ An explanation of all the gaps in your employment record (i.e., to find out whether you have taken time off to have children)

▶ Whether you have any physical or emotional disabilities (but an interviewer can ask whether you have any job-related disabilities)

▶ Provision for child care

▶ Club memberships

▶ Height or weight

▶ Credit rating

▶ Home and automobile ownership

▶ Family planning

A question about whether you smoke is not considered discriminatory.

The following are three suggestions for handling an illegal question:

1. Answer the question and ignore the fact that you know it is illegal.

2. Answer with "I think the question is not relevant to the requirements of this position."

3. Refuse to answer and contact the nearest Equal Employment Opportunity Commission office.

If a question is asked about why you left a previous employer and you had some difficulty in that position, you can state "for personal reasons." This answer can then be discussed in further detail if the interviewer wants to know the particulars.

If the job is offered to you at the time of the interview and you are not sure you want it, you could ask, "May I have some time to think it over?" or "How soon do you need to know?" This reply will give you time to think about the job before you commit yourself.

Be prepared to take terminology tests, transcribing tests, and research skills tests. If you are truly a good prospect, you will be able to tell exactly how you would search for a difficult word, know what the outline would include for an operative report (or discharge summary, history and physical examination report, and so on), be able to answer a question about leaving blanks in transcripts, and be able to tell how you are going to fit this job into your schedule (astute interviewers will be able to determine whether they will be hiring the "leftover" you or the committed you). Be prepared to discuss the last book you read and the last movie you saw—right along with verbatim transcription! Be prepared to discuss working odd hours, odd days, and holidays. When asked to tell something about yourself, be sure it is your professional self, which has nothing to do with your children, spouse, pets, politics, religion, and so on. Be sure to keep good eye contact with your interviewer throughout the interview. Do not rush with your answers to questions.

Some interviews are well run, with knowledgeable experts conducting the survey of your skills and deciding whether you will fit into their organization. You will do well because you have come professionally organized. But what if the interviewer is unskilled? How will you be able to sell your abilities in that case? Come prepared for this possibility, and take a more active position in the interview process by asking more questions about the facility, the type of documents produced, the availability of reference materials, production standards, and so on. Use this situation to your advantage.

It is always a good idea to be interviewed by the department or the person with whom you would be working rather than by personnel from the human resources department, who might not appreciate your understanding of the job requirements or might overlook your school background as a fulfillment of their "must have experience" requirements.

Many organizations have test tapes, timed or not, that are evaluated after you transcribe them. A skills assessment (Figure 16-10) is then completed by the evaluator and discussed with you.

Before you leave your interview, be sure you extend your hand and give a firm handshake to your interviewer as you thank him or her for the time.

MEDICAL TRANSCRIPTION SKILLS ASSESSMENT

Name _____ Test Tape No. _____ Date _____

Your test tape transcript was reviewed and scored as follows:

_____ Omitted medical word x 1.00 _____
_____ Omitted major English word x 0.75 _____
_____ Omitted minor English word x 0.25 _____
_____ Flagged omission (blank) x 0.5 _____
_____ Wrong medical word x 1.00 _____
_____ Wrong English word x 0.50 _____
_____ Misspelled medical word x 0.75 _____
_____ Misspelled English word x 0.50 _____
_____ Typographical medical error x 0.75 _____
_____ Typographical English error x 0.50 _____
_____ Grammatical error x 0.50 _____
_____ Punctuation error, major, changing medical
          meaning x 0.50 _____
_____ Punctuation error, minor x 0.25 _____
_____ Capitalization error x 0.25 _____
_____ Formatting error x 0.25 _____
_____ Style error x 0.00 _____

Additional experience or coursework is recommended in these areas:

❑ Cardiology
❑ Pulmonology
❑ Orthopedics
❑ OB-GYN
❑ Urology
❑ Neurology
❑ Psychiatry
❑ Otorhinolaryngology
❑ Gastroenterology
❑ Surgery
❑ Laboratory medicine
❑ EKG terminology
❑ Abbreviations
❑ Grammar/punctuation
❑ Proofreading skills
❑ Auditory discrimination
❑ General medical knowledge

_____ TOTAL ERROR POINTS

TOTAL LINES *(character count divided by 65)* _____ TOTAL ACCURACY SCORE _____

Your score is calculated by taking the total number of error points and dividing by the total number of transcribed lines to arrive at the error quotient. The error quotient is subtracted from 1.00 to arrive at the accuracy score. This score is then multiplied by 100 to obtain your score. A minimum accuracy of 90% is required for clinic transcriptionists, with 95% or higher required for acute-care transcriptionists. Points are not deducted for common style variations. Evaluation criteria is based on a combination of prior medical transcription experience, education, and skills assessment.

Comments

FIGURE 16-10 A medical transcription skills assessment sheet.

Portfolio

When going for an interview, take along a document file or portfolio. A portfolio gives the interviewer the impression that you are organized and serious about getting the job. The portfolio should contain extra copies of your resumé, school diplomas or degrees, certificates, your Social Security card, a timed typing test certified by an instructor, a few select transcripts or work samples showing knowledge of format, an alphabetical notebook of words, letters of recommendation (from former employers, teachers, family physicians, friends who are MTs, or community leaders), names and addresses of references, and anything else related to your prior education and work experience that is relevant to your current job campaign. Place this information in a manila envelope or report folder with a transparent cover. Do not take a notebook filled with transcripts; they are generally ignored and make unnecessary bulk.

After the Interview

Immediately after a telephone or personal interview, write a note to the interviewer thanking him or her for the interview. Restate your interest in the position, and ask for consideration for employment. Show enthusiasm about the prospect of employment with the company. The example in Figure 16-11 provides an idea of how the letter should appear and what it should contain.

Application Forms

If an organization asks you to fill out an application form, ask for two forms in case you spoil one. Read the application form entirely before you begin. Use a pen to complete the form, and follow the directions carefully, such as "Please print," "Complete in your own handwriting," or "Put last name first." Doing so indicates your ability to follow instructions. Copy from your resumé. Copying helps you to be accurate and consistent. Make the form look exceptionally neat. When you leave, this paper could be all that is left in that office to represent you. Complete all the blanks accurately and honestly; if a question does not apply, write in "NA" (not applicable). Attach additional sheets of paper to answer a question completely, rather than trying to squeeze your answer into a tiny space or answering the question incompletely. Be sure to sign the form. When you are done, reread the form all the way through, word for word, to catch possible errors of omission or commission. You do not want to have to explain or apologize during the interview for a mistake. Remember that misrepresentations could be automatic grounds for firing.

If a question appears on an application form regarding salary, a proper answer might be "negotiable" or "flexible" so that salary can be discussed during an interview. You want to avoid overpricing or underpricing yourself. Before the interview, do some research to see whether the salary (when offered) is acceptable.

5747 Grand View Road
Riddell, XX 09876
January 10, 20XX

Antonia B. Scott-Chang, CMT
Director of Personnel
Medical Transcription Department
St. Anne's Hospital and Medical Center
590 River Road
Riddell, XX 09854

Dear Ms. Scott-Chang:

Thank you for the time and encouragement you gave me during my interview for the position at Saint Anne's in your department. You certainly made me eager to work with you and the rest of your staff. It was very exciting to learn that more than half of your transcription is now being done using back-end speech recognition. As I told you in my interview, speech recognition has been a special interest of mine since I began studying for this career.

Please consider me for the trainee position so that I can prove my abilities and perform the work to your satisfaction. I am eager to try.

I hope to hear from you in the near future (800-476-3939).

Sincerely yours,

"RB" Prabhu

FIGURE 16-11 Example of a thank you letter to use as a follow up after an interview.

In negotiating a salary, you could decide to accept a salary that is lower than what you want with an understanding that after a 3- to 6-month period, your work will be evaluated for an increase of pay.

If you are an immigrant or alien, you will need to establish citizenship with a birth certificate or a Social Security card and your identity with a driver's license with a photograph. If you have a document that establishes both identity and authorization to work, take it with you when you apply for a job (i.e., a U.S. passport, a naturalization certificate, an alien registration card ["green card"], a temporary resident receipt card, or an employment authorization card). Employers must conform to the Immigration Reform and Control Act of 1986 and will request documents from you. If they do not, they can be fined, imprisoned, or both for repeated violations.

PROFESSIONALISM

The dictionary defines *professionalism* as the conduct, aims, or qualities that characterize or distinguish a profession. Because professionalism is intangible, it is difficult to put into words, but "you know it when you see it." *Professional* means more than being proficient at medical transcription. Qualities shared by true professionals are having enthusiasm for work, being courteous and dependable, having the right attitude, and being able to get along with others. As a professional, you want to reflect an image and convey a message that you are bright, alert, capable, and top-notch; therefore, look the part. Professionals are confident, honest, and fair in their dealings with others.

An important aspect of professionalism is a willingness to continue learning even after long experience. To keep abreast of new medical terms, techniques, and procedures, consider joining the AHDI and attending local chapter meetings. Participate in the continuing medical education program by becoming certified. Refer to Chapter 1 for details regarding the requirements to become a CMT or an RMT. Categories of membership include active, associate, institutional, and student.

Aim for personal and professional success.

> 🔧 **MT TOOL BOX TIP:** Professionalism—knowing what it means is a helpful tool toward success.

TIPS FOR HOLDING A JOB

Here are some suggestions on how to keep that job once you have landed it:
- Be punctual in reporting for work.
- Report fit and alert; be absent only when absolutely necessary.
- Be well groomed at all times; dress attractively and appropriately.
- Do not criticize your employer. If you do not like where you are working, find another employer.
- If there are job assignments for which you do not particularly care, accept your share of the responsibility for these without complaints. Every job has its good and bad points.
- Stay within the time limit for coffee breaks and lunch period.
- Limit personal telephone calls made or received to those that are absolutely necessary.
- If you are not busy, offer to assist someone else who is.
- Social visits with other employees should occur only after or before working hours.
- Keep your personal problems to yourself.
- Always do the job the boss's way. Later, when your experience and skills are established, your ideas and suggestions will be welcomed, but not in the beginning.
- Keep a learning attitude. Stay flexible and adjust to new changes.

JOB DESCRIPTION

You might be asked to write a job description listing some of the following:
- What do you actually do when working? If you transcribe, how much do you accomplish per day?
- What are the most complex duties that you perform?
- What skills and experience are required? Since you were hired, have your skills improved?
- To what extent, or in what areas, is independent judgment required?
- What are the likelihood and impact of errors? Since you were hired, have your errors diminished in frequency?
- With whom do you interact? Is the interaction positive or negative, compatible or incompatible?
- What physical effort or manual dexterity is required?
- What unusual working conditions exist?
- What supervisory responsibilities are involved?

The employer must also have developed quantity (productivity) standards and quality standards. From the cost-containment standpoint, this practice is important because a document with content, typographical, grammatical, and punctuation errors may be returned for correction. Redoing the report increases production costs. Proofreading the document while it is on the computer screen instead of when it is printed is the most cost-effective way to ensure quality. Your transcripts will be carefully scrutinized during your 90-day probationary period to see whether you measure up to the employer's standards and whether you are meeting the turnaround time. In addition, your supervisor may take into account your independent action, whether your attendance at work was perfect or whether you missed work due to illness, or whether you stayed overtime to transcribe STAT reports without complaints.

HOW TO LEAVE A JOB

After working several years for one employer, some MTs want to change jobs for a different environment. For example, working in a hospital setting is certainly different from working in a physician's office for one or two dictators. Factors beyond your control could arise, such as illness or a spouse's transfer to another location. Before considering a change in employment, consider all aspects of your total compensation and working environment. It is also wise to obtain a new position before leaving your present one and to give at least 2 weeks' notice, depending on your employer's policy. You can complete the form in Box 16-1 to discover your true earnings before you contemplate a move.

If you know of a well-qualified person to take your place, suggest his or her name to your supervisor. This practice will communicate to your employer that you see the situation from his or her point of view. Make it easy for the replacement to step in. No one is indispensable, but some employees want their presence to be missed so much that they destroy any helpful guides for the new employee. You will be thought of more kindly and will leave a good impression if you leave information that might be helpful to the new employee. Clean out your workstation so that someone else does not have to finish the job before he or she moves in. If you do not like your employer, keep the negative thoughts to yourself and do not make derogatory remarks to your peers. Do not neglect any of your responsibilities or skip any last-minute commitments.

Remember to thank your supervisor, employer, or both and those who helped you in some way or made your job easier and more pleasant. Let your supervisor know what you are doing as your career progresses.

BOX 16-1

DIRECT COMPENSATION

Salary	$ _____
Bonuses	_____
Paid vacation	_____
Sick pay and/or compensation for unused days	_____
Incentive compensation	_____
Parental leave	_____

EMPLOYEE BENEFIT PLANS FULLY OR PARTIALLY PAID BY EMPLOYER—INSURED

Medical/dental insurance	_____
Group term life insurance	_____
Additional accidental death and dismemberment _____	
Long-term disability	_____
Workers' compensation insurance	_____
Federal unemployment taxes (FUTA)	_____
State unemployment taxes (SUI) and employee training tax (ETT)	_____

EMPLOYEE BENEFIT PLANS—UNINSURED

Medical reimbursement	_____
Free medical care for employee	_____
Free medical care for family	_____

RETIREMENT CONTRIBUTIONS

Pension plan	_____
Profit-sharing plan	_____
FICA (Social Security)—employer paid	_____

MISCELLANEOUS

Mileage allowance	_____
Continuing medical education (tuition, registration fees, dues)	_____

TOTAL COMPENSATIONS $ _____

Your paths could cross again directly or indirectly. Perhaps he or she will be in a position to recommend you for a job in the future. Keep your record unblemished, because it can take several years to build a reputation. Be courteous. Be thoughtful. Be professional.

16-1 RESUMÉ ASSIGNMENTS

DIRECTIONS: Prepare your resumé by selecting one of the formats shown in the figures in this chapter or a format of your own design. Use the worksheets if this resumé is your first one. Prepare a rough draft first, and let your instructor read through it. Then prepare a final draft after the constructive criticism.

16-2 SELF-STUDY

DIRECTIONS: The following advertisement appeared in your local newspaper. Compose a cover letter to go with your resumé. Refer to Figure 16-5 for guidance in organizing your thoughts.

FULL TIME

Job No.	Description
1311	Medical transcriptionist. Working in medical records. A thorough knowledge of medical terminology with fast, accurate transcribing required and knowledge of Microsoft Word and Internet research. CMT preferred. Excellent incentive pay program and fringe benefits. Send resumé or call Human Resources Dept., St. Anne's Hospital, 4021 Main Street, Middletown, XX 86868, 800-123-4567.

16-3 CAREER ASSIGNMENTS

DIRECTIONS: Type a list of where you could go for temporary jobs in your locale. Then meet at least three people who have a job that you would like. Obtain their names, places of employment, job titles, and any special skills they needed to obtain the job. Type this list and hand it in to your instructor.

16-4 ONLINE JOB APPLICATIONS

DIRECTIONS: Select the website of one of the medical transcription companies. You can find the names either with a web search or the ads that appear in the professional journals. Access the *employment* section, and fill out the application. Some of the companies have you fill out your experience on different work types, choose specialties and shifts, and apply for full- or part-time employment. You could be offered a test and a chance to post your resumé.

16

CHAPTER

APPENDIX 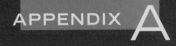 A

Answers to Tests

ANSWERS TO 3-1: SELF-STUDY

Note: Material in parentheses may be included in your answers.

2. **Subject of the sentence:** "I"
   Independent clause: "I appreciate my understanding of medical terminology"
3. **Subject of the sentence:** "You" (this is understood)
   Independent clause: "Please return this to Medical Records (as soon as possible)"
4. **Introductory phrase:** "After spending five hours in the operating room"
   Subject of the sentence: "(the) patient"
   Independent clause: "the patient was sent to the recovery room"
5. **Subject of the sentence:** "(the) patient"
   Independent clause: "The patient is a well-developed, well-nourished black female"
   Second verb clause: "reported that she has been well until this time"
   Appositive: none
   Conjunction: "and"
6. **Subject:** "Joan" and "Beth"
   Independent clause: "Joan and Beth are taking an evening college course in medical ethics"
   Appositive 1: "the emergency department technician"
   Appositive 2: "the admitting clerk"
   Parenthetical expression: none
7. **First subject:** "(the) reception room"
   Independent clause: "The reception room is well lighted and stocked with current literature"
   Second subject: "(the) patients"
   Independent clause: "the patients do not mind their wait to see Dr Jordan"
   Conjunction joining independent clauses: "so"
   Appositive: none
   Nonessential clause: "who never seems to arrive on time"
8. **Independent clause:** "There is overwhelming evidence to prove that the ability to spell is vital to success in this field"
   Parenthetical expression: "however"
   Appositive: none
9. **Subject:** "(the) Association for Healthcare Documentation Integrity"
   Independent clause: "The Association for Healthcare Documentation Integrity has a business and educational meeting every month"
   Appositive: "the national organization for medical transcriptionists"
   Parenthetical expression: none
   Conjunction joining two independent clauses: none

10. **Subject:** "Perfection"
 Verb: "is"
 Independent clause: "Perfection is the key goal in medical transcription skills"
 Appositive: none
 Parenthetical expression: none
 Nonessential phrase: "not speed"
11. **Subject:** "(hospital) transcriptionists"
 Independent clause: This is not a complete sentence; there is no independent clause.
12. **Subject:** the second "you" (understood as occurring just before "please")
 Verb: "have"
 Independent clause: "please have the patient's complete name, address, and telephone number and the admitting diagnosis"
 Nonessential phrase: none
 Introductory clause: "When you telephone the hospital"
 Conjunction joining words in a series: "and"
13. **First independent clause:** "Appointment scheduling requires skill"
 Second independent clause: "it should be a real art"
 Nonessential clause or phrase: "contrary to what you might think" and "and can be"
 Parenthetical expression: "contrary to what you might think"
14. **Independent clause:** "A perfectly typed resume should accompany your letter of application"
 Introductory phrase: none
 Nonessential phrase: "well-planned and prepared"
15. **Independent clause:** "He walks with his heel down (with a varus tendency in the ankle)"
 First dependent group of words: "with no severe problem"
 Second dependent group of words: "with a varus tendency in the ankle"
 Conjunction joining two independent clauses: none
16. **Subject:** "a CBC and sed rate"
 Independent clause: "a CBC and sed rate were carried out today"
 Introductory phrase: "In order to minimize the chance of overlooking a recurrence of infection"
 Nonessential phrase: none

ANSWERS TO 3-2: SELF-STUDY

1. Commas around "your patient." It is a nonessential appositive.
2. Commas after "surgeon" and "opinion." "Whether or not you care for my opinion" is a parenthetical expression.
3. Commas around "not bifocal" to enclose a nonessential expression.
4. Commas around "having been in surgery since two this morning" to enclose a nonessential expression.
5. No commas in this sentence.

ANSWERS TO 3-3: SELF-STUDY

1. No commas are needed; everything here is essential.
2. Place a comma after "prostate." The phrase that follows is nonessential and simply adds further information. This phrase, "one episode of postsurgical hemorrhage," sounds very important. However, if the dictator had wanted to indicate that the information was important (essential), he or she would have dictated it differently. For example, it could have read as follows: "The patient had one episode of postsurgical hemorrhage but otherwise has done well since the transurethral resection of his prostate."
3. Enclose "who is a senior this year" in commas. This phrase is nonessential. "Pat," as a one-word appositive, is not enclosed in commas. Also consider that there could be more than one daughter; the sentence tells us which one.

4. No commas are needed; everything here is essential. The sentence answers the question "*Which* children?"
5. Enclose "Ralph Birch" in commas. It is a nonessential appositive.
6. The phrase "not to operate" is essential and so is not enclosed in commas. It answers the question "*Which* decision?" However, there is a comma after "hasty" to set off "if you ask me," a parenthetical expression.
7. Enclose "which is a photocopy" in commas because it is nonessential.
8. No commas are needed; everything here is essential. The sentence answers the question of *when* to contact the anesthesiologist.
9. Enclose "my textbook" in commas because it is a nonessential appositive.
10. Enclose "Bright disease" in commas because it is a nonessential appositive. How do you know this is an appositive? You consult your dictionary to discover the meaning of any terms you do not know. The position of the words in the sentence will also alert you.
11. Place a comma after "Charles" to set off the nonessential appositive "the new resident."
12. No commas are needed; everything here is essential. The sentence answers the question "*Which* patients?"
13. No commas are needed; everything here is essential.
14. Place a comma in front of "however" to show that it is nonessential. Be sure that you do not enclose "who fail to attend the meeting," because it is essential. You need to know *which* staff members will lose their consulting privileges.
15. Enclose the nonessential "not the pathology department dictation" in commas.
16. Place a comma after "furthermore." It is a parenthetical expression.
17. No commas are needed; "Ethel Clifford" is an essential appositive. You need to know *which* patient because the person being addressed surely has more than one.
18. Place commas around "your patient" because it is a nonessential appositive.
19. No commas are needed; notice the emphasis on "of course."
20. Place a comma after "immediately." The placement and tone of the sentence should help.

ANSWERS TO 3-4: SELF-STUDY

1. Place a comma after "time." This is an introductory phrase.
2. No comma is necessary. Be careful not to separate the subject from the verb by placing a comma after *promotion*. Be alert when you consider placing a comma in front of a verb.
3. Place a comma after "tomorrow." This is an introductory phrase. (The subject, "you," is understood.)
4. Place a comma after "seen." This is an introductory phrase. This phrase is brief, and one might consider omitting the comma; however, the comma does assist the reader and should be included.
5. No comma is necessary. Be careful not to separate the subject from the verb by placing a comma after "billing."
6. Enclose "whom I hired yesterday" in commas. This phrase is nonessential.
7. No comma is necessary. A comma is not needed after "recently," an introductory adverb.

ANSWERS TO 3-5: SELF-STUDY

1. No commas are necessary. Everything is essential, and there is no introductory phrase.
2. No commas are necessary. Everything is essential, and there is no introductory phrase.
3. Enclose the nonessential appositive, "the pathologist," in commas.
4. Enclose the nonessential appositive, "a girl," in commas. Notice that if the sentence read, "The delivery of the baby girl was uneventful," the sentence would have no appositive and thus no comma.
5. Place a comma after "furthermore," a parenthetical expression. The word *furthermore* also serves as a transitional word from whatever was said in a previous sentence.
6. Place a comma after "anesthesia," the final word of an introductory phrase.
7. Place a comma after "safe," the final word of an introductory phrase.
8. It is optional to place a comma after "lunch," the final word of a short introductory phrase. A comma is not really needed with this brief phrase.

9. Place a comma after "home," the final word of an introductory phrase.
10. No commas are necessary. Everything is essential, and there is no introductory phrase. Do not separate the subject from the verb by placing a comma after "word."

ANSWERS TO 3-6: SELF-STUDY

1. "The patient was first seen in my office on Wednesday, July 14, 20XX." *Separate all parts of a complete date.*
2. "Please send this to Natalie Jayne, RN, Chief of Nurses, Glorietta Bay Hospital." *Separate degrees and titles following a person's name.*
3. "Carl A. Nichols Jr was admitted to Ward B." *No comma is used before Jr or Sr unless the user prefers it.*
4. "The blood test included a white blood count, red blood count, hematocrit, and differential." *Separate words in a series. The comma after "hematocrit" is optional.*
5. "There is a history of a mild head injury at age 10, and she was in a moderately severe motorcycle accident about 15 years ago." *Separate two independent clauses with a comma before the conjunction.*
6. "The condition is now stationary and permanent, and he should be able to resume his normal work load." *Separate two independent clauses with a comma before the conjunction.*
7. "She was fully dilated at 2:30 a.m. but did not deliver the second twin until 2:55 a.m." *No comma is necessary, because the second clause is dependent.*
8. "He denies any visual problem, but he uses glasses." *Separate two independent clauses with a comma before the conjunction.*

ANSWERS TO 3-7: SELF-STUDY

1. Rule i. Comma after "time"; some experts would label it optional.
2. Rule i. Comma after "well"; some experts would label it optional.
3. Rule d. Comma after "week."
4. There are no commas in this sentence.
5. Rule i. Comma after "Hospital."
6. There are no commas.
7. Rules g and j. Commas around "MD" and around "Arizona."
8. Rule e. Commas around "2006."
9. Rule f. Optional comma after "Group"; you would have to check with the organization to be sure.
10. Rules d and h. Commas after "examination" and "well-developed."

    Note: There is no comma between *well-nourished* and *white,* the last modifier in the set.

11. Rule h. Comma after "effort" and "breath." (The second comma is optional.)
12. Rules a and e. Commas around "with your concurrence" and "July 1" and a comma after "20XX."
13. Rule d. Comma after "Jones." Note: No comma after "this," because it is the first part of the introductory phrase.
14. Rules a or d, g, b. Commas after "know" and "Briggs" and around "MD" and "partner."
15. Rules e and a. Notice that the expression *which required intravenous antibiotics* simply adds information and does not qualify as being essential. Commas around "20XX" and a comma after "bronchopneumonia."

ANSWER TO 3-8: PRACTICE TEST

September 16, 20XX

Tellememer Insurance Company
25 Main Street, Suite R
Albuquerque, NM 87122

Dear Sir or Madam:

Re: Ron Emerson

I understand from Mr Emerson that the insurance company feels that the charges for my services on June 30, 20XX, are excessive.

Mr Emerson was seen on an early Sunday morning with a stab wound to his chest, which had penetrated his lung, producing an air leak into his chest wall. In addition, he had a laceration of his lung.

After consultation and a review of his x-rays, his laceration was repaired. He was observed in the hospital for 2 days to be sure that he did not have continuing hemorrhage or collapse of his lung.

I feel that the bill given to Mr. Emerson is a fair one. We received on July 31, 20XX, a Tellememer Insurance Company check for $200, and I feel that your payment of $200 is unreasonable. It is doubtful that one could get a plumber to come out early Sunday morning to fix a leaky pipe for $200, and Mr. Emerson's situation, in my opinion, was much more serious than would be encountered by a plumber.

We will bill Mr. Emerson for the remainder $680 balance on his account, but I want you to know that we feel that your payment is insufficient. If he feels that the bill is excessive, we would be glad to submit to arbitration through the County Medical Society Fee Committee. If this fails, I suggest we seek help through the New Mexico Insurance Commission.

Sincerely yours,

William A. Berry, MD

mlo

Enclosed: X-ray report; history and physical report

Copy: Mr. Ron Emerson

ANSWERS TO 3-10: SELF-STUDY

1. Insert periods after the "E" and the "m" at the end of the sentence and optional periods after the "Mr" and the "p." Place a colon between the "4" and the "30."
2. Insert an optional period after "Dr" and a semicolon after "Board." (Periods are not required with MD.) Do not place a period after "Board," which would make two sentences.
3. A period after "Jr" serves both to close the sentence and to punctuate the abbreviation. This is a polite question, and so no question mark is required.
4. A colon is placed after "16" and after "Caution."

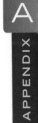

5. A period after "2110" closes the sentence. No punctuation mark used with military time of day. You may add the word "hours" after military time (e.g., "2110 hours").
6. Insert a colon after "problems."
7. A period after "insurance" closes the sentence. No decimal point is needed with the $85.
8. Insert a colon after "General," and a period after "cooperative" to close the sentence.
9. Insert a period after "Good"; no colon is required after "Discharge," but it is not incorrect if it is added.

ANSWERS TO 3-11: SELF-STUDY

1. Rule d. Semicolon after "yet."
2. Rules a and c. Optional period after "Mr" and semicolon after "disease."
3. Rules g and b. Colon after "follows" and decimal point after "$650."
4. Rules g, a, and f. Colon after "staff"; periods after "Dr," "Jr," and "Mrs" period after "A" and "R"; and semicolons after "resident," "director," and "supervisor."
5. Rule h. Colon after "man." (You can't use a semicolon because it is too weak and ignores the invitation in the first clause concerning the "one fact."
6. Rules b and e. Decimal point after "101"; semicolon after "nausea."
7. Rule b. Decimal point after the zero, so that the percentage reads "0.5%."
8. Rule c. Semicolon after "normal."
9. Rule e. Semicolon after "normal." Optional period after Dr.
10. Rule i. Colons after "diagnosis" and "discharge."

ANSWERS TO 3-12: SELF-STUDY

1. Her favorite response is "We've always done it this way."
2. It was an ill-defined tumor mass.
3. The diagnosis is grim—I feel helpless.
4. Her temperature peaked at 106.5 degrees (we were relieved when this occurred), and the seizures subsided. *(Notice that you need to place a comma outside of the parentheses after "occurred.")*
5. There were no 4 × 4s left in the box.
6. Because of his condition (emphysema) and age (88), he is a poor risk for anesthesia at this time.
7. Eighty-five of the patients were seen first in the outpatient department.
8. The patient with the self-inflicted gunshot wound had a poorly applied bandage.
9. The blood pressure ranged from 120/80 to 140/80.
10. This is a very up-to-date drug reference.

ANSWERS TO 3-13: SELF-STUDY

1. Mrs Gail R. Smith-Edwards was hospitalized this morning. She is the 47-year-old woman Dr Blank admitted with a self-inflicted knife wound. Her blood pressure was 60/40. *(Sixty over forty)*
   Rules <u>c and a, *or* b, a, and j. Either set would be correct.</u>

2. Barbara Ness's happy-go-lucky personality was missed when she was transferred from the medical records department.
   Rules <u>e and a, optional h (quotation marks around "happy-go-lucky")</u>

3. Glen Mathews, the well-known trial lawyer, and the hospital's surgeon-in-chief, Dr Carlton Edwards, will appear together (if you can believe that) on TV's latest talk show tonight. It's the only subject on the hospital's "gabfest." *(Note: Make sure your period is placed within the quotation marks.)*
   Rules <u>a, e, c, i, e, f, e, and h</u>

4. I want a stamped, self-addressed envelope enclosed with this letter and sent out with today's mail.
   Rules <u>a and e</u>

5. Dr Davis said his promotion was a good example of "my being kicked upstairs." He obviously didn't want to leave his position in the x-ray department. *(Note: Make sure your period is placed within the quotes.)*
Rules <u>h, f, and b</u>

6. Haven't you ever seen a Z-fixation? Bobbi-Jo will be happy to explain it to you. (*Note:* Do not worry if you overlooked the hyphen in *Bobbi-Jo.* You could not be expected to know that unless you were familiar with her name.)
Rules <u>f, b, and c</u>

7. We're all going to the CCU at 4 o'clock for instructions on mouth-to-mouth resuscitation.
Rules <u>f, f, and a</u>

8. Right eye vision: 20/20.
Left eye vision: 10/400.
Right retinal examination: Normal.
Left retinal examination: Inferior retinal detachment.
Rule <u>j</u>

9. You were seen on September 24 at which time you were having some stiffness at the shoulders, which I felt was due to a periarthritis (a stiffness of the shoulder capsule); however, x-ray of the shoulder was negative. *(Notice that commas would not be a good substitute for the parentheses because of the semicolon needed before however.)*
Rules <u>i and b</u>

10. After he completed the end-to-end anastomosis, he closed with #1 silk through-and-through, figure-of-eight sutures.
Rules <u>a, a, and a</u>

11. Dr Chriswell's diagnosis bears out the assumption that the red-green blindness is the result of an X-chromosome defect. *(Assuming that the examiner's name is Chriswell. If it is Chriswells, then it would be punctuated "Chriswells'.")*
Rules <u>e, a or d, and b</u>

12. After his myocardial infarction (MI), his blood test showed high levels of C-reactive protein.
Rules <u>i and b</u>

ANSWERS TO 3-14: SELF-STUDY

1. Dr Younger couldn't find the curved-on-flat scissors; therefore, "all heck broke loose." *(It would also be correct to just place "heck" in quotation marks.)*
2. The patient's admission time is 3:30 p.m. When he comes in, please call me for a face-to-face confrontation with him about his visitors.
3. This 68-year-old, right-handed, Caucasian retired female telephone operator was well until mid-February. While sitting in a chair after dinner, she had the following symptoms: paralysis of her left arm and left leg, paresthesia in the same distribution, bilateral visual blurring, and some facial numbness.
4. The patient was admitted to the ward at one o'clock in the morning screaming "All's fair in love and lust"; the attending physician sedated him with Thorazine 600 mg/d.
5. The following describes a well-prepared business letter: neat, accurate, well-placed, correctly punctuated, and mechanically perfect. The dictator expects to see an attractive letter with no obvious corrections, smudges, or unevenly inked letters. It is an insult, in my opinion, to place a letter that appears other than described on your employer's desk for signature

ANSWERS TO CHAPTER 3: LET'S HAVE A BIT OF FUN

1. b
2. b
3. a
4. b
5. a
6. b
7. b
8. Both
9. a
10. b
11. b

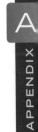

ANSWERS TO 4-1: SELF-STUDY

1. After I finish Medical Transcription 214, I will take a class in medical insurance billing. I want to get a job with Goodwin-Macy Medical Group.
2. All the patients were reminded that the office will be closed on Labor Day, Monday, September 7.
3. Dr Albert K. Shaw's address is One West Seventh Avenue, Detroit, Michigan.
4. Two of the commonly sexually transmitted pathogens are Chlamydia trachomatis and Neisseria gonorrhoeae.
5. It was Mr Geoffry R. Leslie, vice president of Medical Products, Inc., who returned your call.
6. The University Hospital rotation schedule has been posted, and I am assigned to the Emergency Department and you report to Cardiology. (*Specific departments in a teaching hospital.*)
7. Patsy, who works in the Valley View Medical Center, is studying to become a certified medical transcriptionist.
8. The Dorcus Travel Bureau arranged Dr Berry's itinerary through New England last fall.
9. Keep this in mind: Accuracy is more important than speed.
10. The following are my recommendations:
    1. Continuing treatment through the Spinal Defects Clinic.
    2. Evaluations at 2-month intervals during the first year of life.
    3. Physical therapy reevaluation at 6 months of age.
11. The patient has four siblings, all living and well; his mother died of heart disease at age 45 and his father of an automobile accident when he was 24; there is no history of familial disease.
12. We expect Judge Willard Frick to arrive from his home on the Pacific Coast for the Memorial Day weekend.
13. I find *Current Medical Terminology* by Vera Pyle, CMT, to be an excellent reference book for the transcribing station in the Department of Internal Medicine.
14. My uncle, Sam, is a thoracic surgeon in Houston.
15. Mr Billingsgate wrote to say that he had moved to 138 Old Highway Eight, Space 14.
16. We are waiting for confirmation of the diagnosis from the Centers for Disease Control and Prevention; it could be Four Corners virus.
17. Whenever she takes perocet, she develops psychosis and was actually committed to a psych ward after taking it.
18. There is a recent study demonstrating increased benefit of adding bevacizumab (Avastin) monoclonal antibody to the carboplatin and Taxol regimen.

ANSWERS TO 4-2: SELF-STUDY

1. The Right Rev. Michael T. Squires led the invocation at the graduation ceremony for Greenlee County's first paramedic class.
2. Nanci Holloway, a 38-year-old Caucasian female, is scheduled for a cesarean section tomorrow.
3. The internist wanted him to have meprobamate, so he wrote a prescription for Miltown.
4. Johnny Temple had chickenpox, red measles, and German measles his first year in school.
5. I understand that Bob, our p.m. shift MT, is proficient in American Sign Language.
6. The pathology report showed a class IV malignancy on the Pap smear.
7. Some patients have been very sick with Kaposi sarcoma, the rare and usually mild skin cancer that seems to turn fierce with AIDS victims.
8. The Mustard procedure is often used to reroute venous return in the atria.
9. The young man was an alert, asthenic, Indochinese male who was well-oriented to time and place.
10. The gynecologist wrote a prescription for Flagyl for the patient with Trichomonas vaginalis.
11. He was stationed at the Naval Training Center before deployment to the Gulf.
12. Dr Collier recommended a combination of gentamicin and a penicillin, such as Bicillin, for our patient with endocarditis.
13. Barbara, our LPN, is the new membership chairman for the local NOW chapter; she asked me to join.
14. The OD victim was brought to the ER by his roommate.
15. Her right Achilles tendon reflex is +1 compared to the left.
16. She is to begin her first GLAC chemotherapy on June the first.
17. He received an injection of CroFab in the ED after being bitten by a rattlesnake.

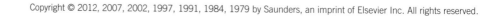

18. The incision was dressed with <u>A</u>daptic, dry gauze, sterile <u>W</u>ebril, and a modified <u>J</u>ones dressing.
19. <u>W</u>e will hold the propranolol, lisinopril, and hydrochlorothiazide, as the patient is on a <u>C</u>ardizem <u>L</u>yo-<u>J</u>ect.
20. <u>P</u>ain management: <u>T</u>ylenol 650 mg p.o. q6 h p.r.n. pain.

ANSWER TO 4-3: SELF-STUDY

<u>FAX</u>   212.555.1247   William A. Berry, MD   <u>Telephone</u> 212.555.0124
3933 Navajo Road
GrandView, XX 00983

1   May 17, 20XX

2   Barbara H. Baker, MD
3   624 South Polk Drive
4   Boothbay Harbor, ME 04538

5   Dear Dr Baker:

6   Re: Mrs Brenda Woodman

7   At the request of Dr Thomas Brothwell, I saw his patient in the office today.
8   He, apparently, felt that her thyroid was enlarged.

9   She stated that she is on Dyflex-G 1/2 tablet q.i.d., SSKI drops 10 t.i.d., Brethine
10   2.5 mg b.i.d., and prednisone 10 mg. She has had asthma for 12 years and,
11   other than a T&A in childhood, has never been hospitalized.

12   On physical examination, her thyroid was 2+ enlarged, especially in the lower
13   lobes, and smooth. The heart was in regular sinus rhythm of 110, and she had
14   findings of moderate bronchial asthma at this time. On pelvic examination, she
15   had a virginal introitus and a moderate senile vaginitis. She had Heberden
16   nodes on the fingers, and vibration sense was decreased by about 25
17   seconds.

18   The laboratory tests, a copy of which is enclosed, showed a normal thyroid
19   function. The urinalysis was negative; and the electrocardiogram, a copy of
20   which is enclosed also, showed some nonspecific ST- and T-wave changes
21   and some positional change, suggestive of pulmonary disease.

22   In summary: I do not feel that the lady has hyperthyroidism but simply an
23   enlarged thyroid due to the prolonged iodide intake.

24   It was my pleasure to see your sister in the office, and I hope that the above
25   findings will reassure her family in the Northeast.

26   Sincerely,

27   William A. Berry, MD

28   ir

29   enclosures

30   cc: Thomas B. Brothwell, MD

ANSWERS TO 5-1: SELF-STUDY

1. The wound was closed in layers with *2-0* and *3-0* black silk sutures.
2. The *3-month-premature* infant was delivered by cesarean section. *(Note hyphens.)*
3. He is a *24-year-old* black male with an admitting blood pressure of *180/100*. *(Note hyphens and slash.)*
4. Paresis is noted in *four-fifths* of the left leg.
5. It was then suture ligated with chromic *#1* catgut sutures. *("No. 1" also correct.)*
6. There were multiple subserous fibroids ranging in size from *0.5* to *2.5 cm* in diameter.
7. There are a *thousand* reasons why I wanted to be a doctor; but at *3 a.m.*, after I have been awakened from a deep sleep, it is hard to think of any. *(Check your commas and semicolon too; capital "AM" also correct.)*
8. My charge for the procedure is *$750*, and the median fee in the community is *$800*. *(Not "$750.00" and "$800.00"; "750 dollars" is also incorrect.)*
9. The patient received *4* units of blood.
10. The bullet traveled through the pelvic plexus into the spinal cord, shattering *S2, S3,* and *S4*. *("S_2, S_3, and S_4" is also correct.)*

ANSWERS TO 5-2: PRACTICE TEST

1. On *September 26, 2010*, she had a left lower lobectomy.
2. Two sutures of *3-0* cotton were placed so as to obliterate the posterior *cul-de-sac*. *(Notice hyphens in the expression "cul-de-sac.")*
3. He smoked *1-1/2* packs of cigarettes a day. *(Leave out the word "and.")*
4. There was a small splinter of glass recovered from just to the right of the iris in the *4 o'clock* area.
5. The resting blood pressure is *76/40*.
6. Please mail this to *Dr Ralph Lavton* at *10 Dublin Street, Bowling Green, Ohio 43402*. *("Ten Dublin Street" is also correct.)*
7. We had *7* admissions *Saturday, 24 Sunday,* and 3 this morning. *(See Rule 5.11; "a.m." is used only with the time of day.)*
8. In the accident, the spine was severed between *C4-5*. *("C_{4-5}" also correct; "C4 and C5" also correct.)*
9. The child was first seen by me in the *Esther Levy Imaging Center* on the evening of *May 11, 2006*. *(Military or European dating is not used in narrative copy except in military documents prepared in the military service.)*
10. I recommend a course of *cobalt-60* radiation therapy. *(Notice the hyphen.)*

ANSWERS TO 5-3: SELF-STUDY

1. Unfortunately, the last biopsy revealed that his carcinoma has changed from a *class I* to a *class III* malignancy.
2. Bleeding was controlled with *2-0* ties.
3. There are well-healed incisions beneath each areolar border from 3 to 9 o'clock.
4. The doctor's callback time is every day at *4 o'clock*. *("Four o'clock" also correct.)*
5. I was called to the *ER* at *three* in the morning, where I performed an emergency tracheotomy on a *4-day-old* male infant. I remained in attendance for *two* hours to be sure he was out of danger. *("2 hours" also correct.)*
6. He came in for a *class III* flight physical. *(A dictator may prefer a capital letter for "Class.")*
7. He has passed the *5-year* mark without any evidence of a recurrence.
8. He has a *grade II* hip dysplasia.
9. The patient had respiratory paralysis due to injury of spinal nerves *C3 through C5*. *("C3-C5" not correct.)*
10. This is her *fourth* admittance this year. *("4th" also correct.)*

ANSWERS TO 5-4: PRACTICE TEST

1. *We must watch Mrs Olsen carefully because she has two stage III decubitus ulcers on her dorsal spine and one stage II on her right heel.*
2. *She was a gravida 6 para 4-1-1-4.*

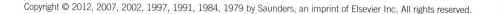

3. *I* can see only *15-20* patients a *day. ("15 to 20" also correct. See Rule 5.10.)*
4. *Please* order *12 two-gauge* needles. *("Twelve 2-gauge" also correct.)*
5. *Use* only *one-eighth* teaspoonful. *(Notice the hyphen; see Rule 5.5. "1/8 teaspoonful" also correct.)*
6. *The* dorsalis pedis pulses were *2+* and equal *bilaterally.*
7. *The* ear was injected with *2% Xylocaine* and *1:6000 Adrenalin.*
8. *Please* check the reading in V_4 again. *("V4" also correct.)*
9. *At* precisely *0730 hours,* she delivered a *3400 g* infant with *Apgar* scores of *9* at *one* minute and *9* at *five minutes.* *(This two-number combination of Apgar scores, evaluation of newborns at one and five minutes after birth, is written in this manner.)*
10. *Please* recheck those *ECG* limb lead readings from lead *I* and lead *II.*

ANSWERS TO 5-6: SELF-STUDY

1. Flexion was limited to *15°,* extension to *10°,* adduction to *10°,* and abduction to *20°. ("Degrees" can also be written out: e.g., "15 degrees.")*
2. By use of a *half-inch* osteotome, *1 cm* of the proximal end of the proximal phalanx was removed.
3. DTRs are *1 to 2+. (Do not use a hyphen when there is a plus-or-minus sign with the number.)*
4. Range of motion of the neck is limited to approximately *70%* of normal. *("70 percent" also correct only if your equipment will not print the percent symbol.)*
5. The date on the cholecystogram was *September 1, 2009.*
6. Estimated blood loss was *100 mL;* none was replaced. *(Note semicolon; see Table 5-1.)*
7. At *2 a.m.,* the patient's temperature was *38.9°C. ("38.9 degrees Celsius" and capital "AM" also correct.)*
8. The *PA* and right lateral roentgenograms show a fracture of the right *3rd* and *4th* ribs. *("Third" and "fourth" also correct.)*
9. Lenses were prescribed, resulting in improvement of his visual acuity to *20/30* in the right eye and *20/45* in the left eye. The visual field examination was normal, and the tension is *17 mmHg* of Schiotz with a *5.5-g* weight. *("17 mm Hg" also correct. Note: The medical office and ED might use the right eye and left eye abbreviations in that sentence so the phrase would appear as follows: "20/30 OD and 20/45 OS.")*
10. She has one sister who is *living and well. (Avoid "L&W" except in chart notes or family history part of a history and physical examination.)*
11. I removed *600 mL* of serosanguineous fluid from the abdomen.
12. We need to use *35 mm* film for this process.

ANSWERS TO 5-7: PRACTICE TEST

1. *Hemoglobin* on *July 27* was *11.2 g;* hematocrit was *37. ("Hb" would be incorrect; "7–27" or "7/27" would be incorrect; and "hct" would be incorrect.)*
2. Did you know that the postal rates were 25 cents for the first ounce and 20 cents for each additional ounce to mail something first class in 1989? *(Not "25¢" and not "oz." "First Class" is, however, also correct.)*
3. The protein was 65 mg%. *(Notice the closed-up spacing of this symbol.)*
4. Electromyography shows a 3+ sparsity in the orbicularis oris.
5. An estimated 0.2 mL of viscid fluid was removed from the middle ear cavity. *(Notice the zero in front of the decimal point.)*
6. He entered the ER at 4 a.m. with a temperature of 99. *("AM" and "99°" are also correct.)*
7. There was a reduction of the angle to within a 2-degree difference.
8. Take 50 mg/day. *("50 mg per day" is also correct.)*
9. I then placed two 4 × 4 sponges over the wound.
10. The TB skin test was diluted 1:100.
11. Drainage amounts to several milliliters a day.
12. He is to take flurazepam HCl 30 mg at bedtime. *(Be sure to change the abbreviation "h.s." to "bedtime." This appears in Table 5.1)*

ANSWERS TO 5-8: SELF-STUDY

1. The urine was negative for sugar, *pH* was *7.0,* and specific gravity was *1.012.*
2. The *BUN* is *45 mg%, 1+* protein.
3. I excised a small, well-circumscribed tumor, *2 mm* in diameter.
4. Use a *3M Vi-Drape* to cover the operative site. *("3-M" might be how you typed it, but this company does not print it that way. "Vi-Drape" is a brand name that you now know. Always expect that words of this sort that are not in the dictionary are brand names. The letter after the hyphen in a brand name is generally capitalized.)*
5. She received her *second dose of 5-FU.* *("2ⁿᵈ dose" also acceptable.)*
6. The culture grew *100,000* colonies of *E. Coli* per milliliter. *(Be sure to change "cubic centimeter" ("cc") to "milliliter" as directed in Table 5-1. Also notice that you do not abbreviate "milliliter" because the term is not used with a number.)*
7. The surgeon asked for a *#7 Jackson* bronchoscope. *("No. 7" also correct.)*
8. There were high serum titers of *IgG* antibodies.
9. The phenotype A_2B was found consistently in the family blood history. *("A2B" also correct.)*
10. Respirations: *16/min.* *("16 per minute" also correct; do not forget to check your punctuation.)*

ANSWERS TO 6-3: SELF-STUDY

1. Notice that paragraph 1 is only one sentence long. What does the dictator do with this sentence? *She introduces the patient with his age, problem, and date first seen.* (Notice that the reference line is the only place that the patient's name is mentioned.)
2. Notice that paragraph 2 is three sentences long. Could the first of these sentences have been placed in the first paragraph? *Yes.* Why or why not? *The other sentences would need to go along with it, however, because they are part of the history of the patient. It is better as it stands.* (This final statement clarifies that *no* is the better answer.)
3. What is the dictator *doing* in paragraph 2? *Giving a brief past history.*
4. Could any part of paragraph 3 logically be part of the second or fourth paragraph? *No.* Why or why not? *This is a definite change from past to present.*
5. What is the author *doing* in paragraph 3? *Giving the physical evidence of the patient's problem.*
6. Again, we have a one-sentence paragraph in paragraph 4. Could the transcriptionist have joined this sentence to paragraph 3? *Yes, but there is nothing wrong with one-line paragraphs.*
7. What did the author *do* in this paragraph? *She explained how she handled the patient's problem.*
8. What is the subject of paragraph 5? *The prognosis (what the expected outcome will be).* Could this paragraph be joined to paragraph 4? *No.* Why or why not? *Because there is a definite shift from "treatment" to "prognosis." It would weaken the impact of each paragraph.*
9. Notice the last line of paragraph 5. Could this have been a paragraph on its own? *Yes.* Why or why not? *It could have stood alone because it is the "plan" to be followed in the treatment program; however, because there are so many brief paragraphs, it is fine where it is.* Could you make it a part of the last paragraph? *Yes.* Why or why not? *It could be done, but there is no reason for it. Actually, doing so would weaken the final paragraph.* Why or why not? *It will weaken the final paragraph. Leave it alone.*
10. What is the dictator doing in the final paragraph? *Saying thank you, which is standard protocol and acknowledges that the recipient of the letter is the patient's primary physician.* Do you think it is appropriate to have this single sentence standing as an entire paragraph? *Yes.* Why or why not? *It provides impact.*

Note: Your words do not have to match the answers exactly, but the ideas expressed should be the same or similar.

ANSWERS TO 6-4: SELF-STUDY

1. Paragraph 1 tells us the type of document this is. What is it? *A final followup letter.*
2. Paragraph 1: What is the subject(s) of this paragraph? *An introduction of the patient about whom the letter is written and a reminder about what has transpired with her. We could call this her "immediate history."*

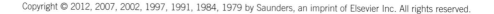

3. Paragraph 2: What is the dictator *doing* in this paragraph? *Stating the patient's present status and proposed plan of treatment.* Could the last two sentences of this paragraph be used to form a new paragraph? *Yes.* Why or why not? *Because it indicates a new subject: the proposed plan. However, that would lead to three very short paragraphs in a row, which is somewhat unattractive. One must think of appearance as well as content when it is possible to do so. (Therefore, "no" would be the better answer.)*

4. Paragraph 3. What is the author saying in this paragraph? *What his involvement with the patient is now.* Could this one have been combined with the last two sentences of paragraph 2? *Yes.* Why or why not? *This would be appropriate because it all pertains to plans for the patient's future care. (Note that the medical transcriptionist's choice here is probably best as a result of the strong opening of paragraph 3: "We will not follow Nora. . . .")*

5. Paragraph 4. What is the subject of this paragraph? *A brief thank-you and close.* Should this be arranged as two short paragraphs? *No. That would not be appropriate.*

Notice that the dictator refers to this patient by name often but, when he does, uses only her first name. This is evidently his solution to avoiding identification of the patient outside of the reference line.

ANSWERS TO 6-6: TYPING PRACTICE TEST

JON L. MIKOSAN, MD
6244 APPLEGATE ROAD
MILWAUKEE, WI 53209
555-234-5678

May 1, 20XX

Ian R. Wing, MD
2261 Arizona Avenue, Suite B
Milwaukee, WI 53207

RE: Mrs Elvira Martinez   (1)

Dear Dr Wing

   I saw your patient Mrs Elvira Martinez in consultation in my office today. She brought the x-rays from your office with her. She was afebrile today but, on questioning, admitted a low-grade fever over the past few days.   (2)

   I removed the fluid, as seen on your film of April 30, from the right lower lung field, and she felt considerably more comfortable. On thoracentesis, there was 50 mL of straw-colored fluid. I am enclosing a copy of the pathology report on the fluid; as you can see, it is negative.   (3)

   Her history is well known to you, so I will not repeat it.   (4)

   On physical examination, I found a well-developed, well-nourished white female with minimal dyspnea. There was no lymphadenopathy. Breath sounds were diminished somewhat on the right; there was dullness at the right base; the left lung was clear to percussion and auscultation. The remainder of the examination was negative.   (5)

   Because of her history of chronic asthma, I suggested she might consider bronchoscopy if this fluid reaccumulates. Because she is a heavy smoker, I insisted she stop smoking completely. If she does not, she will not enjoy continuing good health (although I have no idea of the actual prognosis).   (6)

   Your patient has been returned to you for her continuing care. I will be glad to see her again at any time you think it necessary.   (7)

   Thank you for letting me see this pleasant lady with you.

Sincerely yours,

Jon L. Mikosan, MD

your initials

Enclosure: Pathology report   (8)

ANSWERS TO 7-1: SELF-STUDY

1. <u>sense</u>; *since*
2. <u>naproxyn 4</u>; *Naprosyn/for*
3. <u>Thoracic Surgeon</u>; *thoracic surgeon/<u>setting</u>; sitting/<u>1</u>; one*
4. <u>Paramedics</u>; *paramedics/<u>hospital</u>; Hospital*
5. <u>back</u> *(omit this word)*
6. <u>last year</u>; *20XX (the year date for last year)*
7. <u>patients</u>; *patient's/<u>to read</u>; reading*
8. <u>X-rays</u>; *x-rays/<u>red</u>; read*
9. <u>and ability</u>; *instability*
10. <u>extra ocular</u>; *extraocular (one word)*
11. <u>mad as hell</u>; *very angry; very upset; "mad as heck"; "mad as hell" (Insert the quotation marks for the last two options.)*
12. C (No errors)
13. <u>out</u>; *about (Unless, of course, she has been accused of stealing.)*
14. <u>lady</u>; *leg (Did you notice how easy it was to read "right leg" even with the wrong word there?)*
15. <u>absent</u>; *abstinent*
16. <u>swallowing tires</u>; *swallowing, tires easily (Note comma after "swallowing.")*
17. <u>on changed</u>; *unchanged*
18. <u>for</u>; *with*
19. <u>numb and swollen</u>; *numbness and swelling*
20. <u>H. flu</u>; *H. influenzae; Haemophilus influenzae*
21. C (No errors)
22. <u>Patient has chest pain if she lies on her left side for over a year</u>; *For over a year, the patient has had chest pain if she lies on her left side. (Reword the whole sentence.)*
23. <u>is edentulous, and the teeth are in poor repair</u> *(Check the medical record to see whether the patient is edentulous or the teeth are in poor repair; both conditions cannot exist simultaneously.)*
24. <u>primip whose</u>; *primipara, who is*
25. <u>Sings</u>; *Signs (If you had not been looking for this, would you have seen it?)*
26. <u>is</u>; *was*
27. <u>4-0</u>; *Number 4-0 (Do not begin a sentence with a number. You can also recast the entire sentence to read as follows: "The skin edges of both incisions were secured and reapproximated with 4-0 plain chromic catgut.")*
28. <u>in tact</u>; *intact*
29. <u>in total</u>; *in toto*
30. <u>When three weeks old, his mother first noticed he was not responding to loud noises</u>; *"His mother first noticed that he was not responding to loud noises when he was 3 weeks old" or "When he was 3 weeks old, his mother noticed that he was not responding to loud noises."*

ANSWER TO 7-2: SELF-STUDY

At cystoscopy, there were multiple urethral polyps, small in caliber, and an irritated bladder neck. The urethral orifices were normal, and the remainder of the bladder wall was not remarkable. I will have to presume that the bleeding is coming from the urethral polyps. I do not think this accounts for all of this woman's symptoms, however.

I am returning her to your care and will follow her along for a while to see what we can do about the hematuria.

ANSWER TO 7-3: SELF-STUDY

PATRICK D. QUINN, MD
FAMILY PRACTICE
555 LAKE VIEW DRIVE
BAY VILLAGE, OHIO 44140
(216) 871-4701

July 17, 20XX

T. J. Thompson, Insurance Analyst
Northern Ohio Gas and Electric Company
Post Office Box 1831
Bay Village, OH 44140

Dear Sir:

Re: Richard Wright

Mr Richard Wright was seen in my office on July 9, 20XX.

He was still having considerable pain in the right shoulder area, but there was full range of passive motion, and he felt like he was gradually improving, although he was not nearly as pain-free as before the recent surgery.

The surgical wound was well healed on inspection. There continued to be considerable tenderness to palpation in the depths of the surgical incision site. There was no swelling or increased heat or redness and, as noted above, there was a full passive range of motion of the right shoulder.

Because of the continuing rather excessive pain symptoms, x-rays were obtained, and the findings were thought to be completely within normal limits.

I continue to have no good explanation for the patient's continuing right shoulder symptoms, particularly in their present degree of severity. It would seem to me that he would be much improved over what he was prior to his recent surgery.

I have asked him to use the part as much as possible and to return in two weeks. Hopefully, at that time, some consideration can be given to a return-to-work date. Further reports will be forwarded as indicated.

Thank you for the pleasure of caring for this patient.

Very truly yours,

Patrick D. Quinn, MD

ref

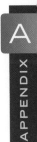

ANSWER TO 7-4: TYPING PRACTICE TEST

Kwei-Hay Wong, MD
1654 Piikea Streeet
Honolulu, Hawaii 96818
Telephone 555-534-0922
Fax 555-534-9512

Diplomat, American Board
Of Otolaryngology

Ear, Nose, Throat
Head and Neck Surgery

September 15, 20XX

Carroll W. Noyes MD
Suite 171
2113 4th Avenue
Houston, TX 77408

RE: Erma Hanlyn

Dear Dr Noyes:

I first saw Erma Hanlyn, your patient, on July 18, 20XX, with a history of a thyroid nodule since March 20XX. This 35-year-old woman had it diagnosed at Alvarado Hospital where they urged her to have surgery, I guess.

She gave a history that the nodule was quite tender when she was seen there and that she was on Synthroid 125 mcg when they took her scan. However when I saw her, the tenderness was gone. I could not feel any nodule.

We have had her stay off the Synthroid so that we could get an accurate reading, and on September 8, 20XX, we had another scintigram done at Piikea General Hospital, which revealed a symmetrical thyroid; it was free of any demonstrable nodules. All of the tenderness is gone, and she feels well. She is elated over the fact that she has avoided surgery.

In my opinion, she probably had a thyroiditis when she was seen at Alvarado, and the radioactive iodine that she was given for the test is responsible for the cure.

Thank you very much for letting me see her with you, and I will be happy to see her again at any time you or she feel it is necessary.

Sincerely,

Kwei-Hay Wong, MD

student's initials

ANSWERS TO 7-5: SELF-STUDY

1. buckle fracture. *(Look under "fracture.")*
2. epididymides *(There are two of these male structures.)*
3. myelodysplastic *(Look under "anemia.")*
4. en bloc *(In one piece)*
5. 0.5 cm *(Use metric and numerals.)*
6. profusion *(Excess.)*
7. CAGE screen *(An acronym for questions about drinking alcohol.)*
8. sloughing
9. plain *(No contrast material used.)*
10. loupe *(A small magnifying glass.)*

11. *aid (An aide is a person who assists.)*
12. *basal (Not a spice!)*
13. *whorl (An arrangement in a circle.)*
14. *fovea*
15. *TRAM (transverse rectus abdominus myocutaneous) flap*
16. *Two plus (spell out a number that begins a sentence) and (was noted).*
17. *C&N (culture and sensitivity)*
18. *led (lead is a metal)*
19. *pearly white*
20. *4 years 5 months old*

ANSWERS TO 8-1: SELF-STUDY

1.	muscle	bipennate
2.	nerve	pilomotor
3.	reflex	myenteric
4.	os	os peroneum
5.	test	Schiller or Schiller's
6.	symptom	labyrinthine
7.	syndrome	Horner or Horner's
8.	paralysis	decubitus
9.	tic	tic douloureux
10.	bandage	Esmarch
11.	maneuver	Pinard's or Pinard
12.	acid	salicylic
13.	pulse	dicrotic
14.	duct	Bartholin's or Bartholin
15.	vas	vas spirale
16.	membrane	diphtheritic
17.	disease	idiopathic
18.	carcinoma	scirrhous or scirrhus
19.	tunica	tunica adventitia
20.	syndrome	POEMS

ANSWERS TO 8-2: PRACTICE TEST

Note: Answers to this test will vary.

1. Colles' First Focus: fracture Second Focus: eponym
   Book: D Section: orthopedic
   Book: I Section: C words
   Book: M Section: Chapter 3
   Comments: Last entry (M) because I don't know if I should use the apostrophe.

2. Albuquerque First Focus: city name Second Focus: none needed
   Book: F Section: A words
   Comments: I will write this in my reference book.

3. Castroviejo First Focus: scissors (surgery) Second Focus: eponym
   Book: K Section: scissors
   Book: I Section: C words
   Book: D Section: eye
   Comments: I knew this one already because I remembered that they are used in eye surgery, but I did not know how to spell it.

4. extirpation

First Focus: surgery
Book: E
Book: K
Book: N

Second Focus: just the word itself
Section: section E or surgery
Section: E words
Section: E words

Comments: I knew this one already.

5. 15 mg or 50 mg

First Focus: drug name
Book: A
Book: B

Second Focus: how drug is delivered
Section: find the name of the drug
Section: find the name of the drug

Comments: I am not sure if the B book will tell about dosage. If it does, this would be my first choice since that is all I need to know.

6. mucous

First Focus: spelling of the word
Book: M
Book: D

Second Focus: noun or adjective
Section: Appendix B: homonyms
Section: skin (get the adjective form)

Comments: (Actually, *mucus* is also a correct word here.)

7. pylorus

First Focus: digestive system
Book: D
Book: E

Second Focus: word itself
Section: digestive system or GI system
Section: P words

Comments: (Answers will vary, of course.)

8. D&C

First Focus: an abbreviation
Book: C
Book: D
Book: M

Second Focus: female reproductive system
Section: D words
Section: D words
Section: Chapter 5

Comments: I had to decide which would be faster: abbreviation list or female word list. Then I had to be sure how to type the abbreviation.

9. aphasia

First Focus: neurology problem
Book: D
Book: M

Second Focus: sound of the word
Section: neurology section
Section: Appendix B: homonyms

Comments: (Answers will vary, of course.)

10. eczema

First Focus: integumentary system
Book: D
Book: M
Book: E

Second Focus: sound of the word
Section: dermatology or integumentary
Appendix B: homonyms
Section: E words

Comments: I have heard this word, but I had no idea how it was spelled.

11. 120 over 80

First Focus: how to write this
Book: M
Book: L

Second Focus: cardiology term
Section: Chapter 5
Section: Numbers

Comments: It is not written correctly. It should be *120/80*.

12. pH

First Focus: abbreviation
Book: C
Book: O (laboratory)

Second Focus: writing the number correctly
Section: P words
Section: abbreviations

Comments: I knew this abbreviation already.

13. Mycobacterium

First Focus: tuberculosis
Book: E
Book: D

Second Focus: disease
Section: tuberculosis
Section: respiratory system

Comments: (Answers will vary, of course.)

14. TMs

First Focus: abbreviations
Book: C
Book: D

Second Focus: ears
Section: T words
Section: sense organs or ears

Comments: (Answers will vary, of course.)

15. PERRLA

First Focus: eyes
Book: D
Book: H

Second Focus: is this an abbreviation?
Section: sense organs or eyes
Section: P words

Comments: I am glad I saw this before I heard it!

ANSWERS TO 8-3: PRACTICE TEST

	Remember the silent letter(s)	Spelling		Remember the silent letter(s)	Spelling
1.	g	gnathodynia	6.	t	Tzanck
2.	p	pterygium	7.	rh	hemorrhage
3.	p	pneumatic	8.	e	cacogeusia
4.	c	cnemial	9.	rh	metrorrhexis
5.	k	knock-knee	10.	rh	menometrorrhagia

ANSWERS TO 8-4: SELF-STUDY

1. femoropopliteal
2. antecardium
3. cerebrovascular accident
4. muscular dystrophy
5. metatarsophalangeal
6. bimanual
7. musculocutaneous/forearm
8. fetal-pelvic
9. vesicocolonic
10. costochondral
11. tracheobronchial
12. in extremis
13. dorsosacral
14. cor pulmonale
15. ileal conduit

ANSWERS TO 8-5: SELF-STUDY

1. (b) nose drops
2. (a) chickenpox
3. (a) reexamine
4. (b) herpesvirus
5. (c) nail plate
6. (c) fingernail
7. (b) lid lag
8. (a) pacemaker
9. (c) eardrum
10. (c) earwax

ANSWERS TO 8-6: PRACTICE TEST

Note: Answers to this test can vary depending on the edition of the *Physicians' Desk Reference (PDR)* used to look for answers. Remember that some generic names have been adopted by drug manufacturers as brand names but the generic form is to be used when transcribing reports unless the employer specifies otherwise. Some generic names sound like a brand name but are spelled differently (e.g., *adrenaline* with an *e* on the end is the generic, and *Adrenalin* without an *e* is the brand name).

1. Depending on the *PDR* edition, the answer may be one of the following:
   Brand and Generic Name Index, Product Name Index, or Alphabetical Index (pink) Brand Names.
2. a. Valium
   b. Soma Compound
   c. Zocor tablets
   d. Altocor (tablets)

A
APPENDIX

   e. Tenormin
   f. Coumadin
3. 50 mg
  Because 15 mg is not a strength indicated.
4. Flumadine; prostatic cancer
5. Flag the report for the dictator.
6. a. Prilosec   omeprazole
   b. Dilantin Kapseals   phenytoin sodium
   c. Plavix tablets   clopidogrel bisulfate
   d. Tofranil   imipramine HCl
   e. Pyridium   phenazopyridine HCl
   f. Fosamax   alendronate sodium
7. What other drug names could be confused with Pyridium: Baridium, Perdiem, Prodium.

ANSWERS TO 9-1: SELF-STUDY

1. medium
2. Media
3. acetabula
4. diverticula
5. ischium

ANSWERS TO 9-2: SELF-STUDY

1. bursa
2. pleurae
3. aorta
4. lamina
5. maxillae

ANSWERS TO 9-3: SELF-STUDY

1. alveoli (Rationale: Lungs have many clusters of air sacs [alveoli].)
2. bronchus
3. calculus
4. fungi (Rationale: Plural because pathologists test for more than one fungus.)
5. malleolus; ilium

ANSWERS TO 9-4: SELF-STUDY

1. anastomosis
2. Diagnoses
3. ecchymosis
4. exostosis
5. prognosis

ANSWERS TO 9-5: PRACTICE TEST

1. bacteria
2. crisis
3. Conjunctivae; sclerae (Rationale: There are two eyes, and so these must be plural.)
4. syllabus
5. metastases (Rationale: Cancer cells have spread to two locations in the liver.)
6. glomeruli (Rationale: A kidney has many filtering units [glomeruli], not just one.)
7. bases

8. viscera; were
9. larvae
10. corpus
11. adnexa; were *(Rationale: The adnexa consist of more than one structure.)*

ANSWERS TO 9-6: SELF-STUDY

1. cervix *(Rationale: Patient has single cervix of the uterus.)*
2. cortex
3. lumina or lumens *(Both are acceptable plural forms.)*
4. epididymides
5. larynx
6. fibromata or fibromas *(Both are acceptable plural forms.)*

ANSWERS TO 9-7: SELF-STUDY

1. acetabulums or acetabula
2. antra or antrums
3. aortas or aortae
4. appendixes or appendices
5. axillas or axillae
6. biopsies
7. carcinomas or carcinomata
8. comedos or comedones
9. conjunctivas or conjunctivae
10. femurs or femora
11. foramens or foramina

ANSWERS TO 9-8: SELF-STUDY

1. noun; singular
2. noun; plural
3. adjective
4. noun; plural
5. noun; singular
6. adjective
7. noun; singular
8. adjective
9. noun; singular
10. noun; singular

ANSWERS TO 10-1: DIAGNOSTIC TEST

1. passed
2. breath
3. C
4. lose
5. principal
6. C
7. then; C
8. whose
9. your; too
10. C
11. course
12. their
13. accept
14. principal; site
15. break
16. correspondence
17. sole
18. They're
19. granted
20. C
21. vary
22. trials
23. oversight
24. incidents
25. context
26. insisted
27. sense
28. loose
29. breech
30. bridle

ANSWERS TO 10-2: SELF-STUDY

1. n; effect
2. n; effects
3. n; affect (E)
4. v; affected
5. v; effected (E)
6. n; effect
7. v; affect
8. v; affect
9. v; affect
10. n; effect

ANSWERS TO 10-3: SELF-STUDY

1. altogether
2. all together
3. anyone
4. anyway
5. any way
6. Although
7. all right *(The word "alright" is misspelled.)*
8. some day
9. someday
10. all ready *(Each is ready.)*
11. already
12. any time
13. anytime
14. everyday
15. some time
16. sometime
17. any more
18. anything

ANSWERS TO 10-4: SELF-STUDY

1. cords
2. as if
3. besides
4. accept; advice *(Meaning "take" and "recommendations.")*
5. discrete (separate and distinct)
6. elicit *(Draw forth.)*
7. Further; imply *(Meaning "additional" and "insinuate," coming from me in contrast to presume as coming from someone else)*
8. lay; lie *(You place a pillow, but you do not ask a patient to "place" himself or herself.)*
9. effected *(Exception to the rule for this verb.)*
10. effects *(Noun form)*
11. bridle
12. etiology (cause)
13. infer *(What I perceive the patient means.)*
14. navel

ANSWERS TO 10-5: SELF-STUDY

1. suprasternal *(If this word was in your transcription and you used your spellchecker, you would not make the incorrect selection here.)*
2. recur *(If this word was in your transcription and you used your spellchecker, you would not make the incorrect selection here; "reoccur" is not a word.)*
3. Regardless *(If this word was in your transcription and you used your spellchecker, you would not make the incorrect selection here; "irregardless" is not a word.)*
4. sitting *(in a particular position)*; lying *(He would not be "placing" down)*
5. sight *(vision)*; affected *(verb)*
6. worst *(Have you noticed that "worst" is preceded by the article "the" in all instances?)*
7. regimen; followup
8. passed *(gone beyond)*
9. root *(source)*
10. Then; some time *(a period of time)*
11. enervated *(exhausted)*
12. nauseated *(sick)*
13. Further *(additional)*
14. imply *(insinuate, coming from me; in contrast to "presume" as coming from someone else; mnemonic device: "I imply")*
15. torturous *(painful, unpleasant)*
16. proceed *(go forward)*
17. effected *("effect" used as a verb in exception to the rule; the sense of power)*
18. effects *(use of the noun form)*

19. affect *("affect" is a noun; used as an exception to the rule)*
20. lain *(stayed)*

ANSWERS TO 10-6: SELF-STUDY

1. whoever *("She" is on call.)*
2. whom; work up *(They called "her" to "work up," a verb.)*
3. whom *(You discharged "him.")*
4. who *("He" fainted.)*
5. supraclavicular *(The prefix "supra-" is used with medical word roots.)*
6. whoever *(You think "he" would arrive.)*
7. Who *(You said she was on call.)*
8. than *(a contrast)*
9. whom *(They consulted "her.")*
10. worse *(very bad)*
11. who *("He" is on call.)*
12. whoever; workup *("He" will complete the "workup," noun form.)*
13. which *("which" introduces a nonessential word group; notice the commas also)*
14. who *("They" had been waiting; "they" had to be told; "which" is not used to refer to persons.)*
15. who *("He" would be available.)*

ANSWERS TO 10-7: PRACTICE TEST

1. aural
2. aura
3. oral
4. ora
5. hypertension
6. hypotension
7. hypotension
8. amenorrhea
9. metrorrhagia
10. aseptic
11. sepsis
12. palpitation
13. palpation
14. tract
15. instillation
16. ileum

ANSWERS TO 10-8: PRACTICE TEST

Your answers do not need to appear exactly as these are written, but all of the elements of the problem need to be corrected with no new incorrect elements added.

1. Q: In the past, she was admitted once and apparently underwent a stress test that was negative in Ohio.
A: She was admitted once in the past and apparently underwent a stress test in Ohio that was reported as negative.

2. Q: He denied any history of angiograms done.
A: According to the patient, no angiograms have been done.

3. Q: It was felt that the afterload reduction would not be significant enough to affect her hemodynamically.
A: Correct. ("affect," the verb, is correct.)

4. Q: She either knocked her head on the fence or she fell to the ground.
A: She knocked her head either on the fence or on the ground when she fell.

5. Q: There was a 35-minute lapse between when the mother called and the arrival of the ambulance.
A: There was a 35-minute lapse between when the mother called and when the ambulance arrived.
also
A: There was a 35-minute lapse between the mother's call and the ambulance's arrival.

6. Q: Neither the patient nor his parents or friends seemed to be aware of the risks involved.
  A: The patient, his parents, and his friends did not seem to be aware of the risks involved.
  also
  A: Neither the patient nor his parents and friends seemed to be aware of the risks involved.

7. Q: Review of systems otherwise is complete but negative.
  A: Correct. ("Review," the subject, is singular.)

8. Q: The teenage patient (that/who/whom) we saw in the office yesterday expired in the emergency department last night.
  A: The teenage patient *whom* we saw in the office yesterday expired in the emergency department last night. *(The answer is the object; you can substitute "him"; "we saw him in the office".)*

9. Q: Dr Jamieson, Dr Gonzales, and (myself/me/I) were selected as new members of the anesthesiology team.
  A: Dr Jamieson, Dr Gonzales, and *I* were selected as new members of the anesthesiology team. *(The reflexive "myself" is not used as the subject, and "me" is used as an object.)*

10. Q: There were 30 patients involved in our double-blind study, and three are being examined each day.
  A: There *are* 30 patients involved in our double-blind study, and *3* are being examined each day. *(Present tense; the study is still going on.)*

11. Q: She (is/was) to be seen in followup but (is/was) unable to keep her appointment.
  A: She was to be seen in followup but was unable to keep her appointment. ("Is" would not be a correct choice because the sentence is speaking of this in the past tense, not writing or speaking about it as going on right at the moment.)

12. Q: The patient was involved in an automobile accident while 5 months pregnant with a taxi.
  A: The patient was 5 months pregnant when she was involved in an automobile accident with a taxi. *(Better, but not nearly as interesting.)*

13. Q: The patient was transferred to the surgery suite with her films in good condition.
  A: The patient was in good condition when she was transferred to the surgery suite with her films. *(You just have to hope that the films were also in good condition!)*

14. Q: The hospital utilization committee reviewed (their/its/it's) discharge policy at yesterday's meeting.
  A: The hospital utilization committee reviewed *its* discharge policy at yesterday's meeting. *(Committee is thought of as a unit.)*

15. Q: On the pathology report, sections 1 through 4 (are/were) labeled "tissue from uterine fundus."
  A: On the pathology report, sections 1 through 4 are labeled "tissue from uterine fundus." (Anyone who caught this one is going to be a terrific proofreader. When the sentence was written without the hints in parentheses, it flew past several proofreaders.)

16. Q: We all wondered about whom the new interns were.
  A: We all wondered about who the new interns were. (The noun clause "who the new interns were" is the object of the preposition "about"; but within the noun clause, you have a form of the verb "to be," which is "were." You learned that objects following this verb form [predicate complement] are treated just as the subject of the sentence. This question is another tricky one, but everything counts toward learning the complex English language.)

17. Q: *Whomever* the physician calls in consultation will have trouble with her.
  A: Correct.

18. Q: The patient will (follow up/followup/follow-up) with (me/myself) next week.
  A: The patient will follow up with me next week. (The verb form is "follow up." For some reason, some dictators like to use the reflexive case "myself," but it does not work here.)

19. Q: A degree of gasping and snoring as well as mouth breathing are further noted.
  A: A degree of gasping and snoring as well as mouth breathing is further noted. (A degree "is" noted; learn to disregard the rest of the words making up the sentence.)

20. Q: The circumflex artery as well as its branches are thought to be free of any irregularities or lesions.
  A: The circumflex artery as well as its branches *is* thought to be free of any irregularities or lesions.

ANSWER TO 11-1: SELF-STUDY

Anthony Frishman   AGE: 12-1/2

October 10, 20XX

HX:	Patient underwent bilateral triple arthrodesis in August 20XX. He is out of splints and doing well. His foot rests are a bit long, and his feet are not touching them. He has no major complaints as far as his feet are concerned.
PX:	He has a long C-curve to the right, which may be slightly increased clinically since last x-rayed in June 20XX, when it was 25°. His feet are in neutral position as far as equinus. There is a slight varus inclination.
X-RAY:	Multiple views of his feet demonstrate fusion bilaterally of the triple staples.
DX:	Limb girdle dystrophy.
RX:	1. Return to clinic in 1–2 months for sitting SP spine x-ray.
	2. Obtain pulmonary function test.

ref

Karl T. Robrecht, MD

ANSWER TO 11-2: PRACTICE TEST

Maryellen Mawson   Age: 6

(Today's date)	This is a 6-year-old who has had a 3-week history of polydipsia, polyuria, polyphagia, and weight loss. The child has become progressively more lethargic over the past 24 hours, and 12 hours ago, the parents noticed she was breathing rapidly.
PX:	Height: 127 cm. Weight: 33 kg. Temp: 99°F. Pulse: 112. BP: 95/70. The child was semicomatose. She has dry mucous membranes but good skin turgor and full peripheral pulses.
STAT Lab:	Sodium 138 mEq/L, potassium 3.3 mEq/L, chloride 97 mEq/L, total CO_2 5 mEq/L, blood glucose 700 mg%.
RX:	Admit STAT to Children's Hospital.

(student's initials)

Eugene W. Gomez, MD

ANSWER TO 11-5: SELF-STUDY

> Brad Philman   Age: 47
>
> 1-13-XX   Pt admitted to Good Sam for bronchoscopy and possible left thoractomy and pleural poudrage. *ren* *right* *2-1-0X* *ren*

APPENDIX A

ANSWERS TO 11-9: SELF-STUDY

The outline or list can be abbreviated or spelled out and can use the SOAP method or the HX-PX method. Answers will vary greatly but should include the following:

▶ Patient's complete name.
▶ The date, and possibly time, of the visit.
▶ Chief Complaint (or CC): Main reason for the patient's visit.
▶ Subjective (or S) or History (or HX): All the details concerning the patient's problem or what has transpired with the problem since the last visit in the office or since the problem first occurred to the present time.
▶ Objective (or O) or Examination (or PX): The details of the examination of the patient, with close attention to the area of the chief complaint.
▶ Assessment (or A) or Diagnosis (or DX) or Impression (IMP): The examiner's assessment of the patient's problem or what may be the patient's problem.
▶ Plan (or P) or Treatment (or RX): Any medication or directions for care given the patient, any laboratory tests ordered, any referrals to consultants, and so on. When and whether the patient should return.
▶ Return-to-work date, if applicable.
▶ The examiner's name or initials and the transcriptionist's initials.

ANSWER TO 12-1: SELF-STUDY

Geoffrey Paul Hawkins
54-98-10

HISTORY

CHIEF COMPLAINT

Abdominal pains and vomiting since 3 a.m.

PRESENT ILLNESS

This 11-1/2-year-old white male, who was perfectly well yesterday and last evening, awoke from his sleep with vomiting at 3 a.m. today. This was followed by nausea, which has been severe, together with a little bile coming up, but no great amount of continued vomiting. There is severe, recurrent, doubling-up type cramping to time of admission at 10 a.m. There has been no recent upper respiratory tract infection, no prior similar episode, no history of recurrent constipation or diarrhea. Patient's last bowel movement was yesterday and of normal quality. His mother reports that he eats sunflower seeds to excess and may have done so yesterday.

PAST HISTORY

Patient was born at home with midwife delivery, uncomplicated. He has had the usual immunizations for childhood. There has been no prior hospitalization, no tonsillectomy, no surgery, no fracture. He has had stitches a couple of times in the office.

FAMILY HISTORY

Mother is 35 and at the present time is under treatment for cancer of the breast. She reports that she had surgery and is on chemotherapy at the present time. She has not been given radiation. Father is age 40, living and well. There are 2 sisters, both older than the patient, both living and well. They both had appendectomies, one of which had ruptured. There are a maternal great niece, uncle, and paternal grandmother who have had diabetes. There is no diabetes in the immediate family and no other history of familial disorders such as bleeding, anemia, tuberculosis, heart disease.

PERSONAL HISTORY

The patient has no known drug allergies, has not been on any medication at the present time. Grade six, but does poorly. Seems to be the class clown according to his mother. He has no hobbies.

SYSTEMIC REVIEW

HEENT*

There has been a muscle in one eye which has been off for years; Dr McMannis is following this. His vision is good. Hearing is normal.

CARDIORESPIRATORY

No known murmurs. No chronic cough, no recent cough, no dyspnea.

GASTROINTESTINAL

No prior GI difficulty. No food allergies. No chronic or recurrent constipation.

GENITOURINARY

No nocturia, no enuresis, no GU infection.

NEUROMUSCULAR

No history of head injury. No history of polio, paralysis, meningitis, or numbness.

Paul R. Elsner, MD

student's initials

D: (yesterday's date)

T: (today's date)

*Subheadings may be abbreviated

ANSWER TO 12-2: PRACTICE TEST (TABULATED BLOCK)

Joseph R. Balentine

423-12-22

Copy: Stuart L. Paulson, MD

HISTORY

CHIEF COMPLAINT:	This patient is a 25-year-old male complaining of recurring epistaxis.
PRESENT ILLNESS:	This patient reports that yesterday he had onset of epistaxis in the left side of his nose. This was intermittent throughout the day, and at 4:30 this morning, he came in to the ER.

PAST HISTORY

ALLERGIES:	None.
ILLNESSES:	The patient had a collapsed lung about 5 years ago and subsequently had surgery but does not know the exact etiology of the problem or the exact name of the surgery. There is no bleeding history except for PI.
MEDICATIONS:	None.

FAMILY HISTORY:	Essentially unremarkable. Father, mother, siblings are all well and healthy.

REVIEW OF SYSTEMS

SKIN:	No rashes or jaundice.
HEENT:	See Present Illness.
CARDIORESPIRATORY:	See Past History. No history of pneumonia, tuberculosis, chronic cough, or hemoptysis. No history of pedal edema.
GASTROINTESTINAL:	Weight is stable. He denies any nausea, vomiting, diarrhea, or food intolerance.
GENITOURINARY:	No history of GU tract infections, dysuria, hematuria, pyuria.
ENDOCRINE:	No polyuria or polydipsia.
NEUROLOGIC:	No history of psychiatric disorder.

Benjamin B. Abboud, MD

Student's initials

D: 11-16-XX

T: 11-16-XX

ANSWER TO 12-5: PRACTICE TEST

Lily Mae Jenkins
5980-A
Copies: Willow Moran, MD
Gordon Bender, MD

HISTORY

CHIEF COMPLAINT
Rectal bleeding, 1 day.

PRESENT ILLNESS
This 90-year-old lady has been looking after her own personal affairs and living with her daughter for the last 3 years. Last night, she had a bowel movement that had some bright-red blood mixed in with it. This morning, she had another bowel movement, and it consisted mostly of bright-red blood. She has a history of gallbladder disease, dating back over 50 years. She refused to have her gallbladder taken out but has been on a low-fat diet ever since that time. Her daughter describes numerous gallbladder attacks, lasting for several days, consisting of severe, right upper quadrant pain. She has had occasional, intermittent right lower quadrant pain that does not seem similar to the gallbladder attacks.

PAST HISTORY
Operations: In 1997, she had enucleation of the left eye. She had surgery in 2005 for glaucoma in the right eye.
Medical: 1986, Colles' fracture, right wrist. 1990s, severe arthritis of her spine. Medications: Patient is presently taking Evista 60 mg per day, Plavix 75 mg every morning, Indocin 1 tablet t.i.d. She takes Bufferin p.r.n. for pain. She takes nitroglycerin 2-3 tablets per week for chest pain and has done so for 5 years.

FAMILY
Both of her parents lived until their 80s. She had 6 children: 1 died at age 3, the result of injuries sustained in an automobile accident; 1 died at age 56 of carcinoma of the breast. Otherwise, the family history is unremarkable. There are 4 children who are alive and well.

FUNCTIONAL INQUIRY
HEENT: Hearing in her right ear is absent. Hearing in her left ear is decreased. There is an artificial eye in the left, and there is only slight vision in her right eye if one comes exactly in the middle of her visual field. Patient has been edentulous for several years.
Chest: Nonsmoker.
Cardiorespiratory: Patient has had angina for over 5 years and abnormal cardiograms for the last 3 years. She is cold all of the time and is constantly bundling herself up in an effort to keep warm.
Gastrointestinal: Her bowel movements have been normal. See Present Illness.
Genitourinary: She has no history of any bladder or kidney infections, despite the fact that she had a history of kidney failure last year.
Neuromuscular: Patient has shooting, severe pains up her spine that are relatively incapacitating, but she manages to keep going by just taking Bufferin.

PHYSICAL EXAMINATION

GENERAL
This is a 90-year-old black woman in no obvious distress, who is hard of hearing but can answer questions.

(continued)

Lily Mae Jenkins
6960-A
History and Physical Examination, page 2

Physical Examination: (continued)

HEENT
Ears: There is wax in both ears. The drums, beyond the wax, appear within normal limits. There is no hearing in the right ear and only slight hearing in the left. Eyes: The left eye is artificial. The right eye is pinpoint. There is no scarring in the right eye, consistent with an iridectomy. She has a cataract in the right eye, as well. Nose: Unremarkable. Mouth: Edentulous.

NECK
There are no carotid bruits. No jugular venous distention. Thyroid is palpable and unremarkable. Range of motion of the neck is generally slightly restricted.

CHEST
Clear to percussion and auscultation.
Heart: The apical beat is not palpable. There is some tenderness over the costochondral cartilages on the left side. Heart size is not enlarged to percussion. There is muffled heart sound. There is no 3rd or 4th heart sound. There are no murmurs heard in the supine position.Breasts: Palpable, and there are no masses noted.

ABDOMEN
Soft. There are marked senile keratoses over the abdominal wall. There is some diffuse tenderness on deep palpation over the cecum in the right lower quadrant. There is no other tenderness noted or abnormal bowel sounds noted in the abdomen. Bowel sounds are within normal limits.

PELVIC
Not done.

RECTAL
Full sigmoidoscopic examination to 25 cm revealed fresh blood in the sigmoid area with no obvious bleeding source noted.

EXTREMITIES
There is essentially no motion in the back. Range of motion of the hips is within normal limits and painless. There is only a +1 dorsalis pedis on the right; otherwise, there are no peripheral pulses present. There is marked coldness of both feet.

CENTRAL NERVOUS SYSTEM
The patient's strength is within normal limits. The reflexes are within normal limits. Coordination is not tested. There is an involuntary shaking, consistent with the diagnosis of old Parkinson disease.

IMPRESSION
1. Acute gastrointestinal hemorrhage, etiology not yet diagnosed.
2. Chronic cholecystitis.
3. Severe osteoarthritis of spine.
4. Arteriosclerotic heart disease with angina pectoris.

Philip D. Quince, MD

student's initials

D: (today's date)

T: (today's date)

ANSWERS TO 12-6: SELF-STUDY

1. To call attention to it.
2. There were no abnormal findings.
3. Because it refers to that major topic in the outline.
4. The "menopause," or end of her regular menstrual cycles.
5. It is a nonessential phrase.
6. The patient did not have a fever or elevated body temperature.
7. No one suffers from or has died of any diseases or conditions that are considered hereditary.
8. How the pupils react to light and accommodation.
9. It was not in keeping with the rest of the format, where topics were spelled out in full. Also, if the outline were dictated, the dictator presumably did not say "NM" but "neuromuscular."
10. It is clear from the transcript that the dictator is referring to both eyes; therefore, the plural form is necessary. English abbreviations are written in capital letters, not lowercase letters, as are Latin abbreviations.
11. This is the custom; it could be called tradition. Some medical transcriptionists prefer the use of the arabic numerals 2 through 12.
12. One must presume that the dictator did not say "T&A"; furthermore, it is not a good idea to abbreviate items of this importance.
13. This is up to you.
14. All three are pretty easy. It is up to you.
15. This is up to you and what you enjoy doing and how you want the end product to appear.

ANSWER TO 13-1: SELF-STUDY

Bacon, Marcia M
52-01-96
Room No. 248-C

DISCHARGE SUMMARY

ADMISSION DATE: May 7, 20XX
DISCHARGE DATE: May 9, 20XX

ADMISSION DIAGNOSIS
Torn medial meniscus, left knee.

HISTORY OF PRESENT ILLNESS
The patient injured her left knee on April 11, 20XX, while playing tennis. She subsequently had difficulty with persistent effusion and pain in the left knee. An arthrogram prior to admission revealed a tear of the medial meniscus.

PHYSICAL EXAMINATION
Absence of tenderness to palpation of any of the joint structures. There was approximately 30-35 mL of fluid within the joint. Range of motion was full.

LABORATORY DATA
Admission hemoglobin was 15.9, hematocrit 47%, with a white count of 7400 with normal differential. Urinalysis was within normal limits. Chem panel 19 showed an elevated cholesterol of 379 mg%. Chest x-ray was reported as negative.

TREATMENT AND HOSPITAL COURSE
The patient was taken to the operating room on the same day as admission, at which time she underwent arthroscopy. This revealed that she had a tear of the medial meniscus. Arthrotomy was performed, with medial meniscectomy. A chondral fracture was noted in the medial femoral condyle, measuring approximately 5 mm in greatest diameter. The edges of this were sheathed. Postoperatively, the patient's course was benign. There was no significant temperature elevation. She became ambulatory with crutches on the first postoperative day, with no difficulty with straight leg raising.

DISPOSITION
The patient is being discharged home, ambulatory, with crutches, and an exercise program. She is to be seen in the office in one week for suture removal.

CONDITION AT THE TIME OF DISCHARGE: Improved.

COMPLICATIONS: None.

MEDICATIONS: None.

DISCHARGE DIAGNOSES
1. Torn medial meniscus, left knee.
2. Chondromalacia, medial femoral condyle.

Henry R. Knowles, MD

(student's initials)
D: 5-10-year
T: 5-11-year

ANSWERS TO 13-4: SELF-STUDY

RADIOLOGY REPORT

Examination Date: June 8, 20XX
Date Reported: June 8, 20XX
Physician: George B. Bancroft, MD
Examination: Mammography, right and left breasts

Patient: Donna Mae Weeser
X-ray No.: 16-A2
Age: 46
Hospital No: 52-80-44

MAMMOGRAPHY,
RIGHT AND LEFT BREASTS: There are retromammary prosthetic devices in position. The anterior parenchyma is somewhat compressed. There is no evidence of neoplastic calcification or skin thickening demonstrated. No dominant masses are noted within the anteriorly displaced parenchyma. No increased vascularity is evident.

IMPRESSION: Mammography, right and left breasts, shows the presence of retromammary prosthetic devices in position. The demonstrated tissue appears within normal limits.

Radiologist _____
Clayton M. Markham, MD

(student's initials)

D: (date)

T: (date)

ANSWERS TO 14-1: SELF-STUDY

1. Please recheck this; it is your responsibility.
2. Remodeling is taking place in the emergency room; therefore, reroute all patient traffic to Ward B until further notice.
3. The new chief-of-staff will take over the first of next month; furthermore, many new physicians will be added to the active staff roster.
   or
   The new chief-of-staff will take over the first of next month, and there will be many new physicians added to the active staff roster. *(Or write two separate sentences.)*
4. To be accurate and to meet your production levels are important here.
   or
   It is important here to be accurate and to meet your production levels.
5. Pull the patient's record; notify the doctor of the emergency; give the record to the doctor; relate any information you have received.
6. Please observe the following:
   a. Enter your department number on each requisition.
   b. Use the preprinted requisitions.
   c. Refer to the patient register, if the preprinted requisition is not available for the record you require.
7. Please include these in the list for duties of the custodian of records:
   a. Keep minimum turnaround time.
   b. Make corrections in the proper way.
   c. Be sure that records are signed or initialed.
   d. Obtain a release before you permit unauthorized persons to see the records.
8. Jogging through the parking lot, I saw many new flowers.
9. My dog stayed at my mother's house while I was on vacation.
10. She was 44 when her first and only child was born.
11. The record, which has been circulated throughout the department, finally was returned.
12. Strike "an attack of."
13. Strike "at a time."
14. Strike "purposes."

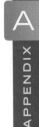

15. Strike "at a" and "date."
16. Strike "engaged in."
17. Strike "during the period."
18. Strike "in duration."
19. Strike "in size."
20. Strike "a period of."
21. I feel *that* the nursing personnel as well as *the* pulmonary medicine staff will benefit from the information and instructions.
22. The *members of the* Advisory Committee and Management Department would like to express their thanks for the time you gave to present the material to us.
23. The medical record might be the physician's only witness in court. For this reason, the medical record must be completely accurate.
24. By writing, one learns to write. *(Just put the comma in the right place!)*

ANSWERS TO 14-2: SELF-STUDY

1. POSSIBLE OUTLINE

▶ Mr Ray Littlefield rlittle@home.net
▶ Consultation appointment with Paul R. Vecchione, MD.
▶ Appointment is February 9, 20XX, at 10:30 a.m.
▶ Dr Vecchione's office is at 984 Briarwood Drive, College Heights, Suite B.
▶ Telephone for Dr Vecchione is 567-3876. His appointment secretary is Brenda.

1. EMAIL

FROM: William A. Berry, MD.
SUBJECT: Consultation with Paul R. Vecchione, MD
DATE: Today at 1:52 p.m.
TO: Ray Littlefield rittle@home.net

This message is to confirm that Dr Berry has arranged an appointment for you to see Dr Paul Vecchione on February 9, 20XX, at 10:30 a.m. Dr Vecchione's office is located in the College Heights Medical Center at 984 Briarwood Drive, Suite B. If this time and date are not convenient for you, please contact Brenda, Dr Vecchione's appointment secretary, at 567-3876.

Please telephone me at College Hospital, 568-3523, or email me if I can be of any further service to you.

Marijane Moss, CMT
Medical Transcription Department
College Hospital and Medical Center
Email: berrymdCHMC@med.com

2. POSSIBLE OUTLINE

▶ Write PTA Program Chairperson, College Heights High School PTA.
▶ Dr Berry will speak to the parents and show a 20-minute film entitled "More Than a Few Beers."
▶ He will need a 35-mm film projector and a meeting room number.
▶ He will be prepared for a question-and-answer period.

2. EMAIL

FROM: William A. Berry, MD.
SUBJECT: College Heights High School PTA
DATE: Today at 4:15 p.m.
TO: PTA program chairperson CollegeHeightsHS@ed.com

This message is to confirm that Dr Berry has agreed to speak on January 10, 20XX, at 6:30 p.m. at the College Heights High School PTA. He plans to show a 20-minute film entitled "More Than a Few Beers" and will need a 35-mm projector and a screen. He will be available for a question-and-answer period after his presentation. Please give me the room number at the school where the meeting is to be held, and telephone me at College Hospital, 568-3523, or email me if I can be of any further service to you.

Marijane Moss, CMT
Medical Transcription Department
College Hospital and Medical Center
Email: berrymdCHMC@med.com

ANSWERS TO 14-3: SELF-STUDY

AGENDA

SAFETY COMMITTEE MEETING

August 22, 20XX

- I. Call to Order
- II. Roll Call and Introduction of guests
- III. Approval of Minutes of July 26, 20XX
- IV. Rotation of Membership
- V. Electrical Safety Program
- VI. Fire Drills
- VII. First Aid
- VIII. Beverage Spilling
- IX. New Business *(This topic might be included on the agenda in case someone at the meeting wants to discuss some new problem to work on.)*
- X. Adjournment

ANSWERS TO 14-4: SELF-STUDY

Here are some possible word choices:

1. Know: perceive, discern, recognize, see, comprehend, understand, realize, appreciate, experience, be aware of.
2. Awful: terrific, tremendous, horrible, dreadful, fearful.
3. Tell: describe, narrate, explain, inform, advise, state.
4. Nice: delicate, fine, pleasing, attractive, accurate.
5. Think: presume, understand, reason, reflect, speculate.

APPENDIX B

Reference Materials

INTRODUCTION

This book is printed on perforated pages so that you can tear out the pages and place them in your personal standard-sized binder or medical transcriptionist (MT) notebook for easy and quick reference. These pages are merely the beginning of your collection. You are encouraged to add to your collection as you encounter new information. Your notebook is an important and valuable tool that you will use as you develop the skills of transcription.

CONTENTS

ABBREVIATIONS COMMONLY USED

This list contains some abbreviations that are commonly used in office chart notes and hospital records. You may want to remove it from this book or photocopy it and place it into your reference book so that you can refer to it at any time. Later, you may want to add new abbreviations and institution-approved lists to your collection. Some abbreviations are pronounced like a word (*cabbage* for *CABG* and *hope* for *HOPE*); others are said as an entire word that is turned into an abbreviation ("milligram" for *mg* and "see section" for *C-section*); and for some, each letter of the abbreviation is spoken (*b.i.d.* and *L & W*).

@*	at
A, B, AB, O	blood types; can also be dictated with subscript numbers
A_1 or A1	first aortic sound
A_2 or A2	second aortic sound
AAMA	American Association for Medical Assistants
AB/ab	abortion
ABGs	arterial blood gases
a.c.	before meals
ACh	acetylcholine
a.d. or AD*	right ear
A&D	ascending and descending (each letter is pronounced: *ay-en-dee*)
ad lib.	freely (usually refers to drug or modality)
ADH	antidiuretic hormone; vasopressin
ADL	activities of daily living
ADT	admission, discharge, transfer
AFB	acid-fast bacillus (tuberculosis organism)
AFIP	Armed Forces Institute of Pathology
Ag	silver
AHDI	Association for Healthcare Documentation Integrity
AIDS	acquired immunodeficiency syndrome (pronounced like a word: "aids")
a.m. or AM	in the morning or before noon
AMA	against medical advice; American Medical Association
AP	anteroposterior (each letter is pronounced: *ay-pee*)
A&P	auscultation and percussion
APC	acetylsalicylic acid (aspirin), phenacetin, and caffeine
Aq	water
ARC	AIDS-related complex (pronounced like a word: "ark")

ARD	acute respiratory disease
ARDS	acute respiratory distress syndrome
a.s. or AS*	left ear
ASAP	as soon as possible (*see* STAT)
ASCVD	atherosclerotic cardiovascular disease
ASD	atrial septal defect *also* Alzheimer senile dementia
Au	gold
AV	atrioventricular
A&W	alive and well
Ba	barium
baso	basophils
BBB	bundle branch block
BCC	basal cell carcinoma
BE	barium enema
bib	drink
b.i.d.	twice a day (each letter is pronounced)
BLE	both lower extremities
BLT	bilateral tubal ligation
BM	bowel movement
BP	blood pressure
BPH	benign prostatic hypertrophy
BRP	bathroom privileges
BS	blood sugar; bowel sounds
BUN	blood urea nitrogen (each letter is pronounced; preferred term is *urea nitrogen*)
BUS	Bartholin urethral and Skene (glands) (this acronym is not generally pronounced like a word)
BVE	bachelor of vocational education
Bx	biopsy
C or °C	Celsius
C1 or C_1	first cervical vertebra (continues through C7 or C_7)
Ca	calcium
Ca or CA	carcinoma (each letter is pronounced)

Ca or Ca²⁺	calcium ion	DOE	dyspnea on exertion
CABG	coronary artery bypass graft (type of surgery) (pronounced like "cabbage")	DPM	doctor of podiatric medicine
		DPT	diphtheria-pertussis-tetanus (vaccine)
CAD	coronary artery disease	DRG	diagnosis-related group
CAT	computed axial tomography	DSM	*Diagnostic and Statistical Manual of Mental Disorders*
CBC	complete blood count		
CC	chief complaint	DTR	deep tendon reflexes
cc	cubic centimeter (pronounced like *see-see*) Use *mL.*	D/W	dextrose and water
		Dx or DX	diagnosis
CCU	coronary care unit; critical care unit	EAC	external auditory canal
		EBL	estimated blood loss
CDC	Centers for Disease Control and Prevention	ECG	electrocardiogram
		ECMO	extracorporal membrane oxygenation (pronounced *ek-moe*)
CF	complement fixation		
CHD	coronary heart disease; chronic heart disease; congestive heart disease	ED	emergency department
		EDC	estimated date of confinement (due date for baby)
CHF	congestive heart failure	EEG	electroencephalogram
cm	centimeter	EENT	eyes, ears, nose, throat
CMA-A	certified medical assistant, administrative	e.g.	example given
		EKG	electrocardiogram
CMA-C	certified medical assistant, clinical	ELISA	enzyme-linked immunosorbent assay (pronounced like a word)
CMT	certified medical transcriptionist	EMG	electromyogram
CNS	central nervous system	EMI	older term for *CAT*
CO	carbon monoxide	EMS	emergency medical services
Co	cobalt	EMT	emergency medical technician or emergency medical treatment
CO₂ or CO2	carbon dioxide		
COD	condition on discharge		
COPD	chronic obstructive pulmonary disease	ENT	ear, nose, throat
		EOM	extraocular movements
CPAP	continuous positive airway pressure (pronounced *see-pap*)	eos	eosinophils
		eq	equivalent
CPR	cardiopulmonary resuscitation	ER	emergency room
CPX	complete physical examination	Esq.	esquire (often attorneys use this after their name)
CR	cardiorespiratory		
C-section	cesarean section	ESR	erythrocyte sedimentation rate
CSF	cerebrospinal fluid	et al.	and others (both words are said)
C&S	culture and sensitivity	F or °F	Fahrenheit
CT	computed tomography	FAHDI	Fellow Association for Healthcare Documentation Integrity
Cu	copper		
CVA	costovertebral angle; cerebrovascular accident	FB	foreign body
		FBS	fasting blood sugar
CXR	chest x-ray	Fe	iron
d	day	FH	family history
DC*	discontinue	FHT	fetal heart tone
D&C	dilation and curettage (each letter is pronounced: *dee-en-see*)	fl oz	fluid ounce
		FSH	follicle-stimulating hormone
DD	differential diagnosis	ft	foot
D₅W or D5W	5% dextrose in water	5-FU	5-fluorouracil (chemotherapy drug)
DNR	do not resuscitate		
DOA	dead on arrival	FUO	fever of unknown origin
DOB	date of birth	Fx	fracture

G	gravida (pregnant)	IVP	intravenous pyelogram
G neg.	gram-negative	K	potassium
G pos.	gram-positive	K^+	potassium ion
GB	gallbladder	kg	kilogram
GC	gonorrhea	km	kilometer
GH	growth hormone	KUB	kidneys, ureters, bladder
GI	gastrointestinal	L	liter
g	gram	L1 or L_1	first lumbar vertebra (continues
GP	general practitioner		through L5 or L_5)
gtt	drop(s)	L&A	light and accommodation
GU	genitourinary	lb	pound
GYN or Gyn	gynecology/gynecologist	LBBB	left bundle branch block
h	hour	LDL	low-density lipoprotein
H	hour or hydrogen	LH	luteinizing hormone
H^+	hydrogen ion	LLQ	left lower quadrant
H_2O or H2O	water	LMP	last menstrual period
Hb or hgb	hemoglobin	LP	lumbar puncture
HCG or hCG	human chorionic gonadotropin	LPN	licensed professional nurse
HCl	hydrochloric acid	LSH	lutein-stimulating hormone
Hct	hematocrit	LTH	lactogenic hormone, prolactin
HDL	high-density lipoprotein	LUQ	left upper quadrant
HEENT	head, eyes, ears, nose, and throat	LVN	licensed vocational nurse
Hg	mercury	L&W	living and well
hgb	hemoglobin	m	meter
H&H	hemoglobin and hematocrit (test on red blood cells)	MDR	minimum daily requirement
		mEq	milliequivalent
HIPAA	Health Insurance Portability and Accountability Act	mg	milligram
		Mg	magnesium
HIV	human immunodeficiency virus	Mg^{2+}	magnesium ion
HOPE	Health Opportunities for People Everywhere (pronounced *hope*)	mg%	milligrams percent
		MI	myocardial infarction
H&P	history and physical (each letter is pronounced: *h-en-pee*)	mL	milliliter
		MM	mucous membrane
HPF or hpf	high-power field	mm	millimeter
HPI	history of present illness	mmHg	millimeters of mercury
Hx or HX	history	mm Hg	millimeters of mercury
I	iodine	monos	monocytes
ibid.	in the same place	MOPP	nitrogen mustard, Oncovin, prednisone, procarbazine (chemotherapy regimen)
ICD-10-CM	*International Classification of Diseases, Tenth Revision, Clinical Modification*		
		mOsm	milliosmole
ICU	intensive care unit	MR	mitral regurgitation
I&D	incision and drainage (each letter is said: *eye-en-dee*)	MRI	magnetic resonance imaging
		MS	master's degree in science; multiple sclerosis
i.e.	that is (each letter is said: *eye-e*)		
IgA	immunoglobulin A (also IgG, IgD, IgB, and IgE)	N	nitrogen
		NA	not applicable
IM	intramuscular	Na	sodium
IMP	impression	Na^+	sodium ion
in.	inch	NG	nasogastric
I&O	intake and output	NKA	no known allergies
IOP	intraocular pressure	NMI	no middle initial
IPPB	intermittent positive pressure breathing	NOS	not otherwise specified
		NPC	near point of convergence (eyes); no previous complaint
IV or I.V.	intravenous		

NPH	no previous history	pO$_2$ or pO2	pressure of oxygen/partial pressure of oxygen
n.p.o.	nothing by mouth	POC	products of conception
NS	not significant	p.r.n.	as required or needed; as the occasion arises (each letter is pronounced)
NSAID	nonsteroidal anti-inflammatory drug		
NSR	normal sinus rhythm	PSA	prostate-specific antigen
NTP	normal temperature and pressure	pt	patient
		PTA	prior to admission
NYD	not yet diagnosed	PVC	premature ventricular contraction
O$_2$ or O2	oxygen		
OB	obstetrics	PX or PE	physical examination
OB-GYN	obstetrics and gynecology	Px	prognosis
o.d. or OD*	right eye	q.	every
O&P	ova and parasites	q.h.	every hour
OR	operating room	q.2 h.	every two hours
o.s. or OS*	left eye	q.3 h.	every three hours
OU*	each eye, both eyes	q.4 h.	every four hours
oz	ounce	q.i.d.	four times a day (each letter is pronounced)
P	phosphorus; pulse		
P$_1$ or P1	pulmonic first sound (P1, P2, and so on)	QRS	complex in electrocardiographic study
P1	para 1 (and so on)	qt	quart
PA	posteroanterior	R	respiration
P&A	percussion and auscultation	r	roentgen
Pap	Papanicolaou test/smear	Ra	radium
PAP	prostatic acid phosphatase	RBBB	right bundle branch block
PBI	protein-bound iodine	RBC	red blood cell count
p.c.	after meals	rbc	red blood cell
pCO$_2$ or pCO2	pressure of carbon dioxide/ partial pressure of carbon dioxide	Rh (factor)	blood type (negative or positive factor antigen on the rbc)
PDR	*Physicians' Desk Reference* (drug reference)	RhoGAM	drug given to Rh-negative women to avoid risk of Rh immunization (pronounced *row-gam*)
PE or PX	physical examination		
PERLA	pupils equal and reactive to light and accommodation	RLQ	right lower quadrant
PERRLA	pupils equal, round, and reactive to light and accommodation	RMT	registered medical transcriptionist
		RN	registered nurse
PET	positron emission tomography	RO	rule out; routine orders
PH	past history	R/O	rule out
pH	hydrogen ion concentration (degree of acidity or alkalinity)	ROS	review of systems
		RUQ	right upper quadrant
PI	present illness	Rx or RX	prescription or treatment
PID	pelvic inflammatory disease	SG	specific gravity
PIP	proximal interphalangeal (joint)	SGOT	serum glutamic oxaloacetic transaminase
PKU	phenylketonuria (test for PKU is given to newborns)	SI	seriously ill
PM or p.m.	after noon	SIDS	sudden infant death syndrome (crib death)
PMH	past medical history		
PMI	point of maximal impulse	sig.	directions
PMS	premenstrual syndrome	SMAC	automated analytic device for testing blood (pronounced smack)
PO	postoperative		
p.o.	by mouth		

SOAP	Subjective, Objective, Assessment, Plan (used for patient notes)	Tx or TX	treatment
		U*	if *unit* is meant, spell it out
		U	uranium
SOB	shortness of breath	UA	urinalysis
SP	status post	URI	upper respiratory infection
sp. gr.	specific gravity	UTI	urinary tract infection
STAT or stat	immediately	UV	ultraviolet
SS	signs and symptoms	VA	visual acuity
STD	sexually transmitted disease	VDRL	Venereal Disease Research Laboratory (test for syphilis)
T1 or T$_1$	first thoracic vertebra (continues through T12 or T$_{12}$)	VF	visual fields
T&A	tonsillectomy and adenoidectomy (pronounced *tee-en-ay*)	viz.	that is; namely
		vs	versus
		VS	vital signs
TAB	therapeutic abortion	VSD	ventricular septal defect
TB	tuberculosis	V&T	volume and tension (pulse)
TIA	transient ischemic attack	WBC	white blood cell count
t.i.d.	three times a day	wbc	white blood cell
TM	tympanic membrane	w-d	well-developed
TNTC	too numerous to count	WF	white female
TPR	temperature, pulse, respiration	WM	white male
TSH	thyroid-stimulating hormone (thyrotropin)	w-n	well-nourished
		WNL	within normal limits
TURP	transurethral resection of the prostate gland	X	times
		X match	cross-match

DRUGS MOST OFTEN PRESCRIBED—TOP 200 DRUG LIST 2009

DRUG*

Accupril (quinapril HCl)
acetaminophen with codeine
Aciphex (rabeprazole sodium)
Actonel (risedronate sodium)
Actos (pioglitazone HCl)
Adderall XR (mixed amphetamines)
Advair Discus (salmeterol xinafoate, fluticasone propionate)
albuterol sulfate
Allegra (fexofenadine HCl)
Allegra-D 12-Hour (fexofenadine HCl, pseudoephedrine HCl)
allopurinol
alprazolam
Altace (ramipril)
Amaryl (glimepiride)
Ambien (zolpidem tartrate)
amitriptyline HCl
amoxicillin
amoxicillin and clavulanate potassium
Amoxil (amoxicillin trihydrate)
Aricept (donepezil HCl)
aspirin
atenolol
Avandia (rosiglitazone maleate)
Avapro (irbesartan)
Avelox (moxifloxacin HCl)
Aviane (levonorgestrel, ethinyl estradiol)
benazepril HCl
Benicar (olmesartan medoxomil)
Bextra (valdecoxib)
Biaxin; Biaxin XL (clarithromycin)
bisoprolol and hydrochlorothiazide
bupropion HCl
buspirone HCl
carisoprodol
Cartia XT (diltiazem HCl)
Celebrex (celecoxib)
Celexa (citalopram hydrobromide)
cephalexin
ciprofloxacin
Clarinex (desloratadine)
clindamycin
clonazepam
clonidine
clotrimazole and betamethasone dipropionate
Combivent (ipratropium bromide, albuterol sulfate)
Concerta (methylphenidate HCl)
Coreg (carvedilol)

Cotrim (trimethoprim, sulfamethoxazole)
Coumadin (warfarin sodium)
Cozaar (losartan potassium)
Crestor (rosuvastatin calcium)
cyclobenzaprine HCl
Depakote (divalproex sodium)
Detrol LA (tolterodine tartrate)
diazepam
diclofenac sodium
Diflucan (fluconazole)
Digitek (digoxin)
digoxin
Dilantin (phenytoin sodium)
diltiazem HCl
Diovan (valsartan)
Diovan HCT (valsartan, hydrochlorothiazide)
doxazosin mesylate
doxycycline hyclate
Duragesic (fentanyl)
Effexor XR (venlafaxine)
Elidel (pimecrolimus)
enalapril maleate
Endocet (oxycodone HCl; acetaminophen)
estradiol
Evista (raloxifene HCl)
famotidine
ferrous sulfate
Flomax (tamsulosin HCl)
Flonase (fluticasone propionate)
Flovent (fluticasone propionate)
fluconazole
fluoxetine HCl
folic acid
Fosamax (alendronate sodium)
fosinopril sodium
furosemide
gemfibrozil
glipizide
glyburide
Humalog (insulin lispro)
Humulin N; Humulin 70/30 (insulin)
hydrochlorothiazide
hydrocodone and acetaminophen
hydroxyzine HCl
Hyzaar (losartan potassium, hydrochlorothiazide)
ibuprofen
Imitrex (sumatriptan succinate)
isosorbide mononitrate
ketoconazole
Klor-Con; Klor-Con M20 (potassium chloride)

---

*Modified from Drake E and Drake R: *Saunders pharmaceutical word book 2010,* St Louis, 2010, Elsevier.

B
APPENDIX

Lamictal (lamotrigine)
Lanoxin (digoxin)
Lantus (insulin glargine)
Lescol XL (fluvastatin sodium)
Levaquin (levofloxacin)
Levothroid (levothyroxine sodium)
levothyroxine sodium
Levoxyl (levothyroxine sodium)
Lexapro (escitalopram oxalate)
Lipitor (atorvastatin calcium)
lisinopril
lisinopril and hydrochlorothiazide
loratadine
lorazepam
Lotrel (amlodipine besylate, benazepril HCl)
lovastatin
meclizine HCl
metformin
methotrexate
methylprednisolone
metoclopramide HCl
metoprolol tartrate
metronidazole
minocycline HCl
MiraLax (polyethylene glycol 3350)
mirtazapine
naproxen sodium
Nasacort AQ (triamcinolone acetonide)
Nasonex (mometasone furoate)
Necon 1/35 (norethindrone, ethinyl estradiol)
Neurontin (gabapentin)
Nexium (esomeprazole magnesium)
Niaspan (niacin)
Norvasc (amlodipine)
nystatin
omeprazole
Omnicef (cefdinir)
Ortho Evra (norelgestromin, ethinyl estradiol)
Ortho Tri-Cyclen; Ortho Tri-Cyclen Lo (norgestimate, ethinyl estradiol)
oxycodone HCl and acetaminophen
OxyContin (oxycodone HCl)
paroxetine HCl
Patanol (olopatadine HCl)
Paxil; Paxil CR (paroxetine HCl)
Penicillin VK (penicillin V potassium)
Pepcid (famotidine)
Plavix (clopidogrel bisulfate)
potassium chloride
Pravachol (pravastatin sodium)

prednisone
Premarin (conjugated estrogens)
Prempro (conjugated estrogens, medroxyprogesterone acetate)
Prevacid (lansoprazole)
promethazine HCl
promethazine with codeine
propoxyphene napsylate and acetaminophen
propranolol HCl
Protonix (pantoprazole sodium)
Pulmicort (budesonide)
quinine sulfate
ranitidine HCl
Rhinocort Aqua (budesonide)
Risperdal (risperidone)
Seroquel (quetiapine fumarate)
Singulair (montelukast sodium)
Skelaxin (metaxalone)
spironolactone
Strattera (atomoxetine HCl)
sulfamethoxazole and trimethoprim
Synthroid (levothyroxine sodium)
temazepam
terazosin HCl
Topamax (topiramate)
Toprol XL (metoprolol succinate)
tramadol HCl
trazodone HCl
triamcinolone acetonide
triamterene and hydrochlorothiazide
Tricor (fenofibrate)
trimethoprim and sulfamethoxazole
Trimox (amoxicillin trihydrate)
TriNessa (norgestimate, ethinyl estradiol)
Tri-Sprintec (norgestimate, ethinyl estradiol)
Ultracet (tramadol HCl and acetaminophen)
Valtrex (valacyclovir HCl)
verapamil HCl, sustained-release form
Viagra (sildenafil citrate)
Vioxx (rofecoxib)
warfarin sodium
Wellbutrin SR (bupropion HCl)
Xalatan (latanoprost)
Yasmin (drospirenone, ethinyl estradiol)
Zetia (ezetimibe)
Zithromax (azithromycin dihydrate)
Zocor (simvastatin)
Zoloft (sertraline)
Zyprexa (olanzapine)
Zyrtec (cetirizine HCl)

B

APPENDIX

GENUS AND SPECIES NAMES COMMONLY USED*

GENUS AND SPECIES	DISEASE CAUSED BY THE ORGANISM/COMMON TERM (IF ANY)	GENUS AND SPECIES	DISEASE CAUSED BY THE ORGANISM/COMMON TERM (IF ANY)
Acanthamoeba keratitis		Chlamydia pneumoniae	
Achromobacter lwoffi		Chlamydia trachomatis	
Acinetobacter lwoffi		Chromobacterium amythistinum	
Acinetobacillus actinomycetem comitans		Cladosporium carrionii	chromomycosis
Actinomyces viscosus		Cladosporium trichoides	cladosporiosis
Aeromonas sobria		Clonorchis sinensis	liver fluke
Afipia felis		Clostridium botulinum	botulism
Alcaligenes bookeri		Clostridium difficile	
Alteromonas putrefaciens		Clostridium histolyticum	
Amoeba proteus		Clostridium perfringens	
Amoeba urinae granulata		Clostridium tetani	tetanus
Ancylostoma duodenale	hookworm	Coccidioides immitis	coccidioidomycosis
Aquaspirillum itersonii		Corynebacterium acnes	
Arcanobacterium haemolyticum		Corynebacterium diphtheriae	diphtheria
Ascaris lumbricoides	ascariasis	Corynebacterium xerosis	
Aspergillus auricularis	aspergillosis	Coxiella burnetii	
Aspergillus fumigatus		Cryptococcus neoformans	
Bacillus cereus	bacillosis	Cysticercus cellulosae	cysticercosis
Bacillus circulans		Cysticercus ovis	
Bacillus coagulans		Cysticercus tenuicollis	
Bacillus proteus		Dermatophagoides farinae	dust mite
Bacteroides fragilis	bacteroidosis	Dermatophagoides pteronyssinus	dust mite
Bacteroides funduliformis		Diplococcus mucosus	
Bacteroides melaninogenicus		Diplococcus pneumoniae	pneumonia
Bartonella bacilliformis		Echinococcus granulosus	echinococcosis/tapeworm
Bartonella elizabethae		Eikenella corrodans	
Bartonella henselae	cat-scratch fever	Endomyces capsulatus	
Bartonella quintana		Entamoeba coli	entamebiasis
Bordetella pertussis		Entamoeba gingivalis	
Borrelia buccalis		Entamoeba histolytica	amebic dysentery
Borrelia burgdorferi	Lyme disease	Enterobius vermicularis	pinworm/enterobiasis
Borrelia recurrentis			
Borrelia vincentii		Enterobacter liquefaciens	
Branhamella catarrhalis		Enterobacter sakazakii	
Brevibacterium linens		Enterococcus faecalis	
Brucella melitensis	brucellosis	Enterococcus faecium	
Brugia malayi		Escherichia coli	
Campylobacter fetus		Escherichia coli O157: H7	
Campylobacter jejuni		Fasciolopsis buski	fluke/fasciolopsiasis
Candida albicans	candidiasis	Franciella tularensis	
Candida glabrata		Friedlander's bacillus	
Cannabis sativa (common term is *marihuana*)		Gardnerella vaginalis	
Cardiobacterium hominis		Giardia lamblia	giardiasis
Cellvibrio fulvus		Haemophilus aegyptius	
Cellvibrio vulgaris		Haemophilus aphrophilus	

*For a more comprehensive list of genus and species names, please visit the Evolve website.

GENUS AND SPECIES	DISEASE CAUSED BY THE ORGANISM/COMMON TERM (IF ANY)	GENUS AND SPECIES	DISEASE CAUSED BY THE ORGANISM/COMMON TERM (IF ANY)
Haemophilus ducreyi		Mycobacterium immunogenum	
Haemophilus influenzae		Mycobacterium interjectum	
Haemophilus pertussis		Mycobacterium intermedium	
Haemophilus vaginalis		Mycobacterium kubicae	
Hafnia alvei		Mycobacterium lentiflavum	
Helicobacter pylori		Mycobacterium leprae	leprosy/Hansen disease
Herellea vaginicola			
Histoplasma capsulatum	histoplasmosis	Mycobacterium mageritense	
Iodamoeba buetschlii		Mycobacterium mucogenicum	
Isopora parasite		Mycobacterium novocastrense	
Ixodes dammini			
Ixodes pacificus		Mycobacterium palustre	
Kingella kingae		Mycobacterium phlei	
Klebsiella oxytoca		Mycobacterium triplex	
Klebsiella pneumoniae		Mycobacterium tuberculosis	tuberculosis
Lactobacillus acidophilus		Mycobacterium tusciae	
Lactobacillus bifidus		Mycobacterium wolinskyi	
Legionella bozemanii		Mycoplasma pneumoniae	pneumonia
Legionella dumoffii		Necator americanus	hookworm
Legionella feeleii		Neisseria gonorrhoeae	gonorrhea
Legionella gormanii		Neisseria meningitidis	cerebrospinal meningitis
Legionella jordanis			
Legionella longbeachae			
Legionella micdadei			
Legionella pneumophila	Legionnaire's disease	Neisseria mucosa	
Leishmania caninum	leishmaniasis	Nocardia asteroides	nocardiosis
Leishmania donovani		Onchocerca volvulus	roundworm/ onchocerciasis
Leptospira interrogans serovar pomona	leptospirosis		
		Paecilomyces variotii	
Malassezia furfur	pustulosis	Pasteurella pseudotuberculosis	
Micrococcus sedentarius			
Microsporum audouinii	ringworm/ microsporosis	Penicillium marneffei	
		Peptococcus magnus	
Microsporum canis	ringworm/ microsporosis	Plasmodium falciparum	
		Plasmodium malariae	malaria
Moraxella lwoffi		Plasmodium vivax	
Morganella morganii		Pneumocystis carinii	
Mycobacterium abscessus		Propionibacterium acnes	
Mycobacterium alvei		Proteus vulgaris	
Mycobacterium avium		Providencia rettgeri	
Mycobacterium bohemicum		Pseudallescheria boydii	
Mycobacterium branderi		Pseudomonas aeruginosa	
Mycobacterium confluentis		Pseudomonas exotoxin	
Mycobacterium conspicuum		Pseudomonas maltophilia	
Mycobacterium genavense		Pseudomonas stutzeri	
Mycobacterium goodii		Psorospermium haeckelii	
Mycobacterium gordonae		Rickettsia akari	
Mycobacterium hassiacum		Rickettsia burnetii	
Mycobacterium heckeshornense		Rickettsia prowazekii	
		Rickettsia quintana	
Mycobacterium heidelbergense		Rickettsia rickettsii	Rocky Mountain spotted fever

GENUS AND SPECIES	DISEASE CAUSED BY THE ORGANISM/COMMON TERM (IF ANY)	GENUS AND SPECIES	DISEASE CAUSED BY THE ORGANISM/COMMON TERM (IF ANY)
Rhizopus nigricans		Strongyloides stercoralis	threadworm/ strongyloidiasis
Rhodococcus equi			
Saccharomyces capillitii		Taenia lata	tapeworm
Salmonella choleraesuis		Taenia saginata	
Salmonella enteritidis	salmonellosis	Taenia solium	
Salmonella typhi	typhoid fever	Torula histolytica	
Schistosoma haematobium		Toxoplasma gondii	toxoplasmosis
Schistosoma japonicum		Treponema buccale	
Schistosoma mansoni		Treponema pallidum	syphilis
Serratia liquefaciens		Treponema vincentii	
Serratia marcescens		Trichinella spiralis	trichiniasis/ trichinosis
Shigella boydii			
Shigella dysenteriae	shigellosis	Trichomonas hominis	trichomoniasis
Shigella flexneri		Trichomonas vaginalis	
Staphylococcus aureus	bacteremia (SAB)	Trichophyton tonsurans	ringworm
Stenotrophomonas maltophilia		Trichophyton violaceum	
		Trichosporon beigelii	
Streptobacillus moniliformis		Trichuris trichiura	whipworm/ trichuriasis
Streptococcus faecalis			
Streptococcus milleri		Trombicula akamushi	
Streptococcus mitis		Trypanosoma cruzi	
Streptococcus pneumoniae		Ureaplasma urealyticum	
Streptococcus pyogenes		Wuchereria bancrofti	

HOMONYMS

Everyday Homonyms

Watch out for these homonyms. They can fool you and your spell-checker and turn up in your voice recognition documents.

abject	object	cell	sell	flee	flea
accept	except	cereal	serial	flow	floe
access	excess	choose	chews	flue	flew/flu
addition	edition	chord	cord	four	for
adverse	averse	cite	sight/site	fowl	foul
advice	advise	click	clique	freeze	frieze
aid	aide	coarse	course	gage	gauge
air	heir	concur	conquer	gaited	gated
ale	ail	confident	confidant	genius	genus
alfa	alpha	cue	queue	graft	graph
allude	elude	current	currant	great	grate
allusion	illusion/elusion	curser	cursor	guarantee	guaranty
alter	altar	dairy	diary	guessed	guest
area	aria	Dane	deign	hail	hale
assistance	assistants	deer	dear	hair	hare
assure	insure/ensure	defuse	diffuse	heal	heel
ate	eight	desert	dessert	hear	here
attendance	attendants	desperate	disparate	heard	herd
aught	ought	devise	device	heart	hart
averse	adverse	die	dye	heir	air
avert	evert/overt	disburse	disperse	him	hymn
awl	all	disc	disk (usually	hole	whole
axis	access		preferred)	holey	holy/wholly
baited	bated	discreet	discrete	hour	our
bale	bail	diseased	deceased	hue	hew
bare	bear	disparate	desperate	illicit	elicit
bases	basis	do	dew/due	illusion	allusion
been	bin	done	dun	illusive	elusive
beet	beat	dough	doe	imminent	immanent
bizarre	bazaar	earn	urn	incidents	incidence
blue	blew	edition	addition	ingenious	ingenuous
bore	boor/boar	ejection	injection	injection	ejection
born	borne	elicit	illicit	insure	assure/ensure
bow	beau, bough	elude	allude	invert	evert/avert
bowl	bole	elusion	allusion/illusion	irasible	erasable
bread	bred	elusive	illusive	its	it's
breadth	breath	eminent	imminent	jewel	joule
break	brake	ensure	assure/insure	kempt	kept
breathe	breath	envelop	envelope	knead	need
bur	burr	erasable	irasible	knew	new
bury	berry	eves	eaves	knot	not
but	butt	evert	avert/invert	know	no
buy	bye/by	ewes	use	knows	nose
callous	callus	excess	access	lacks	lax
canvas	canvass	fair	fare	lapse	relapse
cash	cache	farther	further	latitude	lassitude
casual	causal	faze	phase/phrase	lay	lei
cease	seize	feet	feat	led	lead (the metal)
cede	seed	fir	fur	leek	leak

lessor	lesser	pie	pi	statue	statute
liable	libel	piece	peace	steal	steel/stele
lightening	lightning/	phase	phrase/faze	straight	strait
	lighting	plane	plain	subtle	supple
loop	loupe	pole	poll	sum	some
load	lode	pray	prey	tale	tail
loath	loathe	precede	proceed	tea	tee
loose	lose	president	precedent	team	teem
lye	lie	principle	principal	theirs	there's
made	maid	queue	cue	then	than
mail	male	quite	quiet	there	their/they're
main	mane	rain	reign/rein	tick	tic
maul	mall	real	reel	time	thyme
maze	maize	red	read	tow	toe
mean	mien	reed	read	turn	tern
meet	meat	relapse	lapse	two	too/to
might	mite	rhyme	rime	urn	earn
miner	minor	right	rite/wright/write	vane	vain/vein
mist	missed	road	rode	veil	vale
muse	mews	roll	role	vial	vile
need	knead	root	route	wail	whale
new	knew	row	roe	wait	weight
no	know	rows	rose	waive	wave
nose	knows	rude	rood	ware	wear/where
not	knot	sale	sail	way	weigh
oar	ore	sax	sacks	we	wee
object	abject	seas	seize	week	weak
one	won/Juan	see	sea	wheal	wheel
ought	aught	seed	cede	when	wen
our	hour	seeks	Sikhs	while	wile
overt	evert/avert	seem	seam	whine	wine
owed	ode	seen	scene	whole	hole
pain	pane	sell	cell	wholly	holy/holey
pair	pare/pear	serial	cereal	whose	who's
palate	pallet/palette	sick	sic	wit	whit
pale	pail	sight	cite/site	would	wood
pause	paws	sleigh	slay	write	right/rite
peak	peek	slight	sleight	yolk	yoke
peal	peel	so	sow/sew	you	yew
pearl	purl	sore	soar	your	yore/you're
peer	pier	stationary	stationery		

Medical Homonyms

The following words are commonly encountered in medical transcription. The list is in alphabetical sequence with the homonyms indented and listed below each word. Abbreviated definitions are listed so that you do not have to refer to your medical dictionary unless you want to know a more detailed meaning.

abduction
  addiction
  adduction
  subduction

A drawing away from the midline.

aberrant
  afferent
  apparent
  efferent
  inferent

Wandering or deviating from the normal course.

aberration
  abrasion
  erasion
  erosion
  operation

Deviation from the usual course.

abrasion
  aberration
  erasion
  erosion
  operation

Denudation of skin.

abscess
  aphthous
  absence

A localized collection of pus, caused by infection.

absorption
  adsorption
  sorption

The uptake of substances into tissues.

acetic
  acidic
  ascites

sour, vinegary

acidic

acid forming

addiction
  abduction
  adduction

Dependence on a drug or some habit.

adduction
  abduction
  addiction

A drawing toward the midline.

adherence
  adhered to
  adherent
  adherents

The act or quality of sticking to something.

adsorption
  absorption
  sorption

A collection of a material in condensed form on a surface.

affect
  effect

To have an influence on; the feeling experienced in connection with an emotion.

affective *effective*	Pertaining to a mental state.

afferent
  aberrant
  efferent
	Conveying toward a center.

alveolar
  alveolate
  alveoli
  alveolus
  alveus
  alvus
  areolar
	Pertaining to an alveolus.

alveoli
  alveolar
  alveolate
  alveolus
  alveus
  alvus
  areolar
	Plural of *alveolus.*

alveolus
  alveolar
  alveolate
  alveoli
  alveus
  alvus
  areolar
	A small saclike dilatation.

alveus
  alveolar
  alveolate
  alveoli
  alveolus
  alvus
  areolar
	A trough or canal.

alvus
  alveolar
  alveolate
  alveoli
  alveolus
  alveus
  areolar
	The abdomen with its contained viscera.

amenorrhea
  dysmenorrhea
  menorrhagia
  menorrhea
  metrorrhagia
	Stoppage of the menses.

anecdote *antidote*	amusing story
antidote	remedy

antiseptic
   asepsis
   aseptic
   sepsis
   septic
	Preventing decay or putrefaction.

anuresis *enuresis*	Retention of urine in the bladder.

aphagia
   abasia
   aphakia
   aphasia
	Abstention from eating.

aphakia
   aphagia
   aphasia
	Absence of the lens of the eye.

aphasia
   abasia
   aphagia
   aphakia
   aplasia
	Loss of the power of expression by speech, writing, or signs.

aphthous *abscess*	Adjective form of *aphthae*, referring to small ulcers of oral mucosa.

aplasia
   aphasia
   aphagia
   aphakia
   abasia
	Lack of development of tissue or an organ.

apophysis
   epiphysis
   hypophysis
   hypothesis
	Bony outgrowth or process of a bone.

apposition *opposition*	The placing of things in juxtaposition or proximity.

arrhythmia
   erythema
   eurhythmia
	Variation from the normal rhythm of the heartbeat.

arteriosclerosis
   arteriostenosis
   atherosclerosis
	A disease characterized by thickening and loss of elasticity of arterial walls.

arteriostenosis
   arteriosclerosis
   atherosclerosis
	The narrowing or diminution of the caliber of an artery.

ascites
   acetic
   acidic
	Accumulation of serous fluid in the abdominal cavity.

atherosclerosis
   arteriosclerosis
   arteriostenosis
	A form of arteriosclerosis in which deposits of yellowish plaques containing cholesterol and lipoid material are formed on the inside of the arteries.

B

APPENDIX

atopic
  ectopic
Out of place or allergic.

aural
  aura
  ora
  oral
Pertaining to or perceived by the ear.

auscultation
  oscillation
  oscitation
  osculation
The act of listening for sounds within the body.

axillary
  auxiliary
Pertaining to the armpit.

bare
  bear
Naked.

border
  boarder
  quarter
A rim, margin, or edge.

bolus
  bullous
  bulbous
A rounded mass of food or a pharmaceutical preparation given by IV.

bowel
  bile
  vowel
The intestine.

breath
  breadth
The air taken in and expelled by the expansion and contraction of the thorax.

breathe
  breed
To take air into the lungs and let it out again.

bronchoscopic
  proctoscopic
Pertaining to bronchoscopy or to the bronchoscope.

bruit
  brute
A sound or murmur heard in auscultation.

bulbous
  bolus
  bullous
Bulb-like.

bullous
  bolus
  bulbous
Pertaining to large vesicles.

calculous
  calculus
  caliculus
  callous
  callus
Pertaining to, of the nature of, or affected with calculus.

calculus
  calculous
  caliculus
  callous
  callus
Any abnormal stony mass or deposit formed in the body.

B

APPENDIX

callous
calculous
calculus
callus
talus

Pertaining to a hardened, thickened place on the skin.

callus
calculous
calculus
callous
talus

A hardened, thickened place on the skin; formation of new bone between broken ends of a bone.

cancellous
cancellus
cancerous

Of a reticular, spongy, or lattice-like structure.

cancellus
cancellous
cancerous

Any structure arranged like a lattice.

cancer
canker
chancre

Malignant tumor.

cancerous
cancellous
cancellus

Pertaining to cancer.

canker
cancer
chancre

Ulceration, chiefly of the mouth and lips.

carbuncle
caruncle
furuncle

A cluster of boils; furuncles.

carpus
carpal
corpus

The wrist.

caruncle
carbuncle
furuncle

A small fleshy eminence, either normal or abnormal.

caudal
coddle

Pertaining to the tail.

cellular
sellar
seller

Pertaining to or made up of cells.

chancre
cancer
canker

The primary sore of syphilis.

choleic
colic

Pertaining to bile.

chordae
chordee

Plural form of chorda, a cord or sinew.

chordee *chordae*	Downward bowing of the penis.
choreal *chorial*	Pertaining to chorea.
chorial *choreal*	Pertaining to the outermost layer extraembryonic membrane.
cilium *psyllium*	Eyelash.
cirrhosis *cillosis* *psilosis* *psoriasis* *sclerosis* *serosa* *xerosis*	A degenerative disease of the liver.
coarse *course* *force*	Rough or crude; not fine or microscopic.
colic *choleic*	Pertaining to the colon or acute abdominal pain.
colposcopy *culdoscopy*	Examination of the cervix and vagina with a colposcope.
continence *continents*	Ability to refrain from urination or defecation.
contusion *concussion* *confusion* *convulsion*	A bruise.
cord *chord* *chorda* *cor*	Any long, rounded, flexible structure.
corneal *cranial*	Pertaining to the cornea of the eye.
corpus *carpus* *copious* *core* *corps* *corpse*	A human body; the body (main part) of an organ.
cranial *corneal*	Pertaining to the cranium (skull).
creatine *creatinine*	A compound formed in protein metabolism and found in most living tissue.
creatinine	A compound produced by metabolism of creatine and excreted in the urine.

culdoscopy
colposcopy

Visual examination of the female pelvic viscera by means of an endoscope.

cytology
psychology
sitology

The study of cells.

diaphysis
apophysis
diastasis
diathesis
epiphysis

Shaft of a long bone.

diastasis
diaphysis
diathesis

Dislocation or separation of two bones that are normally attached.

diathesis
diaphysis
diastasis

A predisposition to certain diseases.

dilatation
dilation

A dilated condition or structure.

dilation
dilatation

The process of dilating or becoming dilated.

discission
decision

Incision or cutting into.

dysphagia
dysbasia
dyscrasia
dysphasia
dysplasia

Difficulty in swallowing.

dysphasia
dysbasia
dyscrasia
dysphagia
dysplasia
dyspragia

Impairment of the faculty of speech.

dysplasia
dysbasia
dyscrasia
dysphagia
dysphasia
dyspragia

Abnormality in development of tissues or body parts.

dyspraxia
dystaxia
dystectia

Partial loss of ability to perform coordinated acts.

dystectia

Defective closure of neural tube.

ecchymosis
achymosis
echinosis
echomosis

A bruise.

ectopic
atopic

Located away from normal position.

edema
erythema

Excessive collection of watery fluid in body cavities.

effect
affect
defect

The result; to bring about.

effective
affective

Produce a specific result.

efferent
aberrant
afferent

Conveying away from a center.

efflux
reflex
reflux

Material flowing out.

ejection
injection
rejection

A sudden removal.

elicit
illicit

To cause to be revealed; to draw out.

embolus
bolus
embolism
thrombus

A mass of blood or other formed elements carried in the bloodstream.

eminence
imminence

A slight projection from the surface of the body.

endemic
ecdemic
epidemic
pandemic

Native or restricted to a particular region; an endemic disease.

enervation
denervation
innervation

Lack of nervous energy; removal or section of a nerve.

enteric
icteric

Pertaining to the small intestine.

enterocleisis
enteroclysis

Closure of a wound in the intestine.

enteroclysis

The injection of a nutrient or medicinal liquid into the bowel.

enuresis
anuresis

Involuntary discharge of urine.

epidemic
ecdemic
endemic

The rapid spreading of a contagious disease.

epiphysis
apophysis
hypophysis
hypothesis

Growth center at the end of a long bone.

erythema
   arrhythmia
   erythremia
   eurhythmia
   edema
Redness of the skin due to a variety of causes.

eschar
   a scar
   escharotic
   scar
A slough produced by a thermal burn or by gangrene.

everted
   inverted
Turned outward.

facial
   basal
   fascial
   faucial
   racial
Pertaining to the face.

fascial
   facial
   falcial
   fascia
   fashion
   faucial
Pertaining to fascia.

fauces
   facies
   feces
   foci
   fossa
   fossae
The throat.

fecal
   cecal
   fetal
   focal
   thecal
Pertaining to or of the nature of feces.

fetal
   fatal
   fecal
Pertaining to a fetus.

flanges
   phalanges
The projecting rim, collar, or ribs on an object.

flexor
   flexure
Any muscle that flexes a joint.

flexure
   flexor
A bent position of a structure or organ.

fovea
   phobia
A small depression in the retina of the eye where visual acuity is highest.

fundal
   fungal
Pertaining to the bottom or base.

fund
   fungi
Plural of fundus, a bottom or base.

fungal *fundal*	Of or caused by fungus.
furuncle *carbuncle* *caruncle*	A boil.
gastroscopy *gastrostomy* *gastrotomy*	Inspection of the stomach with a gastroscope.
gastrostomy *gastroscopy* *gastrotomy*	Artificial opening into the stomach.
gavage *lavage*	Feeding by stomach tube.
glands *glans*	Groups of cells that secrete or excrete material not used in their metabolic activities.
glans *glands*	Latin for gland.
hemolysis *homolysis*	Separation of hemoglobin from red blood cells.
heroin *heroine*	A drug, a derivative of morphine.
homolysis *hemolysis*	Destruction of cell by extracts of identical tissue.
humerus *humorous*	Upper arm bone.
hypercalcemia *hyperkalemia* *hypocalcemia*	An excess of calcium in the blood.
hyperinsulinism *hypoinsulinism*	Excessive secretion of insulin by the pancreas; insulin shock.
hyperkalemia *hypercalcemia* *hyperkinemia* *hypokalemia*	Abnormally high potassium concentration in the blood.
hypertension *hypertensin* *hypotension*	High blood pressure.
hypocalcemia *hypercalcemia* *hyperkalemia*	Reduction of the blood calcium level below normal.
hypoinsulinism *hyperinsulinism*	Deficient secretion of insulin by the pancreas.
hypokalemia *hypercalcemia* *hyperkalemia* *hyperkinemia*	Abnormally low potassium concentration in the blood.

hypophysis   Pituitary gland.
   apophysis
   epiphysis
   hypothesis

hypotension   Low blood pressure.
   hypertension

hypothesis   An unproved theory tentatively accepted to explain certain facts or to provide a basis for
   apophysis   futher investigation.
   epiphysis
   hypophysis

icteric   Pertaining to or affected with jaundice.
   enteric
   mycteric

ileac   Pertaining to the small intestine.
   iliac

ileum   Part of the small intestine.
   ilium

iliac   Pertaining to the hip bone.
   ileac

ilium   The flank bone or hip bone.
   ileum

illicit   Illegal.
   elicit

imminence   About to happen.
   eminence

infarction   The formation of an infarct.
   infection
   infestation
   infraction
   injection

infection   Invasion of the body by pathogenic microorganisms.
   infarction
   infestation
   inflection
   inflexion
   in flexion
   injection

infestation   Invasion of the body by small invertebrate animals, such as insects, mites, or ticks.
   infarction
   infection
   injection

injection   Act of forcing a liquid into a body part or organ.
   infarction
   infection
   infestation
   ingestion

innervation   The distribution of nerves to a part.
   enervation

instillation *installation*	Put a liquid into something; gradually establish an idea or attitude.
insulin *inulin*	Protein formed by the islet cells of Langerhans in the pancreas.
inulin *insulin*	A vegetable starch.
inverted *everted*	Turned inside out or upside down.
keratitis *keratiasis* *keratosis* *ketosis*	Inflammation of the cornea.
keratosis *keratitis* *keratose* *ketosis*	Any horny growth, such as a wart or a callosity.
ketosis *keratosis* *keratitis*	Abnormally high concentration of ketone bodies in the body tissues and fluids.
labile *labial*	Easily broken down or altered; emotionally unstable.
labial *labile*	Pertaining to a lip.
laceration *maceration* *masturbation*	Act of tearing; wound made by tearing.
lavage *gavage*	The irrigation or washing out of an organ.
lice *lyse*	Plural form of louse, a parasitic insect that lives on skin and hair.
lichen *liken*	A skin disease composed of small pimples or bumps close together.
lipoma *fibroma* *lipomyoma* *lymphoma*	A benign tumor composed of mature fat cells.
lithotomy *lithotony*	Incision of an organ for removal of a stone.
lithotony *lithotomy*	Creation of an artificial vesical fistula that is dilated to extract a stone.
liver *livor* *sliver*	A large dark-red gland in the upper part of the abdomen on the right side.
livor *liver* *rigor*	Discoloration.

lymphoma
  lipoma

Any neoplastic disorder of the lymphoid tissue.

lyse
  lice

To cause destruction of a cell or substance.

maceration
  laceration
  masturbation

The softening of a solid by soaking.

mastitis
  mastoiditis

Inflammation of the mammary gland (breast).

mastoiditis
  mastitis

Inflammation of the mastoid antrum and cells.

masturbation
  laceration
  maceration

Production of orgasm by self-manipulation of the genitals.

melanic
  melanotic

Pertaining to the unusual darkening of the skin caused by excessive production of melanin.

melanotic
  melanic

Excessive production of melanin in the skin or other tissue.

menorrhagia
  menorrhea
  metrorrhagia

Excessive uterine bleeding during menstruation.

menorrhea
  amenorrhea
  dysmenorrhea
  menorrhagia
  metrorrhagia

The normal discharge of the menses.

metacarpal
  metatarsal

Pertaining to the metacarpus.

metastasis
  metaphysis
  metastases (plural)
  metastasize
  metastatic

The transfer of disease from one site to another not directly connected with it.

metastasize
  metastases
  metastasis
  metastatic

To form new foci of disease in a distant part by metastasis.

metastatic
  metastases
  metastasis
  metastasize

Pertaining to metastasis.

metatarsal
  metacarpal

Pertaining to the metatarsus.

metrorrhagia
  menorrhagia
  menorrhea

Uterine bleeding at irregular intervals, sometimes being prolonged.

B

APPENDIX

modeling
mottling

Making a small representation of a person, thing, or building.

mottling
modeling

An irregular arrangement of spots or patches of color.

mucoid
Mucor
mucosa
mucosal

Resembling mucin.

mucosa
mucosal
mucosin
mucous
mucus

A mucous membrane.

mucosal
mucosa
mucous
mucus

Pertaining to a mucous membrane.

mucous
mucosa
mucosal
mucus

Pertaining to mucus (adjective).

mucus
mucosa
mucosal
mucous

A viscid watery secretion of mucous glands (noun).

myogram
myelogram

A recording or tracing made with a myograph.

necrosis
narcosis
nephrosis
neurosis

Death of tissue.

nephrosis
necrosis
neurosis

Any disease of the kidney.

neurosis
necrosis
nephrosis
urosis

Disorder of psychic or mental constitution.

obstipation
constipation
obfuscation

Intractable constipation.

oral
aura
aural

Pertaining to the mouth.

oscillation
auscultation
oscitation
osculation

A backward-and-forward motion; vibration.

oscitation
  auscultation
  excitation
  oscillation
  osculation

The act of yawning.

osculation
  auscultation
  escalation
  oscillation
  oscitation

To kiss; to touch closely.

osteal
  ostial

Bony.

ostial
  osteal

Pertaining to an orifice or opening.

palpation
  palliation
  palpitation
  papillation

The act of feeling with the hand.

palpitation
  palliation
  palpation
  papillation

Regular or irregular rapid action of the heart.

parasthenia
  paresthesia

A condition of organic tissue that causes it to function at abnormal intervals.

paresthesia
  pallesthesia
  parasthenia
  paresthenia

An abnormal sensation, such as burning or prickling.

parietes
  pruritus

The walls of an organ or body cavity.

parietitis
  parotiditis
  parotitis
  pruritus
  parietes

Inflammation of the wall of an organ.

Paris
  parous
  porous

The capital of France.

parotiditis
  parietitis
  parotitis

Inflammation of the parotid gland.

parotitis
  parietitis
  parostitis
  parotiditis

Inflammation of the parotid gland.

parous
  Paris
  pars
  porous

Having brought forth one or more living offspring.

pedicle	A footlike or stemlike structure.
medical	
particle	
peduncle	
pellicle	
perfusion	The passage of fluid through a membrane.
profusion	
pericardium	The membrane enclosing the heart.
precordium	
perineal	Pertaining to the perineum.
pectineal	
peritoneal	
peroneal	
perineum	The region at the lower end of the trunk between the thighs.
peritoneum	
peritoneum	The serous membrane lining the abdominal walls.
perineum	
peroneal	Pertaining to the fibula or outer side of the leg.
pectineal	
perineal	
peritoneal	
peronia	
phalanges	The bones in the fingers and toes.
flanges	
phobia	An irrational fear of or aversion to something.
fovea	
pleural	Pertaining to the covering of the lung and lining of the thorax.
plural	
pleuritis	Inflammation of the covering of the lung and lining of the thorax.
pruritus	
precordium	The thorax immediately in front of the heart.
pericardium	
prescribe	Advise or authorize the use of medicine or treatment.
proscribe	
profusion	Excess, surplus.
perfusion	
proscribe	Forbid.
prescribe	
prostate	A gland in the male that surrounds the neck of the bladder and the urethra.
prostrate	
prostrate	Lying flat, prone, or supine.
prostate	
pruritus	Severe itching.
parietes	
pleuritis	

psoriasis   Chronic dermatosis.
    cirrhosis
    cillosis
    psilosis
    sclerosis
    serosa
    xerosis

psychology   The science dealing with the mind and with mental and emotional processes.
    cytology
    sitology

psyllium   Plantain seed.
    cilium

pyelonephrosis   Any disease of the kidney and its pelvis.
    pyonephrosis

pyonephrosis   Suppurative destruction of the parenchyma of the kidney.
    pyelonephrosis

pyrenemia   The presence of nucleated red cells in the blood.
    pyoturia
    pyuria

pyuria   The presence of pus in the urine.
    paruria
    pyorrhea
    pyoturia
    pyrenemia

radical   Directed to the source of a morbid process, as radical surgery.
    radicle

radicle   Any one of the smallest branches of a vessel or nerve.
    radical

recession   The act of drawing away or back.
    resection

rectus   abdominal muscles; muscles controlling the movement of the eyeball.
    rhexis
    rictus

reflex   A reflected action; an involuntary muscular movement.
    efflux
    reflux

reflux   A backward or return flow.
    efflux
    reflex

refectory   A place for communal meals.
    refractory

refractory   Not yielding to treatment.
    refectory

resection   Excision of a part of an organ or other structure.
    recession

rhexis   The rupture of an organ or vessel.
    rictus
    rectus

rhonchi
   bronchi
   ronchi
	Plural of *rhonchus:* a rattling in the throat; a dry, coarse rale.

rictus
   rectus
   rhexis
	A fixed grimace or grin.

scar
   a scar
   eschar
   scarf
	A mark remaining after the healing of a wound.

scirrhous
   cirrhosis
   cirrus
   scirrhus
   sclerous
   serious
   serous
	Pertaining to a hard cancer.

scirrhus
   cirrhosis
   cirrus
   scirrhous
   sclerous
   serious
   serous
	Scirrhous carcinoma.

sedentary *sedimentary*	Sitting habitually.
sedimentary *sedentary*	Of, having the nature of, or containing sediment.

sellar
   cellular
   seller
	Pertaining to the sella turcica.

separation
   suppression
   suppuration
	Break; division; gap.

sepsis
   antiseptic
   asepsis
   aseptic
   septic
   threpsis
	The presence in the blood of pathogenic microorganisms or their toxins.

septic
   antiseptic
   asepsis
   a septic
   aseptic
   sepsis
   septal
   septile
   skeptic
	Produced by or resulting from decomposition by microorganisms.

B

APPENDIX

serosa
   cirrhosis
   xerosis
	Any serous membrane (tunica mucosa); tunica serosa; the chorion.

serous
   cirrus
   scirrhous
   scirrhus
   sclerous
   sera
   serious
   serose
	Pertaining to serum.

sheath *sheet*	A close fitting cover for something.
shoddy *shotty*	Badly or poorly made.
shotty *shoddy*	Resembling buckshot or B-Bs, e.g., shotty nodes.

sight
   cite
   -cyte (suffix)
   side
   site
   slight
	The act of seeing; a thing seen.

stasis
   bases
   basis
   station
   status
   staxis
	A stoppage of the flow of blood or other body fluid.

staxis *stasis*	Hemorrhage.

stroma
   soma
   stoma
   struma
   trauma
	The supporting tissue of an organ.

struma
   stoma
   stroma
	Goiter.

suppression
   separation
   suppuration
	The sudden stoppage of a secretion, excretion, or normal discharge.

suppuration
   separation
   suppression
   susurration
	The formation of pus.

sycosis *psychosis*	A disease marked by inflammation of the hair follicles; a kind of ulcer on the eyelid.

B

APPENDIX

tenia
  taenia
  Taenia
  tinea

A flat band or strip of soft tissue.

thenar
  femur
  thinner

The mound on the palm at the base of the thumb.

thrombus
  embolus

A blood clot that remains at the site of formation.

tinea
  linea
  linear
  taenia
  Taenia
  tenia

Ringworm.

trachelotomy
  tracheophony
  tracheotomy

The surgical cutting of the uterine neck.

tracheophony
  trachelotomy
  tracheotomy

A sound heard in auscultation over the trachea.

tracheotomy
  trachelotomy
  tracheophony
  tracheostomy

Incision of the trachea through the skin and muscles of the neck.

track
  tract

Series of marks or pathway (for example, needle track found on drug addicts or patients on dialysis).

tract
  track

A system of organs having some special function (for example, gastrointestinal tract); abnormal passage through tissue.

tympanites
  tympanitis

Distention of the abdomen as a result of gas or air in the intestine or in the peritoneal cavity.

tympanitis
  tenonitis
  tinnitus
  tympanites

Inflammation of the middle ear.

ureter
  ureteral
  urethra
  urethral

The tube that conveys the urine from the kidney to the bladder.

ureteral
  ureter
  urethra
  urethral

Pertaining to the ureter.

urethra
  ureter
  ureteral

The canal conveying urine from the bladder to the outside of the body.

urethral
ureter
ureteral
urethra

Pertaining to the urethra.

urethrorrhagia
ureterorrhagia

A flow of blood from the urethra.

uterus
ureter
urethra
urethral

The womb.

vaccinate
vacillate

Inoculate.

vacillate
vaccinate

To fluctuate.

vagitis
vagitus

Inflammation of the vagal nerve.

vagitus
vagitis

The cry of an infant.

vagus
valgus

The tenth cranial nerve.

valgus
vagus
varus
vastus

Bent outward, twisted, as in knock-knee (genu valgum).

variceal
varicella

Pertaining to a varix (an enlarged artery or vein).

varicella
variceal

Chickenpox.

varicose
verrucose
very close
very coarse

Pertaining to a varix (an enlarged artery or vein).

variolar
variola

Pertaining to smallpox.

venous
Venus

Pertaining to the veins.

Venus
venous

The goddess of love and beauty in Roman mythology; the planet second from the sun.

verrucose
varicose
verrucous
vorticose

Rough; warty.

verrucous
varicose
verrucose
vorticose

Rough; warty.

vesical
fascicle
vesica
vesicle
vessel

Pertaining to the bladder.

vesicle
fascicle
vesica
vesical
vessel

A small bladder or sac containing liquid.

vessel
vesical
vesicle

A tube or duct containing or circulating a body fluid.

villous
villose
villus

Shaggy with soft hairs.

villus
villose
villous

A small vascular process or protrusion.

viscera
visceral
viscus

Plural of *viscus*.

viscus
discus
vicious
viscera
viscose
viscous

Any large interior organ in any one of the three great cavities of the body.

womb
wound

The uterus.

wound
womb

An injury to the body caused by physical means.

xerosis
cirrhosis
serosa

Abnormal dryness.

B

APPENDIX

LABORATORY TERMINOLOGY AND NORMAL VALUES

Laboratory Terms and Symbols

The following are some of the more common laboratory terms and symbols.

TERM OR SYMBOL	MEANING
10^1	"Ten to the power of one"; shorthand for 10
10^2	100
10^3	1000
10^4	10,000 (If you cannot write superscript, you can write 10 exp 4.)
10^9	1,000,000,000
ABG	Arterial blood gases
ALT	Alanine aminotransferase, also known as serum glutamic pyruvic transaminase
C&S	Culture and sensitivity
cm^3	Cubic centimeter
cu cm	Cubic centimeter
cu mm	Cubic millimeter
dL (dl)	Deciliter
dm^3	Cubic decimeter
ESR	Erythrocyte sedimentation rate
IU	International units
MCH	Mean corpuscular hemoglobin
MCHC	Mean corpuscular hemoglobin concentration
MCV	Mean corpuscular volume
mm^3	Cubic millimeter
pH	Alkalinity or acidity of a solution; hydrogen ion concentration
PT	Prothrombin time, the test to check for one of the blood-clotting factors
RBC	Red blood cell count
rbc	Red blood cell
SGPT	See ALT
WBC	White blood cell count
wbc	White blood cell
μg	Microgram (1/1,000,000,000 gram)
μL (μl)	Microliter
μm	Micrometer
acid-fast bacilli	Organisms that cause tuberculosis and leprosy; bacteria from which acid does not wash out stain (e.g., Mycobacterium tuberculosis and Mycobacterium leprae)
agar	Stiffening agent in media
agglutination	Clumping together, as of blood cells that are incompatible
anisocytosis	Erythrocytes that are unequal in size and shape
assay	Measure of biologic activity
baseline	Denotes a test result obtained before onset of symptoms
basocyte	Undifferentiated or basophilic leukocyte
basophil(e)	Leukocyte that readily takes up basic (alkaline) dyes
battery	A group of tests performed together
blood gas analysis	Measure of the exchange and transport of gases in the blood and tissues
borderline	Result that is on the margin between normal and abnormal
buffy coat	A layer of white blood cells found between the plasma and the red blood cells in centrifuged samples of anticoagulated blood
concentration	Amount of a substance per unit volume
critical level	See panic level
electrolytes	Sodium, potassium, chloride, and bicarbonate (also called HCO_3)
en bloc	In one piece
erythrocytosis	Increase in the number of red blood cells
false-negative	Denotes the absence of a condition or disease that is actually present

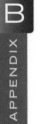

false-positive	Denotes the presence of a condition or disease that is not actually present
Gram stain	The standard staining procedure for the classification of bacteria (notice capital letter)
gram-negative	The characteristic of losing the stain
gram-positive	The characteristic of taking up the stain
granulocyte	A granular leukocyte
greater	Technical jargon for "more" or "higher"
in vitro	In the laboratory
in vivo	In the body
inoculation	Introduction of material into a medium or into a living organism
level	See concentration
medium	Substance in which a culture is grown
negative	Showing no reaction
normal range	Based on its own previous test results
normal	Within the normal range or limits
panel	A group of tests performed together
panic level	Markedly abnormal test result
parameter	Anything capable of being measured
plasma proteins	Albumin, globulin, fibrinogen, and prothrombin
plating	Placing material onto a solid medium in a Petri dish
positive	Having a reaction
profile	A group of tests performed together
rate	Change per unit of time
reference range	See normal range
serology	Study of antigen-antibody reaction with a variety of immunologic methods
shift to the left	An increase in the percentage of band cells
smear	Thin, translucent layer of material spread on a microscope slide and stained
STAT/stat	Immediately
streaking	See plating
therapeutic range	The range for medication that results the in best health benefits
time	Interval required for reaction to take place
titer	Highest dilution in a series that yields a positive result
turnaround time	Time that elapses between the ordering of a test and receiving the report of the results (abbreviated TAT)
value	Quantitative measurement of the concentration, activity, and other characteristics of specific substances

Note: Remember the following when you transcribe laboratory data and values: Some physicians dictate the word *lab* as a short form for *laboratory*, which is acceptable except in headings and subheadings.

Computerized Examinations

When laboratory tests are ordered, it is common to hear, for example, "Dr. Mendez ordered a SMAC test on Mrs. Garcia." The equipment that is used, the Sequential Multiple Analyzer Computer, can be abbreviated and typed as "SMAC," "SMA," or "Chem" (for chemistry). This study is a panel of chemistry tests; from 4 to as many as 22 tests can be performed on the blood specimen (e.g., SMAC-8, SMA-5, Chem-9).

Writing Laboratory Values

Use numbers to express laboratory values, but avoid beginning a sentence with a number. As discussed in Chapter 5, always place a zero (0) before a decimal (e.g., 0.6, not .6). Do not use commas to separate a laboratory value from the name of the test (e.g., hemoglobin 14.0). When typing several laboratory tests, separate related tests by commas, and separate unrelated tests by periods. If you are uncertain whether the tests are related, use periods. Use semicolons when a series of internal commas is present.

EXAMPLES

Red blood cell count 4.2, hemoglobin 12.0, hematocrit 37. Urine specific gravity 1.003, pH 5.0, negative glucose.

Differential showed 60 segs, 3 bands, 30 lymphs, 5 monos, and 2 basos; hemoglobin 16.0; and hematocrit 46.1.

Normal Values

Because normal values vary slightly from one laboratory to another depending on the type of equipment that is used, the values given throughout this section are approximate. Many values increase from threefold to tenfold during pregnancy. The brief forms and abbreviations given in parentheses throughout the section are acceptable for use in laboratory data sections of medical documents. The normal values shown here are expressed in conventional units. It is preferred to express a value as *normal for age* rather than as simply *normal*.

The following material concerns the tests and interpretations of the results of the tests on the specimens of blood (plasma, red blood cells, white blood cells, and platelets), urine, and stool.

Hematology Vocabulary

Various methods are used to collect blood samples, including capillary tubes and venipuncture (phlebotomy, the usual method).

Blood consists of the following components:

▶ Formed elements: red blood cells (erythrocytes that carry oxygen), white blood cells (leukocytes that fight infection), and platelets or thrombocytes (cells that aid in blood coagulation)

▶ Fluid part: plasma contains 90% to 92% water and 8% to 10% solids (e.g., carbohydrates, vitamins, hormones, enzymes, lipids, salts)

Hematology Tests and Values

The following information introduces you to laboratory terms used in medical reports that contain patient blood data.

TEST OR COMPONENT	NORMAL VALUES	CLINICAL SIGNIFICANCE OR PURPOSE
Haptoglobin	16 to 200 mg/dL	Decreases in hemolytic anemia; increases with certain infections
Hemoglobin (HG, Hgb, HGB)	Male: 14.0 to 18.0 g/dL Female: 12.0 to 16.0 g/dL 10-year-old: 12 to 14.5 g/dL	Increases with polycythemia, high altitude, chronic pulmonary disease; decreases with anemia, hemorrhage
Methemoglobin	0% to 1.5% of total hemoglobin	Used to evaluate cyanosis
Hematocrit (crit, HCT)	Male: 40% to 54% Female: 37% to 47% Newborn: 50% to 62% 1-year-old: 31% to 39%	Increases with dehydration and polycythemia; decreases with anemia and hemorrhage
White blood cell count (leukocyte count, WBC)	4,200 to 12,000/mm^3 Birth: 9.0 to 30.0 x 1000 cells/mm^3	Increases with acute infection, polycythemia, and other diseases; extremely high counts in leukemia; decreases in some viral infections and other conditions
Red blood cell count (erythrocyte count, RBC)	Male: 4.6 to 6.2 million/mm^3 Female: 4.2 to 5.4 million/mm^3	Increases with polycythemia and dehydration; decreases with anemia, hemorrhage, and leukemia

Corpuscular Values of Erythrocytes (Indices)

Note: Normal values are different at different ages.

TEST OR COMPONENT	NORMAL VALUES	CLINICAL SIGNIFICANCE OR PURPOSE
Mean corpuscular volume (MCV)	80 to 105 μm	Increases or decreases in certain anemias
Mean corpuscular hemoglobin (MCH)	27 to 31 pg/rbc	Increases or decreases in certain anemias
Mean corpuscular hemoglobin concentration (MCHC)	32% to 36%	Increases or decreases in certain anemias

Blood Gases

Blood gas values are used to measure the exchange and transport of the gases in the blood and tissues. Many disorders cause imbalances, such as diabetic ketoacidosis.

MEASUREMENT	ARTERIAL	VENOUS
pH	7.35 to 7.45	7.33 to 7.43
Oxygen (O_2) saturation	94% to 100%	60% to 85%
Carbon dioxide (CO_2)	23 to 27 mmol/L	24 to 28 mmol/L
Oxygen, partial pressure (PO_2 or pO_2)	80 to 100 mm Hg	30 to 50 mm Hg
Carbon dioxide, partial pressure (PCO_2 or pCO_2)	35 to 45 mm Hg	38 to 55 mm Hg
Bicarbonate (HCO_3)	22 to 26 mmol/L	23 to 27 mmol/L
Base excess	-2 to $+2$ mEq/L	—

Coagulation Tests

TEST OR COMPONENT	NORMAL VALUES	CLINICAL SIGNIFICANCE OR PURPOSE
INR (international normalized ratio) with PT (prothrombin time)	PT: 12 to 14 seconds INR range: 1.5-3.5	Most laboratories report PT results that have been adjusted to the INR for patients on anticoagulant drugs. These patients should have an INR of 2.0 to 3.0 for basic "blood-thinning" needs.
Sedimentation rate (ESR or sed rate)	*Wintrobe method* Male: 0 to 5 mm/hr Female: 0 to 15 mm/hr *Westergren method* Male: 0 to 15 mm/hr Female: 0 to 20 mm/hr	Increases with infections, inflammatory diseases, and tissue destruction; decreases with polycythemia and sickle cell anemia
Prothrombin time (PT)	12.0 to 14.0 seconds	Indicates ability of blood to clot for patients receiving anticoagulant drugs (e.g., warfarin [Coumadin] or heparin). These patients should have an INR of 2.0 to 3.0 for basic "blood-thinning" needs
Partial thromboplastin time (PTT)	35 to 45 seconds	Used to monitor heparin therapy
Fibrin split products (fibrin)	Negative at 1:4 dilution	Increases with disseminated intravascular coagulopathy
Fibrinogen	200 to 400 mg/100 mL	Increases with disseminated intravascular coagulopathy
Fibrinolysis	0	Increases with disseminated intravascular coagulopathy
Coombs test	Negative	Used to test infants born to Rh-negative mothers
D Dimer (a fibrin degradation fragment)	0-300 ng/mL	Used to help diagnose deep venous thrombosis (DVT), pulmonary embolism (PE), or disseminated intravascular coagulation (DIC)
Bleeding time Duke Ivy SimPlate	 1 to 5 min <5 min 3 to 9.5 min	 Used to test platelet function Used to test platelet function Used to test platelet function
Clot lysis time	None in 24 hr	Used to test for excessive fibrinolysis
Clot retraction time	30 to 60 min	Used to test platelet function
Coagulation time (Lee-White test)	5 to 15 min	Used to test for abnormalities in clotting
Factor VIII	50% to 150% of normal	Becomes deficient in classic hemophilia
Tourniquet test	Up to 10 petechiae	Used to detect vascular abnormalities

B

APPENDIX

Differential

This blood smear study determines the relative number of different types of white blood cells present in the blood; the total should equal 100%. A blood smear contains red blood cells, platelets, and white blood cells. The size and shape (structure) of these cells are also reported.

TEST OR COMPONENT	NORMAL VALUES	CLINICAL SIGNIFICANCE OR PURPOSE
Polymorphonuclear neutrophils	45% to 80%	Increases with appendicitis, myelogenous leukemia, and bacterial infections (polyps, segs, stabs, bands)
Lymphocytes (lymphs)	20% to 40%	Increases with viral infections, whooping cough, infectious mononucleosis, and lymphocytic leukemia
Eosinophils (eos or eosin)	1% to 3%	Increases with allergenic reactions, allergies, scarlet fever, parasitic infections, and eosinophilic leukemia
Monocytes (monos)	1% to 10%	Increases with brucellosis, tuberculosis, and monocytic leukemia
Basophils (basos)	0% to 2%	Increases in myeloproliferative diseases and inflammation. Basophils produce histamine during inflammatory reactions.
Myelocytes (myelos)	0%	Increases can indicate a malignancy such as chronic myelogenous leukemia. Not normally seen in the peripheral blood smear.
Platelets	150,000 to 350,000/mm^3	Increases with hemorrhage. Low platelet counts can result in uncontrolled bleeding. Very high platelet numbers can contribute to a blood clot forming in a blood vessel and can be involved in atherosclerosis.
Reticulocytes	25,000 to 75,000/mm^3	Decreases with leukemias

Morphology

The shape of the cells can be described with the following abbreviations: aniso (anisocytosis), poikilo (poikilocytosis), macro (macrocytic), micro (microcytic), and hypochromia.

Chemistry

TEST OR COMPONENT	NORMAL VALUES	CLINICAL SIGNIFICANCE OR PURPOSE
A1c levels	5% (6.5% or greater means a diagnosis of diabetes)	Measures average blood sugar levels over a three-month period by taking a sample of hemoglobin A1c molecules.
Albumin/globulin (A/G) ratio	1.1 to 2.3	This ratio is the calculation of serum albumin compared to serum globulin levels to determine whether there is an overproduction or underproduction of gamma globulin. A low A/G ratio could be multiple myeloma or other autoimmune disorder.
Globulin	1.5 to 3.7 g/dL	A type of protein found in the serum. Used in the calculation of the A/G ratio.
Albumin	3.0 to 5.0 g/dL	Decreases with kidney disease and severe burns.
Blood urea nitrogen (BUN)	10.0 to 26.0 mg/dL	Used to diagnose kidney disease, liver failure, and other diseases.
BMP (basic metabolic panel)	See individual tests	This frequently ordered panel of tests gives the physician important information about the current status of kidneys, BUN, creatinine, and acid/base balance. A group of 8 specific tests: glucose, calcium, sodium, potassium, CO_2, chloride, blood sugar, and electrolyte.
Calcium (Ca)	8.5 to 10.5 mg/100 mL	Used to assess parathyroid functioning and calcium metabolism and to evaluate malignancies.
Cholesterol, total serum	Normal: 200 mg/dL High: 200 to 240 mg/dL Borderline: 200-239 mg/dL High risk: >240 mg/dL	Increases with diabetes mellitus and hypothyroidism; decreases with hyperthyroidism, acute infections, and pernicious anemia.

Chemistry—cont'd

TEST OR COMPONENT	NORMAL VALUES	CLINICAL SIGNIFICANCE OR PURPOSE
High-density lipoproteins (HDL)	30 to 85 mg/dL	Has best correlation with development of coronary artery disease; decreased level indicates increase risk.
Low-density lipoproteins (LDL)	62 to 186 mg/dL	Greater than normal levels may be associated with increased risk of heart disease.
Creatinine, serum	0.7 to 1.5 mg/100 mL	Used to screen for abnormalities in renal function
Electrolyte panel		
Bicarbonate, serum (bicarb or HCO_3)	23 to 29 mEq/L	Bicarbonate is not usually tested by itself. The test actually measures the blood level of CO_2. During laboratory testing, HCO_3 is converted to CO_2. HCO_3 is important in neutralizing acids. Its concentration in the blood gives an idea of how well the kidneys and lungs can control acid/base balance.
Carbon dioxide (CO_2)	23 to 29 mEq/L	Most of the carbon dioxide in the blood is in the form of bicarbonate. Either term can be used.
Chloride (Cl)	96 to 106 mEq/L	Used to diagnose disorders of acid/base balance.
Potassium (K)	3.5 to 5.0 mEq/L	Used to diagnose disorders of water balance and acid/base imbalance.
Sodium (Na)	136 to 145 mEq/L	Used to diagnose acid/base imbalance.
Fasting blood glucose	70 to 110 mg/100 mL	Used to screen for abnormalities in carbohydrate metabolism.
Gamma-glutamyl transpeptidase (GGTP)	Male: <40 IU/L Female: <30 IU/L	A liver/biliary enzyme that is especially useful in the diagnosis of obstructive jaundice, intrahepatic cholestasis, and pancreatitis.
Glucose-tolerance test (GTT), fasting blood glucose	70 to 100 mg/dL 30 min: 120 to 170 mg/dL 1 hr: 120 to 170 mg/dL 2 hr: 100 to 140 mg/dL 3 hr: <125 mg/dL	Used to detect disorders of glucose metabolism.
Glycated hemoglobin (HbA1c) or A1c test	5% considered normal 6.5% or greater means diagnosis of diabetes	This blood test measures average blood sugar levels over several weeks and reports the result as a number. This number represents the percentage of damaged hemoglobin, which occurs as a result of consistently high blood sugars. Glycated hemoglobin is recommended for both checking blood sugar control in people who might be prediabetic and monitoring blood sugar control in patients with more elevated levels, termed diabetes mellitus.
Magnesium, serum	1.5 to 2.5 mEq/L	Essential for function of variety of enzymes and body processes. Hypomagnesemia (<1.5mEq/L) or deficiency states of Mg have been found in increased insulin resistance and have been shown to correlate with a number of chronic cardiovascular diseases, including hypertension, diabetes mellitus, and hyperlipidemia. Hypermagnesemia: Increased magnesemia (>2.5mEq/L) acute and chronic renal failure.
Phosphate	2.5 to 4.5 mg/dL	The body needs phosphorus to build and repair bones and teeth, help nerves function, and make muscles contract. Most (about 85%) of the phosphorus contained in phosphate is found in bones. The rest of it is stored in bones throughout the body. A high level of phosphate in the blood is usually caused by kidney disease, hypoparathyroidism, untreated diabetic ketoacidosis, or certain bone diseases. Low values can be caused by hyperparathyroidism, certain bone diseases, lack of vitamin D, severe burns, severe malnutrition or starvation.
Troponin Troponin complex	<0.4 ng/mL Peaks in 10-24 hours, begins to fall off after 1-2 weeks	Ordered for patients who have chest pain to see if they have had a heart attack or other damage to their heart.

B

APPENDIX

Immunoglobulins (Ig), Serum

TEST OR COMPONENT	NORMAL VALUES	CLINICAL SIGNIFICANCE OR PURPOSE
IgA	60 to 333 mg/dL	Involved in antibody responses.
IgD	0.5 to 3.0 mg/dL	Involved in antibody responses.
IgE	>300 ng/mL	Involved in antibody responses.
IgG	550 to 1900 mg/dL	Involved in antibody responses.
IgM	45 to 145 mg/dL	Involved in antibody responses.
Iron, serum	75 to 175 µg/dL	Ordered when physician is concerned about iron deficiency and anemia. Test measures amount of iron circulating bound to transferrin. TIBC and transferrin usually ordered with total serum iron.
Lipid panel (includes total cholesterol, triglycerides, HDL, and LDL)	See separate tests for normal values	Group of tests for determining risk of coronary heart disease.
Liver functions		
Acid phosphatase (ACP)	0 to 0.8 IU/L	Used to diagnose whether prostate cancer has spread to other parts of the body and to check the effectiveness of treatment. The test has been largely supplanted by the prostate specific antigen test (PSA).
Alkaline phosphatase, serum (ALP or alk. phos.)	30 to 130 IU/L	Used to diagnose liver and bone diseases.
Bilirubin (total)	0.3 to 1.1 mg/dL	Increases with conditions causing red blood cell destruction or biliary obstruction.
Direct bilirubin	<0.2 mg/dL	
Lactate dehydrogenase (LDH)	25 to 175 IU/L	Used to diagnose myocardial infarction and in differential diagnosis of muscular dystrophy and pernicious anemia
Alanine-aminotransferase (ALT [SGPT*])	10 to 45 IU/L	Used to detect liver disease; increases with acute pancreatitis, mumps, intestinal obstructions.
Aspartate aminotransferase (AST [SGOT†])	10 to 45 IU/L	Used to detect tissue damage; increases with myocardial infarction; decreases in some diseases; becomes elevated in liver disease, pancreatitis, excessive trauma of skeletal muscle.
Total protein	6.0 to 8.0 g/dL	Increases with liver diseases.
Triglycerides (TG), serum	10 to 170 mg/dL	Become elevated in atherosclerosis, liver disease, hypothyroidism, and diabetes mellitus.
Uric acid	2.2 to 7.7 mg/dL	Used to evaluate renal failure, gout, and leukemia.

*The abbreviation SGPT (serum glutamic pyruvic transaminase) is an older term and has been replaced by ALT (alanine aminotransferase). Both are transaminases and are used for liver function tests.

†The abbreviation SGOT (serum glutamic oxaloacetic transaminase) is an older term. AST (aspartate aminotransferase) may be used instead. Used for liver function tests.

Radioassays for Thyroid Functions

TEST OR COMPONENT	NORMAL VALUES	CLINICAL SIGNIFICANCE OR PURPOSE
Triiodothyronine (T3)	25% to 38%	Measures the amount of T3 hormone in the blood, part of a thyroid function evaluation.
Thyroxine (T4)	4.4 to 9.9 µg/100 mL	Can be ordered as a Total T4 and free T4. Can help evaluate thyroid function, either hyper- or hypothyroidism.
Thyroid-stimulating hormone (TSH)	0 to 3 ng/mL or 2 to 8 µIU/mL	Evaluates thyroid function and/or symptoms of hyper- and hypothyroidism. Usually ordered along with T4.

B

APPENDIX

Serology

TEST OR COMPONENT	NORMAL VALUES	CLINICAL SIGNIFICANCE OR PURPOSE
Antinuclear antibody (ANA)	Negative	Used to diagnose certain autoimmune diseases
C-reactive protein (CRP)	Negative	Increases in inflammatory diseases
Rheumatoid arthritis (RA) latex	Negative	Used to detect arthritis
Rapid plasma reagin (RPR)	Negative	Used to diagnose venereal disease
Venereal Disease Research Laboratory (VDRL)	Nonreactive	Used to diagnose venereal disease (syphilis)

Urinalysis Vocabulary

In a routine urinalysis, four types of examinations are performed:
1. Physical examination to measure volume, color, character, and specific gravity.
2. Chemical examination for determining alkalinity or acidity (pH), glucose, and albumin (protein) content.
3. Chemical tests, including tests for acetone, diacetic acid, urobilinogen, and bilirubin.
4. Microscopic examination for counting the white and red blood cells and identifying casts, cylindroids, epithelial (skin) cells, crystals, amorphous urates and phosphates, bacteria, and parasites.

Urinalysis Tests and Values

The following are laboratory terms used in medical reports that contain data on results of urinalysis.

Physical Examination and Chemical Tests

TEST OR COMPONENT	NORMAL VALUES	CLINICAL SIGNIFICANCE OR PURPOSE
Color	Yellow, straw-colored, or colorless	Redness could mean blood
Turbidity (clarity)	Clear	Cloudiness could mean bacteria or pus
Specific gravity (spec. grav.)	1.002 to 1.030	Measure of concentration depends on state of hydration
pH	4.5 to 8.0	Indicates the acidity or alkalinity of the urine
Nitrite	Negative	Indicates whether a bacterial infection is present
Protein or albumin	Negative	Indicates whether the kidneys are functioning properly
Glucose (sugar)	Negative	Indicates whether carbohydrates are being metabolized properly
Hemoglobin	Negative	Indicates whether the kidneys are functioning properly
Acetone or ketones	0 or negative	Indicates whether fats are being metabolized properly
Blood, occult	Negative	Indicates whether the kidneys are functioning properly
Bilirubin (bili)	0.02 mg/dL; negative	Indicates whether the liver is functioning properly
Urobilinogen	0.1 to 1.0 Ehrlich units/dL	Indicates whether the liver is functioning properly

Microscopy

TEST OR COMPONENT	NORMAL VALUES	CLINICAL SIGNIFICANCE OR PURPOSE
CELLS		
Red blood cells per high-power field (rbcs/hpf)	0 to 2/hpf	Increases with infections
White blood cells per high-power field (wbcs/hpf)	5/hpf	Increases with infections
Epithelial cells per high-power field (renal, caudate cells of renal pelvis, urethral, bladder, vaginal)	Few or moderate	Increases with infections
Bacteria per low-power field (yeast and bacteria)	Few or moderate	Increases with infections

Continued

Microscopy—cont'd

TEST OR COMPONENT	NORMAL VALUES	CLINICAL SIGNIFICANCE OR PURPOSE
CASTS (AND ARTIFACTS)		
Casts per low-power field (granular, fine, coarse, hyaline, leukocyte, epithelial, waxy, blood)	Negative	May form from kidney disorders
CYLINDROIDS		
Mucous threads	Few or moderate	In most cases, presence is benign
Spermatozoa	None	Presence indicates recent intercourse
Trichomonas vaginalis	None	Presence indicates infection with this organism
Cloth fibers and bubbles	None	Presence indicates poor collection

Crystals Found in Acid Urine

Note: Most crystals are normal; a few are considered abnormal and can be associated with diseases (e.g., cystine, tyrosine, leucine, and some drug crystals).

TEST OR COMPONENT	NORMAL VALUES
Crystals per low-power field (uric acid, amorphous urates, hippuric acid, calcium oxalate, tyrosine needles, leucine spheroids, cholesterin plates, cystine)	Few

Crystals Found in Alkaline Urine

TEST OR COMPONENT	NORMAL VALUES
Crystals per low-power field (triple phosphate, ammonium and magnesium, triple phosphate going in solution, amorphous phosphate, calcium phosphate, calcium carbonate, ammonium urate)	Few

PLURAL FORMS

The following list contains commonly used foreign or non–English-based singular and plural forms.

Singular	Plural	Singular	Plural
acetabulum	acetabula	cranium	crania
addendum	addenda	criterion	criteria
adnexum	adnexa	crux	cruxes
alga	algae	datum	data
alto	altos	dens	dentes
alumna	alumnae	diagnosis	diagnoses
alumnus	alumni	dialysis	dialyses
alveolus	alveoli	dictum	dicta
ameba	amebas	diverticulum	diverticula
amicus curiae	amici curiae	ecchymosis	ecchymoses
analysis	analyses	embolus	emboli
anastomosis	anastomoses	embryo	embryos
antrum	antra	encephalitis	encephalitides
apex	apices	exegesis	exegeses
aponeurosis	aponeuroses	enteritis	enteritides
appendix	appendices, appendixes	epididymis	epididymides
areola	areolae	exostosis	exostoses
artery	arteries	femur	femurs, femora
arthritis	arthritides	fetus	fetuses
atrium	atria	femoris	femora
axilla	axillae	fibula	fibulas
bacillus	bacilli	fimbria	fimbriae
bacterium	bacteria	fistula	fistulae, fistulas
base	bases	focus	foci
basis	bases	foramen	foramina, foramens
bona fide	bona fides	fornix	fornices
bon vivant	bons vivant	fossa	fossae
bronchus	bronchi	fundus	fundi
brucellosis	brucelloses	ganglion	ganglia
bulla	bullae	genius	geniuses
bursa	bursae	genu	genua
calculus	calculi	genus	genera
calix	calices	glandula	glandulae
calyx	calyces	glans	glandes
canthus	canthi	gyrus	gyri
caput	capita	haustrum	haustra
carcinoma	carcinomata, carcinomas	helix	helices
catharsis	catharses	hernia	herniae, hernias
cervix	cervices, cervixes	hilum	hila
cicatrix	cicatrices	humerus	humeri
chorda	chordae	ileum	ilea
coccus	cocci	ilium	ilia
comedo	comedones	index	indexes, indices (for numeric expressions)
compendium	compendiums		
conjunctiva	conjunctivae	iris	irides
cornea	corneae, corneas	ischium	ischia
cornu	cornua	keratosis	keratoses
corpus	corpora	labium	labia
cortex	cortices	lacuna	lacunae
crisis	crises	lamina	laminae

Seldom used.

Singular	Plural	Singular	Plural
larva	larvae	psychosis	psychoses
larynx	larynges	pubis	pubes
leiomyoma	leiomyomata	pudendum	pudenda
lentigo	lentigines	pupa	pupae
locus	loci	quantum	quanta
lumen	lumina, lumens	quorum	quorums
madam	mesdames	radius	radii
matrix	matrices	ratio	ratios
maxilla	maxillae	residuum	residua
maximum	maxima	rhinoplasty	rhinoplasties
meatus	meatuses, meatus	rhonchus	rhonchi
media	mediae (middle)	ruga	rugae
medium	media	sarcoma	sarcomata, sarcomas
medulla	medullae, medullas	sclera	sclerae
meningitis	meningitides	sclerosis	scleroses
meniscus	menisci	sepsis	sepses
metastasis	metastases	septum	septa
miasma	miasmas	sequel	sequels
milieu	milieux, milieus	sequela	sequelae
millennium	millennia	serum	sera
mitosis	mitoses	sinus	sinuses
mucosa	mucosas, mucosae	spermatozoon	spermatozoa
musculus	musculi	sputum	sputa
neurosis	neuroses	sternum	sternums
nucleus	nuclei	stigma	stigmata
mycelium	mycelia	stimulus	stimuli
naris	nares	stoma	stomata, stomas
nevus	nevi	stratum	strata
nucleus	nuclei	sulcus	sulci
oculus	oculi	syllabus	syllabuses, syllabi
optimum	optima	symposium	symposia
opus	opera	synopsis	synopses
os	ora (meaning mouths)	testis	testes
os	ossa (meaning bones)	therapy	therapies
ovary	ovaries	thesis	theses
ovum	ova	thorax	thoraces, thoraxes
papilla	papillae	trachea	tracheae
paralysis	paralyses	ulcus	ulcera
paries	parietes	ulna	ulnas
pars	partes	ultimatum	ultimatums
pelvis	pelves	umbilicus	umbilici
petechia	petechiae	ureter	ureters
phalanx	phalanges	urethra	urethras
phenomenon	phenomena	urinalysis	urinalyses
placebo	placebos	uterus	uteri
placenta	placentae	uvula	uvulas
pleura	pleurae	vas	vasa
plexus	plexuses	vena cava	venae cavae
pollex	pollices	verruca	verrucae
pons	pontes	vertebra	vertebrae, vertebras
prognosis	prognoses	vesicle	vesicles
prospectus	prospectuses	villus	villi
prosthesis	prostheses	virus	viruses
protozoon	protozoa	viscus	viscera
proviso	provisos	zygion	zygia

SHORT FORMS, BRIEF FORMS, AND MEDICAL SLANG

Throughout the following list, an asterisk (*) indicates that the short form should be written out. The remainder can be used as is, with site approval.

Short Form	Means
abd*	abdomen
abs*	abdominal muscles
adm*	admission
afib*	atrial fibrillation
alb*	albumin
alk*	alkaline
amb*	ambulatory
amp*	ampule
amp and gent*	ampicillin and gentamicin
amt*	amount
anes*	anesthesia
ant*	anterior
approx*	approximately
appy*	appendectomy (also *hot appy,* meaning an acute appendicitis)
art*	arterial line
bact*	bacteria (pronounced *back-tee*)
bands	band neutrophils
basos	basophils (a type of white blood cells)
benzos*	benzodiazepine
bili*	bilirubin
bili light*	bilirubin light
bio*	biology
brady*	bradycardia
cap gas*	capillary blood gas
caps	capsules
cath*	catheter
cathed*	catheterized
cauc*	Caucasian
chemo*	chemotherapy
coags*	coagulation studies
consult	consultation
cords*	vocal cords
cric*	cricothyrotomy
crit*	hematocrit
crypto*	cryptosporidium
C-section	cesarean section
cysto*	cystoscopy
DC*	discontinue or discharge; always write this out.
decub*	decubitus
defib*	defibrillated
dex*	dexamethasone
diff*	differential
dig* or dij*	digitalis
doc*	doctor
echo*	echocardiogram

Short Form	Means
echs*	ecchymoses (bruises)
emerg*	emergency
eos	eosinophils (a type of white blood cells)
epi*	epidural anesthesia or epinephrine
equiv*	equivalent
esp*	especially
e-stim*	electrical stimulation
eval*	evaluation
ex lap*	exploratory laparotomy
exam	examination
flu	influenza
fluoro*	fluoroscopy
frac*	fracture
frag*	fragment
freq*	frequency or frequent
glob*	globulin
H. flu*	Haemophilus influenzae, H. influenzae
H&H*	hemoglobin and hematocrit
head post*	examination of brain
hep lock*	heparin lock
hosp*	hospital
hot appy*	acute appendicitis
hypo*	hypodermic or injection
imp*	impression
infarct	infarction
inoc*	inoculate (pronounced *in-ock*)
inop*	inoperable (pronounced *in-op*)
kilo*	kilogram (kg; e.g., 6 kg, not 6 kilos)
lab	laboratory
lap*	laparotomy
lap chole*	laparoscopic cholecystectomy
lymphs	lymphocytes (a type of white blood cell)
lytes*	electrolytes
mag plus*	magnesium plus
max*	maximum
meds*	medications
mets*	metastases
metz*	Metzenbaum scissors
mikes*	microgram
monos	monocytes (a type of white blood cell)
multip*	multipara (a woman who has borne more than one child)

Short Form	Means	Short Form	Means
narcs*	narcotics	pulse ox*	pulse oximetry
neg*	negative	quads*	quadriceps muscle
nick you*	NICU (neonatal intensive care unit)	reg*	regular
		rehab*	rehabilitation
nitro*	nitroglycerin	romied*	ROMI (rule out myocardial infarction)
norm	normal		
nullip*	nullipara (a woman who has never borne a child)	Rx	prescription
		sats*	oxygen saturations
ODd*	overdosed	satting*	oxygen saturations
Oh neg*	O-negative blood	scrim*	discrimination
Ox sat*	oxygen saturation	script*	prescription
Pap smear/test	Papanicolaou smear or test	sec*	second or secondary
path*	pathology	sed rate	sedimentation rate
path lab*	pathology laboratory or department	segs	segmented neutrophils
		sick you*	SICU (surgical intensive care unit)
pecs*	pectoral muscles	sinus tack*	sinus tachycardia
peds*	pediatrics	snif unit*	SNF (skilled nursing facility)
plates*	platelets	spec*	specimen
pneumo*	pneumothorax	stabs	stab cells (band cells)
polys	polymorphonuclear leukocytes/granulocytes	staph	Staphylococcus (a bacterium)
		strep	Streptococcus (a bacterium)
pos*	positive	succs and fent*	succinylcholine and fentanyl
post*	postmortem examination or autopsy	subcu*	subcutaneous (usually referring to an injection)
postop*	postoperative	surg*	surgery or to perform surgery
preemie	premature infant	T max*	maximum temperature
preop*	preoperative	tabby*	therapeutic abortion
prep	to prepare	tabs*	tablets
prepped	prepared	tachy*	tachycardia
pressors	vasopressors (blood pressure medications)	temp*	temperature
		tibs, fibs, pops*	tibial, fibular, and popliteal
primip*	primipara (a woman who is bearing her first child)	tics*	diverticula
		t max*	maximum temperature
pro time	prothrombin time (blood clotting time)	tox screen*	toxicology screen test
		trach*	tracheostomy
procto*	proctoscopy	V fib*	ventricular fibrillation
psych*	psychology or psychiatry or mental health unit	V tach*	ventricular tachycardia
		vanc*	vancomycin
psych eval*	psychiatric evaluation	vitals*	vital signs

SOUND AND WORD FINDER TABLE

The following are some common examples of how English and medical terms sound phonetically and clues as to how the terms would be spelled to help you locate them in the medical dictionary. If you cannot find a word when you look it up, refer to this table and use another combination of letters that has the same sound.

IF THE PHONETIC SOUND IS LIKE	TRY THE SPELLING	EXAMPLES
a in *fat*	ai	plaid
	al	half
	au	draught
a in *sane*	ai	pain
	ao	gaol
	au	gauge
	ay	pay, x-ray, Tay-Sachs
	ue	suede
	ie	piedra
	ea	break
	ei	vein
	eigh	weigh
	et	sachet
	ey	they, peyote
a in *care*	ai	air, clairvoyant
	ay	prayer
	e	there
	ea	wear
	ei	their
a in *father*	au	aural, auricle, auscultation
	e	sergeant
	ea	heart
a in *ago*	e	agent
	i	sanity
	o	comply
	u	focus
	iou	vicious
aci in *acid*	acy	acystia
ak	ac	accident
	ach	achromatic
	acr	acromegaly
ark	arch	archicyte
b in *big*	bb	rubber
	pb	cupboard
bak in *back*	bac	bacteremia
bee	by	presbyopia
ch in *chin*	c	cello
	Cz	Czech
	tch	stitch
	ti	question
	tu	denture, fistula
d in *do*	dd	puddle
	ed	called
die	di	diagnosis, diarrhea
dis	dis	discharge
	dys	dyspnea

IF THE PHONETIC SOUND IS LIKE	TRY THE SPELLING	EXAMPLES
dew	deu	deuteropathy
	dew	dewlap
	du	dura
e in *get*	a	any
	ae	aesthetic
	ai	said
	ay	says
	e	edema
	ea	head
	ei	heifer
	eo	leopard
	ie	friend
	oe	roentgen
	u	burial
e in equal	ae (British spelling)	haemoglobin
	ay	quay
	ea	lean
	ee	free
	ei	deceit
	eo	people
	ey	key
	i	hemicardia
	ie	siege
	oe	amoeba
	y	tracheotomy
e in *here*	ea	ear
	ee	cheer
	ei	weird
	ie	bier
ek	ec	lectotype, eczema
	ek	ekphorize
er in *over*	ar	liar
	ir	elixir
	or	author, labor
	our	glamour
	re	acre
	ur	augur
	ure	measure
	yr	zephyr
eri, ere, aire	ery	erythrocyte, erythema
you	eu	euphoria, eugenic
ex	ex	extravasation
	x	x-ray
f in *fine*	ff	cliff
	gh	laugh, slough
	lf	half
	ph	physiology, prophylactic
fizz	phys	physical
floo, flu	flu	fluoride, fluoroscopy
g in go	gg	egg
	gh	ghost
	gu	guard
	gue	prologue
gli in *glide*	gly	glycemia

B

APPENDIX

IF THE PHONETIC SOUND IS LIKE	TRY THE SPELLING	EXAMPLES
grew	grou	group
guy (also see *jin*)	gy	gynecomastia
h in *hat*	g	Gila monster
	wh	who, whooping (cough)
he	he	hematoma
	hae (British spelling)	haematology
hi in *high*	hy	hydrocele
i in *it*	a	usage
	e	English
	ee	been
	ia	carriage
	ie	sieve
	o	women
	u	busy
	ui	built
	y	laryngeal, nystagmus
i in *kite*	ai	guaiac
	ay	aye
	ei	height, meiosis
	ey	eye
	ie	tie
	igh	nigh
	is	islet (of Langerhans)
	uy	buy
	y	myograph
	ye	rye
ik or ick	ich	ichthyosis
ink	inc	incubator
j in *jam*	d	gradual
	dg	judge
	di	soldier
	dj	adjective
	g	register, fungi
	ge	vengeance
	gg	exaggerate
gin	gyn	gynecology
k in *keep*	c	eczema
	cc	account
	ch	chronic tachycardia
	ck	tack
	cq	acquire
	cu	biscuit
	lk	walk
	qu	liquor
	que	plaque
key	che	chemotherapy
	chy	ecchymosis
ko	cho, co	cholecyst, colon
kon	chon	chondroma
	con	condyloma
kw in *quick*	ch	choir
	qu	quintuplet
l in *let*	ll	call
	sl	isle

IF THE PHONETIC SOUND IS LIKE	TRY THE SPELLING	EXAMPLES
la in *lay*	lay	layette
	le	lei
lack	lac	lacrimal
loo	leu	leukocyte
	lew	lewisite
m in *me*	chm	drachm
	gm	phlegm
	lm	balm
	mb	limb
	mm	hammer toe
	mn	hymn
mass	mac	macerate
mix	myx	myxedema
n in *no*	cn	cnemial
	gn	gnathic
	kn	knife
	mn	mnemonic
	nn	tinnitus
	pn	pneumonia
ng in *ring*	ngue	tongue
new	neu	neurology
	pneu	pneumococcus
o in *go*	au	mauve
	eau	beau
	eo	yeoman
	ew	sew
	oa	foam
	oe	toe
	oh	ohm
	oo	brooch
	ou	shoulder
	ough	dough
	ow	row
o in *long*	a	all
	ah	Utah
	au	fraud
	aw	thaw
	oa	broad
	ou	ought
off	oph	exophthalmos, ophthalmology
oi in *oil*	oy	boy
oks	occ	occiput
	ox	oxygen
oo in *tool*	eu	leukemia
	ew	drew
	o	move
	oe	shoe
	ou	group
	ough	through
	u	rule, tularemia
	ue	blue
	ui	bruise

IF THE PHONETIC SOUND IS LIKE	TRY THE SPELLING	EXAMPLES
oo in *look*	o	wolffian
	ou	would
	u	pull, tuberculosis
ow in *out*	ou	mouth
	ough	bough
	ow	crowd
p in *put*	pp	happy
pack	pach	myopachynsis, pachyderma
pi in *pie*	py	nephropyosis
r in *red*	rh	rhabdocyte
	rr	berry
	rrh	cirrhosis, hemorrhoid
	wr	wrong, wrist
re in *repeat*	rhe	rheostosis
	ri	malaria
	rrhe	otorrhea
rew	rheu	rheumatism
	rhu	rhubarb
rom	rhom	rhomboid
rye	rhi	rhinoplasty
s in *sew*	c	cyst, foci
	ce	rice
	ps	psychology
	sc	sciatic, viscera
	sch	schism
	ss	miss
	sth	isthmus
sh in *ship*	ce	ocean
	ch	chancre
	ci	facial
	s	sugar
	sch	Schwann cell
	sci	fascia
	se	nauseous
t in *tea*	pt	pterygium, ptosis
zh in *azure*	ge	garage, massage, curettage
	s	vision
	si	fusion
	zi	glazier
zi (rhymes with *sigh*)	zy	zygoma, zygote, enzyme
	x	xiphoid
zz	ss	scissors
	zz	buzz

B

APPENDIX

As an additional spelling aid, here are groups of letter combinations that can cause problems when you are trying to locate a word.

If You Have Tried...	*Then Try...*
pre	per, pra, pri, pro, pru
per	par, pir, por, pur, pre, pro
is	us, ace, ice
ere	ear, eir, ier
wi	whi
we	whe
zi	xy
cks, gz	x
tion	sion, cion, cean, cian
le	tle, el, al
cer	cre
si	psi, ci
ei	ie
x	eks
z	xe
dis	dys
ture	teur
tious	seous, scious
air	are, aer
ny	gn, n
ance	ence
ant	ent
able	ible
fizz	phys

STATE NAMES AND OTHER US POSTAL SERVICE ABBREVIATIONS

Two-Letter State Abbreviations for the US and Its Dependencies

Alabama	AL	Kentucky	KY	Ohio	OH
Alaska	AK	Louisiana	LA	Oklahoma	OK
Arizona	AZ	Maine	ME	Oregon	OR
Arkansas	AR	Maryland	MD	Pennsylvania	PA
California	CA	Massachusetts	MA	Puerto Rico	PR
Canal Zone	CZ	Michigan	MI	Rhode Island	RI
Colorado	CO	Minnesota	MN	South Carolina	SC
Connecticut	CT	Mississippi	MS	South Dakota	SD
Delaware	DE	Missouri	MO	Tennessee	TN
District of Columbia	DC	Montana	MT	Texas	TX
Florida	FL	Nebraska	NE	Utah	UT
Georgia	GA	Nevada	NV	Vermont	VT
Guam	GU	New Hampshire	NH	Virginia	VA
Hawaii	HI	New Jersey	NJ	Virgin Islands	VI
Idaho	ID	New Mexico	NM	Washington	WA
Illinois	IL	New York	NY	West Virginia	WV
Indiana	IN	North Carolina	NC	Wisconsin	WI
Iowa	IA	North Dakota	ND	Wyoming	WY
Kansas	KS				

Two-Letter Abbreviations for Canadian Provinces and Territories

Alberta	AB	Nova Scotia	NS
British Columbia	BC	Ontario	ON
Manitoba	MB	Prince Edward Island	PE
New Brunswick	NB	Quebec	QC
Newfoundland and Labrador	NL	Saskatchewan	SK
Northwest Territories	NT	Yukon Territory	YT

B

APPENDIX

TRADEMARKED FORMS (PACKAGING, DOSAGE FORMS, AND DELIVERY SYSTEMS) USED WITH DRUG NAMES*

Abbo-Pac
Accu-Pak
Act-O-Vial
ADD-Vantage
Adria-Oncoline Chemo-Pin
ADT
AeroChamber
Aerolizer
Aerotrol
Appli-Kit
Appli-Ruler
Appli-Tape
Arm-A-Med
Arm-A-Vial
Aspirol
Atrigel
Atrigel Depot
Autoject2
Back-Pack
Betaject 3
bidCAP
Brik-Paks
Bristoject
Capsulets
Carpuject
Carpuject Smartpak
Cartrix
Chemo-Pin
Chronosule
Chronotab
click·easy
Clinipak
Compack
ControlPak
cool.click
CycloTech
Delcap
Detecto-Seal
Dey-Dose
Dey-Lute
Dialpak
Dis-Co Pack
Diskets
Diskhaler
Diskus
Dispenserpak
Dispertab
Dispette
Dispos-a-Med

Divide-Tab
Dividose
D-Lay
Dosa-Trol Pack
Dosepak
Dosette
Dospan
Drop-Dose
Dropperettes
Drop-Tainers
Dulcet
Duracaps
DuraSite
DuraSolv
Dura-Tab
DUROS
EasyInjector
Enduret
Enseal
EN-tab
Entri-Pak
Expidet
Extencap
Extentab
Faspak
Fast-Trak
Filmlok
Filmseal
Filmtabs
FlashDose
FlexPen
Flo-Pack
Gelseal
Glossets
Gradumet
Gy-Pak
Gyrocap
HandiHaler
HumaPen
HumatroPen
Hyporet
Identi-Dose
Infatab
Inhal-Aid
Inject-all
Inlay-Tabs
InspirEase
Intensol
Iofoam

Isoject
Kapseal
Kronocap
KwikPen
Lanacaps
Lanatabs
Lederject
Linguets
Liqui-Gels
Liquitab
Lozi-Tabs
Luer-lock
Lyo-Ject
MDI
Memoir
Memorette
Microcaps
Min-I-Mix
Mistometer
Mix-O-Vial
Mono-Drop
Monovial
NewPaks
NordiPen
Nu-knit
Nursette
Ocudose
Ocumeter
OptiPen One
Oralet
OROS
Ovoid
Partaject
Pastilles
PenFill
PenInject
Perles
Pilpak
Plateau Cap
Pockethaler
Prefill
PulsePak
Pulvule
Quicklets
Rapimelt
RapiTabs
Redi Vial
Rediject
Redipak

*Compiled from Drake E: *Saunders pharmaceutical word book 2010,* St Louis, 2010, Saunders.

RediTabs
Repetab
Rescue Pak
Respihaler
RespiPak
Respirgard II
Respules
Robicap
Robitab
Rotacaps
Rotadisk
RxPak
SandoPak
Sani-Pak
Secule
Select-A-Jet
Sequels
SeraJet
SigPak
SingleJect
Slocaps
SmartMist
SnapTab
Softabs
SolTabs
Soluspan
Solvet
Spancaps

Spansule
Sprinkle Caps
STATdose
Stat-Pak
Steri-Dose
Steri-Vial
Sterules
Supprette
Supule
Tabloid
Tabules
Tamp-R-Tel
Taperpak
Tel-E-Amp
Tel-E-Dose
Tel-E-Ject
Tel-E-Pak
Tel-E-Vial
Tembid
Tempule
Ten-Tab
TetraBriks
TetraPaks
Thera-Ject
Tiltab
Timecap
Timecelle
Timespan

Timesules
Titradose
Traypak
T-Tabs
Tubex
Turbinaire
Turbuhaler
UDIP
U-Ject
Ultra Vent
Uni-Amp
Unimatic
Uni-nest
Unipak
Uni-Rx
Unisert
Univial
Vaporole
Veridate
Viaflex
Vision
Visipak
Wallette
WOWtabs
Wyseal
Z-Pak
Zydis

UNUSUAL MEDICAL TERMS COMMONLY DICTATED IN MEDICAL REPORTS

After mastering a beginning terminology course and embarking on a transcription career, you will probably be taken aback when you hear the physician or dictator giving you an unusual expression, such as "coffee-ground stools." The dictation could be quite clear and you could probably type the expression without difficulty but with a question in your mind concerning what you "really" heard. Or it could be that the dictation is not clear, and you forge ahead looking for the words in a medical or English reference. Chances are that you will not find the expression. More than 100 unusual terms commonly dictated in medical reports are listed here to help you with puzzling dictation.

acorn-tipped catheter
Adam's apple
aerobic deafness
airborne gap
ALARM
alligator clamp
Ambu bag
anal wink
anchovy
angle of Louis
apple peel syndrome
argyle tube
ash leaf spots (eye)
BABYbird respirator
BabyFace ultrasound
BackBiter
bagged
balloon-on-a-wire
banana blade knife
banjo-string adhesions
baseball stitch
basement membrane
Battle's sign
batwing arms
beat knee syndrome
beaver fever
berry aneurysm
Best clamps
bikini bottom
Billroth II (procedure)
birdcage splint
Bird machine (on the Bird)
Bird's Nest filter
bird-like facies
bishop's nod
black comet's artifact
black doggie clamps
black hairy tongue
black heel
Blessed-Dementia Information-Memory-
  Concentration Test
blown pupil
blowout fracture
blue bloaters

blue diaper syndrome
blue dot sign
blue toe syndrome
blueberry muffin baby
boat hook
boggy uterus
bone wax
bony thorax
bookoo
boss (surface)
bow-tie sign
boxer's nose
bread-and-butter heart
bronze diabetes
bubble boy disease
bubble hair
bucket-handle tear
buffalo hump
buffy coat
bulldog clamp
bull's eye lesion
Bunny boot
buried bumper syndrome
butcher's broom
butterfly bumper syndrome
butterfly needle
CABG (pronounced "cabbage")
CAT scan
café au lait spots
cake mix kit
chain cystogram
Chance fracture
chandelier sign
charley horse
cherry angioma
chocolate agar
chocolate cyst
choked disc (or disk)
Christmas disease
cigarette (or cigaret) drain
circle of death
clap (gonorrhea)
clergyman's knee
clog (clot of blood)

clue cell
cobblestoning mucosa
cobra head plate
Coca-Cola–colored urine
coffee-ground stools or emesis
cogwheel breathing
cogwheel gait
cogwheel rigidity or motion
coin test
collar-button abscess
collar-button appearance
comb sign
corn cockle
corn picker's pupil
cottonoid patty
cowboy collar
COWS
cracked pot sound
cracker test
cradle cap
crick
currant jelly stools
DAD
Dandy scissors
dawn phenomenon
devil's bones
devil's pinches
Dis-Co Pack
dog-boning complication
doll's eye movements
DOOR syndrome
double bubble sign
double whammy syndrome
drawer sign
dripping candle appearance
duck waddle test
dumbbell tumor
dumping syndrome
echo sign
fat depot
fat pad
fat towels (wound towels)
fern test (an estrogen test)
finger clubbing
finger dissection
fish fancier's finger
fish tank granuloma
fish-mouthed cervix
flashers and floaters (eye examination)
49er brace (a knee brace)
frank breech position
frown incision
gallops, thrills, and rubs
game leg
Gelfoam cookie

gift wrap suture
gimpy (lame)
glitter cells
glove-juice technique
Goodenough test
goose egg (swelling caused by blunt trauma)
gull-wing sign
gulper's gullet
gum ball headache
guy suture
haircut (syphilitic chancre)
hair-on-end sign
hammock configuration
hanging drop test
hedgehog molecule
HELLP syndrome
hickey
Hickey-Hare test
His (bundle)
hot cross bun deformity
hot potato voice
incidentaloma
in-the-bag lens implantation
jackstone calculus
jogger's nipples
joint mice
joker (instrument)
kangaroo care
Kerley's B lines (costophrenic septal lines)
Kerley's C lines
keyhole surgery
kick counts
kink artifact
kissing spine
kissing-type artifact
lacer cock-up (splint)
leather bottle stomach
lemon squeezer (instrument)
listing gait
little leaguer's elbow
Little lens
locked-in syndrome
locker room syndrome
loofah folliculitis
loose body
maple syrup urine disease (MSUD)
march fracture
mare's tail
meat wrapper's asthma
Mercedes sign
Mill-house murmur
moth-eaten appearance
mouse (periorbital ecchymosis)
mouse units
MUGA

mulberry molars
Mule vitreous sphere
musical bruit
Mustard procedure
mute toe sign
napkin-ring obstruction
nutcracker esophagus
nutmeg liver
octopus test
onion peel sensory loss
orphan drug
outrigger (orthopedic)
ox cell hemolysin test
oyster (mass of mucus coughed up)
pantaloon hernia
pants-over-vest (technique)
parrot beak tear
past-pointing test
patient flat lined ("expired" is preferred)
pawpaw
peanut (a small surgical gauze sponge)
pencil-in-cup deformity
PERLA or PERRLA
piggyback probe
pigtail catheter
piles (hemorrhoids)
pill esophagitis
pill-rolling (tremor)
pink puffer
pins and needles (paresthesias)
pizza lung
plus disease
polly-beak
pollywogs
POP (plaster of paris)
pop-off needle
porcelain gallbladder
port-wine stain
postage stamp type skin graft
prep or prepped (from the word "prepared")
prostate, boggy
proudflesh (granulation tissue)
prune belly syndrome
puddle sign
pulmonary toilet
purse-string mouth
purse-string suture
pyknic habit (short, stocky body build)
rabbit nose
rabbit stools
raccoon eyes
rice-water stools
rocker-bottom foot
rooting reflex
rubber booties

Rufus and Ruby
rugger jersey sign
runner's rump
running off (diarrhea)
sago spleen
salmon flesh excrescences
sand (encrusted secretions about the eyes)
saucerize (refers to suturing a cyst inside out so that it will heal)
sausage fingers
Scotty dog's ear
sea bather's eruption
seagull bruit
setting sun sign
shiner
shoelace suturing
shotty nodes
sick building syndrome
silhouette sign or Golden's S sign
silver fork deformity
simian crease (seen in Down syndrome)
Sippy diet
skin wheals
skinny needle or Chiba needle
sky suture
sleep (inspissated mucus about the eyes)
Slinky catheter
smile or smiling incision
smoker's face
snowball opacities
snowbanks
snuff box
SOAP note
speed dissection
spoon nails
starry-sky pattern
steeple sign (on chest x-ray)
stick-tie
stonebasket
stoved (of a finger), means stubbed
strawberry gallbladder
strawberry hemangioma
strawberry tongue
string sign
sucked candy bone
sugar-tong plaster splint
sugar-tongs (instrument)
"surf" test (surfactant test of amniotic fluid)
sundown syndrome
swan-neck catheter
swimmer's view
tailor's bunion
tailor's seat
tennis elbow
ThumZ' up (thumbs)

tincture of time
Tomocat
trick (of a joint), means unstable
trigger finger
tumor plot
two-flight dyspnea
two-pillow orthopnea
vaginal candle
walking pneumonia
washerwoman's skin
watermelon stomach

weaver's bottom
wet mount
whistletip catheter
wing suture
witches' milk
wrinkle artifact
yoga foot drop
yuppie flu
ZEEP (zero end-respiratory pressure)
zit (comedo)

APPENDIX C

Medical Documents

This appendix is a collection of figures showing the formats of various documents found in medical records or in medical institutions. This collection gives you the opportunity to see that the styles vary considerably. All of the documents included are authentic in every way; only the patient data, names of physicians, dictators, place names, and institutions have been fictionalized. The documents were not edited to conform to the style or formats taught in the text. The examples are provided to give you an idea of the variety that exists in executing documents and to encourage you to streamline your own formats. Some of the documents are consistent in organization. A few are very "busy," with the use of underlining, boldface, and full capital letters to no clear purpose. As stated in the chapter work, have a reason for the style you use. Some medical transcriptionists (MTs) who provided these documents remarked that they are required by the client to use the certain style shown in their documents. Some liked it; others did not. The idea that the institution is working to simplify and coordinate the style and format of all documentation is great as long as the format chosen is clean, easy to read, and not cumbersome to follow. At this time, there is no standard for formats, but work is being done on the issue. With the advent of the electronic medical record, it is vital that documents be consistent.

The second reason for this collection is to provide you with some experience with medical record documents themselves. The documents range from the initial visit to the discharge summary. The MTs and others who so graciously provided these documents knew that you would be able to benefit, and that is why they took the time to carefully remove any identifying data from a record before it left the facility and became available for reproduction here. Approximately 20 facilities participated in this endeavor, including hospitals, large and small transcription services, emergency departments, acute care facilities, private medical offices, specialty clinics, insurance companies, and medical record documentation experts. Please take the time to read the list of contents for a short discussion of medical records.

CONTENTS

FIGURE C-12 Emergency department report in the HX, PX, DX format, spelling out the headings. (HX, history; PX, physical examination; DX, diagnosis).

FIGURE C-13 Urgent care center chart note.

FIGURE C-14 Mental health clinic chart note.

FIGURE C-15 Clinic chart note. Because so many capital letters are used and no boldface or underlining is used, the positive allergy response does not stand out. Be alert for this problem.

FIGURE C-16 History and physical examination report (H&P), full block style.

FIGURE C-17 History and physical examination report (H&P), full block style. Good use of bold for headings.

FIGURE C-18 History and physical examination report (H&P), dictated from the emergency department, two pages.

FIGURE C-19 History and physical examination report (H&P).

FIGURE C-20 History and physical examination report (H&P).

FIGURE C-21 History and physical examination report (H&P), modified block format with boldface and underlining, two pages.

FIGURE C-22 History and physical examination report (H&P). Notice the header, which is entered onto the screen when the MT downloads the dictation.

FIGURE C-23 Discharge summary transcribed for a facility that uses the bottom of the page for identifying material.

FIGURE C-24 Discharge summary transcribed by the medical office MT. (See Figure C-21 for this patient's history and physical examination report [H&P].)

FIGURE C-25 Hospital discharge summary. If you wonder why it is so brief, read the final sentence.

FIGURE C-26 Discharge summary, hospice care. Notice the header, which was discussed in Figure C-22.

FIGURE C-27 Operative report, modified block style. The bottom of the page is used for the identifying material.

FIGURE C-28 Operative report, modified block style.

FIGURE C-29 Operative report.

FIGURE C-30 Operative report, full block style.

FIGURE C-31 Radiology report, modified block style.

FIGURE C-32 Radiology report, unknown style. Notice that the footers on this document are somewhat different. Actually, the MT's full name was used on the original; it was removed along with the other actual names of persons and places.

FIGURE C-33 Bone density report. Notice the unusual use of the bullets and superscript.

FIGURE C-34 Pathology report. When the transcription is downloaded, these headers and footers are embedded.

FIGURE C-35 Dermatopathology report, full block style.

FIGURE C-36 Histopathology report, full block style.

FIGURE C-37 Electroencephalogram (EEG) report, full block style.

FIGURE C-38 Magnetic resonance imaging (MRI) report, modified block style. Nice use of boldface.

FIGURE C-39 Radiation therapy report, run-on style.

FIGURE C-40 Hospital consultation, full block style.

FIGURE C-41 Hospital consultation. Notice that all the drug names are typed in full capital letters. This format is not easy to read.

FIGURE C-42 Medicolegal document typed in full block letter format.

FIGURE C-43 Hospital nursing staff policy.

FIGURE C-44 Memo followed in subsequent figures. This contains some interesting information on medical records; also, see the format for transcribing policies. The outline format is used on the policy.

FIGURE C-45 Three pages of an operational policy concerning medical records.

FIGURE C-46 Pathology macros: fallopian tubes, prostate, and placenta.

FIGURE C-47 Exercise treadmill stress test macro.

FIGURE C-48 Complete macro for confidential psychiatric report, including compliance statement; three pages.

FIGURE C-49 Disclosure statement macro.

To access the collection of figures, please go to the Evolve website: http://evolve.elsevier.com/Diehl/transcription

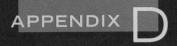

APPENDIX D

Rules and Helpful Hints for Transcribing

DICTATION SETS FOR STUDENTS

1. Beginning practice dictation in electronic format (55 documents)
2. Speech recognition (SR) dictated reports in electronic format (10 documents)
3. Authentic dictation in electronic format (99 documents)

Set 1: Reference Notes for Beginning Transcription on the Evolve Website

The material is authentic medical dictation. The facts in the examples have been altered only to the extent necessary to prevent identification of the cases or parties involved. No evaluations of medical practice, medical advice, or recommendations for treatment are to be inferred from the selections. Both male and female dictators have been used, and both foreign and American regional accents have been included.

Initially, the letters are dictated slowly with some punctuation and paragraphing indicated. Directions for punctuation and style are provided with each letter or report to test your knowledge of mechanics. The dictator instructs you to place the letter style and type of punctuation used in the upper-right corner of the page. Later in the program, a more natural dictating speed is used, and you are asked to employ your own skills in paragraphing and punctuation.

Dates you transcribe should be the date dictated with the year *20XX* following.

Throughout the dictation you will hear doctors' names, a few drug names that are no longer in the drug formulary, and place names that are not spelled when dictated. A list of these follows.

The following names constitute the roster of names used in the dictation. Unless otherwise dictated, it is assumed that all of the dictators are physicians, which necessitates the use of "MD" after the name dictated. You might use mailing addresses throughout by selecting that of a local medical center.

DOCTOR NAMES

Ashby, Francis S.	Fisher, David C.	Michaelson, Philip B.
Barton, Ralph R.	Frick, Malcolm A.	Miller, Kenneth E.
Benson, Robert T.	Garcia, Frank R.	Mills, Lorraine F.
Black, Nelson Gunter	Garcia, Raymond C.	Morgan, Julia L.
Brown, Richard L.	Gomez, Carl J.	Mosley, Mark M.
Camp, John M.	Hartman, Daniel O.	Northway, Mary Elizabeth
Cane, Florence C.	Hoffman, Renee B.	Norton, Mary A.
Cheung, Kim	Horowitz, Frank E.	O'Brien, Moira
Cummings, Arthur B., Jr.	Huber, Ralph P.	O'Connor, Brian M.
Day, Randolph T.	Jacobs, Irene L.	Ottavio, Patricia B.
Delaney, Scott P.	Johnson, Elizabeth F.	Paolini, Violetta O.
Denton, Charles E., III	Kraft, David C.	Pierce, Andrew G.
Dorunda, Helen Davidson	Larkin, Edward A.	Redman, Norman B.
Douglas, Martin P.	Livingston, Stephanie K.	Richards, Joan R.
Drexler, Elvera P.	Macdonald, Winthrop G.	Richmond, Lawrence M.
Drummond, Frank C.	Mason, Lester J.	Roseman, John T.

Rutterman, Fernando A.
Sachs, Bernice D.
Sharp, Preston W.
Shaw, Phillip N.
Sklar, Aaron B.
Sloan, Terence W.
Smith, Jeremy T.
Smith, Maureen J.
Stanford, Raymond N.
Swensen, Erik M.
Takashima, Toshiro
Templeton, Barry O.
Tu, Thomas
Wagner, Charles M.

Walsh, Felix W.
Walter, Jane A.
Waxman, Fred M.
Waxman, Howard T.
Waxman, William B.
Wilcox, David B.
Wilson-Layton, Justin
Woodman, Kenneth R.
Zatts, Percy R.

PLACE NAMES

Chambers Hospital
Encino

DRUG NAMES (THAT MIGHT NOT BE FOUND IN CURRENT DRUG REFERENCE BOOKS)

Atromid-S
Regular (insulin)
Tedral
Mellaril 15 mg
Butazolidin

Set 2: Speech Recognition Dictated Reports in Electronic Format on the Evolve Website

There are ten SR dictated reports with the answers to the first two in Appendix A. Your instructor will score the remaining eight. Each one consists of two parts: the audio portion and the SR portion. You will listen to the audio and correct the SR portion.

▶ Use the style you have been learning in your textbook to write numbers, place punctuation, use abbreviations, select capitalization, and so on.
▶ Remember to expand abbreviations appropriately. Your instructor will be using a key that will indicate which abbreviations can be used and which need to be expanded. This is very important when transcribing diagnoses/assessments.
▶ Follow the appropriate sequence and expansion for document headings. Many are dictated out of sequence. Format outlines follow. It is probably easier to transcribe what you hear and adjust the format with cut and paste when you are finished.
▶ Use the following sequence for dates that are written as figures: two-digit month, two-digit day, four-digit year.

EXAMPLE

08/09/2011

▶ If you are able to refer to the key, please notice that there are some words in the key that were not dictated but are part of document requirements. These are shown in italics. Notice also that there are some words, also shown in italics, that were dictated but not transcribed. They could be expanded or they were deemed redundant.
▶ Remember to expand platelet counts so they are in the hundred thousand.

EXAMPLE

Dictated: "platelet count 146."

Transcribed: "platelet count 146,000."

Facility and Place Names

The following is a list of place names and physician names that occur in both set 1 and set 3 documents. Keep this list handy so that you may refer to it to enable you to spell them properly.

FACILITY AND PLACE NAMES

Asbury Heights Skilled Nursing Facility
Bethany Clinic of Skeet Club
Bethany College
BJC ER
Bruning, PA
Dominican Emergency Department
Dominican Hospital
Felton, California
Fort Bragg

Gainesville
Greensboro
High Point Regional
High Point Surgery Center
Kaiser Hospital
Landmark
Lawrenceville
Lehigh Valley Hospital
Moses Cone
MPC
Regional First Care

Santa Cruz Medical Foundation
Scotts Valley
Seabright Facility
Sewickley Hospital
Sutter Maternity and Surgery Center
UCSC
UCSF
UPMC Mercy
Watsonville

DOCTOR NAMES

Dr Adelstein
Dr Allen
Dr Altschuler
Dr Arvind
Dr Bashore
Dr Beerel
Dr Biesecker
Dr Bonacorsi
Dr Brunelli
Dr Butler
Dr Caudry
Dr Cedar
Dr Colatrella
Dr Conroy
Dr Crevello
Dr de la Pena
Dr Dorn
Dr Edwards
Dr Eisendorf
Dr Fleagle
Dr Fletcher
Dr Gill
Dr Gonzalez

Dr Griggs
Dr Hurray
Dr John
Dr Joseph
Dr Kuhn
Dr Kumasaka
Dr Lane
Dr Larson
Dr Leach
Dr Lee
Dr Luzanna
Dr MacDonald
Dr Martin
Dr Massie
Dr McQuillan
Dr Mejias
Dr Mlik
Dr Monahan
Dr Mullins
Dr Neave
Dr Nguyen
Dr Patel
Dr Perryman
Dr Philbin

Dr Piepgrass
Dr Pinto
Dr Roberts
Dr Rosen
Dr Rothenberg
Dr Safyan
Dr Samhouri
Dr Sawhney
Dr Seftel
Dr Sell
Dr Sepesi
Dr Shieh
Dr Shields
Dr Singh
Dr Sirhen
Dr Taylor
Dr Theodoran
Dr Tilles
Dr Ventura
Dr Wainer
Dr Walsh
Dr Ward
Dr Westberry
Dr Ziembicki

Format Requirements

The order of the various formats when transcribed in the Set 1 documents is as follows:

OPERATIVE REPORT
  PREOPERATIVE DIAGNOSIS
  POSTOPERATIVE DIAGNOSIS
  PROCEDURES
  INDICATION FOR PROCEDURE
  OPERATIVE SUMMARY
  ESTIMATED BLOOD LOSS
  COMPLICATIONS

DISCHARGE SUMMARY
  PRIMARY DIAGNOSIS
  SECONDARY DIAGNOSES
  SERVICE
  CONSULTATIONS
  PROCEDURES
  HISTORY AND PHYSICAL
  DISPOSITION
  DISCHARGE CONDITION
  DISCHARGE MEDICATIONS
  DISCHARGE INSTRUCTIONS AND FOLLOWUP

D

APPENDIX

HISTORY AND PHYSICAL
    HISTORY OF PRESENT ILLNESS
    EMERGENCY DEPARTMENT COURSE (When applicable)
    PAST MEDICAL HISTORY
    PAST SURGICAL HISTORY (When applicable or dictated)
    ALLERGIES
    MEDICATIONS
    FAMILY HISTORY
    SOCIAL HISTORY
    REVIEW OF SYSTEMS
    PHYSICAL EXAMINATION
    LABORATORY
    IMPRESSION AND PLAN

CONSULTATION
    HISTORY
    REVIEW OF SYSTEMS
    PAST MEDICAL HISTORY
    SOCIAL HISTORY
    FAMILY HISTORY
    ALLERGIES
    CURRENT MEDICATIONS
    PHYSICAL EXAMINATION
    LABORATORY DATA
    ASSESSMENT AND PLAN

Set 3: Electronic Dictation of 99 Actual Medical Reports on the Evolve Website

- Refer to the list of place names and doctor names given with Set 2 instructions.
- Download your dictation as your instructor directs.
- Follow the format as dictated unless the dictator has dictated a part out of order. You may refer to your textbook or Set 2 instructions for the correct order of documents.

Index

Page numbers followed by *f* indicate figures; *t,* tables; *b,* boxes.

Fibrinolysis, 503t
Fibrin split products, 503t
Fidelity, 56b–58b
Figures, numbers as, 124–130
File
   defined, 56b–58b
   maintenance of, 50–52
   transcriptionist's, 27–28, 28f
File notation for letter, 163
File server, 56b–58b
File transfer protocol (FTP), 56b–58b
Final progress notes, 334–335
Finances in home-based business, 409
Flagging, 179, 181, 187–188, 189f
Flash drive, 43, 43f, 56b–58b
Flow sheet, 50
Flyers for marketing, 407, 408f
Folding of letter, 170, 170f
Followup, 257–258
Follow up, 257–258
Follow-up, 257–258
Font, 56b–58b
Foot control, 49, 49f
Foreign accent, 51t, 187
Forensic pathology, 347
Formal agenda, 378f
Formally, 258
Formerly, 258
For The Record, 217
Fractions
   decimal, 130
   slash in, 93
   spelling out of, 123
   whole numbers with, 130
Fracture, Roman numerals with, 132t
Fragments, sentence, 366
Fraud, 16b–17b
French terms, 221
   plural, 240
Front-end speech recognition (FESR), 46
FTP. *See* File transfer protocol (FTP)
Full block format
   for hospital documents, 377f
   for letters, 149–150, 149b, 150f–153f
   for minutes, 380f
   for reference line, 161
Functional inquiry. *See* Review of systems (ROS)
Functional resumé, 415
Further, 257

G

Gamma-glutamyl transpeptidase (GGTP), 504t–505t
Garbled words, 51t
Gastrointestinal (GI) system in review of systems, 313
GearPlayer, 49f
"General" topic in physical examination, 317

Generic drugs, 221–222
   capitalization and, 107
Genitalia, physical examination of, 320
Genitourinary (GU) system in review of systems, 313
Genus, 473–475
   capitalization of, 107
   periods with, 82
Geographic locations, capitalization of, 109
GGTP. *See* Gamma-glutamyl transpeptidase (GGTP)
GI. *See* Gastrointestinal (GI) system in review of systems
Global search and replace, 56b–58b
Globulin, 504t–505t
Glucose
   fasting blood, 504t–505t
   urine, 507t
Glucose-tolerance test (GTT), 504t–505t
Glycated hemoglobin, 504t–505t
Goals, production, 7
Government agencies, capitalization of, 109–110
Grade, Roman numerals with, 132t
-gram, 241t–242t
Gram (g), 120t
Grammar, 247
   for adjective modifiers, 265
   for antecedents, 265
   for collective nouns, 265–266
   correcting errors of, 184
   for dangling constructions and misplaced modifiers, 266
   for homonyms and other confusing word pairs, 248–250
   for indefinite pronouns and verbs, 266
   in letter transcription, 149
   for parallel structure, 266–267
   for personal pronouns, 267–268
   for plural pronouns with singular antecedents, 268–269
   for plurals and singulars, 268
   for proper terms for persons, 270
   for sentence structure, 269
   for verb tense, 269–270
   for word-choice pairs, 250–265
-graph, 241t–242t
-graphy, 241t–242t
Gravida, 132, 313
Greek derivation, medical terms of, 217–218
   plural endings for, 234–238
Gross description of specimen, 337–340
Gross negligence, 16b–17b
GTT. *See* Glucose-tolerance test (GTT)
GU. *See* Genitourinary (GU) system in review of systems
Guide to Internet Job Searching 2008-2009, 415

GYN. *See* Gynecologic (GYN) system in review of systems
Gynecologic (GYN) system in review of systems, 313
Gynecologic history, 312

H

Habits, history of, 311
Hacking, computer, 38–39
Hair, in review of systems, 312
Hand/foot control, 49, 49f
Handhelds, 36
Handwritten chart entries, 36
Haptoglobin, 502t
Hard copy, 44, 56b–58b
Hard drive, 39, 42, 56b–58b
Hardware for computer systems, 37–39, 56b–58b
HDL. *See* High-density lipoproteins (HDL)
Head and neck
   physical examination of, 318
   in review of systems, 313
Head crash, 56b–58b
Heading
   in hospital reports, 376
   in memos, 371
   in minutes, 381
Headset, 56b–58b
Healthcare directive, 16b–17b
Health Data Matrix, 8, 217
Health information assistant, 4
Health Insurance Portability and Accountability Act of 1996 (HIPPA), 12–15, 55
Health Professions Institute, 10, 11f–12f, 414
Health record, electronic, 20–21
Heart
   physical examination of, 319
   in review of systems, 313
Heart murmurs, Roman numerals with, 132t
HEENT
   in physical examination, 318
   in review of systems, 312–313
Height
   of workstation, 44, 45f
   writing of, 125
Hematocrit (crit, HCT), 502t
Hematology
   tests and normal values, 502–507
   vocabulary for, 502
Hemoglobin (HG, Hgb, HGB), 502t
   glycated, 504t–505t
   urinary, 507t
High complexity medical decision making, 276
High-density lipoproteins (HDL), 504t–505t
Hints, 51b, 176, 290–294, 529
HIPPA. *See* Health Insurance Portability and Accountability Act of 1996 (HIPPA)

Iron, serum, 506t
Irregardless, 261
-is, 236
-ism, 241t–242t
-ist, 241t–242t
IT. *See* Information technology (IT)
Italian words, plural, 240
-itis, 241t–242t
-ity, 241t–242t
-ive, 242t
-ix, 237

J

Jargon, errors associated with, 185
JC. *See* Joint Commission (JC)
Job
    career *versus,* 27
    leaving of, 426, 426b
Job description, 4–5, 6f, 425–426
Job opportunities, 3
    temporary, 417–420
Joint Commission (JC)
    abbreviations, acronyms, and slang
        requirements and, 18
    signature requirements of, 18
Journals, 217
Jump drive, 43, 56b–58b
Justification, 56b–58b

K

Ketones, urinary, 507t
Keyboard, 38
    ergonomic, 44, 45f
    Magic Wand, 53
    shortcut commands, 403t
kilo- (k), 120t
K (Potassium), 504t–505t

L

Laboratory findings in medicolegal
    reports, 348–349
Laboratory terminology, 229, 500–501
Laboratory values
    critical errors associated with, 178
    hematologic, 502–507
    normal, 502
    writing, 501
Lactate dehydrogenase (LDH), 506t
LAN. *See* Local-area network (LAN)
Languages, capitalization of, 106
Laser printer, 43–44
Last, 258
Latest, 258
Latin abbreviations, periods with, 82
Latin medical terms, plural endings
    for, 234–238
Lay, 258–259
LDH. *See* Lactate dehydrogenase
    (LDH)
LDL. *See* Low-density lipoproteins
    (LDL)
Lee-White test, 503t
Legal responsibilities, 10–17, 13f–14f
Let it stand, proofreader's marks for,
    196, 197f–198f

Letterhead, 151–153, 155f
Letter(s), 147. *See also* Capital letters;
        Lowercase letters
    address of
        city and state, 156
        inside, 155–156
        street, 156
    attention line of, 160
    body of, 157, 158f
    complimentary close of, 157
        capitalization of, 104
        comma after, 78
    copies of, 163
        blind, 160
    date line of, 153
        comma in, 79
    envelope preparation for, 169–170
    file notation for, 163
    formats of, 149–160, 149b,
        150f–154f
    hyphen after, 88
    introduction to, 148–149
    letterhead for, 151–153, 155f
    mailing of, 170, 170f
    notations in
        distribution, 159–160
        enclosure, 159
    in outline, 381, 382f
    paper for, 151
    paragraphing of, 165–169
    parentheses around, 93
    personal or confidential notations
        in, 162
    placement of, 163–165
    plural, apostrophe for, 92
    postscript of, 160
    to prospective clients, 410, 411f
    qualities of, 149
    reference initials in, 159
    reference line of, 161–162
    salutation of, 156–157
        capitalization of, 104
        colon after, 83
    signature line of, 157–159
        capitalization in, 105
    signing of, 170
    sizes of stationary for, 170–172
    thank you following job interview,
        424, 424f
    "to whom it may concern" in,
        160–161
    two-page, 162–163
    typing techniques, 149
    vocabulary associated with, 149b
Leukocyte count, 502t
Level, Roman numerals with, 72t
Level 1 examination, 9–10
Libel, 16b–17b
Licensure abbreviations, 8–10
Lie, 258–259
Life-sustaining procedure, 16b–17b
Like, 259
Limb leads, Roman numerals
    with, 72t
Line count, 7, 411

Lipid panel, 506t
Lists
    colons with, 83
    in hospital reports, 376–377
    in minutes, 381
Literary works, quotation marks for,
    92
Liter (L), 120t
Liver function tests, 506t
Local-area network (LAN), 36–37,
    41–42, 56b–58b
Loose, 259
Lose, 259
Low complexity medical decision
    making, 276
Low-density lipoproteins (LDL),
    504t–505t
Lowercase letters, 104
    proofreader's marks for, 196,
        197f–198f
Ltd., commas following, 74
Lungs
    physical examination of, 319
    in review of systems, 313
Lymphocytes (lymphs), 504t

M

-ma, 237
Macros, 41
    defined, 56b–58b
    errors associated with, 180
    history and physical examination
        report, 301
    memo, 370
Magic Wand Keyboard, 53
Magnesium, serum, 504t–505t
Magnetic resonance imaging (MRI)
    report, 342, 343f
Mailing(s)
    of letter, 170, 170f
    for marketing, 407
Maintenance
    of cassette tape transcriber, 52
    of computer systems, 39
    file, 50–52
Major errors, 179, 179f
Majority, 259
Malpractice, 16b–17b
Manual signature, 18
Marketing, 407, 408f
Marks, proofreader's, 195–202,
    196f–198f
-mata, 234t, 237
Mathematical abbreviations, 137
Maybe, 259
May be, 259
Mean corpuscular hemoglobin
    concentration (MCHC), 502t
Mean corpuscular hemoglobin
    (MCH), 502t
Mean corpuscular volume (MCV),
    502t
Measurements
    abbreviations of, 82
    plural, 239

Media
defined, 56b–58b
dictation, 48–49, 48f–49f
disposal of electronic, 55
Medical administrative assistant, 4
Medical coding, 275–276
Medical communication, 3
Medical decision making, 276–277
Medical dictation editor, 4
Medical dictionary, 207–208
cross-references in, 208–211,
210f
line-drawing illustration in,
209f
typical word entry from, 208f
Medical office administrator, 4
Medical questions, websites for,
228–229
Medical record notes. *See* Chart notes
Medical record number, 311
Medical records/reports, 16b–17b,
17–25, 527
abbreviations in, 135–136
authentication of, 18
autopsy protocol, 346–348,
346f–347f
capitalization in, 108
chart or progress notes in, 273
(*See also* Chart notes)
completeness of, 19–20
consultation report, 345, 345f
correction of, 20
dates on, 19
deadlines for, 19
discharge summary, 334–335, 335f,
337f
electronic, 21
history and physical examination
report, 299 (*See also* History and
physical examination [H&P]
report)
medicolegal reports, 348–350,
349f–350f
metric system in, 120–121
operative report, 335–336,
338f–340f
ownership of, 20
pathology report, 336–341,
341f
privileged communication and,
21
psychiatric report, 350–351,
352f–353f
quality assurance regarding (*See*
Quality assurance [QA])
radiology and imaging reports,
341–345, 342f–344f
release of, 21–24, 22f, 24f, 26f
retention of, 25
right to privacy and, 21
signatures on, 18
turnaround time for, 19
Medical scribe, 4
Medical spellers, 211–212
Medical spelling, 217–218

Medical transcription
interests and, 3
introduction to, 2–3
job description, 4–5, 5f
job opportunities, 3
preparation for, 52
rules and helpful hints for, 176,
529
skills needed for, 3, 5–7
speed of, 7
*Medical Transcription Guide Do's &
Don'ts,* 221
Medical Transcription Industry
Alliance (MTIA) Code of ethics,
10, 13f
Medical transcriptionist (MT)
Bill of Rights for, 9f
certification for, 8–10
certified, 8–10
finding employment as, 3, 412–420
application forms in, 424–425
cover letter for, 417, 420f
electronic job search for, 415
follow-up letter in, 424, 424f
interview skills in, 420–425,
423f
introduction to, 406
job *versus* career, 27
portfolio for, 424
resumé for, 415–417, 416f–419f
skills assessment sheet in, 423,
423f
temporary, 417–420
home-based, 406–411
business and, 409–410
developing clientele in, 410,
411f–412f
emotional needs in, 409
equipment for, 409
home-based entrepreneur,
406–407
office space for, 407–409
professional considerations and
work ethics in, 409
professional fees in, 410–411
qualities needed in, 410
records and finances in, 409
remote-based work site, 406
subcontracting in, 411
terminology associated with,
407
initials of in letter, 159
job description, 4–5, 5f, 425–426
leaving job as, 426, 426b
marketing yourself as, 407, 408f
notebook or file for, 27–28, 28f
physically challenged, 7–8
equipment for, 52–53
professionalism of, 25–27, 425
professional levels of, 388–389
registered, 4, 8
tips on holding job as, 425
Medical word books, 211–212
Medicare, signature requirements of,
18

Medicolegal reports, 348–350,
349f–350f
Membership in Association for
Healthcare Documentation
Integrity, 8
Memoranda (memos), 370–373,
371f
Memory, 56b–58b
Men, salutations used for, 157
Mentally deficient client, psychiatric
report for, 350
Mentally retarded, 350
Menu, 56b–58b
Merge, 56b–58b
Merriam-Webster's Collegiate Dictionary,
207
-meter, 241t–242t
Meter (m), 120t
Methemoglobin, 502t
Metric measurements/system
abbreviations of, 82, 136
in medical records, 120–121
typing of drugs and, 138
-metry, 241t–242t
Microscopic description of specimen,
337–340
Microscopy, urinary, 507t–508t
Military address, 169
Military ranks, capitalization of,
105
Military time, 127, 348
milli- (m), 120t
Minor errors, 179, 179f
Minus symbol, 129, 134t
Minutes, 380–381, 380f
capitalization in, 109–110
Misplaced modifiers, 266
Misunderstandings, errors associated
with, 186–187
Mixed numbers, 130
Mixed punctuation, 149b,
150f–154f
Modem, 38–39, 56b–58b
Moderate complexity medical decision
making, 276
Modified block format style
consultation report in, 345f
history and physical examination
report in, 304–306, 305f,
320f
with indented paragraphs, 150
letters in, 149, 149b, 154f
operative report in, 340f
for reference line, 161–162
run-on, 306–307, 307f
short-stay report in, 328f
Modifier(s)
adjective, 265
compound, hyphen with, 87
misplaced, 266
Monocytes (monos), 504t
Months, capitalization of, 109
Morphology of cells, 504
Most, 259
Mouse, 38

PUNCTUATION RULE SYNOPSIS

PUNCTUATION	RULE	PAGE
Use a Comma or Pair of Commas		
To set off a nonessential word or words from the rest of the sentence	3.1a	69
To set off nonessential appositives	3.1b	70
To set off a parenthetical expression	3.1c	70
To set off an introductory phrase or clause (See also Rule 3.2b)	3.2a	73
To set off the year in a complete date	3.3	74
To set off the name of the state when the city precedes it	3.4	74
To set off *Inc.* or *Ltd.* in a company name	3.5	74
To set off titles and degrees after a person's name	3.6	74
To separate elements of words in a series	3.7	75
To separate two independent clauses	3.8	75
To set off the name of a person in a direct address	3.9	78
To separate certain modifiers	3.10	78
To avoid confusion	3.11	78
After the complimentary close	3.12	78
In certain long numbers	3.13	79
To separate the parts of a date in the date line of a letter	3.14	79

PUNCTUATION	RULE	PAGE
Use a Period		
At the end of a sentence	3.15	81
With single capitalized word abbreviations	3.16	82
When the genus is abbreviated	3.16	82
In certain lowercase Latin abbreviations	3.16	82
To separate a decimal fraction from whole numbers	3.17	82

PUNCTUATION	RULE	PAGE
Use a Semicolon		
Between two independent clauses when there is no conjunction	3.18	82
Between independent clauses if either or both are already punctuated	3.19	82
Before a parenthetical expression when it is used as a conjunction	3.20	83
Between a series of phrases or clauses when any item in the series has internal commas	3.21	83

PUNCTUATION	RULE	PAGE
Use a Colon		
To introduce a list or series of items	3.22	83
After the salutation in a business letter when "mixed" punctuation is used	3.23	83
Between the hours and minutes indicating the time	3.24	83
In ratios and dilutions	3.24	83
After the introductory word or words in a history and physical examination report	3.25	84
With the introductory words in an outline	3.25	84
To introduce an example or clarify an idea	3.26	84

PUNCTUATION	RULE	PAGE
Use a Hyphen		
When two or more words have the force of a single modifier	3.27	86
Between conflicting terms	3.28	87
In a series of modifiers	3.29	87
When numbers are compounded with words	3.30	87
Within compound numbers 21 to 99 when they are written out	3.31	87
Between a prefix and a proper noun	3.32	87
After prefixes *ex, self,* and *vice;* to avoid awkward combinations of letters	3.33	87
After a prefix when the unhyphenated word would have a different meaning (Exceptions, see Rule 3.35)	3.34	87
	3.35	88
In certain chemical expressions	3.36	88
To take the place of the words *to* and *through*	3.37	88
After a single letter joined to a word that together form a coined term	3.38	88
Between compound nouns and compound surnames	3.39	89

PUNCTUATION	RULE	PAGE
Use a Dash		
For a forceful break	3.40	89
For summary	3.41	89

PUNCTUATION	RULE	PAGE
Use an Apostrophe		
To show singular or plural possession	3.42	89
In contractions	3.43	91
In possessive expressions of time, distance, and value	3.44	91
To form the plural of some letters	3.45	92

PUNCTUATION	RULE	PAGE
Use Quotation Marks		
To enclose the exact words of a speaker	3.46	92
To enclose the titles of minor literary and artistic works	3.47	92
To single out words or phrases	3.48	92
To set off slang, coined, awkward, or whimsical words	3.49	92

PUNCTUATION	RULE	PAGE
Use Parentheses		
To set off clearly nonessential words or phrases	3.50	93
Around figures or letters that indicate divisions in narrative copy	3.51	93

PUNCTUATION	RULE	PAGE
Use a Slash		
In certain technical terms	3.52	93
To offer a word choice	3.53	93
To write fractions	3.54	93

PUNCTUATION	RULE	PAGE
Spacing with Punctuation Marks		
No space	3.55	94
One space	3.56	94
Two spaces	3.57	94